Essentials of Child and Adolescent Psychiatry

Edited by

Mina K. Dulcan, M.D.
Jerry M. Wiener, M.D.

D1231247

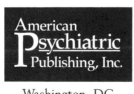

Washington, DC
London, England

If you would like to buy **between 25 and 99 copies** of a this title or any other APPI title, you are eligible for a 20% discount; please contact APPI Customer Service at appi@psych.org or 800-368-5777. If you wish to buy **100 or more copies** of the same title, please email us at bulksales@psych.org for a price quote.

Copyright © 2006 American Psychiatric Publishing, Inc.
ALL RIGHTS RESERVED

Manufactured in the United States of America on acid-free paper
10   09   08   07   5   4   3   2

Typeset in Adobe's New Baskerville and Goudy Sans Medium

American Psychiatric Publishing, Inc.
1000 Wilson Boulevard
Arlington, VA 22209-3901
www.appi.org

Library of Congress Cataloging-in-Publication Data
Essentials of child and adolescent psychiatry / edited by Mina K. Dulcan, Jerry M. Wiener.
        p. ; cm.
    Includes bibliographical references and index.
    ISBN 1-58562-217-6 (pbk.: alk. paper)
    1. Child psychiatry. 2. Adolescent psychiatry.   I. Dulcan, Mina K.   II. Wiener, Jerry M., 1933–   .
    [DNLM: 1. Mental Disorders—Child. 2. Adolescent Psychiatry. 3. Child Psychiatry. WS 350 E778 2006]
    RJ499.E744 2006
    618.92'89—dc22

                                                                      2005026052

British Library Cataloguing in Publication Data
A CIP record is available from the British Library.

Contents

Part I

Assessment and Diagnosis

Part II

Developmental Disorders

Part III

Psychiatric Disorders

Part IV

Disorders Affecting Somatic Function

Part V

Special Issues

Part VI

Treatment

Contributors

Chelsea M. Ale, B.A.
Clinical Research Assistant, The Pediatric Anxiety Research Clinic (PARC), Bradley/Hasbro Children's Research Center, Providence, Rhode Island

Lisa Amaya-Jackson, M.D., M.P.H.
Director, Trauma Treatment Service, Department of Psychiatry, Duke University Medical Center, Durham, North Carolina

Eugene V. Beresin, M.D.
Director, Child and Adolescent Psychiatry Residency Training Program, Massachusetts General Hospital/McLean Hospital; Co-Director, Harvard Medical School Center for Mental Health and Media; Associate Professor of Psychiatry, Harvard Medical School, Boston, Massachusetts

Gail A. Bernstein, M.D.
Endowed Professor in Child and Adolescent Anxiety Disorders; Head, Program in Child and Adolescent Anxiety and Mood Disorders, Division of Child and Adolescent Psychiatry, University of Minnesota Medical School, Minneapolis, Minnesota

Joseph Biederman, M.D.
Chief, Clinical and Research Program in Pediatric Psychopharmacology, Massachusetts General Hospital; Professor of Psychiatry, Harvard Medical School, Boston, Massachusetts

Héctor R. Bird, M.D.
Professor of Clinical Psychiatry, Columbia University College of Physicians and Surgeons; Deputy Director, Department of Child Psychiatry, New York State Psychiatric Institute, New York, New York

Bruce Black, M.D.
Director, Comprehensive Psychiatric Associates, Wellesley, Massachusetts; Assistant Professor of Psychiatry, Tufts University School of Medicine, New England Medical Center, Boston, Massachusetts

Donna J. Champine, M.D.
Clinical Assistant Professor of Psychiatry, Department of Psychiatry, University of Michigan Medical School, Ann Arbor, Michigan

Brent Collett, Ph.D.
Acting Assistant Professor, University of Washington School of Medicine, Attending Psychologist, Department of Child Psychiatry and Behavioral Pediatrics, Children's Hospital and Regional Medical Center, Seattle, Washington

Martha E. Crotts, M.D.
Private practice, Rockford, Illinois

Peter T. Daniolos, M.D.
Residency Training Director and Medical Director, Center for Autism Spectrum Disorders, Department of Psychiatry and Behavioral Sciences, Children's National Medical Center; Assistant Professor of Psychiatry, Behavioral Sciences, and Pediatrics, George Washington University School of Medicine, Washington, D.C.

Craig L. Donnelly, M.D., M.A.
Director, Pediatric Psychopharmacology, Associate Professor of Psychiatry and Pediatrics, Section of Child and Adolescent Psychiatry, Department of Psychiatry, Dartmouth Medical School, Lebanon, New Hampshire

Mina K. Dulcan, M.D.
Margaret C. Osterman Professor of Child Psychiatry; Head, Department of Child and Adolescent Psychiatry, Children's Memorial Hospital; Director, Warren Wright Adolescent Program, Northwestern Memorial Hospital; Professor of Psychiatry and Behavioral Sciences and Pediatrics; Chief, Child and Adolescent Psychiatry, Northwestern University, Feinberg School of Medicine, Chicago, Illinois

Kamryn T. Eddy, M.A.
Center for Anxiety and Related Disorders, Department of Psychology, Boston University, Boston, Massachusetts

Carl Feinstein, M.D.
Professor of Psychiatry and Behavioral Sciences and Director, Division of Child and Adolescent Psychiatry, Stanford University School of Medicine, Stanford, California

Jennifer B. Freeman, Ph.D.
Assistant Professor (Research), Department of Psychiatry and Human Behavior, Brown Medical School; Co-Director/Staff Psychologist, The Pediatric Anxiety Research Clinic (PARC), Bradley/Hasbro Children's Research Center, Providence, Rhode Island

Abbe M. Garcia, Ph.D.
Assistant Professor (Research), Department of Psychiatry and Human Behavior, Brown Medical School; Staff Psychologist, The Pediatric Anxiety Research Clinic (PARC), Bradley/Hasbro Children's Research Center, Providence, Rhode Island

Laurence L. Greenhill, M.D.
Professor of Psychiatry, Division of Child Psychiatry, New York State Psychiatric Institute, Columbia University College of Physicians and Surgeons, New York, New York

XiaoYan He, M.D.
Assistant Professor of Clinical Psychiatry, University of California, Davis; Child and Adolescent Psychiatrist, Kaiser Permanente—South Sacramento, Sacramento, California

Robert L. Hendren, D.O.
Professor of Psychiatry; Executive Director, M.I.N.D. Institute; Chief, Child and Adolescent Psychiatry, University of California–Davis, Sacramento, California

David B. Herzog, M.D.
Director, Eating Disorders Unit, Child Psychiatry Service, Massachusetts General Hospital; Professor of Psychiatry (Pediatrics), Harvard Medical School, Boston, Massachusetts

Steven L. Jaffe, M.D.
Professor of Child and Adolescent Psychiatry, Emory University School of Medicine, Atlanta, Georgia; Clinical Professor, Morehouse School of Medicine, Atlanta, Georgia

Paramjit T. Joshi, M.D.
Endowed Chair, Department of Psychiatry and Behavioral Sciences, Children's National Medical Center; Professor of Psychiatry, Behavioral Sciences, and Pediatrics, George Washington University School of Medicine, Washington, D.C.

Lawrence C. Kaplan, M.D.
Director, Division of Genetics and Child Development, Children's Hospital at Dartmouth, Lebanon, New Hampshire; Associate Professor of Pediatrics, Dartmouth Medical School, Hanover, New Hampshire

Clarice J. Kestenbaum, M.D.
Professor of Clinical Psychiatry and Director of Training Emerita, Division of Child and Adolescent Psychiatry, Columbia University College of Physicians and Surgeons, New York, New York

Deepa Khushlani, M.D.
Assistant Professor of Psychiatry and Behavioral Sciences, George Washington University School of Health Sciences, Washington, D.C.

Robert A. King, M.D.
Professor of Child Psychiatry and Medical Director, Tourette's/OCD Clinic, Yale Child Study Center, Yale University, New Haven, Connecticut

Angelica L. Kloos, D.O.
Department of Psychiatry, Thomas Jefferson University Hospital, Philadelphia, Pennsylvania

Ann E. Layne, Ph.D.
Assistant Professor, Division of Child and Adolescent Psychiatry, University of Minnesota Medical School, Minneapolis, Minnesota

James F. Leckman, M.D.
Neison Harris Professor of Child Psychiatry and Pediatrics, Yale Child Study Center, New Haven, Connecticut

Henrietta L. Leonard, M.D.
Professor and Director of Training, Child and Adolescent Psychiatry, Rhode Island Hospital and Brown Medical School; Director, The Pediatric Anxiety Research Clinic (PARC), Bradley/Hasbro Children's Research Center, Providence, Rhode Island

Bennett L. Leventhal, M.D.
Professor of Psychiatry and Director, Center for Child Mental Health and Developmental Neuroscience, Institute for Juvenile Research, The University of Illinois at Chicago College of Medicine; Irving B. Harris Professor of Child and Adolescent Psychiatry, Emeritus, The University of Chicago, Chicago, Illinois

Melvin Lewis, M.B., B.S., F.R.C.Psych., D.C.H.
Professor Emeritus of Child Psychiatry and Pediatrics, Yale Child Study Center, Yale University, New Haven, Connecticut

John S. March, M.D., M.P.H.
Chief, Division of Childhood and Adolescent Psychiatry, and Professor of Psychiatry, Departments of Psychiatry and Psychology: Social and Health Sciences, Duke University Medical Center, Durham, North Carolina

Jon McClellan, M.D.
Associate Professor, Department of Psychiatry, University of Washington, Seattle, Washington

Edgardo Menvielle, M.D.
Assistant Professor of Psychiatry and Behavioral Sciences, George Washington University School of Health Sciences, Washington, D.C.

David J. Mullen, M.D.
Associate Professor of Psychiatry, University of New Mexico; Executive Medical Director, UNM Children's Psychiatric Hospital, Albuquerque, New Mexico

Kathleen Myers, M.D., M.P.H.
Associate Professor, University of Washington School of Medicine; Director, Consultation-Liaison Psychiatry, Department of Child Psychiatry and Behavioral Pediatrics, Children's Hospital and Regional Medical Center, Seattle, Washington

Janet S. Ng, B.A.
Clinical Research Assistant, The Pediatric Anxiety Research Clinic (PARC), Bradley/Hasbro Children's Research Center, Providence, Rhode Island

Cynthia R. Pfeffer, M.D.
Professor of Psychiatry and Director, Childhood Bereavement Program, Weill Medical College of Cornell University, White Plains, New York

Jennifer M. Phillips, Ph.D.
Staff Psychologist, Department of Psychiatry and Behavioral Sciences, Division of Child and Adolescent Psychiatry, Stanford University School of Medicine, Stanford, California

David Pruitt, M.D.
Professor, Psychiatry and Pediatrics, and Division Director, Child and Adolescent Psychiatry, University of Maryland College of Medicine, Baltimore, Maryland

Judith L. Rapoport, M.D.
Chief, Child Psychiatry Branch, National Institute of Mental Health, National Institutes of Health, Bethesda, Maryland

Gloria Reeves, M.D.
Assistant Professor, Division Child and Adolescent Psychiatry, University of Maryland College of Medicine, Baltimore, Maryland

Jay A. Salpekar, M.D.
Director of Outpatient Services, Department of Psychiatry and Behavioral Sciences, Children's National Medical Center; Assistant Professor of Psychiatry, Behavioral Sciences, and Pediatrics, George Washington University School of Medicine, Washington, D.C.

John E. Schowalter, M.D.
Albert J. Solnit Professor of Child Psychiatry and Pediatrics; Chief, Child Psychiatry, Yale Child Study Center, Yale University, New Haven, Connecticut

Ramon Solhkhah, M.D.
Director, Child and Adolescent Psychiatry, St. Luke's–Roosevelt Hospital Center; Assistant Professor of Clinical Psychiatry, Columbia University, New York, New York

Thomas Spencer, M.D.
Assistant Director, Pediatric Psychopharmacology, Massachusetts General Hospital; Professor of Psychiatry, Harvard Medical School, Boston, Massachusetts

Susan E. Swedo, M.D.
Chief, Pediatrics and Developmental Neuropsychiatry Branch, National Institute of Mental Health, National Institutes of Health, Bethesda, Maryland

David Szydlo, M.D., Ph.D.
Associate Research Scientist, Yale Child Study Center, Yale University School of Medicine; Director of Education and Curriculum Development, National Center for Children Exposed to Violence, Yale University School of Medicine, New Haven, Connecticut

Ludwik S. Szymanski, M.D.
Director Emeritus of Psychiatry and Center for Autism and Related Disorders, Institute for Community Inclusion, Children's Hospital Boston; Associate Professor of Clinical Psychiatry, Harvard Medical School, Boston, Massachusetts

Luke Y. Tsai, M.D.
Professor of Psychiatry and Pediatrics, University of Michigan Medical School; Director, Developmental Disorders Clinic, University of Michigan Medical Center, Ann Arbor, Michigan

Thomas Walsh, M.D.
Clinical Associate Professor of Psychiatry and Behavioral Sciences, George Washington University School of Health Sciences, Washington, D.C.

Bruce Waslick, M.D.
Professor, Department of Psychiatry, Tufts University School of Medicine, Boston, Massachusetts

Elizabeth B. Weller, M.D.
Professor of Psychiatry and Pediatrics, Department of Psychiatry, University of Pennsylvania; Department of Child and Adolescent Psychiatry, The Children's Hospital of Philadelphia, Philadelphia, Pennsylvania

Ronald A. Weller, M.D.
Senior Lecturer, Department of Psychiatry, University of Pennsylvania, Philadelphia, Pennsylvania

Jerry M. Wiener, M.D. (deceased)
Leon Yochelson Professor of Psychiatry and Behavioral Sciences, and Professor of Pediatrics, Department of Psychiatry, George Washington University School of Medicine, Washington, D.C.

Timothy Wilens, M.D.
Director of Pediatric Substance Abuse Unit, Pediatric Psychopharmacology, Massachusetts General Hospital; Associate Professor of Psychiatry, Harvard Medical School, Boston, Massachusetts

Joseph L. Woolston, M.D.
Professor, Child Psychiatry and Pediatrics, Yale Child Study Center, Yale University School of Medicine, New Haven, Connecticut

Preface

The first edition in this series of comprehensive textbooks on clinical child and adolescent psychiatry was published in 1991, with Jerry Wiener, M.D., as Editor, in collaboration with the American Academy of Child and Adolescent Psychiatry. The *Textbook* has changed and expanded as our field has developed and research has blossomed, and I was honored to pick up the reins after Jerry's untimely death while chapters were being written and edited. In 2004 *The American Psychiatric Publishing Textbook of Child and Adolescent Psychiatry,* Third Edition, was published.

As growing knowledge has led to more substance and greater detail in each successive edition of the *Textbook,* a need emerged for a shorter, less expensive book that would focus on the "essentials." This is that abbreviated version. Jerry Wiener's name remains on this book as co-editor, because he selected so many of the authors and directed so much of the content from which this current book derived. The key principles in organizing this book and revising the

chapters have been to update where important new information has emerged and to focus on the practical information that is essential for a non–child psychiatrist who is evaluating and treating children and adolescents with psychiatric disorders. As a result of the national shortage of child and adolescent psychiatrists, mental health care for youth often is provided by other professionals or not at all. Our primary target audience for this book is the general psychiatrist, but we hope it will be useful to a broad range of physician and nonphysician mental health, pediatric, and neurological clinicians in their efforts to care for youth with emotional and behavioral problems and their families.

In order to produce an abbreviated, more accessible text, approximately half of the chapters were selected as those most important to the intended readership. Some excellent chapters could not be retained and still meet our goal of a shortened, more tightly focused book. Chapters or sections directed more toward subspecialists were not included.

The retained chapters were pruned to various degrees, and all were updated in content and references. Historical material and reports on research for which clinical implications are not yet known were reduced, with a constant eye on retaining what would be immediately useful in the clinician's office. The organization of the chapters is similar to that in the larger *Textbook*. Some chapters were combined, but no new ones have been added.

Of the seven chapters in the Treatment section of the *Textbook*, only one remains: Psychopharmacology. This is the chapter that required the most revision to remain current with the rapidly changing field of pediatric psychopharmacology. We surely do not want to imply that pharmacotherapy is indicated and psychotherapy is not. Each of the book's chapters on specific disorders covers a variety of treatments, both psychosocial and pharmacological. For each disorder, a different combination of treatments is emerging from research as the best for a specific category of patients. Of course, each youth and family is unique and may benefit from different types, amounts, and combinations of treatments. We chose to retain only the single treatment chapter on psychopharmacology because most non–child psychiatrist physicians (general psychiatrists, pediatricians, neurologists, family physicians) treating child psychiatric disorders will be providing evaluation and pharmacotherapy, not psychotherapy. In those cases, the psychotherapy will likely be done by psy-

chologists, social workers, or family therapists, for whom very brief chapters on therapy would not be useful because of their much more extensive training. For those physicians, nurses, and nonmedical mental health professionals who do conduct therapy, many entire books are available that address the various modalities. For the reader seeking an overview of psychotherapeutic treatments for youth, *The American Psychiatric Publishing Textbook of Child and Adolescent Psychiatry*, Third Edition, contains chapters summarizing psychodynamic therapy, cognitive-behavior modification, family and group psychotherapies, hypnosis, and milieu treatment.

John McDuffie and Bob Hales provided sage advice and valuable assistance in the preparation of this book, as in the others I have done with American Psychiatric Publishing. Tina Coltri-Marshall was indispensable in keeping track of authors, chapters, communications, and revisions as we updated, revised, and cut and pasted to produce this trimmed-down current summary of the field.

My husband, Richard Wendel, graciously interrupted his own scholarly pursuits in his neighboring study to provide support and encouragement as this book took shape.

Onward and upward!

Mina K. Dulcan, M.D.
Children's Memorial Hospital
Northwestern University
Feinberg School of Medicine
Chicago, Illinois

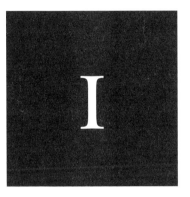

Assessment and Diagnosis

Overview of Development From Infancy Through Adolescence

Melvin Lewis, M.B., B.S., F.R.C.Psych., D.C.H.

Human development starts with genetic potential and blossoms through the interaction between the individual and the caring others in the individual's environment. Certain species characteristics may strongly influence the emergence and form of particular patterns of functioning. For example, the prolonged relative biological helplessness of the human infant is associated with characteristic patterns of attachment behavior, which presumably have great survival value. Furthermore, functions that are closely tied to central nervous system maturation (e.g., motor development) appear to be more robust and resistant to environmental influences than, for example, the capacity to develop relationships, which is exquisitely sensitive to environmental influences, particularly the competence of the mothering person.

For convenience, we tend to focus on discrete elements within disciplines. However, development is a complex process, and ultimately all the discrete elements must be integrated. As yet, no single theory is completely satisfactory.

Theories of developmental stages imply the development of a mental structure. Thus, psychoanalysis (Freud), psychosocial development (Erikson), and cognitive development (Piaget)—which together can be called the structural theories—postulate a genetically determined capacity for the development of patterns or systems of behavior in which the child acts on the environment from the very beginning. The overall behavior patterns

Sections of this chapter were modified from Lewis M, Volkmar F: *Clinical Aspects of Child and Adolescent Development*, 3rd Edition. Baltimore, MD, Lea & Febiger, 1990.

that then emerge are qualitatively different from one another but also exhibit continuity. The clinical implication of such structural theories is that some kind of reorganization within the child is required (e.g., resolution of intrapsychic conflict, alteration of the family homeostasis, and acquisition of new schema).

On the other hand, some theories of function and behavior do not appear to have a strong developmental point of view and rely instead on certain principles of reaction. Such reactive theories postulate that the child reacts in particular ways to environmental stimuli. Major examples of this type of theory are stimulus-response theory, learning theories, classical conditioning theory, and operant conditioning theory. The clinical implication of such reactive theories is that because it is regarded as learned behavior, the symptom is removed (i.e., the symptom is the disorder) and the disorder is cured through relearning or environmental change.

Although development is a complex process involving biological, psychological, cultural, and social factors, for convenience the study of development is usually approached along the lines of its major functional components.

The maturational and developmental lines discussed below include motor sequence, the senses, emotions, language development, cognitive development, memory and information processing, moral development, attachment, psychosexual phases, and temperament. A summary of developmental tasks and an account of developmental concepts concerning body image and psychological aspects of illness and death are also provided.

Motor Sequence

Gesell and Amatruda (1941/1964) observed that most children creep, can be pulled to their feet, and have a crude prehensile release by the time they are 10 months old. Within the next 2 months, they can walk with help and can grasp a small pellet. By age 2 years, they are running with ease, although not with great skill.

A steady increase in motor skills can be observed in most children. By age 3 years, a child can stand on one foot, dance, and jump, and he or she is also more dexterous than before and can build a tower of 10 cubes. Ambidexterity gives way to lateralization sometime during the third year, although handedness may not be firmly established for several years. Leg, eye, and ear dominance also may not become firmly established until the seventh, eighth, or ninth year, respectively, or even later. *Laterality* is a measurable, specialized, central function of a paired faculty such as eyes, ears, hands, and feet. *Preference* is the subjective, self-reported experience of an individual and need not be the same as objectively measured laterality. The preference of an individual may be related more to the acuity of the peripheral organ (e.g., the ear) than to anything else. *Dominance* is the term used for the concept of cerebral hemisphere specialization (e.g., information processing, language, and speech lateralization). Hemispheric lateralization appears to proceed sequentially from gross and fine motor skills to sensorimotor skills to speech and language (Leong 1976). Handedness is commonly consolidated around age 5 years; footedness, around age 7 years; eye preference, around age 7 or 8 years; and ear preference, around age 9 years (Touwen 1980).

Children become increasingly agile during the period of early childhood (e.g., learning to skip on alternate feet). Perceptual-motor skills also improve: a child at age 2 years can copy a circle; by age 3 years, a cross; by age 5 years, a square; and by age 7 years, a diamond. Memory also improves with brain maturation: by age 6 years, the child can count five digits forward and three digits backward. Between ages 6 and 11 years, the child not only learns new motor skills, such as balancing on a bicycle, but at some point, perhaps around age 9 years, does so with ease.

The Senses

Within a few hours after birth, the infant pays most attention to high-contrast visual stimuli (Kessen 1967). By 1 week of age, infants prefer to look at strongly patterned shapes, for example, a face, especially one in motion (e.g., nodding) (Fantz et al. 1975). With a "visual cliff" procedure, depth perception can be demonstrated by age 2 months (Campos et al. 1970). Color perception can also be demonstrated at this time (Bornstein 1975). The newborn can discriminate the particular smell of the mother (Engen et al. 1963) and can also discriminate the four basic tastes—sweet, acidic, salty, and bitter (Kobre and Lipsitt 1972). The newborn clearly experiences pain (e.g., on circumcision) (Porter et al. 1988). Infants hear at birth and respond preferentially to the mother's voice (Mills and Melhuish 1974).

Emotions

Emotions are complex phenomena having subjective, perceptual, and cognitive—as well as neurophysiological, expressive, and motoric—components interacting with one another and with the environment. The development of emotions appears to proceed through a progressive differentiation from more or less global affective states (e.g., generalized excitement) to more specific emotions such as anger or delight, depending in part on the infant's experience of social interaction and increasing maturation. Attempts to control emotions are seen in children in nursery school (age 3 years).

The expression of pleasure occurs early. Whole-face smiles in response to positive social interaction occur at about age 4–6 weeks (Sroufe and Waters 1976) and increasingly become involved in the attachment behaviors of infants that promote social reciprocity. Smiling is also seen when the infant seems to have mastered a task. Laughter is the next expression of pleasure to appear, usually around age 4 months, and is often seen in response to peek-a-boo games.

Anxiety occurs in infants in response to sudden stimulus changes. Fear and anxiety in response to the sight of a stranger (Kagan 1984) occur at age 8 months, followed by separation anxiety when the security provided by the presence and proximity of an attachment figure is threatened. Anger is often seen in response to frustration and restraint, perhaps peaking in the second year. However, it may also be seen in school-age children and adolescents when the same conflict occurs. Guilt, which involves awareness of a transgression and a feeling of remorse, may be observed in 2-year-olds.

Preschool children fear animals, frightening dreams, and natural phenomena such as thunder and lightning. School-age children fear harm to the body, and adolescents may exhibit social anxiety. Most of these fears tend to diminish with age.

Presumably, all affects can serve adaptive and protective functions. However, excessive affects can be disorganizing.

Language Development

The sequence for the making of sounds is broadly the same in all children everywhere (Lenneberg 1967). Children vocalize and respond to sounds from birth, possibly even prenatally. The infant can be soothed specifically by the voice of his or her mother (primary caregiver) as early as the first few weeks. By age 6 weeks, the infant begins to utter repetitive strings of sound called *babbling*. In doing so, the infant finds satisfaction in producing at will sounds that at first occurred involuntarily. Skill is acquired in making sounds, and the sounds of others are imitated as nearly as possible.

Up to about 5 months the infant tends to use "filler syllables," which are usually nasals and which gradually decrease as multiple syllable utterances occur (Aoyama 2001). Thus, the number of filler syllables increases up through 20 months, after which it drops dramatically.

The nearer the approximation of the infant's sounds to those of the parents, the more marked will be the parents' approval and the greater will be the infant's incentive to repeat such sounds. In this way, the phonetic pattern of the child's mother tongue is acquired. Inadequate stimulation in these early weeks may restrict the frequency and variety of sounds.

The capacity to discriminate among different sounds is present in the newborn (Friedlander 1970). Almost from the beginning, the infant seems to be programmed to move in rhythm to the human voice (Condon and Sander 1974) and will orient with eyes, head, and body to animate sound stimuli (Mills and Melhuish 1974). Subsequent language development correlates most closely with motor development. Crying, which is present during fetal life, soon becomes differentiated during the first few months into recognized cries related to hunger, discomfort, pain, pleasure, and other stimuli (Wolff 1969). As crying decreases, cooing increases, and vowel sounds (e.g., "ooh")

begin to dominate. Consonants begin to appear at about age 5 months and words at about age 1 year, with a range of 8–18 months (Morley 1965). At the same time, by age 1 year, the infant discriminates between and responds to differences in language, depending on who is speaking and how that person is speaking (e.g., the intonation and the amount of repetition used). Vocabulary gradually increases to approximately 200 words by age 2 years. Nouns appear first, then verbs, adjectives, and adverbs. Pronouns appear by the time the child is age 2 years, and conjunctions, after age 2½ years. By this time, too, the child's understanding of language has increased immensely. Between the ages of 2 and 4 years, the child has acquired, or learned, most of the fundamental (as opposed to the academic) rules of grammar.

Early schemas of experience precede symbolic language, and language comprehension precedes language production (children understand words and sentences long before they can say them).

It is very likely that the mother's spoken words are initially experienced by the infant as tones and rhythms rather than as words with meanings, and as such they are part of the kinesthetic, tactile, visual, auditory, olfactory, and gustatory bombardment that the infant tries to assimilate and organize. Eventually, the child's percept of mother, for example, already linked to the word *mother*, becomes better defined. In this sense, mothers are sensitive language teachers of their children (Moerk 1974). The sensitive timing, repetition, and associated pleasurable affects with which mothers uses words for labeling, shaping, and so on serve to stimulate the development of language in their children. (Curiously, mothers seem to talk more to their baby girls than to their baby boys [Halverson and Waldrop 1970].)

Children continue to learn phonology, syntax, and semantics throughout the school years. The utterances of young children appear to depend on the support of the nonlinguistic environment. For example, if one asks a child a question out of context, the child often "draws a blank" (Bloom 1975). Young children tend to respond more readily when they are asked to talk about events that are in a more immediately perceived context.

Cognitive Development

■ Piaget's Theory

The beginning of thinking is in the body. The infant reacts to a sensory stimulus with a motor reaction: when a finger is placed in the infant's hand, the infant will grasp; when a nipple is placed in the infant's mouth, he or she will begin sucking; when a pattern is placed in front of the infant's eyes, he or she will respond by looking. This sensorimotor pattern is the earliest kind of thinking, and it starts with innate patterns of behavior such as grasping, sucking, looking, and gross body activity.

The basic element in Piaget's theory of the child's cognitive development is the *schema*, which consists of a pattern of behavior in response to a particular stimulus from the environment. However, the schema is more than just a response, because the child also acts on the environment. For example, the infant sucks in response to a nipple. The schema of sucking then becomes increasingly complex as the child reacts to and acts on a wider range of environmental stimuli. Thus, when the thumb is put into the mouth, the schema of sucking evoked by a nipple is gradually broadened to include this new and similar but not identical stimulus, the thumb. The new object (the thumb) is said to be *assimilated* into the original schema. At the same time, sucking behavior has to be slightly modified because the thumb is different in shape, taste, and other characteristics from the nipple. This act of modification, which Piaget called *accommodation*, results in a new equilibrium. These two processes, assimilation and accommodation, proceed in ever-increasing complexities.

Four major stages of development are described in Piaget's theory:

1. Sensorimotor stage (from birth to 2 years)
2. Preoperational stage (from 2 years to 7 years)
3. Concrete operational stage (from 7 years to adolescence)
4. Formal operational stage (adolescence)

In the sensorimotor stage (birth to 2 years), six substages are discernible:

1. In the first month, the infant exercises a function, such as looking or grasping, simply because the function exists.
2. During the next 3–4 months (from age 1 to 4½ months), new schemas are acquired that usually center on the infant's own body (e.g., his or her thumb).
3. Sometime between ages 4½ and 8 or 9 months, the infant tries to produce an effect on the object he or she sees or grasps. That is, he or she now includes events or objects in the external environment (e.g., a rattle).
4. By ages 8 to 11½ months, the infant begins to be aware of the existence of unperceived objects hidden, for example, behind a pillow or in peek-a-boo games. This is also the time of so-called stranger anxiety. The mental image of the object has now achieved some degree of permanence in the infant's mind (*object permanence*).

5. In the first half of the second year (age 11 or 12–18 months), the child explores an object and its spatial relationship more thoroughly, for example, by putting smaller objects into and taking them out of larger ones.

    a. The child initiates changes that produce variations in the event itself, for example, dropping bread and then toys from different heights or different positions.
    b. The child actively searches for novel events.

6. By the end of the second year (ages 18–24 months), the child shows some evidence of reasoning; mental trial and error replaces trial and error in action.

The use of toys and play for a child is essentially a form of thinking. External objects (play items) are organized in such a way as to represent the child's internal symbolization of events and fantasies. Piaget called this evocation of past events and fantasies in the present play *deferred imitation,* a characteristic of symbolic thought.

The preoperational stage, occurring approximately between the ages of 2 and 7 years, clearly reflects progress over the preceding stage of sensorimotor intelligence. Two substages are described: 1) *symbolic activity* and make-believe play and 2) *decentration.*

The substage of symbolic activity and make-believe play occurs between the ages of 2 and 4 years. In this substage, symbolic thought and representation develop. Language becomes increasingly important as the child learns to distinguish between actual objects and the labels used to represent them. As a result, the child gradually becomes able to reason symbolically rather than motorically. However, despite these significant ad-

vances, there are striking cognitive limitations to preoperational thinking. The child's judgments in the early preoperational stage are dominated by the child's perceptions of events, objects, and experiences. Furthermore, the child can attend to only one perceptual dimension or attribute at a time. The concept of time is also not available to a child at this preoperational stage. Sequences and daily routines can be recognized (e.g., mealtime, playtime, sleep time, day and night, and Daddy's or Mommy's going and coming), but the child has no concept of an hour, a minute, a week, or a month.

The preoperational child is also extremely egocentric. By that, Piaget did not mean that the child is selfish. Rather, Piaget used the term *egocentric* to refer to a certain cognitive limitation during the preoperational stage, namely, that the young child is conceptually unable to view events and experiences from any point of view but his or her own. The child is clearly the center of his or her own representational world. Similarly, the child is unable to differentiate clearly between the self and the world, between the subjective realm of thoughts and feelings and the objective realm of external reality.

In addition, at the preoperational stage, the child's reasoning is neither inductive nor deductive but what Piaget termed *transductive.* That is, the young child tends to relate the particular to the particular in an alogical manner. Events may be viewed as related not because of any inherent cause-and-effect relationship but simply on the basis of spatial or temporal contiguity or juxtaposition. Furthermore, the child at this stage is unaware of and therefore unconcerned about possible logical contradictions.

The substage of decentration occurs between ages 4 and 7 years. In this substage, an increased accommodation to reality gradually takes over, and the child's own interests, perception, and points of view progressively decenter. The decentering comes about partly because of the child's increased social involvement (e.g., at school). Social interaction virtually demands that the child use language, and the child discovers that what he or she thinks is not necessarily the same as what the child's peers think. The child begins to recognize other points of view.

The concrete operational stage usually occurs between ages 7 and 11 years. The child at this stage is no longer bound by the configuration perceived at a given moment. Two variables (e.g., height and width) can now be taken into account at once. Piaget (1952) performed what is now a classic experiment. One form of Piaget's experiment follows. The child is first asked to make sure that the amounts of water in two identical beakers are the same. The water from one of the beakers is then transferred into a tall, narrow cylinder. The child is asked whether the remaining beaker contains the same amount of water as the cylinder. A child who is in the preoperational stage may say "no" and, if asked why, may say either that the cylinder contains more water "because it's higher" or that the beaker contains more water "because it's wider." A child who is at the concrete operational stage will be able to say, "Yes, the amount of water is the same" and, if asked why, will be able to say, "because it's narrower in the cylinder and wider in the beaker" and (perhaps) "because it's the same water that had been in the other beaker."

The child has mastered what Piaget called the concept of *conservation*. The child learns to apply the concept of conservation not only to volume but also to number, class, length, weight, and area.

These types of conservation occur at different ages. The conservation of objects occurs quite early, usually by the end of the sensorimotor period. Quantity is conserved at ages 6–8 years and weight at ages 9–12 years. Probably the variation in age at which different conservations are achieved is related to how easily the property can be dissociated from the child's own action. According to Piaget (1958), "It is more difficult to…equalize…objects whose properties are less easy to dissociate from one's own action, such as weight, than to apply the same operation to properties which can be objectified more readily, such as length" (p. 249).

Age 6 or 7 years marks a key turning point in the child's thinking. After age 6 or 7 years, the child is no longer bound by his or her perception and can apply reasoning. It is the age at which the child starts first grade. It also corresponds in psychoanalytic theory to the time when the oedipal struggle is thought to be resolved and the superego consolidated. Feelings can be distanced, thought about, and put into context. Also, the child can more readily distinguish between fantasy and reality.

In short, the major advance in the concrete operational stage is that the child can apply basic logical principles to the realm of concrete experiences and events without being bound by his or her perceptions. Gradually, logical thought processes become organized into an increasingly complex and integrated network through which the surrounding world is confronted and responded to systematically.

Piaget (1969) observed that in the formal operational stage, "the great novelty that characterizes adolescent thought and that starts around the age of 11 to 12, but probably does not reach its point of equilibrium until the age of 14 or 15,…consists in the possibility of manipulating ideas in themselves and no longer in merely manipulating objects" (p. 23). The young adolescent can now use hypotheses, experiment, make deductions, and reason from the particular to the general. The adolescent is no longer tied to the environment. He or she in essence can now make theoretical statements independent of specific content and can apply this way of thinking to many kinds of data.

The result is a further release from the concrete world: "The most distinctive property of formal thought is this reversal of direction between reality and possibility; instead of deriving a rudimentary type of theory from the empirical data, as is done in concrete inferences, formal thought begins with a theoretical synthesis implying that certain relations are necessary and this proceeds in the opposite direction" (Piaget 1958, p. 251).

Pragmatically, Piaget provided a set of cognitive developmental norms that are useful to the clinician. For example, preschool children are often preoccupied with superpowerful and giant figures such as dinosaurs and doll-figure heroes and heroines that represent the perceived powerful and idealized human figures in the child's life. This representation is evident in the symbolic play of young children. The clinician can then use this information as a means of understanding the concerns, conflicts, wishes, and anxieties of a child. Piaget's system also offers an explanation of the preoperational child's difficulties in resolving emotional as well as intellectual problems. For such a child, fantasy and reality may be poorly differentiated and affects more difficult to conceptualize.

The school-age child in the concrete operational stage is trying to construct an orderly and lawful world and is becoming socialized. These processes can be seen, for example, in the child's use of rules in games, such as checkers and Monopoly, and in the child's acceptance of symbols such as paper money and the hierarchical implications in games like checkers (e.g., "king").

■ Memory and Information Processing

Memory is increasingly viewed as a highly complex process consisting of numerous interacting systems that function at different levels. Such systems include attention (Mirsky et al. 1991) and motivation systems, as well as the actions of neurotransmitters and hormones.

During fetal development an astonishing, orderly, massive migration of cells occurs, starting in a proliferative zone near the cerebral ventricle and ending in various locations of the cerebral cortex. This migration was found to continue throughout the middle third of gestation, at which time neurogenesis appeared to be complete; that is, no further neurogenesis was found to occur (Rakic 1996; Rakic et al. 1994).

However, Gould et al. (1999) asserted that the neocortex in primates continues to acquire a large number of new neurons and in fact does so on a daily basis throughout the life cycle. Specific memory functions may be confined to specific domains. According to Squire (1987):

> Each specialized system has its own specific, short-term, working-memory capacity and also the capacity to retain in long-term memory specific features or dimensions of information. Each specialized system thereby stores the product of its own processing. Long-term memory of even a single event depends on synaptic change in a distributed ensemble of neurons, which themselves belong to many different processing systems, and the ensemble acting together constitutes memory for the whole event. (p. 241)

Information processing theories view cognition as a data processing system analogous to a computer (Newell et al. 1958). The mental processes are defined in terms of a sequence of problem-solving steps that transform sensory or perceptual input into cognitive or behavioral output.

"Chunking" is regarded as a central strategy for managing (processing) information (Miller 1989). Chunks are aggregates of related facts, concepts, or precepts that enlarge with experience. These chunks become hierarchically integrated, one within another. In essence, chunking is the process by which representations, procedures, and memories that occur together are automatically accessed simultaneously.

Chunking occurs in what is now called *short-term memory*. For example, a child perceives an auditory sensation, which is instantaneously scanned for pattern recognition (e.g., it may immediately be recognized as speech). Information processing theory suggests that this speech pattern is then transferred into short-term memory, where it may last for about a minute or two and then evaporate, or it may undergo some other process and last longer. Other processes might include a rehearsal strategy such as repetition (e.g., as one repeats a telephone number aloud to enable remembering it). One of three things may then happen to the item:

1. It may be emitted or discharged in a behavioral–affective response (e.g., one makes the telephone call).
2. It may be stored (i.e., remembered) in long-term memory.
3. It may remain temporarily in short-term memory for further processing of the kind mentioned above. Within the context of short-term memory, new information may also interact with relevant information retrieved from long-term memory.

Working memory is the term used when all of the active processes described above (chunking, rehearsal, discharge, and storage) are taking place.

Long-term memory appears to involve two types of knowledge:

1. *Declarative knowledge* (a "knowing that" kind of memory), which is knowledge of facts, concepts, and ideas that are nodal, with links between nodes representing associations between ideas. This kind of knowledge is accessible to consciousness and can be declared. Amnesia due to brain damage usually results in a loss of this kind of declarative knowledge.
2. *Procedural knowledge* (or "how-to" implicit knowledge), which is knowledge of how to perform certain skills—such as riding a bicycle, reading, certain conditioned responses, and perhaps subliminal sound or image retention—all of which soon become automatized. This kind of knowledge is usually unconscious and is usually not lost in the amnesia commonly found in brain damage. However, because procedural memory is mediated by the basal ganglia, lesions of the basal ganglia will consequently disrupt procedural memory and will cause impairment of motor memory and deficits in learning new motor skills, as in Huntington's disease and parkinsonism.

In essence, information theory proposes a number of networks that are called forth for various tasks—a model that is in contrast to, for example, the Piagetian developmental structural concept of a hierarchical organization of mental operations (e.g., concrete operations and formal operations).

Memory seems to develop in spurts. For example, there seems to be a developmental shift and enhancement of memory between ages 8 and 12 months, perhaps in relation to central nervous system maturation (Kagan 1971, 1984). Clinically, this also corresponds to the time when one commonly sees children become anxious when around strangers.

Very soon after birth, an infant recognizes and remembers the mother's voice, smell, taste, and touch; as mentioned earlier, the infant can remember the mother's smell virtually at birth. From an evolutionary perspective, these capacities can be understood in terms of their value for attachment and survival. However, initially, memory is short. A 1-month-old infant can remember a mobile for about 24 hours (Weizmann et al. 1971). By age 5 or 6 months, an infant can remember for several weeks an object seen only for a few minutes (L.J. Cohen and Gelber 1975). Memory subsequently increases in duration as memories accumulate and as memory becomes less context dependent. Evidence of early memory is seen in phenomena such as object permanence, object constancy, stranger reaction, attachment behaviors, and separation anxiety. Memories of the past gradually lead to predictions of the future (e.g., the infant anticipates that the mother is about to leave by observing her preparatory actions).

During the school-age years, children quickly acquire a wider repertoire of metacognitive strategies to improve memory, and today, good teachers help each child identify his or her best metacognitive strategy.

Children's short-term memory for things that they understand may be as good as, if not better than, adults' short-term memory (Johnson and Foley 1984; Loftus and Davies 1984); however, such memories are vulnerable because of children's susceptibility to suggestions. Some researchers (R.L. Cohen and Harnick 1980; Dale et al. 1978; S. Murray, "The Effect of Post-Event Information on Children's Memories for an Illustrated Story," unpublished manuscript, 1983) found in the laboratory that asking leading questions increased the likelihood that subjects of all ages would incorporate the memory of specific information contained in those questions into answers given 2 weeks later (R.L. Cohen and Harnick 1980; S. Murray, unpublished manuscript, 1983). In an attempt to observe children in a more realistic setting, Goodman et al. (1987) studied children receiving inoculations in their doctors' offices. The researchers found the children to be highly accurate in their recall of events, but they also found that 3- and 4-year-olds were more suggestible than 5- and 6-year-olds. The latter showed some suggestibility but mostly in regard to detail about the room rather than to information about persons or actions. Children seem to notice items that adults might consider irrelevant, but they also make more errors of omission than do adults (Neisser 1984). Sometimes children try to fill gaps in their memories by confabulating, although in some instances the apparent confabulation may be the result—neurobiologically speaking—of faulty or inaccurate recall. And perhaps because children lack previous knowledge, they may have difficulty relating events and organizing disparate elements into a cohesive whole (Johnson and Foley 1984). However, as noted by Kobasigawa (1974), if given external prompts or cues, children can perform quite well on recall, a fact that a clever attorney might use when he or she asks leading questions of a child witness.

Recall in children may be confounded by a number of factors related to cognitive and emotional development. For example, children younger than age 6 years may, in some situations, confuse fact with fantasy. Johnson and Foley (1984) found that young children had some difficulty in discriminating between what they had done and what they had thought of doing. However, the researchers concluded that children at this age were able to differentiate their own thoughts from another person's actions. Young children are also often concrete in their thinking.

Young children may quite correctly describe events in relation to holidays, seasons, birthdays, meals, or television programs (Hudson 1990). Older children have been shown in some studies to be quite accurate with regard to frequency of occurrence or temporal sequence of events (A.L. Brown 1975; Hasher and Zacks 1979). Recent studies have reported that some children as young as 16 months can remember sequentially (i.e., temporally). In general, however, young children, ages 4–6 years, are able to locate events spatially but have difficulty dating events in real time compared with children age 10 years and older, who generally have acquired the concept of time units and sequences and therefore can more easily order events temporally (Goldstone and Goldfarb 1966).

It is very likely that what we call a memory is not just the simple recall of a thing or an event but the representation of multiple processes—including perceptions, fantasy formation, and affects—that are aroused by, or that come to be associated with, an "event" (or even a nonevent). From the point of view of psychopathology and treatment, still other processes are involved, including defenses that are subsequently mobilized against the anxiety that arises when a memory and its associated affects emerge during treatment.

Moral Development

Moral behavior derives in part from the basic cultural rules governing social action that the child assimilates and internalizes, and moral development is the increase in the degree to which the internalization and accommodation of these

basic cultural rules have occurred.

Fear of punishment is prominent in young children. The next attribute to develop is an urge to confess. By age 12 or 13 years, most children seem to react directly with guilt and internal self-criticism when faced with the fact of their transgression, although this reaction often occurs at a much younger age.

Piaget's (1965) view on the moral development of the child can be conceptualized in the context of the major stages of cognitive development:

- *Preoperational stage:* The morality is one of constraints—rules of behavior are viewed as natural laws handed down by the child's parents. Violation brings retribution or unquestioned punishment, and no account is taken of motives.
- *Concrete operational stage:* The morality is one of acceptance—rules of behavior become a matter of mutual acceptance, with complete equality of treatment, but no account is taken of special circumstances.
- *Formal operational stage:* The morality is one of cooperation—rules can be constructed as required by the needs of the group as long as they can be agreed on. Motives are now taken into account, and circumstances may temper the administration of justice.

As the child advances through these stages, progressive decentering occurs. Building on Piaget's views, Kohlberg (1964) suggested three major levels of development of moral judgment (Table 1–1).

Numerous criticisms of Kohlberg's (1964) work have been made. Some of the stages, especially the later stages, have not been reliably substantiated, and many believe that descriptions of some stages are too politicized in favor of a liberal viewpoint. Others think that the

Table 1–1. Kohlberg's three major levels of development of moral judgment

Level I: Premorality (or pre–conventional morality)

Type 1. Punishment and obedience orientation (i.e., obedience to parents' superior force)

Type 2. Naive instrumental hedonism (i.e., agreement to obey only in return for some reward)

Level II: Morality of conventional role conformity

Type 3. Good-boy morality of maintaining good relations, approval of others (i.e., conformity to rules in order to please and gain approval)

Type 4. Authority-maintaining morality (i.e., adherence to rules for the sake of upholding social order)

Level III: Morality of self-accepted moral principles

Type 5. Morality of social contract, of individual rights, and of, for example, democratically accepted law (with a reliance on a legalistic "social contract")

Type 6. Morality of individual principles of conscience (there is voluntary compliance based on ethical principles; this level is probably not reached until early adolescence, and it may not be reached at all)

stages described are, in any event, bound by culture, the historic moment, middle-class status, and male gender of the subjects. As a result of these criticisms, Kohlberg attempted some revisions. For example, Kohlberg (1978) and Colby (1978) subsequently identified two types of reasoning at each stage: type A emphasizes literal interpretation of the rules and roles of society, whereas type B is a more consolidated form and refers to the intent of normative standards. However, in general, Kohlberg (1978) essentially held to the same hierarchical sequence and idealized end point.

More recently, Gilligan (1982) offered a different view of moral development in which an expanding connection with and concern for others was thought to represent an alternative developmental pathway and goal. This alternative and equally valid pathway has been demonstrated more often in girls than in boys; that is, in general, girls seem to have "a greater sense of connection and concern with relationships more than with rules" (p. 202).

Attachment Behavior

Attachment is an affectional tie that one person forms with another person, enduring over time. Attachment is discriminating and specific. One may be attached to more than one person, but there is usually a gradient in the strength of such multiple attachments (Schaffer and Emerson 1964). Attachment implies affect, predominantly affection or love.

Bonding implies a selective attachment (L.J. Cohen 1974) that is maintained even when there is no contact with the person with whom the bond exists.

Attachment behavior is behavior that promotes proximity to or contact with the specific figure or figures to whom the person is attached. Attachment behavior includes signals (crying, smiling, vocalizing), locomotion (looking, following, and approaching), and contacts (clambering up, embracing, and clinging). Sucking, clinging, following, crying, and smiling are used by the time a child is age 8 or 9 months. Attachment behavior is strongest in toddlers; bonding is most secure in older children (Rutter 1976b).

Bowlby (1969) proposed that the biological function of attachment behavior is to protect the infant from danger, especially the danger of attack by predators. The system may be activated by hormonal state, by environmental stimulus, and by central nervous system excitation.

The system is terminated in response to a specific terminating signal (e.g., attachment achieved) or by habituation. The attachment behavior system is in equilibrium with other important behavior systems (e.g., exploratory behavior, which is elicited by stimuli that have novelty and complexity or change and may draw the infant away from the mother).

At least 15 kinds of attachment behavior have been described (Ainsworth 1963), including differential crying, smiling, and vocalization; greeting responses, such as lifting of arms and hand clapping; crying when the mother leaves; scrambling over the mother; following the mother; clinging and kissing; and exploration away from the mother when the mother is a secure base, with rapid return to the mother as a haven of safety.

Spitz (1965) talked of three "organizers" as a concept to account for the factors that govern the process of transition from one level of development to the next:

1. The first organizer is the smiling response, which is the visible manifestation of a certain degree of organization in the psychic apparatus.
2. The second organizer is the 8-month anxiety, which marks a new stage in development.
3. The third organizer is the achievement of the sign of negation and of the word *no*. In Spitz's view, it is the first abstraction, or symbol, formed by the child, usually at the beginning of the second year (around 15 months), when the infant turns his or her head away to refuse food (a response that has its origins in the rooting reflex).

■ Factors That Influence the Development of Attachment

Four factors influence the development of attachment. The first factor concerns sensitive phases in the development of infant–mother attachment. The sensitive phase during which attachments are most readily formed spans a period of months in the middle of the first year. It probably starts in the neonatal period. Provence and Lipton (1962) showed that infants kept in an institution until they are ages 8–24 months find it difficult to become attached to a foster mother later and that 24 months seems to be the upper limit of the sensitive phase for becoming attached for the first time. The second factor concerns infant-care practices such as feeding practices. The third factor concerns maternal care, infant behavior, and mother–infant interaction. The mother's contribution to attachment is affected by factors such as her hormonal state, her parity and experience, and her personality. The infant's contribution is affected by factors such as wakefulness and activity level, crying, temperament, genetic makeup, and organic makeup. The final factor influencing the development of attachment concerns maternal deprivation.

Several clinical types of attachment have been described, including *secure, insecure-avoidant, insecure-resistant,* and *insecure-disorganized/disoriented* (Main and Solomon 1986).

Clinically, attachment theory is useful as a basis for providing appropriate care of premature infants and very young children in the hospital, deciding on adoption practices and child placement, and understanding certain aspects of child abuse.

Although a full discussion is beyond the scope of this chapter, it is important to note an increasingly large body of research involving the roles of oxytocin and vasopressin in relation to social memory and social attachment. The genes involved appear to have been robustly conserved throughout evolution—from fish, reptiles, birds, and mammals—in complex neural pathways that extend from olfactory bulbs through to the amygdala and cortex (Insel 1997; Leckman and Herman 2002).

Psychosexual Development

By age 2 years, children know their own sex (i.e., boy or girl) and recognize clearly whether others are boys or girls. By age 5 years, the child knows that one's sex is (more or less) permanent. Sex role behaviors are shaped and influenced through interactions with others, beginning at birth. Self-stereotyping and further socialization increase with peer relationships and are manifested in play and toy preferences. However, play in children is not necessarily predictive of adult sexual identity. Green (1987) reported that boys who persistently play more like girls, who cross-dress, and who prefer or wish to be a girl *may* be more likely to become homosexual but are not definitely so. Some boys also may have a genetic predisposition to homosexuality (Bailey and Pillard 1991).

■ Psychoanalytic Views

In psychoanalytic theory, the sexual aim of a young infant is said to be to obtain pleasure and relief from discomfort by the most immediate means possible. The infant draws pleasure from a wide variety of visual, tactile, kinesthetic, and auditory stimuli.

Oral Phase

By far the most sensitive region in the infant—and apparently the greatest source of pleasure—is the mouth. The object of the sexual instinct is thought to be the body of the infant, seen in *autoerotic* (self-stimulating) activities such as mouthing and sucking. It is important to note that certain genetic factors and biological orienting patterns are in operation before

any psychological mechanisms. For example, the suck reflex is coordinated to the cyclical flow of breast milk (Dubignon and Campbell 1969), and by age 6 days the infant can selectively orient to smell, preferring mother's milk (Macfarlane 1975).

Anal Phase

As the infant develops and as speech and the capacity for symbol formation emerge, the child begins to experience feelings about separateness and worth. A sense of autonomy develops that has to be reconciled with ambivalent feelings, all at about the same time that new skills are acquired, only one of which is sphincter control. During this process, according to psychoanalytic theory, the anal mucosa is said to become "erotogenized" and may serve in part the aims of the ambivalent feelings just mentioned. Indeed, the young child may express his or her ambivalence in the (pleasurable) holding in and letting go of feces during bowel movements. However, this ambivalence may also be expressed in the controlling and clinging behaviors seen in some 2- and 3-year-old children. This suggests that the alleged central role of the anal mucosa at this stage has probably been exaggerated, reflecting perhaps the practices that prevailed at the time Freud made his observations.

Phallic-Oedipal Phase

When the child is between ages 3 and 6 years, behavior that is more clearly recognizable as sexual appears. The child at this stage is very much aware of the anatomical differences between the sexes and is curious about pregnancy, childbirth, and death. Sometimes this interest is represented in the play of the child. For example, play with toys that involves filling and emptying, opening and shutting, fitting in and throwing away, and building up and knocking down blocks has been interpreted as representing a curiosity about the body and sexual functions.

Opportunities for the sequential development of play in childhood thus become as important for the sexual development of the child as they are for other purposes (e.g., problem solving, mastery of body skills, functional pleasure in play, coping with anxiety, facilitating relationships, and communication purposes). The child at this stage is said to experience intense sexual and aggressive urges toward both parents, but the aim is less well defined. Boys and girls may become absorbed by fairy-tale or television characters that serve to represent the children's own fantasies. Such fantasies also emerge in the dreams of children. Children at this age may also play at being mothers and fathers or doctors and nurses—working toward a partial fulfillment of their sexual aims, which at this time may be partially fused with their aggressive fantasies. Boys and girls may be quite exhibitionistic and possessive, especially of the parent of the opposite sex. Hostility toward the same-sex parent seems to be influenced by certain characteristic family patterns of relationships present in a particular society (Honigmann 1954).

Latency Phase

Between ages 6 and 12 years, during the elementary-school years, concepts of inevitability regarding birth, death, and sex differences become clarified, and the sense of time and the ability to differentiate between fantasy and reality become established. Defense mechanisms, which in general bar from consciousness certain unacceptable impulses and fantasies and at the same time provide some substitute gratification, are strengthened. The child consolidates earlier reactions, such as shame against exhibitionistic urges, disgust against messiness, and a sense of guilt that serves to contain sexual and aggressive wishes. The child's play at this time is usually characterized by organization, whether in a board game or a team game. Sex play, far from being dormant, continues actively, especially with voyeuristic tendencies and the urge to touch. The sex play often may be more discreet at this age (i.e., adults may see it less often); however, it also may be quite overt, with much interest and curiosity (Reese 1966). The object of the sexual instinct may be a peer, but the actual playmate may be of either sex.

■ Puberty and Adolescence

Pubertal Maturation

Physical pubertal maturation proceeds in predictable sequences that differ by sex and vary considerably in timing among individuals (Marshall and Tanner 1970; Tanner 1962). Early-maturing females and late-maturing males are more likely to receive negative peer and adult evaluations than on-time females and early-maturing males (Tobin-Richards et al. 1983). Physically attractive adolescents are stereotyped more extensively than unattractive adolescents (Langlois and Stephan 1981), and unattractive adolescents seem to have more adjustment and behavioral problems than their attractive counterparts (Lerner and Lerner 1977).

Cultural Perspectives on Adolescence

Adolescence as a phase of development existed in some form long before it was recognized and conceptualized in the United States by G. Stanley Hall in 1904. For example, at the time of the Sumerian culture of 4000 to 3000 B.C., the first case of juvenile delinquency was recorded on clay tablets (Kramer 1959). The *Oxford English Dictionary* traces the word itself to the fifteenth century.

In all cultures and in all times the period has been marked by rites of passage. In simple cultures where young men and women are needed to do adult work, the period of initiation is short. The initiation rites vary from culture to culture, but they often involve periods of fasting or other ordeals.

During puberty, the young adolescent struggles to achieve body mastery, to control sexual and aggressive urges, to separate from the family, to find new and appealing sexual relationships, and to achieve a sense of identity. In the course of this struggle, the sexual behavior of the adolescent may include petting and mutual masturbation (which may be heterosexual or homosexual) and, eventually, intercourse. Sometimes, earlier aims and objects are temporarily gratified and used (e.g., in isolated acts of fellatio or in exhibitionistic behavior).

Other Views

Rutter (1971, 1976a) reviewed the scientific literature on normal psychosexual development. He concluded that Freud's description of the oral and anal stages is too narrow and somewhat misleading, that the oedipal situation is not universal, that Freud's description of the latency period is wrong in most respects, and that Freud's concept of an innate sex drive that has a quantifiable energy component is only a half-truth. Rutter noted that current evidence is insufficient to decide among the various psychological theories of sexual development.

Temperament

In the course of their clinical observations and research for their New York Longitudinal Study, Thomas and Chess (1977) became fascinated with what they perceived as the individual styles that characterized each child—or rather, the peculiar shaping and reshaping of these styles as the child and his or her family develop. This phenomenon came to be known as the *temperament* of the child.

Chess and Thomas (1986) identified nine categories of behavior that constitute the individual's temperament: 1) activity level, 2) rhythmicity (hunger, elimination, sleep–wake), 3) approach or withdrawal response, 4) adaptability to a change in the environment, 5) threshold of responsiveness, 6) intensity of any given reaction, 7) mood (quality, quantity), 8) degree of distractibility, and 9) persistence in the face of obstacles.

About 1 child in 10 was found to have a so-called difficult temperament, and about 1 in 6 was in a slow-to-warm-up group. About two-fifths of the children studied were found to have a so-called easy temperament.

The New York Longitudinal Study showed, among other things, that the consistency of the interactional process between temperament and environment constituted a kind of continuity. This continuity also allowed some plasticity in development. Although this plasticity in turn might make some kinds of predictions uncertain, it also suggested that early parental errors and even specific emotional trauma to the child do not necessarily have fixed, inevitable consequences and that therapeutic intervention could help at any stage of development. It also suggested that subsequent improved and positive experiences following a therapeutic intervention might in themselves have a further therapeutic effect.

These ideas challenged some previously held views on the causes of various developmental and clinical phenomena. In particular, Thomas and colleagues (1968) added the important idea that the child, far from being a passive recipient or simply a responder to various stimuli, is an active initiator and contributor to his or her own experience and development. They also found that this activity on the part of the child was determined to an extent by the child's temperament and that the child's particular developmental characteristics contributed in important ways to some of the behavior disorders seen in children.

Also new was the notion of variations in style originating in the genotype of an individual and brought out and modified by the individual child's active interaction with the environment, with each strain modified and capable of being shaped by experience, teaching, and learning.

A practical and central concept devised by Thomas and Chess (1977) to study and understand the child's struggle for mastery was the "goodness of fit" in the complex interactions over time between the child's temperament and the environment.

In this clinical perspective, temperament is not seen as a theory of development; rather, it is regarded as but one attribute of an individual—albeit an important one. Clinically, these concepts and findings of temperament studies are useful in understanding and relieving certain parent–child problems.

For an account of other research contributions on the topic of temperament, see Kagan 2002.

Developmental Tasks

Finally, development can be thought about in terms of its meaning for the individual from infancy through adolescence, as outlined by Erikson (1959).

The developmental task of the very young infant is to achieve adaptation to the outside world. Sometime between ages 1½ and 3 years it becomes clear that a child is tackling several other develop-

mental tasks. First, a fundamental task is to achieve greater physical independence. The maturation of the child's neuromuscular system is central to feelings of self-worth. The child also makes a shift from a passive to an active position. Furthermore, the child now can think instead of act by using language with symbols and concepts. Whereas the young child at first uses few words, mostly in the service of direct discharge of feelings (primary process), the child as he or she ages begins to use language more independently of immediate need. In concert with this development, definite attitudes toward people are formed, especially toward those who set limits. It is toward such persons that the child may behave in a "negativistic" manner. For example, the child may say, "I don't want to" and "No!" when a parent makes a request or sets a limit. It is as though the child is defining autonomy through oppositional behavior. However, in some instances, the behavior may be a manifestation of anxiety, as the child struggles against a regressive pull. In other instances, the behavior may be a direct discharge of aggression against the parent, especially if the parent–child relationship is an ambivalent one.

Perhaps the crux of the school-age period of development is the child's move toward greater separation, independence, and autonomy at a time when he or she is still capable of being demanding, intrusive, and negativistic. The extent to which the child successfully emerges from this stage depends on many factors, including the degree to which the parents facilitate or hinder the child's progress.

When adolescence arrives, at least four major groups of developmental tasks can be defined: 1) defining oneself (identity), 2) achieving separation and coming to terms with specific feelings about one's family, 3) developing love relationships, and 4) achieving mastery over one's impulses, body functions, and capacities.

Developing Concepts of Body, Illness, and Death

■ Concept of Body

Judging from the infant's facial expressions and vocal sounds, in the beginning, the infant seems to be aware of and react to pleasurable body states and feelings and states of discomfort arising from hunger, thirst, wetness, pain, temperature extremes, fatigue, and illness. The infant soon learns that his or her body has a separate existence but does not initially appear to recognize any well-defined boundary.

The infant clearly sees and touches his or her body, at first randomly and then intentionally. For example, as early as age 3 weeks, the infant can reliably put his or her thumb in the mouth. The infant also experiences a wide range of sensory stimuli, including those accompanying being fed, burped, bathed, diapered, cuddled, tickled, whirled in the air, spoken and sung to, and confronted almost nose to nose by strange, seemingly contorted faces.

By ages 3–6 months, the infant can smile appreciatively when shown a moving mask consisting of forehead, eyes, and nose, indicating the infant's capacity for pattern recognition—in this case, the elements of a face. The infant also begins to discriminate between sensations that come from within and those that come from the outside (what is me and what is not me). Gradually, the infant perceives, constructs, and recognizes the mothering person's face, and the mothering person's face becomes associated with all the actions of the mother that satisfy the infant. Meanwhile, the infant is further exploring and differentiating among the parts of his

or her own body. The infant takes pleasure in peek-a-boo games, which help the child begin to acquire object permanence—the sense of what is here, what is hidden but continues to exist, and what is absent. The infant begins to change from watching his or her image in a mirror as though it were some other child to recognizing his or her own image. The infant remembers this image and, usually by 8 or 9 months, has at least a rudimentary sense of self. All these developments—leading up to a firm sense of self and body and to the child's attachment to the important figures in his or her life—flourish in the context of reliable, predictable, loving, responsive, and stimulating parenting and the advent of language.

By the time a child is age 2 or 3 years, the child's image of his or her body is more defined. The typical 3-year-old can name body parts such as eyes, nose, and mouth, and a 4-year-old usually can draw a simple representation of the body—usually a single circle with dots for eyes and nose, a curved line for the mouth, hair (by which the child usually identifies the sex), lines representing limbs that spring from the circle, and an indeterminate number of digits at the end of each limb. The child also often seems to have the idea that the body is a kind of sac filled with fluid that sometimes oozes out. If the child skins his or her knee and some blood oozes out, the 3-year-old may become upset at the loss of fluid. The child at this age is often readily reassured by the application of a bandage strip, which seems to seal the leak and hides the wound from view.

Later, the child will acquire some concept of internal organs, usually from the conversations of older persons. However, the internal organs are usually stereotyped (e.g., hearts that look like the representations on valentine cards). At this stage, the child's drawings depict bodies with floating organs, and the child has no clear idea of their function or physiology. By age 5 or 6 years, the child represents the body more accurately in his or her drawings, with distinct head and torso; more body parts, such as eyebrows and ears; and more detail, such as clothing.

Sometimes the child's inner mental image of his or her body is represented in play, especially play that involves toys that can be filled and emptied, open and shut, fitted together and pulled apart, messed and cleaned, and hoarded or discarded. As the child's cognitive development, learning, and experience increase, the child's knowledge of his or her body gradually becomes increasingly accurate, although gaps in knowledge and misconceptions may persist through adolescence and even adulthood.

■ Concepts of Illness

Although neonates have no concept of illness, they feel and react to painful attacks on the body (e.g., circumcision of a newborn requires that the infant be anesthetized). Perhaps the earliest idea of illness in the child at age 2 or 3 years is as a form of punishment (*immanent justice*) that has been visited on the child for misdeeds, committed or imagined, which also may be a source of guilt. Next the child develops a primitive concept of contagion: illness is caused by a bug or germ, which you might catch. As the child imagines it, the germ is caught by touching something dirty or by eating something that is bad for you. How the germ brings about the symptoms of the illness remains a mystery to the child, who may nonetheless invent a theory. By age 5 or 6 years, the child can and will ask questions and should receive simple, straightforward, truthful answers.

■ Psychological Reactions to Illness

Every child has a psychological reaction to his or her own illness and to illness in siblings and parents. The intensity of the reaction may vary with the child's developmental level and premorbid psychological state, the seriousness of the illness, and the reactions of the family. Factors that increase the child's likelihood of having an intense psychological reaction to illness can be divided into those that are specific to the child and those that are specific to the family and the child's relationship with his or her parents.

Possible stressful factors specific to the child include 1) age; 2) premorbid psychopathology; 3) severe illness; 4) chronic illness and multiple hospitalizations; 5) difficult, painful treatment; and 6) poor preparation for hospitalization or treatment.

Possible stressful factors specific to the child's relationship with his or her parent or parents include 1) relationships characterized by parental neglect, abuse, ambivalence, hostility, rejection, unpredictability, or inconsistency; 2) psychiatric disturbance in either parent; and 3) maladaptive parental reactions to illness, such as unrealistic expectations or feelings of helplessness and pessimism.

Additional risk factors that may intensify the child's psychological reactions to illness include exposure to illness factors (e.g., disfigurement, loss of autonomy, and immobilization) and parents' reactions of loss, grief, guilt, depression, anxiety, exhaustion, isolation, marital strain, financial drain, and secrecy about the illness (often found in families with acquired immunodeficiency syndrome [AIDS]).

Manifestations of the child's normal psychological reactions to illnesses may include the following:

- *Biopsychological symptoms,* such as malaise, reduced threshold for pain, irritability, loss of appetite, and sleep disturbance.

- *Increased attachment behaviors,* such as clinging and demanding behavior and intensified separation anxiety.
- *Regression,* expressed as thumb sucking, returning to baby speech, and wetting or soiling.
- *Passivity,* with marked feelings of helplessness and powerlessness.
- *Frightening fantasies* about the illness and treatment, fear of mutilation and bodily harm, and overwhelming guilt.
- *Excessive anxiety,* with intense mobilization of psychological defense mechanisms, such as denial, or symptoms of phobic reactions or conversion disorder.
- *Reactivation* of premorbid psychiatric symptoms.

These reactions may also appear when children are exposed to serious illness in a parent or sibling.

■ Psychological Reactions to Chronic Illness

Most chronically ill children seem to cope adequately and do not develop mental health, social, or school adjustment problems. Certain risk factors associated with chronic illness of any kind may nevertheless adversely affect the child's and the family's coping capacities, and these factors may also affect the child who is exposed to stresses brought on by chronic illnesses in a family member.

Factors that must be considered in any assessment of psychological risk for the child include the strengths or weaknesses of the adaptive capacities of the child, including the child's temperament and cognitive-developmental stage; the adaptive capacities of the parents; how well the child and his or her parents fit together; the positive or negative aspects of the sociocultural context of the hospitalization; and the depth and duration of discomfort and pain experienced or observed. Other general psychosocial factors that may affect, but not necessarily cause, an adverse psychological outcome are lower socioeconomic status, poor diet, unhygienic living conditions, and violent environment.

Chronic illness in a child sometimes entails recurrent or long-term hospitalization. When this occurs, new stresses arise, including loss of autonomy and a sense of decreased competence, relative immobilization, impaired functioning, body intrusion, invasion of privacy, and disfigurement. Parents of a chronically ill child are likely to experience fatigue, guilt, depression, and anxiety, as well as marital stress and economic loss. The whole family may become isolated. Children who are younger than 5 years may experience difficulty in attachments as a result of recurrent hospitalization. Sometimes, staff members who are caring for a chronically ill child—particularly one who is inexorably deteriorating—may become discouraged, frustrated, and angry and may displace these feelings onto the child, with undesirable effects on the child and his or her family.

■ The Child's Cognitive Understanding of Death

Very young children may see, experience, and understand the death of someone they know and love as an abandonment, which, the child may reason, has come about because of his or her own misbehavior. This cognitive idea is similar to the child's initial immanent justice concept of illness. This experience and reasoning may evoke feelings of guilt, anger, sadness, and loss. These thoughts and feelings are important to the young child, who needs help in understanding that the death of the loved person is not the child's fault.

School-age children who have acquired or are acquiring the concepts of universal inevitability, finality, irreversibility, and the causality of death can mourn more successfully and can use their increased cognitive and emotional maturity to deal more effectively with the feelings of sadness, anger, and guilt that are aroused by the experience of a death in the family. At the same time, the death of a loved person may exacerbate the school-age child's concerns about harm to his or her body. These concerns may continue until the normative developmental tasks of adolescence are resolved.

Many other risk factors may adversely influence the psychological outcome for a child when a death occurs (Osterweis et al. 1984):

- Loss to a child before age 5 years or during early adolescence
- Loss of a mother for a girl before age 11 years or loss of a father for an adolescent boy
- Premorbid psychological difficulties in the child or lack of prior knowledge about death
- A conflictual relationship with the deceased or a poor subsequent relationship between the child and the step-parent
- A surviving parent who is psychologically vulnerable and excessively dependent on the child, or an environment that is unstable and inconsistent
- Lack of adequate family or community support, or a surviving parent who lacks access to available supports
- A death that was not expected or prepared for (e.g., the result of suicide or homicide)

■ Mourning

Children and adolescents have a wide range of reactions to the illness and death—from whatever cause—of a parent or sibling. It is important to recognize this individuality, especially during the mourning process (Furman 1974; Krementz 1981).

Young children may believe that the family member did not really die (especially if the death was sudden and in a remote hospital) and will one day come back from some faraway place, or the child may have a fantasy of being seen by or reunited with the absent parent, who the child may believe is now in heaven. Young children tend to mourn on a piecemeal basis, extended over time; thus, a child will most feel the loss when a fun time previously shared with the parent (e.g., a birthday celebration or a vacation) does not happen. This event becomes a time for more mourning. Later, a child may pretend the dead parent is just "away" and will daydream or recall memories of past times with the parent. It is not unusual for a child to want to keep something that belonged to the now-dead parent as a way of holding on to the memory of the parent or a token of identification with the lost parent.

Children usually hesitate to share fantasies or memories of the dead parent with other children for fear of being teased. A child may feel embarrassed, ashamed, or uncomfortably unique, gripped by the sense that he or she alone has a dead parent. These feelings—along with emotions such as anger, anxiety, sadness, and loneliness—may also be kept secret. If a child becomes caught in the web of a family's secret, he or she will avoid expressing feelings and opinions for fear of upsetting the living parent.

Children work to overcome grief in part by expressing to themselves or to others—sometimes during play—their feelings of sadness. A child may also exhibit various mechanisms of defense, including denial. Children who lack sufficient opportunity to share feelings, or whose opportunity is actively blocked, may resort unconsciously—or even consciously—to behavioral manifestations of their anxiety, frustration, and anger, engaging in disruptive behaviors such as marked oppositionality, temper tantrums, antisocial conduct, and high-risk behavior.

The child or adolescent also must deal with the grief reactions of the surviving parent, including withdrawal, avoidance, denial, and anger. Roles in the family may change. The child may become the substitute for the lost parent and may take on some parental or even marital roles—perhaps caring for siblings or comforting the surviving parent. The child may feel a sense of urgency and desperation as well as guilt in striving to perform the parental role while still being in need of parenting himself or herself.

Children and adolescents must also deal with the many changes that may occur in the family, including new partners for the surviving parent, sometimes through remarriage. The surviving parent may have to change jobs or locations, and the family's standard of living may decline.

The child or adolescent may become fearful that the surviving parent may die. A child who fears being left alone may react by becoming oversolicitous of the surviving parent, by being angry, or by acting out anxieties and guilt about the safety of the surviving parent by courting precarious or dangerous situations. Such displacement of fears, anxieties, and guilt at the same time gives the child a transient feeling of being in control instead of suffering passively the anxiety of an anticipated and dreaded abandonment.

In short, children and adolescents react to the death of a parent in a variety of ways: some cry a lot, some deny the death, some try to avoid thinking about it in the hope of continuing with their lives, and some clamor for attention through their behavior. These and other reactions may be determined in part by the previous relationship with the now-dead parent, the relationship with surviving family members, and the inner life and temperament of the child. In any event, the young person's unique way of reacting to the death of a parent should be respected and understood by those trying to help the child or adolescent deal with his or her feelings.

References

Ainsworth MDS: The development of infant-mother interaction among the Ganda, in Determinants of Infant Behavior, Vol 2. Edited by Foss BM. London, Methuen, 1963, pp 67–112

Aoyama K: Filler syllables in early language development. Paper presented at the Yale Child Study Center, November 21, 2001

Bailey JM, Pillard RC: A genetic study of male sexual orientation. Arch Gen Psychiatry 48:1089–1096, 1991

Bloom L: Language development review, in Review of Child Development Research, Vol 4. Edited by Horowitz FR. Chicago, IL, University of Chicago Press, 1975, pp 245–303

Bornstein MH: Qualities of color vision in infancy. J Exp Child Psychol 19:401–419, 1975

Bowlby J: Attachment (Attachment and Loss, Vol 1). New York, Basic Books, 1969

Brown AL: The development of memory: knowing about and knowing how to know. Adv Child Dev Behav 10:104–152, 1975

Campos JJ, Langer A, Krowitz A: Cardiac responses on the visual cliff in prelocomotor human infants. Science 170:196–197, 1970

Chess S, Thomas A: Temperament in Clinical Practice. New York, Guilford, 1986

Cohen LJ: The operational definition of human attachment. Psychol Bull 81:107–217, 1974

Cohen LJ, Gelber E: Infant's visual memory, in Infant Perception: From Sensation to Cognition, Vol 1: Basic Visual Processes. Edited by Cohen L, Salapatek P. New York, Academic Press, 1975, pp 347–403

Cohen RL, Harnick AH: The susceptibility of child witnesses to suggestion. Law Hum Behav 4:201–210, 1980

Colby A: Evolution of a moral-developmental theory, in New Directions for Child Development: Moral Development. Edited by Damon W. San Francisco, CA, Jossey-Bass, 1978, pp 89–104

Condon WS, Sander LW: Neonate movement is synchronized with adult speech: interactional participation and language acquisition. Science 183:99–101, 1974

Dale PS, Loftus E, Rathbun R: The influence of the form of the question of eyewitness testimony on preschool children. J Psycholinguist Res 7:269–277, 1978

Dubignon J, Campbell D: Sucking in the newborn during a feed. J Exp Child Psychol 7:282–298, 1969

Engen T, Lipsitt LP, Kaye H: Olfactory responses and adaptation in the human neonate. J Comp Physiol Psychol 56:73–77, 1963

Erikson E: Identity and the Life Cycle. New York, International Universities Press, 1959

Fantz RL, Fagan JF, Miranda SB: Early visual selectivity, in Infant Perception: From Sensation to Cognition, Vol 1: Basic Visual Processes. Edited by Cohen L, Salapatek P. New York, Academic Press, 1975, pp 249–345

Friedlander BZ: Receptive language development in infancy: issues and problems. Merrill Palmer Q 16:7–51, 1970

Furman E: A Child's Parent Dies: Studies in Childhood Bereavement. New Haven, CT, Yale University Press, 1974

Gesell AO, Amatruda CS: Stages and sequences of development (1941), in Developmental Diagnosis, 11th Edition. New York, Harper & Row, 1964, pp 8–14

Gilligan C: In a Different Voice: Psychological Theory and Women's Development. Cambridge, MA, Harvard University Press, 1982

Goldstone S, Goldfarb JL: The perception of time by children, in Perceptual Development in Children. Edited by Kidd AH, Rivoire JL. New York, International Universities Press, 1966, pp 445–486

Goodman GS, Aman C, Hirschman J: Child sexual and physical abuse: children's testimony, in Children's Eyewitness Memory. Edited by Ceci S, Toglia MP, Ross D. New York, Springer-Verlag, 1987

Gould E, Reeves AJ, Graziano MS, et al: Neurogenesis in the neocortex of adult primates. Science 286:548–552, 1999

Green A: The "Sissy" Boy Syndrome and the Development of Homosexuality. New Haven, CT, Yale University Press, 1987

Halverson CF, Waldrop MF: Maternal behavior towards own and other preschool children: the problems of "ownness." Child Dev 41:839–845, 1970

Hasher L, Zacks RT: Automatic and effortful process in memory. J Exp Psychol Gen 108:356–388, 1979

Honigmann JJ: Culture as Personality. New York, Harper, 1954

Hudson JA: The emergence of autobiographical memory in mother-child conversation, in Knowing and Remembering in Young Children. Edited by Fivush R, Hudson JA. New York, Cambridge University Press, 1990

Insel TR: A neurobiological basis of social attachment. Am J Psychiatry 154:726–735, 1997

Johnson MK, Foley MA: Differentiating fact from fantasy: the reliability of children's memory. J Soc Issues 40:33–50, 1984

Kagan J: Change and Continuity in Infancy. New York, Wiley, 1971

Kagan J: The Nature of the Child. New York, Basic Books, 1984

Kagan J: The contribution of temperament to developmental profiles, in Child and Adolescent Psychiatry: A Comprehensive Textbook, 3rd Edition. Edited by Lewis M. Philadelphia, PA, Lippincott Williams & Wilkins, 2002, pp 211–220

Kessen W: Sucking and looking: two organized congenital patterns of behavior in the newborn, in Early Behavior: Comparative and Developmental Approaches. Edited by Stevenson HW, Hess EH, Rheingold HL. New York, Wiley, 1967

Kobasigawa A: Utilization of retrieval cues by children to recall. Child Dev 45:127–134, 1974

Kobre KR, Lipsitt LP: A negative contrast effect in newborns. J Exp Child Psychol 14:81–91, 1972

Kohlberg L: Development of moral character. Review of Child Development Research 1:400–404, 1964

Kohlberg L: Revisions in the theory and practice of moral development, in New Directions in Child Development: Moral Development. Edited by Damon W. San Francisco, CA, Jossey-Bass, 1978, pp 83–88

Kramer SN: History Begins at Sumer. Garden City, New York, Doubleday, 1959

Krementz J: How It Feels When a Parent Dies. New York, Knopf, 1981

Langlois JH, Stephan CW: Beauty and the beast: the role of physical attraction in peer relationships and social behavior, in Developmental Social Psychology: Theory and Research. Edited by Brehm SS, Kassin SM, Gibbons SX. New York, Oxford University Press, 1981, pp 152–168

Leckman JF, Herman AE: Maternal behavior and developmental psychopathology. Biol Psychiatry 51:27–43, 2002

Lenneberg EH: Biological Foundation of Language. New York, Wiley, 1967, pp 128–130

Leong C: Lateralization in severely disabled readers in relation to functional cerebral development and synthesis of information, in The Neuropsychology of Learning Disorders. Edited by Knights RM, Baker DJ. Baltimore, MD, University Park Press, 1976, pp 221–231

Lerner RM, Lerner JV: Effects of age, sex, and physical attractiveness on child–peer relations, academic performance, and elementary school adjustment. Dev Psychol 13:585–590, 1977

Loftus EF, Davies GM: Distortion in memory of children. J Soc Issues 40:51–67, 1984

Macfarlane A: Olfaction in the development of social preference in the human neonate. CIBA Found Symp (33):103–117, 1975

Main M, Solomon J: Discovery of an insecure, disorganized/disoriented attachment pattern: procedures, findings and implications for the classification of behavior, in Affective Development in Infancy. Edited by Yogman M, Brazelton TB. Norwood, NJ, Ablex, 1986, pp 95–124

Marshall WA, Tanner JM: Variations in the pattern of pubertal changes in boys. Archives of Disease in Childhood 45:13–23, 1970

Miller PH: Theories of Developmental Psychology, 2nd Edition. New York, WH Freeman, 1989

Mills M, Melhuish E: Recognition of mother's voice in early infancy. Nature 252:123–124, 1974

Mirsky AF, Anthony BJ, Duncan CC, et al: Analysis of the elements of attention: a neuropsychological approach. Neuropathol Rev 2:109–145, 1991

Moerk E: Changes in verbal child-mother interactions with increasing language skills of the child. J Psycholinguist Res 3:101–116, 1974

Morley ME: The Development and Disorders of Speech in Childhood, 2nd Edition. Edinburgh, Churchill Livingston, 1965

Neisser Y: The control of information pickup in selective looking, in Perception and Its Development. Edited by Pick AD. Hillsdale, NJ, Lawrence Erlbaum, 1984, pp 201–219

Newell A, Shaw J, Simon HA: Elements of a theory of human problem solving. Psychol Rev 65:151–166, 1958

Osterweis M, Solomon F, Green M (eds): Bereavement: Reactions, Consequences and Care. Washington, DC, National Academy Press, 1984

Piaget J: The Child's Conception of Number. Translated by Gattegno C, Hodgson FM. London, Routledge & Kegan Paul, 1952

Piaget J: The Growth of Logical Thinking. New York, Basic Books, 1958

Piaget J: The Moral Development of the Child. New York, Free Press, 1965

Piaget J: The intellectual development of the adolescent, in Adolescence: Psychosocial Perspectives. Edited by Caplan G, Lebovici S. New York, Basic Books, 1969, pp 22–26

Porter FL, Porges SQ, Marshall RE: Newborn pain cries and vagal tones: parallel changes in response to circumcision. Child Dev 59:495–505, 1988

Provence S, Lipton RC: Infants and Institutions. New York, International Universities Press, 1962

Rakic P: Development of the cerebral cortex in human and nonhuman primates, in Child and Adolescent Psychiatry: A Comprehensive Textbook. Edited by Lewis M. Baltimore, MD, Williams & Wilkins, 1996, pp 9–30

Rakic P, Cameron RS, Komura H: Recognition, adhesion, transmembrane signaling and cell motility in guided neuronal migration. Curr Opin Neurobiol 4:63–69, 1994

Reese HW: Attitudes toward the opposite sex in late childhood. Merrill Palmer Quarterly 12:157–163, 1966

Rutter M: Normal psychosexual development. J Child Psychol Psychiatry 11:259–283, 1971

Rutter M: Other family influences, in Child Psychiatry. Edited by Rutter M, Hersov L. Oxford, Blackwell, 1976a, pp 74–108

Rutter M: Separation, loss and family relationships, in Child Psychiatry. Edited by Rutter M, Hersov L. Oxford, Blackwell, 1976b, pp 47–73

Schaffer HR, Emerson PE: Patterns of response to physical contact in early human development. J Child Psychol Psychiatry 5:1–13, 1964

Spitz R: The First Year of Life. New York, International Universities Press, 1965

Squire LR: Memory and Brain. New York, Oxford University Press, 1987

Sroufe LA, Waters E: The ontogenesis of smiling and laughter: a perspective on the organization of development in infancy. Psychol Rev 83:173–189, 1976

Tanner JM: Growth at Adolescence, 2nd Edition. Oxford, England, Blackwell Scientific Publications, 1962

Thomas A, Chess S: Temperament and Development. New York, Brunner/Mazel, 1977

Thomas A, Chess S, Birch HG: Temperament and Behavior Disorders in Children. New York, New York University Press, 1968

Tobin-Richards MH, Boxer AM, Peterson AC: The psychological significance of pubertal change: sex differences in perception of self during early adolescence, in Girls at Puberty. Edited by Brooks-Gunn J, Peterson AC. New York, Plenum, 1983, pp 127–154

Touwen BCL: Laterality, in Scientific Foundations of Developmental Psychiatry. Edited by Rutter M. London, Heinemann, 1980, pp 154–164

Weizmann F, Cohen L, Pratt J: Novelty, familiarity and the development of infant attention. Dev Psychol 4:149–154, 1971

Wolff P: The natural history of crying and other vocalizations of early infancy, in Determinants of Infant Behavior, Vol 4. Edited by Foss BM. London, Methuen, 1969, pp 88–295

Self-Assessment Questions

Select the single best response for each question.

1.1   Theories of development formulated by Freud, Erikson, and Piaget share which of the following characteristics?

   A.   They postulate a genetically determined capacity for the development of patterns or systems of behavior by the child.

   B.   They propose that the overall behavior patterns that emerge are qualitatively similar to one another.

   C.   They are all structural theories of development that imply that reorganization within the child is unnecessary.

   D.   They postulate that the child reacts in particular ways to environmental stimuli.

   E.   None of the above.

1.2   By age 5 years, a child will have attained all of the following motor developmental milestones *except*

   A.   Can stand on one foot.

   B.   Can dance and jump.

   C.   Manifests firmly established leg, eye, and ear dominance.

   D.   Can copy a square.

   E.   Can build a tower of 10 cubes.

1.3   Piaget conceptualized four major stages of cognitive development. Which of the following states the correct sequence in which these stages normally occur, from birth to adolescence?

   A.   Preoperational, sensorimotor, concrete operational, formal operational.

   B.   Concrete operational, sensorimotor, preoperational, formal operational.

   C.   Sensorimotor, concrete operational, formal operational, preoperational.

   D.   Formal operational, concrete operational, sensorimotor, preoperational.

   E.   Sensorimotor, preoperational, concrete operational, formal operational.

1.4   *Chunking* is

   A.   A process by which representations, procedures, and memories that occur together are automatically accessed simultaneously.

   B.   A type of long-term memory.

   C.   A form of procedural knowledge.

   D.   All of the above.

   E.   None of the above.

1.5   According to Spitz (1965), organizers that govern the process of transition from one level to the next in the development of attachment include all of the following *except*

   A.   Sustained eye contact in response to an interaction.

   B.   The smiling response.

   C.   Eight-month anxiety.

   D.   Achievement of the sign of negation.

   E.   None of the above.

1.6 In psychoanalytic theory, the *anal phase* of psychosexual development is characterized by

A. The child's focus on autoerotic activities.
B. The child's experience of intense sexual and aggressive urges toward both parents.
C. The child's development of concepts of inevitability regarding birth, death, and sex differences.
D. The child's experience of feelings of separateness and worth.
E. The child's sequential development of play.

Classification of Child and Adolescent Psychiatric Disorders

Mina K. Dulcan, M.D.

Jerry M. Wiener, M.D.

Diagnostic classification of childhood psychiatric disorders had its formal beginning with the publication by Leo Kanner (1935) of the first English-language textbook of child psychiatry. Kanner placed all disorders in categories of "personality difficulties." In the third (and final) edition of his textbook, Kanner (1957) addressed the limitations of then available diagnostic classifications. Personality problems were categorized as related to physical illness, psychosomatic problems, and behavior problems. By that edition, the influence of psychoanalytic theory was considerably in evidence, as was a wealth of astute observation, clinical wisdom, and sound advice. The classification system was largely phenomenological, with little conceptual framework.

The first edition of DSM (American Psychiatric Association 1952) was published in 1952. There were only four categories for which childhood or adolescence was a specific condition: 1) chronic brain syndrome associated with birth trauma; 2) schizophrenic reaction, childhood type; 3) special symptom reactions such as learning disturbance, enuresis, and somnambulism; and 4) adjustment reactions (habit disturbance, conduct disturbance, neurotic traits) of infancy, childhood, and adolescence.

The Group for the Advancement of Psychiatry (GAP) Committee on Child Psychiatry published its classification in 1966 (Group for the Advancement of Psychiatry 1966). The GAP classification provided a broad, inclusive biopsychosocial and developmental framework within which to include interactive, etiological, and phenomenological considerations. Innovations in the GAP classification were new categories of healthy response and developmental deviations in maturational rate or sequence, use of a symptom list, and modifying of diagnoses as acute or chronic and mild, moderate, or severe.

DSM-II

DSM-II (American Psychiatric Association 1968) was intended to coincide with the *International Classification of Diseases,* 8th Revision (ICD-8; World Health Organization 1969). DSM-II tried to avoid terms that carry with them implications regarding either the nature of a disorder or its causes and to be "explicit about causal assumptions when they are integral to a diagnostic concept" (p. viii). DSM-II reflected the growing importance of biological theories and research findings in understanding mental disorders and the growing challenge to psychoanalytic theory as either sufficiently or even predominantly explanatory. Descriptive phenomenology assumed a larger role than it had previously.

DSM-II did represent progress in the classification of child and adolescent disorders. Mental retardation was placed as the first category. Schizophrenia, childhood type, remained, as did an expanded section of "special symptoms" and transient situational disturbances. The major change was the addition of "behavior disorders of childhood and adolescence," including the following:

- Hyperkinetic reaction
- Withdrawing reaction
- Overanxious reaction
- Runaway reaction
- Unsocialized aggressive reaction
- Group delinquent reaction

DSM-III

DSM-III (American Psychiatric Association 1980) became the hallmark of the dramatic changes that had occurred in psychiatry during the previous 20 years. Except when etiology was clearly known, as in organic mental disorders, no assumptions as to etiology were included. DSM-III was comprehensively categorical, provided specific diagnostic criteria for each disorder, and introduced a five-part multiaxial system that allowed for the coding of physical disorders, psychosocial stressors, and the highest level of adaptive functioning in the past year (in addition to the coding of disorders on Axis I and Axis II).

DSM-III introduced the Axis I category "Disorders Usually First Evident in Infancy, Childhood, or Adolescence," which included the following:

- Mental retardation
- Attention-deficit disorder (with and without hyperactivity)
- Conduct disorder (with five subtypes)
- Anxiety disorders (separation anxiety, avoidant, and overanxious disorders)
- Other disorders of infancy, childhood, or adolescence (reactive attachment, schizoid, oppositional, and identity disorders, and elective mutism)
- Eating disorders
- Stereotyped movement disorders (tic disorders and Tourette's disorder)
- Other disorders with physical manifestations (stuttering, enuresis, encopresis, and sleepwalking and sleep terror disorders)
- Pervasive developmental disorders (including infantile autism)

"Specific developmental disorders" were to be coded on Axis II. Diagnoses such as schizophrenia, affective disorders, organic disorders, and anxiety disorders were to be made in children and adolescents by applying the same criteria required for adults.

The major principles guiding DSM-III-R (American Psychiatric Association 1987) were the same as for DSM-III. Because developmental disorders usually begin in childhood and persist into adulthood, a new category was created on Axis II that included 1) mental retardation, 2) pervasive developmental disorders (autistic disorder), and 3) specific developmental disorders (including academic, language, and motor skills disorders).

DSM-IV

Relevant disorders in DSM-IV (American Psychiatric Association 1994) and its Text Revision (DSM-IV-TR; American Psychiatric Association 2000) are listed both under disorders "usually first diagnosed in infancy, childhood, or adolescence" and in subsequent sections that are applicable to all age groups and use the same diagnostic criteria as for adults (e.g., affective, schizophrenic, and anxiety disorders). "The provision of a separate section for disorders that are usually first diagnosed in infancy, childhood, or adolescence is for convenience only and is not meant to suggest that there is any clear distinction between 'childhood' and 'adult' disorders.... For most (but not all) DSM-IV disorders, a single criteria set is provided that applies to children, adolescents, and adults" (p. 37).

"Disorders Usually First Diagnosed in Infancy, Childhood, or Adolescence" include

- Mental retardation
- Learning disorders (LDs)
- Motor skills disorder
- Communication disorders
- Pervasive developmental disorders (PDDs)
- Attention-deficit and disruptive behavior disorders (DBDs)
- Feeding and eating disorders of infancy or early childhood
- Tic disorders
- Elimination disorders
- Other disorders of infancy, childhood, or adolescence

A number of changes in DSM-IV apply to childhood. The overarching category of developmental disorders coded on Axis II is dropped. PDDs and LDs, motor skills disorder, and communication disorders have been moved to Axis I from Axis II. PDDs in DSM-IV now include

- Autistic disorder
- Rett's disorder
- Childhood disintegrative disorder, also termed *Heller's syndrome* and *infantile dementia*
- Asperger's disorder
- PDD not otherwise specified

The diagnostic criteria for LDs allow for the presence of a neurological condition. LDs now include

- Reading disorder
- Mathematics disorder
- Disorders of written expression
- LD not otherwise specified

The communication disorders category now includes both language and speech disorders and is subdivided into

- Expressive language disorder
- Mixed receptive–expressive language disorder
- Phonological disorder
- Stuttering
- Communication disorder not otherwise specified

The category attention-deficit and disruptive behavior disorders replaces the previously simplified category of DBDs. This category now is subdivided into

- Attention-deficit/hyperactivity disorder (ADHD), which is subclassified into
  1. Combined type
  2. Predominantly inattentive type
  3. Predominantly hyperactive–impulsive type

- ADHD not otherwise specified
- Conduct disorder—childhood-onset or adolescent-onset type
- Oppositional defiant disorder
- DBD not otherwise specified

The category of anxiety disorders of childhood or adolescence is eliminated, being subsumed under the disorders of infancy, childhood, or adolescence (see below) and anxiety disorders.

The new category of feeding and eating disorders of infancy or early childhood includes

- Pica
- Rumination disorder
- Feeding disorder of infancy or early childhood—the persistent failure to eat adequately, with weight loss or failure to gain weight

Gender identity disorders (GIDs) have been removed from "Disorders Usually First Diagnosed in Infancy, Childhood, or Adolescence" and reclassified under "Sexual and Gender Identity Disorders," with the categories "in children," "in adolescents or adults," and "not otherwise specified." Transsexualism has been dropped and is now subsumed under GID with specifiers.

The tic disorders category is essentially unchanged in DSM-IV, with a drop in the upper limit of age at onset from 21 to 18 years, and includes

- Tourette's disorder
- Chronic motor or vocal tic disorder
- Transient tic disorder
- Tic disorder not otherwise specified

The elimination disorders category (encopresis and enuresis) has minor changes in duration specifiers and terminology.

The DSM-III-R category of other disorders of infancy, childhood, or adolescence has been reorganized and now includes

- Separation anxiety disorder
- Selective mutism
- Reactive attachment disorder of infancy or early childhood, for which two subtypes have been added—the inhibited type and the disinhibited type (indiscriminate and diffuse attachments)
- Stereotypic movement disorder; the specifier "with self-injurious behavior" is added if the behavior results in self-damage requiring treatment
- Disorders of infancy, childhood, or adolescence not otherwise specified

Eating disorders now constitute a separate category in DSM-IV incorporating anorexia nervosa and bulimia nervosa. Anorexia nervosa is now subdivided into restricting and binge-eating/purging types. Subtypes of bulimia nervosa include purging and nonpurging types.

In the DSM-IV section on anxiety disorders, social phobia subsumes the DSM-III-R category of avoidant disorder. DSM-IV includes criteria for and discussion of childhood onset. Generalized anxiety disorder in DSM-IV now subsumes DSM-III-R overanxious disorder of childhood and requires "excessive" anxiety and worry rather than "unrealistic" worries. The DSM-IV discussion of diagnostic features, age features, and criteria includes considerations relevant to childhood onset.

Finally, DSM-IV conceptualizes Axis IV as "psychosocial and environmental problems" (Table 2–1). These problems affect the diagnosis, treatment, and prognosis of Axis I and Axis II disorders and play a role in the onset or exacerbation of a psychiatric disorder.

Table 2–1. DSM-IV Axis IV Psychosocial and Environmental Problems

Problems with primary support group

Problems related to the social environment

Educational problems

Occupational problems

Housing problems

Economic problems

Problems with access to health care services

Problems related to interaction with the legal system/crime

Other psychosocial and environmental problems

DSM-IV-TR

DSM-IV-TR (Text Revision) was published by the American Psychiatric Association in 2000 to reflect new research since the publication of DSM-IV. With very few exceptions, changes were made only in the text of the manual, not in the criteria themselves. The goals were to correct errors and ambiguities and to use empirical data to update and clarify sections of the manual describing symptoms, associated features, etiology, comorbidity, course, and prognosis. An exception to the rule of not changing criteria was made in the "Tic Disorders" section (including Tourette's disorder): "Clinically significant distress or impairment" is no longer required for the diagnosis.

Other Diagnostic Criteria Sets

A collaboration between the American Academy of Pediatrics and the American Psychiatric Association (including representatives of the American Academy of Child and Adolescent Psychiatry) developed the *Diagnostic and Statistical Manual for Primary Care* (DSM-PC), Child and Adolescent Version (American Academy of Pediatrics 1996). This is designed to be used by pediatricians and family physicians to classify emotional and behavioral prob-

lems seen in office practice. It includes a system for coding "Situation" that might be producing a child's symptoms and three clusters of "Child Manifestations": Developmental Variations, Problems Requiring Intervention, and Disorders (for those children who meet DSM-IV criteria for a disorder).

The DSM system has very limited utility for infants and toddlers. The Zero to Three/National Center for Clinical Infant Programs (1994) published a diagnostic classification system specifically tailored for very young children.

Toward DSM-V

Because each new version of DSM disrupts clinicians' work, clinical administrative systems, and research, a decision has been made that DSM-V will be published no sooner than 2011. The American Psychiatric Association has convened work groups to develop white papers setting out the issues to be considered for various age groups and diagnoses and to specify what new research is required to clarify and improve our diagnostic system.

References

American Academy of Pediatrics: The Classification of Child and Adolescent Mental Diagnoses in Primary Care: Diagnostic and Statistical Manual for Primary Care (DSM-PC) Child. Chicago, IL, American Academy of Pediatrics, 1996

American Psychiatric Association: Diagnostic and Statistical Manual: Mental Disorders. Washington, DC, American Psychiatric Association, 1952

American Psychiatric Association: Diagnostic and Statistical Manual of Mental Disorders, 2nd Edition. Washington, DC, American Psychiatric Association, 1968

American Psychiatric Association: Diagnostic and Statistical Manual of Mental Disorders, 3rd Edition. Washington, DC, American Psychiatric Association, 1980

American Psychiatric Association: Diagnostic and Statistical Manual of Mental Disorders, 3rd Edition, Revised. Washington, DC, American Psychiatric Association, 1987

American Psychiatric Association: Diagnostic and Statistical Manual of Mental Disorders, 4th Edition. Washington, DC, American Psychiatric Association, 1994

American Psychiatric Association: Diagnostic and Statistical Manual of Mental Disorders, 4th Edition, Text Revision. Washington, DC, American Psychiatric Association, 2000

Group for the Advancement of Psychiatry: Psychopathological Disorders in Childhood: Theoretical Considerations and a Proposed Classification, Vol 6. New York, Group for the Advancement of Psychiatry, 1966

Kanner L: Child Psychiatry. Baltimore, MD, Charles C Thomas, 1935

Kanner L: Child Psychiatry, 3rd Edition. Baltimore, MD, Charles C Thomas, 1957

World Health Organization: International Classification of Diseases, 8th Revision. Geneva, World Health Organization, 1969

Zero to Three/National Center for Clinical Infant Programs Diagnostic Classification Task Force: Diagnostic Classification of Mental Health and Developmental Disorders of Infancy and Early Childhood. Arlington, VA, The Zero to Three/National Center for Clinical Infant Programs, 1994

Self-Assessment Questions

Select the single best response for each question.

2.1 A number of changes were made in DSM-IV (American Psychiatric Association 1994) that apply to childhood. Which of the following is one of these changes?

A. A new category of pervasive developmental disorders was to be coded on Axis II.
B. Motor skills disorders were moved from Axis II to Axis I.
C. Learning disorders were moved from Axis I to Axis II.
D. Communications disorders were moved from Axis I to Axis II.
E. None of the above.

2.2 Pervasive developmental disorders include all of the following *except*

A. Childhood schizophrenia.
B. Autistic disorder.
C. Rett's disorder.
D. Asperger's disorder.
E. Childhood disintegrative disorder.

2.3 In DSM-IV, the new category *feeding and eating disorders of infancy or early childhood* included all of the following *except*

A. Feeding disorder of infancy or early childhood (persistent failure to eat adequately, with weight loss or failure to gain weight).
B. Pica.
C. Anorexia nervosa.
D. Rumination disorder.
E. None of the above.

2.4 The tic disorders category of DSM-IV was left essentially unchanged from that in DSM-III-R (American Psychiatric Association 1987) except for which of the following?

A. The addition of Tourette's disorder.
B. The elimination of chronic motor or vocal tic disorder.
C. The lowering of the upper limit of age at onset to 18 years.
D. The addition of transient tic disorder.
E. None of the above.

2.5 In DSM-IV, the category *other disorders of infancy, childhood, or adolescence* was reorganized to include which of the following disorders?

A. Separation anxiety disorder.
B. Selective mutism.
C. Reactive attachment disorder of infancy or early childhood.
D. Stereotypic movement disorder.
E. All of the above.

The Clinical Interview of the Child

Clarice J. Kestenbaum, M.D.

The clinical interview always has been the sine qua non of the psychiatric evaluation. As MacKinnon and Michels (1971) observed in *The Psychiatric Interview in Clinical Practice,* a "clear understanding of the psychopathology and psychodynamics is the foundation of the psychiatric interview" (p. 1). The foremost goal of the clinical interview is to establish a diagnosis. The interviewer may begin an intake session with a particular hypothesis about the nature of the patient's problem, but with each new piece of evidence the patient presents, the hypothesis formulation may change in mid-interview. For example, the therapist may view an overactive child as possibly having attention-deficit/hyperactivity disorder but soon discover that nightmares and phobias point to an anxiety disorder.

Despite advances in molecular genetics, breakthroughs in cellular pathology, and new knowledge about mind–brain synergy, our understanding of the etiology of disorders has not changed very much. "Clinical syndromes continue to be defined by patterns of symptoms and

course of illness, using the methods of Hippocrates, Sydenham, and other great physicians," according to McClellan and Werry (2000, p. 19). They stated, furthermore, that "the lack of understanding regarding the exact nature and etiology of psychiatric disorders requires that diagnoses be made based solely on recognized patterns or clusters of symptoms. Although helpful, this has all the diagnostic precision of 'fever.'…Although the clinical interview remains the accepted standard of psychiatric assessment, research suggests that clinicians' diagnoses are fraught with numerous biases" (p. 20).

Thus, a variety of structured interviews have been developed so that evidence-based research designs can be both reliable and valid (see Chapter 6, "Diagnostic Interviews," in this volume). For an in-depth understanding of the complex factors that constitute an integration of psychopathology and psychodynamics inherent in any given individual, however, the clinical interview remains the best instrument we have.

In the assessment of an adult, the

chief informant is the patient. Additional information may, of course, be requested from other physicians, hospital records, or psychological tests, but usually the skilled interviewer can obtain a psychiatric history and perform a mental status examination in one or two sessions if the adult is reasonably cooperative. The task facing the child psychiatric interviewer, however, is far more complex. The interviewer first must take into account the child's age, cognitive level of development, and willingness to discuss problems. The examination of the child alone rarely, if ever, can serve as the only source of information sufficient for making a diagnosis, but the examiner can certainly form a valuable diagnostic impression.

Children between ages 3 and 6 years can usually provide correct information when questions are asked in a way commensurate with their developmental level (Bjorklund and Muir 1988; Ornstein et al. 1991). The interviewer must be careful about making assumptions about the validity of a child's report in highly charged situations, such as custody cases or cases involving child abuse allegations. Younger children are suggestible and may repeat information fed to them by a hostile parent involved in an angry divorce, despite their own observations to the contrary (Ceci et al. 1987). However, additional information is also needed that the child cannot supply: a developmental history (including genetic background), a broad understanding of the home environment, and some knowledge of the significant people in the child's life. A thorough assessment from the school and other aspects of the child's world often is needed for a comprehensive evaluation, including current or past events (e.g., the death of a parent, effects of divorce, or a traumatic event such as a fire or automobile accident) that may have a lasting impact on future development.

School reports as well as pediatric records (including a neurological examination when indicated) may be sent to the diagnostician before the first visit. A psychological evaluation may already have been obtained or may be requested by the evaluator. Evaluation of family functioning is important. A family interview at some point in the evaluation process helps to determine the quality of the parent–child "fit"; for example, depression in the mother, alcoholism in the father, and a disruptive home environment may become more apparent.

The clinical interview with the child should be considered as one piece of a puzzle that is ready to be assembled when all other data are gathered. In presenting a detailed method of approaching a child and the child's family, from the initial telephone call to the final presentation of the findings, Gardner (1985) observed that "the initial interview and intensive evaluation should provide an in-depth understanding of the child's problems and also establish a good relationship or at least communication with the child and family members…without which the likelihood of a successful psychotherapy is minimal" (p. 371).

To make a valid diagnosis, one needs a thorough familiarity with child development, psychopathology, and the current DSM-IV-TR (American Psychiatric Association 2000) diagnostic criteria. Structured interviews do not allow for gathering data on the full range of feelings, personality organization, and coping mechanisms as does the free-range clinical interview. For these reasons, a semistructured clinical interview—the Mental Health Assessment Form (MHAF; Kestenbaum and Bird 1978)—was developed to provide a bridge between the structured questionnaire and the open-ended clinical interview. The MHAF may be used with children between ages 6 and

12 years. (There is a supplement for adolescents.) It can be performed within a relatively brief period, 45 minutes, or extended for several sessions, depending on the clinical situation.

Cards or questionnaires are not used. The "structure" is in the mind of the examiner. The examiner must be familiar with child developmental principles and psychopathology because the MHAF was designed to be used by clinicians with a certain level of training and experience.

The interview itself involves inquiry into all areas of a child's life and functioning, including specific questions about 1) the child in his or her family (a description of home and family life problems in family relationships), 2) the child in school (including sports, hobbies, homework, and relationships with teachers and peers), 3) the child's fantasy life (quality and content of fantasies and dreams, as well as problem-solving ability), and 4) the child's personality organization (self-concept, overall mood, perceptions, coping mechanisms).

The MHAF consists of 189 items divided into two major sections (Table 3–1). Part I is scored according to observable data and is primarily a mental status examination. It is subdivided into five major areas: 1) physical appearance, 2) motoric behavior and speech, 3) relatedness during the interview, 4) affect, and 5) language and thinking. Part II scores information derived from the content of the interview. Both historical and developmental data elicited from the child during the interview are included. Part II also deals with the child's self-concepts and perceptions in his or her world. It is divided into six major areas: 1) feeling states, 2) interpersonal relations, 3) symbolic representation (fantasies and dreams), 4) self-concept, 5) conscience/moral judgment, and 6) general level of adaptation.

General level of adaptation includes positive attributes: personality characteristics such as skills or talents, interests (e.g., hobbies), perseverance (stick-to-itiveness), frustration tolerance, creativity, imagination, sense of humor, empathy, ability to cope with stress (e.g., actual events by history such as separations, hospitalizations, illnesses), and problem-solving ability (when given an imaginary situation).

The rater must use both clinical experience and theoretical knowledge to determine whether the particular item is to be scored within the expectable range or to determine the degree of deviance from age-group norms. There is a section at the end of the form for descriptive information as well as a global assessment score for the current level of function (Shaffer et al. 1983).

The questions designed specifically for the MHAF interview can be geared toward younger or older children and take into account degrees of cooperation and resistance. Suggested questions are presented in an open-ended manner. The examiner is advised to follow the child's lead and not stay rigidly within a given framework. He or she may return at any time to topics that were brushed aside or ignored the first time around (Bird and Kestenbaum 1988).

Interviewing the Younger Child (Ages 5–9 Years)

There is no "best way" to interview children. Various techniques are derived from practicing a variety of established approaches with a number of children and adding new approaches that have proved helpful in establishing rapport with young children in a relatively brief period (no checklists). What follows is a distillate of my clinical experience.

In most circumstances, the clinician interviews one or both parents, before meeting with the child, to ascertain the

Table 3–1.   Outline of the Mental Health Assessment Form

Part I—Mental status

I.   *Physical appearance*
   A.   General attractiveness
   B.   Physical characteristics
   C.   Physical maturation
   D.   Observable deviations in physical characteristics
   E.   Grooming and dress
   F.   Gender differentiation

II. *Motoric behavior and speech*
   A.   Motor activity
   B.   Motor coordination
   C.   Presence of unusual motoric patterns, habit patterns, and mannerisms
   D.   Speech

III. *Relatedness during interview*
   A.   Quality of relatedness as judged by nonverbal behavior
   B.   Quality of relatedness as judged by verbal behavior
   C.   Social interaction

IV. *Affect*
   A.   Inappropriate affect
   B.   Constriction of affect
   C.   Elated affect
   D.   Depressed affect
   E.   Labile affect
   F.   Overanxious affect
   G.   Angry affect
   H.   Histrionic affect

V.   *Language and thinking*
   A.   Overall intelligence
   B.   Cognitive functions
   C.   External reality testing
   D.   Use of language
   E.   Thought process
   F.   Attention span

Part II—Content of the interview

VI. *Feeling states*
   A.   Depression
   B.   Elation
   C.   Mood disturbance (other)
   D.   Anger
   E.   Anxiety
   F.   Irritability
   G.   Impulsivity

Table 3–1.   Outline of the Mental Health Assessment Form *(continued)*

VII. *Interpersonal relations*
   A.   The child's relationship with his or her family
   B.   The child's relationship with other adult authority figures
   C.   The child's relationship with peers
   D.   The child's relationship with pets
   E.   Modes of interaction with others
   F.   Aggressive behavior
   G.   Sexual behavior

VIII. *Symbolic representation*
   A.   Fantasies
   B.   Dreams

IX. *Self-concept*
   A.   Dissatisfaction with self
   B.   Comparison of self with peers
   C.   Comparison of self with ideal self

X.   *Conscience/moral judgment*
   A.   Deficit in development of conscience
   B.   Antisocial behavior

XI. *General level of adaptation*
   A.   Personality characteristics
   B.   Defense mechanisms
   C.   Maladaptive solutions in dealing with anxiety

nature of the presenting problem, to obtain pertinent information, and to suggest ways of informing the child about the nature of the psychiatric examination. In those instances when the child refuses to leave the parent (usually a manifestation of separation anxiety), the parent is invited into the consultation room. Otherwise, the child is interviewed alone.

Most children spend a few minutes examining the strange surroundings, such as children's books, drawing materials, a dollhouse with simple furniture and little dolls, several hand puppets in full view, and a few standard games. An explanation may be given about the nature of the interview, with some reassurance if necessary.

The interview can begin with a question about why the child has been brought to see the psychiatrist. For example, this is how the interview with Marjorie, age 7 years, began:

Marjorie: I don't know.
Dr. K: Did your mother explain that I am the kind of doctor who helps children with their feelings and troubles?
Marjorie: No.
Dr. K: Well, I am. Some children have the kind of troubles everyone can see. For instance, if there's a child in school who bullies other children, or yells or throws things in class, or gets into fights…
Marjorie: Billy's like that. He's always in the principal's office.
Dr. K: Yes, exactly. I might see someone like Billy to help him with his problem controlling himself. But I also see children who have problems no one can see—worries about their parents going away, bad dreams, sad feelings.

Marjorie said nothing, but her solemn nod let me know my words made an impression.

After such an introduction, I shift gears and ask neutral questions about the child's home, family members, and pets. I might ask the child to draw a floor plan of his or her house or apartment—his or her room, the distance from the parents' room, the approximate distance to the school—and perhaps a rough sketch of his or her family. In 5 minutes, I will have already observed the child enough to score (mentally) the first part of the MHAF: general attractiveness, motor activity and coordination, presence or absence of tics, quality of speech, and relatedness to me (usually determined by eye contact, shyness, withdrawal, and general affect). I can estimate the child's overall level of intelligence by his or her vocabu-

lary and comprehension, ability to follow directions, and graphomotor skill in drawing. Of course, if there seems to be a problem in cognitive functioning, I will order a psychological examination if one has not already been obtained. I usually turn the conversation to the subject of favorite activities, friends, playmates, and sleepovers.

In my experience, for a child with school problems, nothing so readily establishes the distinction between a learning disability and attention-deficit or conduct disorder as fantasy play. In Marjorie's case, further testing and appropriate academic intervention coupled with brief psychotherapy may be extremely helpful.

Another technique that can be used with younger children is asking projective make-believe questions. For example, the same question brought forth very different responses from a dysthymic 8-year-old and a psychotic child of the same age:

Dr. K: Billy, make believe you are looking out the window and you hear an enormous crash. What do you see?
Billy: Two cars crash into each other.
Dr. K: And then what happens?
Billy: The ambulance comes.
Dr. K: And then what?
Billy: Nothing. Everyone is dead.

Most nondepressed children, unlike Billy, manage to get the passengers to a hospital where everyone is eventually saved. In response to the same question, Mark, a psychotic child, gave a very bizarre answer:

Mark: A monster from outer space throws a bomb and the whole world is killed and all the people in it and you and me too and then he eats all the pieces up and the ocean is all bloody and he drinks it and it's delicious.

Another projective technique is a variant of Winnicott's (1971) "squiggles" game—that is, drawing a scribbled design and asking the child to use his or her imagination, to complete the drawing by turning it into anything he or she thinks of, and to tell a story about the completed picture.

Overall mood can be elicited by the appearance of the "mood machine." Facing the child, I extend one arm, bent 90 degrees at the elbow:

> *Dr. K:* John, pretend my arm is a pendulum. On one side we have "happiness," on the other side "sadness," and straight up is "neutral." [I swing my arm slowly.] Now, when my arm reaches the place that describes how you feel most of the time, yell, "Stop!"

I then ask the child to describe the happiest and saddest events in his or her life. I often inquire about dreams and, when possible, ask the child to draw a picture of the dream. This drawing can lead to inquiry about perceptual distortions, such as familiar objects taking on frightening aspects, illusions at night, hypnagogic phenomena, or hallucinations.

Interviewing the Older Child (Ages 10–12 Years)

There is no explicit age cutoff at which the interviewer knows with certainty whether to begin with the version of the MHAF designed for younger children or to shape questions according to the presumed cognitive level of the preadolescent or adolescent youngster. Some 10-year-olds do far better when interviewed with the use of techniques usually reserved for younger children; others conduct themselves like teenagers. A sensitive interviewer will know when to shift gears. In general, I begin with the chief complaint. Frequently, the older child also will deny having any problems:

> *James (age 10):* My parents said I had to come or I could not watch TV.
> *Dr. K:* Boy, they must really think there's a problem. What do you think about it?
> *James:* Nothing. Ask them!
> *Dr. K:* I did already, but you know, I'm not so interested in their opinion as I am yours. The fact that they think there's a problem and even insist on your coming when you think there's no problem at all…well, even that's a problem! Besides, whatever you tell me is a one-way street. I want to hear all sides, but I don't repeat back to them what you say. I like to form my own opinion.

Usually this type of opening is sufficient to establish some degree of rapport.

After inquiries about interests and school activities, children are asked to describe their friends (or enemies). Then I might inquire about peer relationships; for example, "If I asked your best friend about you, what would he (she) say?"

For preadolescents, self-esteem is very much connected to body image. When asked "If there was anything you could change about yourself, what would it be?" most very young adolescents discuss their pimples, hair color, braces, or unsightly blemishes. If the answer is "everything," depression is a major diagnostic consideration.

It is important to obtain some idea about the development of empathy. Exploring feelings about animals is usually a useful approach. The clinician should inquire about family pets—their names, personality characteristics, and children's identifications with their pets. Other questions probing for empathic feelings bring forth a variety of responses:

Dr. K: What would you do if a new girl appeared in class one day in the middle of the term?

Jill (age 11): Well, I'd go over to her and tell her my name and introduce her to my friends and show her where the bathroom is and all.

Dr. K: Why would you do that?

Jill: Well, I went to a new school once, and I felt all scared and alone, and so I'd know how she feels.

George (age 10, responding to the same question, except that the newcomer is a boy): Well, I wouldn't hit him or anything…not on the first day.

Most children find the type of interview I have described reassuring and nonpressured. I usually try to end the session on an upbeat note with a statement such as "I think we can put our heads together and figure out what we want to do." If psychotherapy is indicated and the evaluating psychiatrist is not available for treatment, the child should be told that as the consultant, you will find the right person to help with the problem. The consultant should always explain what the next step will be, whether it is further testing, a second interview, a family interview, or a visit with the parents alone.

Summing-Up Session

When all information has been gathered and a diagnostic impression is made, a treatment plan is formulated. Next, an appointment is set up with the parents to discuss options.

Often several treatment modalities may be indicated: psychotherapy with parental counseling, psychoanalysis, pharmacological intervention combined with therapy, family therapy, tutoring, or language and learning therapy. The recommendation could be a change of school, residential placement, or hospitalization. It is important that parents are helped to feel comfortable discussing their finances and the range of possibilities so that the best arrangement can be instituted, taking individual circumstances into account. When acting as a consultant, one must be available for helping with the disposition and facilitation of treatment, particularly in the event that the child or family is not satisfied with the referral. Setting the fee, establishing rules, discussing vacations, and the like take place during the summing-up session. Once a treatment plan has been selected, the child is invited to participate in the subsequent planning (for instance, the session time should not compete with a regular after-school activity) and to discuss the reasons for the type of treatment offered.

Conclusion

The semistructured interview I describe in this chapter is only one aspect of the total evaluation. It provides a reliable and comprehensive assessment of the signs and symptoms of psychiatric disorder, as well as positive attributes and strengths of the patient. Moreover, such an interview is therapeutic in that a relationship is established from the outset, an important factor if further psychotherapy is the recommended intervention. Used together with the information based on physical examination, history, and cognitive functioning, in addition to the problems reported by patients and their parents, it provides a valid psychiatric diagnosis that can result in an optimal psychotherapeutic intervention.

References

American Psychiatric Association: Diagnostic and Statistical Manual of Mental Disorders, 4th Edition, Text Revision. Washington, DC, American Psychiatric Association, 2000

Bird H, Kestenbaum CJ: A semi-structured approach to clinical assessment, in Handbook of Clinical Assessment of Children and Adolescents, Vol 1. Edited by Kestenbaum CJ, Williams DT. New York, New York University Press, 1988, pp 19–30

Bjorklund DF, Muir JE: Children's development of free recall memory: remembering on their own. Annals of Child Development 5:79–123, 1988

Ceci SS, Ross DF, Tuglia MP: Suggestibility of children's memory: psychological implications. J Exp Psychol Gen 116:338–349, 1987

Gardner RA: The initial clinical evaluation of the child, in The Clinical Guide to Child Psychiatry. Edited by Shaffer D, Ehrhardt AA, Greenhill LL. New York, Free Press, 1985, pp 371–392

Kestenbaum CJ, Bird HR: A reliability study of the Mental Health Assessment Form for school-age children. J Am Acad Child Psychiatry 17:338–347, 1978

MacKinnon R, Michels R: The Psychiatric Interview in Clinical Practice. Philadelphia, PA, WB Saunders, 1971

McClellan JM, Werry SM: Introduction: research psychiatric diagnostic interviews for children and adolescents. J Am Acad Child Adolesc Psychiatry 39:19–27, 2000

Ornstein PA, Larus DM, Clubb PA: Understanding children's testimony: implications of research on the development of memory. Annals of Child Development 8:145–176, 1991

Shaffer D, Gould MS, Brasic J, et al: A Children's Global Assessment Scale (C-GAS). Arch Gen Psychiatry 40:1228–1231, 1983

Winnicott DW: Therapeutic Consultations in Child Psychiatry. New York, Basic Books, 1971

Self-Assessment Questions

Select the single best response for each question.

3.1   The Mental Health Assessment Form (MHAF)

   A. May be used with children between the ages of 3 and 6 years.
   B. Usually requires about 3 hours to complete.
   C. Employs questionnaires.
   D. Consists of 54 items.
   E. Obtains information on all areas of a child's life and functioning.

3.2   The MHAF consists of two parts. Part II ("Content of the Interview") deals with all of the following areas *except*

   A. Motoric behavior and speech.
   B. Interpersonal relations.
   C. Self-concept.
   D. Feeling states.
   E. Symbolic representation.

3.3   When interviewing the younger child (ages 5–9 years), the examiner should do all of the following *except*

   A. Interview one or both parents before meeting the child.
   B. Allow the child to examine the environment.
   C. Explain the nature of the interview to the parents.
   D. Refrain from explaining the reason for the interview to the child, because such information may be upsetting.
   E. Provide reassurance if necessary.

3.4   When interviewing the older child (ages 10–12 years), the examiner should

   A. Begin with general questions to avoid having a child get defensive about the chief complaint.
   B. Start by using the MHAF designed for older children.
   C. Obtain some idea about the child's development of empathy.
   D. End with the chief complaint.
   E. Refrain from having a parents-only meeting after the initial interview so that the child will not feel excluded.

3.5   The MHAF semistructured interview can be used to accomplish all of the following *except*

   A. Assess for the signs and symptoms of a psychiatric disorder.
   B. Identify positive attributes of the patient.
   C. Conduct a formal assessment of the patient's cognitive functioning.
   D. Establish a relationship with the patient.
   E. Evaluate the strengths of the patient.

The Clinical Interview of the Adolescent

Robert A. King, M.D.

John E. Schowalter, M.D.

The psychiatric evaluation of an adolescent is intended to obtain as full a picture as possible of the current difficulties in the overall context of the strengths and weaknesses of the adolescent and his or her family (King et al. 2005). Although formal psychological testing, structured instruments, laboratory data, and information gathered from school may be useful adjuncts, the heart of this clinical endeavor is the diagnostic interview with the adolescent and family.

The Prologue

It is important early on to clarify who is the moving force in seeking consultation and what is the adolescent's attitude toward the process. By seeking out a therapist, an adult patient acknowledges, at least implicitly, a problem and a desire for assistance. In contrast, the primary school–age child most often is simply brought by the parents. The adolescent's situation lies somewhere in between. Many adolescents take a cautious and ambiguous stance as to whether there is any problem for which help is wanted, or instead there is mere passive compliance with a parental initiative.

Several considerations must guide the clinician in deciding whether the first interview should be with the adolescent, the parents, or all together. Seeing the adolescent first underlines his or her active participation in the process and serves to allay anxiety that the therapist and parents will collude against or gang up on the youngster. However, some adolescents will protest that this casts them in the role of being the problem or the patient, when in their view the difficulty lies instead with their parents or between family members. The clinician must make clear that he or she is not out to assign blame but rather to help understand the difficulties the adolescent and the family have been confronting and to hear the views of all concerned. This usually requires both individual and family interviews. In most cases, the adolescent should be seen before the parents, but the parents may have to be seen first if they have difficulty getting their child to come for the first appointment.

The parents also should be seen alone to hear their concerns, to assess their explicit and implicit reasons for seeking assistance at this time, and to obtain a developmental and family history. The interview with the parents also yields valuable data concerning their view of the role played by the adolescent and the symptomatology in the psychic economy of the parents as individuals, as a couple, and in the family as a whole.

It often is useful at some point during the evaluation to interview the adolescent and parents together. The clinician frames the meeting's purpose as a forum in which family members can talk together; active structuring of this meeting may be needed to prevent the session from deteriorating into a "you hold him while I hit him" session in which the parents tell the therapist what is wrong with their child. Without the interviewer's active intervention, the adolescent may become very guarded or adversarial when seen with the parents. A family interview provides a useful opportunity to see how family members interact and to scrutinize overt and covert alliances and conflicts, shared family assumptions, coping patterns, and convergent and divergent areas of concern, as well as the family's ability to work together therapeutically and to make constructive use of the clinician's skills.

Confidentiality

Adolescents generally are very sensitive to the extremity of some of their thoughts and actions. Many fear that this information might be divulged by the clinician to their parents or to other authority figures. It is important from the outset for the parents and the adolescent to know that therapist–patient interactions are confidential. The exception is when the therapist believes that the patient or someone else is in danger. This rule should be spelled out at the beginning not only for general clarity but also to emphasize that it is a generic and not a specific response to a particular patient or disclosure. Patients sometimes want the clinician to tell something to parents or others "because you can say it much better than I can." Such a spokesperson role occasionally may be indicated, but its use should be preceded by a careful discussion and should occur in the adolescent's presence.

Developmental Issues and Interview Behavior

The clinician's approach to the interview with the adolescent is informed by an understanding of the developmental tasks and dynamics of adolescence and by the characteristic patterns used by adolescents to relate to adults and to manage their conflicts and anxiety (King 2002; Meeks and Bernet 2001). In the process of reworking and loosening dependent and libidinal ties to parents, adolescents turn, at times with a vengeance, to peers as objects of support and longing. Although some nonparental adults may be admired and turned to for guidance or identification, the adolescent's relationship with most adults is colored by a strong push toward autonomy and a great wariness of feeling vulnerable, dependent, or controlled. Even many adolescents who consciously want help approach a clinical evaluation with anxiety about revealing problems that they may regard as shameful weaknesses and with concerns about being criticized, controlled, or overwhelmed or becoming regressively dependent. These apprehensions may take the form of bland denials of any difficulties or insistence that either "everything is okay" or "I can handle it by myself."

Narcissistic vulnerability and difficulty tolerating ambivalence, internal conflicts, or painful feelings lead many adolescents to portray their problems as arising from outside rather than from within themselves. Adolescents often externalize one side or another of their conflicted feelings. A youngster may focus on bitter complaints of parental overprotectiveness while ignoring inner insecurities or wishes to be taken care of. Many adolescents deal with anxiety, guilt, shame, and other painful affects by means of counterphobic maneuvers or reversal of affect. For example, frightened teenagers may pick fights rather than take flight, and it is not unusual for sad adolescents to feel primarily angry during an interview. The clinician must learn to look beyond the adolescent's surface behavior and develop a capacity to notice when the youngster "doth protest too much."

An unrealistic faith in the "omnipotence of thought" is also characteristic of many adolescents who want to believe that even long-standing maladaptive patterns can be overcome simply by resolving to do things differently. Exploration of a problem area may thus be resisted with the sincere protestation, "Oh, I don't do that anymore" (i.e., not since yesterday). Adolescents' moods are labile, and their time perspective is short. Today's insoluble crisis, eternal passion, or irreversible decision may be forgotten by next week. Therefore, it is useful to evaluate an adolescent over time to assess which issues are transient and which are enduring. Of course, a propensity to fre-quent, albeit transient, upsets is in itself an important vulnerability to note.

Personal Issues for the Interviewer

Work with adolescents makes special demands on the clinician and is not to everyone's taste. Recall of and comfort with one's own adolescence are an enormous advantage. Enjoying teenagers is a prime prerequisite, followed by tact, flexibility, and a sense of humor. Schopenhauer once described friendship as "the art of distances." The same might be said of interviewing adolescents. Conveying a genuine and benign interest in the adolescent is essential. Condescension, aloofness, or excessive passivity in the interviewer is likely to be fatal. On the other hand, most adolescents will be frightened by overfamiliarity, seductiveness, or failure of the clinician to maintain an adult role.

Adolescents' narcissism is exquisitely tender, and one must learn how to talk frankly yet tactfully about vulnerable areas in such a way that adolescents do not feel they are being criticized. In the face of some adolescents' insistence that "you are either for me or against me," the clinician's task is to convey a genuine empathic interest in the adolescent's own view of the situation without collusively implying uncritical acceptance of that view.

Clinicians who work with adolescents need a good knowledge of their own adolescence and what they have made of that experience. Clinicians also must be aware of their feelings and biases about parenting. For example, at moments, the clinician may feel tempted to identify strongly with patients' struggles against authority or feel a twinge of envy at their seeming freedom of sexual or aggressive expression; on the other hand, the clinician may find that certain adolescents or situations stir censorious or confrontational impulses or an identification with beleaguered or embattled parents. In short, the interviewer may feel either pressured to regress to an adolescent's viewpoint or propelled into a defensive parental stance.

The Interview

In the interview, the clinician is interested in several aspects of the presenting problem (King et al. 2005). What is the nature of the difficulty the adolescent is experiencing, and what areas of adaptive functioning are affected and to what degree? How does the adolescent think about the problem—as one lying entirely within, as a problem between himself or herself and others, or as a difficulty coming solely from without? Is the difficulty acute or long-standing? Which elements of the problem seem reactive, and which appear related to intrapsychic conflict or character? Do the symptoms provide important secondary gains for the patient or family? If chronic medical illness or constitutionally based developmental difficulties (such as dyslexia) are present, what has the adolescent made of them?

Beyond the manifest problem, the clinician also must assess the adolescent's personality structure and level of psychosexual development. Of particular importance are ego functions such as the capacity to tolerate frustration or anxiety, the degree of psychological-mindedness, the quality of mood regulation, and vulnerability to regression or impulsivity. This broader assessment of the adolescent's strengths and weaknesses is best accomplished in the course of reviewing how the adolescent is coping with the major adaptive tasks in the various realms of his or her life: school, family, and friends. It is important to inquire matter-of-factly about sadness, suicidality, eating habits, drug and alcohol use, and the presence of possible legal difficulties.

The degree to which one performs a formal, as opposed to an informal, mental status examination depends on variables such as the severity of the disorder, the reason for the evaluation, the time available, and the experience of the interviewer. A more formal approach is likely to be used when a disorder is severe, when precise documentation is required, or when there are concerns about the possibility of psychosis, dementia, or an organic brain syndrome. Basic areas to be covered in both formal and informal mental status examinations include the adolescent's general appearance, behavior, ability to relate, mood perceptions, thought content and coherence, memory, general information, intelligence, judgment, and insight.

To obtain a full picture, it is important not to limit the interview to areas of difficulty (King et al. 2005). The adolescent should know that the interviewer is interested in learning about him or her as a whole person, including areas of strength, enjoyment, and accomplishment. Adolescents may become defensive or blandly deny difficulties in the face of a too-exclusive focus on pathology. The experienced and empathic diagnostician conveys a genuine interest in learning about the nature, quality, and depth of the young person's interests, hobbies, and recreations. Rather than demonstrating or feigning one's familiarity with the latest rock group, sports cars, or athletic team, it is preferable to let the adolescent teach one about his or her particular interests. In so doing, the adolescent can enjoy a sense of mastery and control and some sense of parity with the adult examiner. At the same time, the clinician can learn what blend of interests, identifications, sublimations, and direct instinctual and narcissistic gratifications animates the adolescent. The temptation to make early interpretations is best resisted. Even, perhaps especially, if accurate, they are more likely to scare the patient away than to impress him or her with the interviewer's sagacity.

A closely related area is that of values, ideals, and aspirations. What are the adolescent's values, and who are the adolescent's models for emulation or disidentification? Are these values congruent or in conflict with those of the patient's family, subculture, or larger society? What is the adolescent's sense of the future, and what aspirations, realistic or not, does the adolescent have for it?

The world of friends and peers is another related area for exploration. With whom does the patient "hang out"? What do they do for fun? How do they get along? Friends may be chosen on many grounds, including shared interests, admired virtues, or repudiated aspects of the adolescent's self. Friends may function as sources of support or admiration, as partners for sexual or aggressive exploitation, as collusive companions in regression or delinquency, as targets for projection, and so on. Asking the adolescent to tell one what a close friend is like provides an opportunity to learn how the adolescent thinks about people and relationships and to assess his or her capacity for empathy. Adolescents' own concerns are often more readily revealed in displacement: "I have a friend who is always…" It is sometimes helpful to ask whether a friend is bothered by or involved with something the adolescent has denied but is likely involved in himself or herself.

The topic of peer friendships leads naturally to the topic of dating and sexual relationships. This area requires tact and a good measure of rapport with the patient. Even so, one may not always receive a fully candid response during the diagnostic phase. Beyond the usual issues of privacy, this area of adolescents' lives is usually filled with concern and uncertainty, no matter how enlightened they may consider

themselves to be. Does the teenager date, and is there anyone of either sex with whom he or she is close? What is the other person like, and what attracted each to the other? How has the relationship gone? Are there patterns in regard to the type of person found attractive and to the course of past relationships? When the patient has romantic daydreams (as we all do), what are they like? What is the script? Have any of the patient's relationships developed into sexual ones? Has the adolescent had other sexual experiences? Here one wants to be open to hearing about possible episodes of sexual abuse and concerns about sexual orientation. The goal goes beyond assessing the patient's popularity, experience, and ease with intimacy. Rather, the clinician is interested in the patient's "preconditions for loving" and the influences guiding object choice, as well as the extent to which recurrent anxiety, envy, ambivalence, sadomasochism, or issues of exploitation or narcissistic gratification interfere with the capacity for intimacy.

The Epilogue

Because of the adolescent's natural concern, it is important that the clinician summarize the findings at the end of the initial interviews. This summary should occur after the patient has been invited to add anything about which the interviewer has not asked and to say what he or she believes to be the best approach to be taken. Although this response may be quite different from what the clinician plans to propose, it is better to know areas of disagreement and resistance earlier than later.

Almost always, it is better first to share the recommendations and the reasons for them with the adolescent alone. An exception is when hospitalization is mandatory and parental support and quick action are required. Otherwise, it is useful to get the adolescent's reactions, to discuss any potential confidentiality questions, and to make any adjustments that seem indicated for the initial plan. The subsequent summarization for the parent or parents should be in the adolescent's presence.

References

King RA: Adolescence, in Child and Adolescent Psychiatry: A Comprehensive Textbook, 3rd Edition. Edited by Lewis M. Baltimore, MD, Lippincott Williams & Wilkins, 2002

King RA, Schwab-Stone M, Peterson B, et al: Psychiatric assessment of the infant, child, and adolescent, in Kaplan and Sadock's Comprehensive Textbook of Psychiatry, 8th Edition, Vol 2. Edited by Kaplan HI, Kaplan VA. Baltimore, MD, Lippincott Williams & Wilkins, 2005, pp 3044–3075

Meeks JE, Bernet W: The Fragile Alliance: An Orientation to Psychotherapy of the Adolescent, 5th Edition. Malabar, FL, Krieger Publishing, 2001

Self-Assessment Questions

Select the single best response for each question.

4.1   Which of the following statements concerning the initial interview of an adolescent is *false?*

A. Seeing the adolescent first highlights the patient's active participation in the process.

B. Seeing the adolescent first may allay fears that the parents and therapist will gang up on the patient.

C. The therapeutic alliance between the clinician and adolescent may be harmed if the clinician meets alone with the parents; such an approach is therefore discouraged.

D. The clinician should make clear to the adolescent that he or she is not out to assign blame.

E. None of the above.

4.2   Characteristic adolescent patterns of responding to interviews with a therapist include which of the following?

A. Anxiety about revealing problems that they may regard as weaknesses.

B. Externalization of one side or another of conflicted feelings.

C. Counterphobic measures to deal with painful affects.

D. An unrealistic faith in the "omnipotence of thought."

E. All of the above.

4.3   To interview an adolescent effectively, which of the following are important qualities for a clinician?

A. Having experienced similar problems in adolescence.

B. Possessing a sense of humor.

C. Being informal and familiar.

D. Being close in age to the adolescent so that he or she can identify with the clinician.

E. All of the above.

4.4   When should a formal mental status examination be conducted with an adolescent?

A. When there is a concern about psychosis.

B. When the disorder may be severe.

C. When precise documentation is required.

D. When there is a possibility of dementia.

E. All of the above.

4.5   In interviewing adolescents, the therapist should

    A. Limit the interview to areas of difficulty.

    B. Demonstrate his or her familiarity with any topic that the adolescent may bring up, such as rock groups.

    C. Make early interpretations to assist the adolescent with the session.

    D. Avoid asking about dating or sexual relationships.

    E. Ask about friends and peers.

The Parent Interview

Bennett L. Leventhal, M.D.

Martha E. Crotts, M.D.

The most commonly performed procedure in all of medicine is the clinical interview. The capacity to perform this critical clinical procedure is inherent to good practice, and in no other specialty is it more significant than in child and adolescent psychiatry. The clinical interview must be adapted to accommodate the effective examination of both individuals who present with vastly different developmental capacities and third parties who are unique sources of information about the identified patient. The parents of the child or adolescent patient are usually the most important of these third parties. By providing information about the child and family, the parents enable the clinician to understand not only the child's behavior but also the functioning of the family, the individuals, the environment, and the whole system in which the child exists.

Rutter and Cox (1985) emphasized the importance of children's experiences in their family lives. They clearly identified not only the role of parents in modifying children's behaviors but also the role of children in shaping parental behaviors.

Additionally, they pointed out that there are different types of parenting that interact in a unique way with a particular child's development, behaviors, and other characteristics, thus implying the necessity for interviewing parents in any evaluation or treatment process.

The parent interview is an essential part of an evaluation or other clinical process involving children and adolescents. However, clinicians must be concerned about the utility of the information acquired from the parent interview. Does the parent interview provide a valid account of the information necessary to formulate a diagnosis, establish a treatment plan, and monitor the treatment of a given child? When one thinks broadly about ways to interview parents—that is, the use of structured interviews, unstructured interviews, and parent report scales—one recognizes that there is enormous variability in the quantity and quality, and therefore in the reliability and validity, of the information obtained. Indeed, studies have shown that parental reports often are temporally distorted and that parents may

57

deny a particular problem or may be unable to recall pertinent past behavior (Chess et al. 1966). Mednick and Shaffer (1963) arrived at similar conclusions as a result of their studies of mothers' retrospective reports collected in a pediatric setting. Maternal interviews were compared with pediatric records, and the mothers' reports were found to be discrepant 21%–62% of the time for facts about discrete experiences, such as breastfeeding, childhood illnesses, and the age at completion of toilet training.

Kashani et al. (1985) also found low agreement between parents and children on all DSM-III-R (American Psychiatric Association 1987) Axis I disorders. Interestingly, the patterns of disagreement were generally consistent in that children reported more anxiety and depressive symptoms, whereas parents stressed more externalizing symptoms, such as oppositional behavior and short attention span. The authors concluded that multiple sources of information might help the clinician arrive at a clearer clinical picture. Weissman et al. (1987) reviewed numerous studies and identified discrepancies between parent and child reports on the nature, extent, and severity of children's symptoms. Irrespective of the interview setting, the diagnostic criteria, the method of interview, or the symptom scales, the authors found that children reported far more information about all their disorders. Indeed, Weissman et al. recommended that at least in certain types of studies, one should consider interviewing only the child if a choice has to be made. In contrast, Orvaschel et al. (1981) found that parents were more accurate in providing factual time-related information. Using an early version of the Diagnostic Interview Schedule for Children (DISC) and the Diagnostic Interview Schedule for Children, Parents' Version (DISC-P, the parent interview), Edelbrock et al. (1985) studied age differences in the reliability of interviews of children. Not surprisingly, these investigators found that the reliability of a child's report increased with the child's age and with the presence of overt behaviors such as aggression and hyperactivity. The importance of parental collaboration was most evident in the results of structured parent interviews for younger children. In general, parents were believed to be more reliable than their children until the children reached age 10 years, after which there was little or no difference in the reliability of parent and child reports.

Despite reported discrepancies, parents can and do provide essential information about a child's birth, development, medical history, and current functioning and symptoms, as well as marital and family history.

Simmons (1987) warned the clinician to identify clearly who is the patient. The child may be presented as the identified patient. However, careful discussion with the parents and child and examination of each parent, the marital couple, the family, the child's school, and the family's community are necessary to assess the child and to develop an intervention plan. Therefore, most clinicians agree that the parent interview is but one component of an evaluation that must be placed into the clinical context. Data gathered from the parents and from other parties may be affected greatly by the attitude parents hold toward a referral for therapy, toward the child, and toward other matters in the child's life. Furthermore, it appears essential, in most clinical settings, to evaluate features such as parental temperament, personality organization, and psychopathology to place the data that the parents provide into a clinical context that also includes the child's role in the parents' struggles, unconscious and conscious wishes for the child, and other dynamic issues (Greenspan and Greenspan 2003).

What, then, is the function of the parent interview? Certainly the gathering of information about the child's history and the child's present functioning is crucial. Equally important, however, is the opportunity for the clinician to develop an alliance. This alliance may be the key to sustaining the evaluation and treatment process and to fostering the child's relationship with the clinician. Developing an alliance with parents during the interview process is not simply a matter of collecting information; it is also important to give them information. The clinician can and should identify strengths and weaknesses in the child and help the parents clarify what they already know. The clinician also can give parents information about normal child development and the clinical process. In this way, the parent interview becomes a collaborative effort.

Parent interviews are conducted in a variety of settings; therefore, it is important for the clinician to identify the purpose of the interview beforehand. Some interviews are part of a diagnostic process, whereas others are a component of individual, family, or parent-oriented treatment. Furthermore, some interviews take place under scheduled circumstances, whereas others are in an acute setting, such as an emergency room, or are part of the inpatient, pediatric, or psychiatric consultation. Each of these interviews has a different tone and a separate set of goals.

Depending on the purpose of the interview, a variety of formal, partially or fully structured instruments could be used as part of the interviewing process. Although formal interviewing instruments can never replace the parent interview conducted by an experienced clinician, these instruments can provide supplemental information. Instruments are generally divided into two types: 1) those that are administered by the clinician or trained staff and 2) those that are self-administered. Instruments administered by the clinician may be either semistructured or structured. For more information on these child psychiatric diagnostic instruments, see Chapter 6 ("Diagnostic Interviews").

Self-administered instruments or rating scales can be completed by the parent before or after the in-person interview. Some rating scales assess a wide range of symptoms. Others are used to evaluate specific symptom clusters or diagnoses. Rating scales are discussed in detail in Chapter 7 ("Rating Scales").

An additional option is to use family measurement instruments for data collection from parents. These instruments are numerous and varied with regard to their emphases. Areas in which they can be of assistance include exploration of parental roles and parent–child interactions, among other aspects of family functioning. Family assessment measures are covered in more detail in the American Psychiatric Association's *Handbook of Psychiatric Measures,* specifically the chapter entitled "Family and Relational Issues Measures" (Messer and Reiss 2000).

Whether self-administered or administered by staff or the clinician, formal instruments can be completed and their results available for use at the time of the interview. They may serve as efficient tools in the current health care environment, in which time is of the essence.

Components of an Interview

All good parent interviews incorporate some degree of structure, which is ultimately the responsibility of the interviewer; therefore, all parent interviews require careful thought and planning. Each interview has five components: 1) preliminaries, 2) prologue, 3) interview proper, 4) closing, and 5) epilogue.

The clinician must establish the goals for each particular interview and set a tentative agenda in advance. The beginning of the interview sets the tone for the balance of the process.

■ Preliminaries

The preliminary phase is the planning for the interview process. The first tasks of this phase are to identify the patient and the purpose of the interview, in order to determine the interview type and goals. For example, if the interview is to be diagnostic, then the collection of information may be the most critical component of the interview; if the interview is to be therapeutic, then the means of intervention and the goals of the treatment must be clearly understood before the intervention is to begin. The content of the interview differs significantly according to the age and diagnostic category of the identified patient. Once these preliminary tasks have been completed, the clinician must ascertain that the amount of time available and other conditions are suitable to meet the interview objectives.

■ Prologue

The prologue is the introductory phase. It begins with introductions, which must be respectful of the parental role and competence, and details the circumstances of the interview. Similarly, introductions must clearly identify the clinician and his or her role while also setting the ground rules regarding matters such as confidentiality. During this portion of the interview, it is useful to assess both the parents' and the clinician's expectations for the interview and to get some indications about, for example, parental defensiveness, shame, guilt, and embarrassment:

> It is never easy to think of a child as having these sorts of problems. You may even be embarrassed or scared. Despite this, you have been able to come for help. Now I would like to help you understand what is happening so we can make a plan to solve the problems facing both you and your child.

■ Interview Proper

The interview proper is the opportunity to establish an alliance with the parents while collecting data and making the appropriate interventions. Even in a parent interview, it is important to attend to the more traditional elements of the psychiatric evaluation. Transference, countertransference, resistance, defenses, strengths, weaknesses, and similar matters that specifically relate to the parents require careful assessment. The clinician simultaneously must assess family matters, including traditions, locus of control, discipline, family dynamics, communication, and other matters that more commonly are associated with parent and family functioning. At the same time, the interviewer must help parents to manage their anxiety and to maintain an appropriate sense of responsibility for the child.

■ Closing

The closing portion of the parent interview is the clinician's opportunity to reassure the parents and reinforce their control and competence. It is also a time for answering questions that the parents may have and articulating the next step in the clinical process:

> At this point, there are several possibilities to explain the current situation. These are 1)…, 2)…, 3)…, and 4)…. I would like to suggest that we do the following to answer the remaining questions and establish a treatment plan. I realize that this may seem a bit overwhelming or confusing, so please be sure that I have satisfactorily answered your questions before we proceed.

■ Epilogue

Finally, each clinician must allow some time to review the interview. By carefully reconsidering the data that have been acquired and the response to interventions, the clinician can review the validity of the plans and the next step. Similarly, planning for future clinical activity can be assessed before the report of the interview is generated. Although the epilogue may be the end of the parent interview, it also may be the beginning of further clinical activity with the parents and the child.

Source of Referral

It is always useful to assess parental attitudes about the referral and the source of referral and why parents have accepted the referral for an evaluation at a particular time. This information not only may guide the clinical process but also may help identify problems that are of particular interest to the patient and the family. For example, a family that is forced into an evaluation by an outside agency or the legal system may perceive the evaluation very differently from a family in which there is an extensive history of psychiatric illness that is being manifested by the child, who is the identified patient. It is also important to consider the relationship between the clinician and the referral source as the clinical process unfolds.

Impression of Parents

It is important to derive a general impression of the parents. This allows the clinician to develop a preliminary conceptual framework in which to place the child's and the parents' functioning in a family context. It is also important to gain some appreciation not only of the parents' role in shaping the lives of their children but also of the children's capacity to shape the parental role (Rutter and Cox 1985).

Types of Interviews and Settings

■ Diagnostic Interview

In the diagnostic or history-taking interview, the information to be collected from parents is both factual and impressionistic. It is important, whenever possible, to review additional sources of information—for example, medical and school records and records from previous evaluations or testing. A detailed outline of historical information to guide the interviewer is provided in Table 5–1.

■ Medical Consultation Setting

In medical consultation settings, the parents are important informants about the child's premorbid functioning and the impact of the child's illness on the child and the family. Even in this setting, it is important to identify who is the patient and what is the agenda of the person requesting the consultation. For example, an adolescent patient may be identified as noncompliant with the treatment when, in fact, the source of conflict originates in ambivalent relationships between the primary treating physician and the parents, who are highly involved and may try to control the medical treatment process. Therefore, the focus during the parent interview, although manifestly directed toward the child's medical care, may be more directly related to the parents' sense of control, frustration, and incompetence in the clinical situation.

■ Emergency Setting

In emergency settings, where the clinician must make rapid decisions about assessment and treatment, entirely different forms of parent interviews are necessary to evaluate whether there is a risk of self-injury or of injury to others, or whether the child is a possible victim of physical or sexual

Table 5–1.   Outline of biopsychosocial history

Chief symptom and reasons for referral

History of present illness

Development of the symptoms

Attitudes of child and parents toward the symptoms

Effects of the symptoms on child and family

Stressors

Prior psychological or psychiatric evaluations

Prior treatment

Psychotherapy: type, frequency, duration, effects

Medication: exact dosages, schedule, beneficial and adverse effects

Environmental changes and effects

Current developmental status

Habits

Motor abilities and activity level

Attention

Speech and language

Academic performance

Relationships with peers

Risk-taking behaviors

Sexual development and behavior

Hobbies, activities, athletic interests and skills

Relationships with family members and other significant adults

Review of behavioral and psychological symptoms

Medical review of systems

Past history

Psychiatric

Medical

Neurological

Developmental history

Pregnancy and delivery

Neonatal period, infancy, early childhood

Temperament

Milestones

Motor

Cognitive

Speech and language

Social

School history

Traumatic events

Table 5–1.   Outline of biopsychosocial history *(continued)*

Psychosocial and psychiatric history of each parent

Developmental history of the couple/family life cycle

Family medical history

Current family circumstances, concerns, liabilities, resources

abuse. In the emergency setting, the focus of the interview must be on assessing the risk of danger and establishing a safe and protective environment for the child. In some circumstances, extraordinary levels of parental defensiveness, anxiety, guilt, and avoidance of conflict may be present. In addition, because legal culpability for the events may be in question, careful attention must be given to details such as evasiveness of the parents.

■ Medication Consultations

Commonly, clinicians are asked to consult with pediatricians, family practitioners, or other mental health professionals concerning psychopharmacological interventions. Before the consultation, a great deal of information may be provided by other professionals, and often the parents arrive in these settings with strong feelings that they are being criticized or that the situation is rapidly becoming desperate. Still others approach the medication consultation seeking a medication to definitively treat their child. The medication consultation with parents requires not only careful gathering of a child history and family history but also careful assessment of parental expectations. These expectations must be dealt with directly, along with provision of detailed information about the treatment process. The parents must be carefully and accurately informed about the types of medications to be used, the potential side effects and serious consequences related to these medications, and the real therapeutic potential. Because medication consultations are often stressful and the information itself is critical, the parent interview in this case often takes on an instructive format.

Conclusion

Fundamentally, the parent interview is a pedagogic process. It is an opportunity for the parents to teach the clinician about themselves, their roles as parents, the child, and the family. The parent interview also is an opportunity for the clinician to teach parents about the clinical process and perhaps about the parents themselves and their child. For all of this teaching to take place, each party must be open to the process.

References

American Psychiatric Association: Diagnostic and Statistical Manual of Mental Disorders, 3rd Edition, Revised. Washington, DC, American Psychiatric Association, 1987

Chess S, Thomas A, Birch HG: Distortions in developmental reporting made by parents of behaviorally disturbed children. J Am Acad Child Psychiatry 5:226–234, 1966

Edelbrock C, Costello AJ, Dulcan MK, et al: Age differences in the reliability of the psychiatric interview of the child. Child Dev 56:265–275, 1985

Greenspan SI, Greenspan NT: The Clinical Interview of the Child, 2nd Edition. Washington, DC, American Psychiatric Publishing, 2003

Kashani JH, Orvaschel H, Burk JP, et al: Informant variance: the issue of parent-child disagreement. J Am Acad Child Psychiatry 24:437–441, 1985

Mednick SA, Shaffer JBP: Mothers' retrospective reports in child-rearing research. Am J Orthopsychiatry 33:457–461, 1963

Messer SC, Reiss D: Family and relational issues measures, in Handbook of Psychiatric Measures. Washington, DC, American Psychiatric Association, 2000, pp 239–260

Orvaschel H, Weissman MM, Padian N, et al: Assessing psychopathology in children of psychiatrically disturbed parents: a pilot study. J Am Acad Child Psychiatry 20:112–122, 1981

Rutter M, Cox A: Other family influences, in Child and Adolescent Psychiatry: Modern Approaches. Edited by Rutter M, Hersov L. London, Blackwell, 1985, pp 58–81

Simmons JE: Psychiatric Examination of Children. Philadelphia, PA, Lea & Febiger, 1987

Weissman MM, Wickramaratne P, Warner V, et al: Assessing psychiatric disorders in children: discrepancies between mothers' and children's reports. Arch Gen Psychiatry 44:747–753, 1987

Self-Assessment Questions

Select the single best response for each question.

5.1 Mednick and Shaffer (1963) found that when maternal interviews were compared with pediatric records, the mothers' reports were discrepant what percentage of the time?

   A. 0–6%.
   B. 7%–15%.
   C. 16%–20%.
   D. 21%–62%.
   E. 63%–75%.

5.2 A number of investigators have studied the parent interview. Which of the following descriptions of their findings is *incorrect*?

   A. Weissman et al. (1987) found that parents reported far more information about their children's disorders than did the children themselves.
   B. Orvaschel et al. (1981) found that parents were more accurate in providing factual time-related information.
   C. Edelbrock et al. (1985) found that the reliability of a child's report increased with the child's age.
   D. Edelbrock et al. (1985) found that in children 10 years of age and older, parent and child reports showed little or no difference in reliability.
   E. None of the above.

5.3 Which of the following is a function of the parent interview?

   A. Gathering information about the child's history.
   B. Assessing the child's present functioning.
   C. Identifying the child's strengths and weaknesses.
   D. Giving parents information about normal child development.
   E. All of the above.

5.4 The parent interview may be divided into five phases: preliminaries, prologue, interview proper, closing, and epilogue. What is the primary purpose of the *closing* phase?

   A. Assess the parents' and the clinician's expectations for the interview.
   B. Establish an alliance or empathetic relationship with the parents while collecting data and making the appropriate interventions.
   C. Reassure the parents and reinforce their control and competence.
   D. Review the interview, the validity of the plans, and the next step.
   E. None of the above.

5.5   In emergency settings, the focus of the parent interview is

   A. Directly related to the parents' sense of control, frustration, and incompetence in the clinical situation.
   B. To assess the risk of danger and to establish a safe and protective environment for the child.
   C. To assess the child's medical care.
   D. To obtain factual and impressionistic information.
   E. All of the above.

Diagnostic Interviews

Jon McClellan, M.D.

Psychiatric syndromes continue to be defined by consensus-based diagnostic categories (which incorporate defined symptom criteria) rather than by etiological mechanisms (which for the most part are unknown). The field has not shared the enormous scientific and technological advances affecting other medical specialties, primarily because the complex mechanisms underlying brain function and mental illness remain elusive. Disease-causing genetic mutations have been identified for only a few psychiatric disorders (e.g., Alzheimer's type dementia, fragile X syndrome, Rett's disorder). The complexity of brain development suggests that most psychiatric disorders emanate from multifactorial processes involving an interplay between genetic, biological, and/or environmental risk and protective factors. Unraveling such complex processes is an enormous challenge and is in part dependent on the presence of a valid diagnostic schema to characterize meaningful phenotypes.

The DSM (beginning with the third revision, DSM-III [American Psychiatric Association 1980]) and ICD (*International Classification of Diseases and Related Health Problems*) systems commenced the epoch of psychiatric diagnostic classification. Although syndromes such as schizophrenia, depression, manic depression (now called bipolar disorder), and autism were well described prior to these classification schemas, the application of diagnoses was often variable and unreliable. The atheoretical basis of the DSM and ICD systems—emphasizing clinically defined syndromes, with criteria based on symptomatology and pattern of illness—moved the field away from diagnostic formulations grounded in unproven theoretical doctrines and ill-defined constructs. Criteria-based diagnoses improve reliability and ensure that similar definitions are used by different clinicians and across sites, thereby enhancing communication for clinical, administrative, and research purposes. However, despite the utility of criteria-based diagnostic categories, the validity of many of these categories remains unknown, especially for those specific to child psychiatry.

Psychiatric Interviews

The clinical interview, the primary diagnostic tool for psychiatry, has evolved over time. Early formulations were often based on indirect observations of discourse and

67

play (in children) without direct questioning. With the advent of the DSM and ICD diagnostic systems, interview strategies shifted to a more disease-oriented approach, a change prompted in part by the recognized lack of clinician reliability in diagnosing recognized illnesses (e.g., schizophrenia, autism) and in part by the recognized lack of an etiological model on which to base a diagnostic system.

The subjective and variable nature of the symptom reports used to generate psychiatric diagnoses remains a limitation. Information derived from patients, their families, and other observers (e.g., teachers) is subtle, complex, and often conflicting (Achenbach et al. 1987). Clinicians' diagnoses are potentially fraught with numerous biases (Angold and Fisher 1999), including the following:

- Making diagnoses before all relevant information is collected
- Collecting information selectively when confirming and/or ruling out a diagnosis
- Neglecting to be systematic in collecting and organizing information
- Allowing the clinician's particular expertise (e.g., a physician in a mood disorders clinic diagnosing most patients' disorders as depression, regardless of each patient's clinical presentation) to influence diagnosis assignment
- Assuming correlations between symptoms and illnesses that in reality are spurious or nonexistent (e.g., equating all irritability with mania)

The creation of diagnostic criteria helped structure the diagnostic process. However, even when the same diagnostic criteria are used, disagreement may occur for any of the following reasons (Costello 1996):

- Differences in wording of the questions used to identify symptoms
- Differences in how clinicians interpret the responses
- Differences in responses the patient may make to different interviewers or to the same interviewer at different times

Structured Diagnostic Interviews

Two types of diagnostic tools, questionnaires and interviews, have been developed for clinicians and researchers to enhance the reliability of the information gathered and improve the diagnostic process. Questionnaires are usually completed by patients, parents, or other significant individuals (e.g., teachers) and generally focus on broader domains of psychopathology but may focus more narrowly on specific illness states or symptoms. For a thorough discussion of questionnaires and checklists pertinent to child and adolescent psychopathology, see Chapter 7 ("Rating Scales").

Structured diagnostic interviews are designed to elicit information from children and/or their parents about various aspects of functioning and mental health, including specific inquiries about symptom criteria for different psychiatric disorders. They are primarily used for psychiatric research, both in epidemiological surveys and in clinical studies. The instruments vary as to whether they are administered by clinicians or trained interviewers (although some researchers use research assistants to administer measures originally designed for clinician administration). Structured interviews were first developed to examine mental health problems in adults; interviews for use with children and adolescents and their families were subsequently developed. Many of the available measures have evolved over several versions, dating back to DSM-III.

■ Interview Characteristics and Relevant Concepts

There are several characteristics and concepts relevant to the development, choice, use, and interpretation of structured diagnostic interviews.

Validity

Validity reflects the degree to which a measure or classification system accurately characterizes the entity it is examining. Descriptors of various types of validity include *face validity* (how well a category as defined appears to describe a recognized illness), *predictive validity* (how well the category predicts a pertinent aspect of care, such as treatment needs or prognosis), and *construct validity* (whether the category has meaning in terms of what it is designed to describe).

Childhood psychiatric disorders generally have face validity but not necessarily construct or predictive validity, categories that are less extensively studied and more difficult to examine. Diagnostic validity is difficult to assess in psychiatry. Because of the lack of biological markers, diagnoses made with a structured interview are often compared with those made by experienced clinicians. This practice is problematic, given that clinician diagnoses are notoriously unreliable and thus may not represent the "gold standard." Furthermore, because the same diagnostic criteria define both methods of diagnosis, the validity of a diagnostic tool is not independent from the diagnostic criteria it assesses.

Some authors assess the construct validity of their diagnostic instruments as a method of inferring validity. Comparison is often made with a series of other measures that assess predictive and/or concurrent features of the disorder, using a strategy referred to as a nomological network (Cronbach and Meehl 1955). For example, the results of a diagnostic interview are compared with several pertinent theoretically related attributes, such as patterns and stability of diagnoses, independent ratings of psychopathology, service utilization, and family psychiatric history. Thus, by a process akin to triangulation, researchers examine the validity of a measure by determining its proximity to that of other theoretically related measures or attributes. The inferred validity of each measure supports the validity of the entire construct.

This method avoids the problems associated with defining a diagnostic gold standard. However, the diagnostic construct is only as valid as the measures or attributes used to define it. Validity of diagnostic concepts and constructs is often examined by comparing the results of diagnostic interviews with related questionnaires (e.g., determining the association between a diagnosis of major depressive disorder on a structured interview and the score on a depression rating scale). Because the same symptoms are assessed by both measures, the instruments are not truly independent. This type of validity test is commonly used, but it represents a circular logic that simply reifies the diagnostic criteria rather than establishing the validity of the disorder or the measure.

Another challenge is distinguishing between syndrome specificity and severity. Many measures used to predict validity assess functional impact (e.g., academic or social impairment). Although a diagnosis may be a good indicator of impairment, this is not unexpected, given that impairment is usually one of the diagnostic criteria. Furthermore, although functional impairment is an important health issue, it does not imply specificity. The actual validity of the disorder itself—or the diagnostic criteria that define it—remains illusory.

Reliability

Reliability reflects agreement, including how often different interviewers assign the same diagnosis (interrater reliability), how consistently respondents report the same symptoms or diagnoses over time (test–retest reliability), and how internally consistent the measure is (i.e., the degree to which different sections of the measure give similar information).

Differences in diagnostic reliability may be due to 1) differences in the information collected, 2) theoretical biases held by diagnosticians, and/or 3) variations in symptoms that individuals with disorders will experience over time. Diagnostic tools must be reliable to be useful, but reliability does not ensure validity. A diagnostic category may be reliably defined but not valid. Conversely, a disorder may be valid, but the diagnostic criteria, or the instruments used to assess for its presence, may not be reliable.

The methods used by investigators to establish reliability for a diagnostic interview raise some interesting questions. For example, establishing reliability at one site often means establishing agreement with the senior investigator. Many studies simply have other examiners watch and score the same interviews. There is no guarantee that the same results would be obtained at another program. Research is needed to establish the reliability of measures across different sites.

Interview Type

The available diagnostic interviews are often described in terms of their degree of structure—that is, how closely interviewers must follow an outlined script (Costello 1996). In a highly structured interview, the interviewer asks set questions using specified wording, and the subject's responses are recorded as given. Semistructured interviews allow interviewers to use their own probe questions and/or incorporate other sources of information to assess symptoms and interpret the subject's responses. Angold and Fisher (1999) questioned this distinction, suggesting that it is the degree of decision-making process allowed by the interviewer that is structured rather than the questions themselves. Using this model, interviews can be characterized as 1) respondent-based, in which the interviewer follows a set script without interpreting the subject's response, and/or 2) interviewer-based, in which the interview serves as a tool to guide the interviewer's questioning, including definitions of symptoms and patterns of disorders that the interviewer uses to decide whether a symptom is present. These two methods are not necessarily mutually exclusive, and many interviews have elements of both.

■ Defining Cases

The goal of the psychiatric interview is to identify whether an individual has an illness. Theoretically, using the current categorical model, psychiatric disorders are either present or absent. However, in practice, how cases are defined will depend on the nature and application of diagnostic criteria. Therefore, in any sample, individuals will be either disordered or nondisordered (reflecting the true population prevalence rates) and will be classified as either cases or noncases (depending on the diagnostic criteria). Although it is hoped that these two concepts are related, being a case is not necessarily the same as being truly disordered (Zarin and Earls 1993). This model assumes that the disorder actually does exist in nature, an assumption that may not hold true for any given illness.

In assessing a diagnostic instrument's utility in identifying cases, the following concepts are important:

- *Sensitivity:* The percentage of individuals in a sample who have the disorder who are accurately identified by the interview

- *Specificity:* The percentage of individuals in a sample who do not have the disorder who are accurately identified by the interview as being nondisordered

- *Predictive value positive:* The percentage of individuals in the defined sample positively identified by the interview who actually have the disorder

- *Predictive value negative:* The percentage of individuals in the defined sample identified by the interview as not having the disorder who are in fact nondisordered

Psychiatric "caseness" is determined by whether a patient's illness meets a specified number of symptom criteria. It is important to remember that diagnostic categories were created largely by consensus and that in reality, a single cutoff (i.e., number of criteria met) is unlikely to accurately categorize every individual with a given disorder. Diagnostic systems attempt to find a balance between using broader criteria so as to identify all cases (thereby risking overdiagnosis [false positives]) and using more conservative criteria (thereby risking underdiagnosis [false negatives]). The trade-off between false positives and false negatives is unavoidable.

The positive predictive value and negative predictive value are influenced by the overall prevalence of the condition being investigated, whereas sensitivity and specificity are theoretically independent of prevalence rates (Robins 1985). Therefore, the probability of correctly diagnosing a rare condition using a given diagnostic tool may be low, even if the tool has acceptable sensitivity and specificity ratings. This fact also holds true for predicting other types of rare events, such as suicides or acts of isolated violence in adolescents.

■ Structured Diagnostic Interviews in Common Use

Table 6–1 outlines characteristics of the structured diagnostic interviews most often used with children and adolescents. The choice of interview generally depends on the purpose (e.g., epidemiological versus treatment study), the diagnoses to be assessed, the type of interviewer (clinician versus lay interviewer), the training requirements, the researcher's familiarity with or previous use of the instrument, the time required for administration, and the costs.

Respondent-based interviews capture the patient's response without interpretation by the interviewer. This limits variability in how information is obtained. They are typically used in epidemiological surveys, where trained lay interviewers, not clinicians, administer the measure. The National Institute of Mental Health (NIMH) Diagnostic Interview Schedule for Children (DISC) (Shaffer et al. 2000) is the most widely tested measure, having undergone several multicenter field trials to establish its use for the NIMH epidemiological study. It is generally administered by trained lay interviewers, which lowers the cost, making it useful for large epidemiological studies examining for prevalence rates of disorder within a population.

In interviewer-based interviews (Angold and Fisher 1999), the concepts to be explored are defined with a range of possible answers, but interviewers are allowed to phrase questions in their own words and/or develop their own probes to elicit further information. Depending on the methods being used, the interviewer may also incorporate information obtained from other sources (e.g., other

Table 6–1.   Structured diagnostic interviews most often used with children and adolescents

Instrument	Disorders covered	Informant	Age range (years)	Type	Time (minutes)	Interviewer qualifications	Special issues
NIMH Diagnostic Interview Schedule for Children, Version IV (NIMH DISC-IV; Shaffer et al. 2000)	ANX, BEH, EAT, ELIM, MOOD, SCH, SUB, TIC	Child, parent	6–17	Respondent	70–120	Trained lay interviewer	Computerized voice and Spanish versions available
Versions							
DISC-Y (Youth)			9–17				
DISC-P (Parent)			6–17				
Child and Adolescent Psychiatric Assessment (CAPA; Angold and Costello 2000)	ANX, BEH, EAT, ELIM, MOOD, SCH, SOM, SUB, TIC	Child, parent	9–17	Interviewer	60–150	Bachelor's degree plus training program	Glossary used to define symptoms and severity ratings; Spanish version available
Related Instruments							
YAPA (Young Adult Psychiatric Assessment)		Patient	18+				
PAPA (Preschool Age Psychiatric Assessment)		Parent	3–6				

Table 6–1. Structured diagnostic interviews most often used with children and adolescents (*continued*)

Instrument	Disorders covered	Informant	Age range (years)	Type	Time (minutes)	Interviewer qualifications	Special issues
Schedule for Affective Disorders and Schizophrenia for School-Age Children (K-SADS; Ambrosini 2000) Versions K-SADS-E (Epidemiological) K-SADS-P/L (Present and Lifetime) K-SADS-P (Present state) Washington University K-SADS	ANX, BEH, EAT, MOOD, SCH, SUB Also assesses ELIM and TIC Expands definitions of mania	Child, parent	6–18	Interviewer	75–90	Trained clinician	Although designed for clinicians, many researchers use trained interviewers
Diagnostic Interview for Children and Adolescents (DICA; Reich 2000)	ANX, BEH, EAT, ELIM, MOOD, PSYCH, SOM, SUB, TIC	Child, parent	6–17	Respondent/ interviewer	60–120	Trained lay interviewer	Used as both structured and semistructured interview
Structured Clinical Interview for DSM-IV, Childhood Diagnoses (KID-SCID) (Matzner et al. 1997)	ANX, BEH, MOOD, SCH, SOM, SUB	Child, parent	7–17	Interviewer	60–120	Clinician	Only preliminary data available

Table 6–1. Structured diagnostic interviews most often used with children and adolescents *(continued)*

Instrument	Disorders covered	Informant	Age range (years)	Type	Time (minutes)	Interviewer qualifications	Special issues
Interview Schedule for Children and Adolescents (ISCA; Sherrill and Kovacs 2000)	ANX, BEH, EAT, ELIM, MOOD, PSYCH, SOM, SUB, TIC	Child, parent	8–17	Interviewer	120 (parent), 60 (child)	Clinician	Organized around symptom reports
Children's Interview for Psychiatric Syndromes (ChIPS; Weller et al. 2000)	ANX, BEH, EAT, ELIM, MOOD, SCH, SUB	Child, parent	6–18	Respondent	40	Trained lay interviewer	Primarily a screening tool
Dominic-R (Valla et al. 2000)	ANX, BEH, DEP	Child	6–11	Pictorial	15–25	Trained lay interviewer	Pictorial depiction of DSM-III-R symptoms; versions for African American and French-speaking children available

Note. ANX=anxiety disorders (often includes posttraumatic stress disorder); BEH=disruptive behavior disorders; DEP=depressive disorders; EAT=eating disorders; ELIM=encopresis and enuresis; MOOD=mood disorders (depressive and bipolar); NIMH=National Institute of Mental Health; PSYCH=nondiagnostic screen for psychotic symptoms; SCH=schizophrenia and psychotic disorders; SOM=somatoform disorders; SUB=substance abuse/dependence; TIC=tic disorders. Type of interview: respondent=answers coded on the basis of responses (also described as structured); interviewer=interviewer allowed to make clinical judgments regarding respondent's answers (also called semistructured). Interview times are approximate and may vary depending on the case and interviewer.

informants, medical records) prior to making a decision about a particular symptom or diagnosis. Some of the interviews have screening questions so that entire topics can be skipped if the initial inquiry is negative. Interviewer-based interviews require some clinical decision making on the part of the interviewer, are often used in studies of clinical populations, and are presumably more tolerable to clinicians.

Among the interviewer-based instruments, the Child and Adolescent Psychiatric Assessment (CAPA; Angold and Costello 2000), the Schedule for Affective Disorders and Schizophrenia for School-Age Children (K-SADS; Ambrosini 2000), and the Diagnostic Interview for Children and Adolescents (DICA; Reich 2000) have been most studied. The CAPA has an extensive glossary to aid decision making and provides separate ratings of symptomatology and psychosocial impairment. The K-SADS has been used extensively in child psychiatry research, especially in the area of mood disorders, and includes individual ratings of symptom impairment. The DICA can be used either by clinicians as an interviewer-based instrument or by lay interviewers as a respondent-based measure.

The Interview Schedule for Children and Adolescents (ISCA; Sherrill and Kovacs 2000); the Children's Interview for Psychiatric Syndromes (ChIPS; Weller et al. 2000); and the Structured Clinical Interview for DSM-IV, Childhood Diagnoses (KID-SCID; Matzner et al. 1997) have less research supporting their reliability and validity and are not used as widely. All, however, are promising tools. The ISCA has been used to study mood and anxiety disorders in youth. There is a version for young adults, which is potentially useful for longitudinal follow-up studies. Because the ISCA is structured around symptom reports rather than

diagnostic categories, it can be used to explore alternative ways of defining disorders. The ChIPS is respondent-based and can be administered in a relatively short period of time. Therefore, it may be useful as a screening tool in, for example, a clinic setting. The KID-SCID is an adaptation of the adult SCID (First et al. 1996), which is widely used for studies of mood and psychotic disorders.

The Dominic-R (Valla et al. 2000, 2002) uses pictures as cues to inquire about symptoms. Each picture has an accompanying question the interviewer uses to prompt the child for a response. This measure was developed because younger children may not provide reliable responses with standard question-and-answer interviews. However, the pictorial methods entail difficulties in assessing certain concepts important to diagnosis, such as duration and severity. The Dominic-R is computerized and highly structured but does not include inquiries about frequency, duration, or age at onset of symptoms.

Discussion

Structured diagnostic interviews are useful tools that have improved the reliability of diagnostic assignment. Although most often used by researchers, these instruments would likely enhance practice if adopted by clinicians in community settings. A number of structured diagnostic interviews are available for assessment of psychiatric illness in youth. When using these instruments, it is important to recognize their limitations.

All diagnostic tools involve error, and use of even those with excellent ratings of sensitivity and specificity will result in misdiagnosis. Slight variations in wording, or in how the instrument is scored, may produce significant changes in prevalence estimates (Robins and Cottler

2004). There is a paucity of research comparing one structured diagnostic interview with another or examining which instruments are superior for certain diagnoses or clinical issues.

In addition, the presence of a diagnosis may not adequately characterize clinical significance, as defined by either treatment needs or level of impairment (Frances 1998; Regier et al. 1998). One difficulty is in the ability to discriminate between individuals with actual disorders and individuals with typical yet problematic responses to some type of event or stimulus. Human beings have a fairly consistent repertoire of responses to stress, regardless of the source (a final common pathway). Symptoms may represent transient adaptive changes in mood, behavior, and/or physiological measures rather than evidence for a distinct pathological state (Regier et al. 1998). Many symptoms are not necessarily specific to any single disorder (e.g., irritability, sleep problems, aggression).

Another difficulty is that children may overreport rare or unusual phenomena, such as obsessive-compulsive, psychotic, or manic symptoms, with structured diagnostic interviews (Breslau 1987; Weller et al. 1996). This is likely due to the child's either misinterpreting the question or not being aware of the concept being described. In general, younger children lack the prerequisite attention span, abstract awareness (including time lines for duration criteria), and verbal skills necessary to understand the concepts involved (Valla et al. 2000). Clinical judgment generally is touted to be the mechanism for differentiating nonspecific experiences or problems from qualitatively specific psychiatric symptoms. Yet the lack of reliability across clinicians challenges this notion. Glossary-based interviews (e.g., CAPA, K-SADS) address this by developing clear definitions and training the interviewers to recognize the distinctions.

The noted low rates of agreement between different informants (e.g., parent–child, parent–teacher) represent another challenge (Achenbach et al. 1987; Rutter 1997). It is generally taught that youth are thought to be better at describing their own internalizing states, whereas adults are better at describing acting-out behaviors in children. Research is needed to clarify when and if this is the case. Poor agreement does not necessarily imply error. Some differences are expected, because children's behavior depends to some extent on the setting and situation (Achenbach et al. 1987).

Psychiatric decision making is dependent on the integration of information from diverse sources and perspectives, including the patient and family interviews, the mental status examination, collateral informants (e.g., teachers), and other treatment providers. These decision-making processes must be quantified in a manner that translates to different settings and situations

There are no universally accepted algorithms dictating how to combine different types of information. For example, are both child and parent reports of symptoms necessary for diagnosis? If not, which informant's information takes precedence? How do the responses of other informants, such as teachers, influence the findings? These are complex processes normally characterized as clinical judgment.

The utility of diagnostic interviews in clinical settings outside of academic centers must be examined. By compelling clinicians to follow standard diagnostic and interviewing methods, structured interviews promote more consistent diagnostic practices and help justify therapeutic interventions and outcomes. These are important issues as the field moves toward evidence-based practices. Computerized instruments and medical records allow the integration of clinical care and information management systems, thus promoting the inclusion of standardized assessments and treatment protocols into routine care.

The validity of a diagnostic interview is no greater than the validity of the diagnoses themselves. Although children and adolescents with psychiatric disorders can be reliably differentiated from control subjects without disorders, the distinction between disorders is less clear (Reeves et al. 1987). The lack of a definitive gold standard for identifying disorders remains a significant impediment. If structured diagnostic interviews are to be the gold standard, how can their validity be examined? Diagnostic criteria were originally created in an attempt to describe recognized disorders, yet unwittingly, they have become the disorders. The same criteria used to define a disorder are used to validate its existence. The challenge is distinguishing between the validity of a disorder and the criteria or measure that defines it. Ultimately, making that distinction will require the identification of external markers for disorders, separate from phenomenological criteria.

References

Achenbach TM, McConaughy SH, Howell CT: Child/adolescent behavioral and emotional problems: implications of cross-informant correlations for situational specificity. Psychol Bull 101:213–232, 1987

Ambrosini PJ: Historical development and present status of the Schedule for Affective Disorders and Schizophrenia for School-Age Children (K-SADS). J Am Acad Child Adolesc Psychiatry 39:49–58, 2000

American Psychiatric Association: Diagnostic and Statistical Manual of Mental Disorders, 3rd Edition. Washington, DC, American Psychiatric Association, 1980

American Psychiatric Association: Diagnostic and Statistical Manual of Mental Disorders, 4th Edition, Text Revision. Washington, DC, American Psychiatric Association, 2000

Angold A, Costello E: The Child and Adolescent Psychiatric Assessment (CAPA). J Am Acad Child Adolesc Psychiatry 39:39–48, 2000

Angold A, Fisher PW: Interviewer-based interviews, in Diagnostic Assessment in Child and Adolescent Psychopathology. Edited by Shaffer D, Lucas CP, Richters JE. New York, Guilford, 1999, pp 34–64

Breslau N: Inquiring about the bizarre: false positives in Diagnostic Interview Schedule for Children (DISC), ascertainment of obsessions, compulsions and psychotic symptoms. J Am Acad Child Adolesc Psychiatry 26:639–655, 1987

Costello AJ: Structured interviewing, in Child and Adolescent Psychiatry, A Comprehensive Textbook, 2nd Edition. Edited by Lewis M. Baltimore, MD, Williams & Wilkins, 1996, pp 457–464

Cronbach L, Meehl P: Construct validity in psychological tests. Psychol Bull 52:281–302, 1955

First MB, Gibbon M, Spitzer RL, et al: User's Guide for the Structured Clinical Interview for DSM-IV Axis I Disorders—Research Version. New York, Biometrics Research Department, New York State Psychiatric Institute, 1996

Frances A: Problems in defining clinical significance in epidemiological studies. Arch Gen Psychiatry 55:116, 1998

Matzner F, Silva R, Silvan M, et al: Preliminary test-retest reliability of the KID-SCID. Scientific proceedings, American Psychiatric Association meeting, 1997. Available at: http://cpmcnet.columbia.edu/dept/scid/kidscid.htm. Accessed April 16, 2003

Reeves JC, Werry JS, Elkind GS, et al: Attention-deficit conduct, oppositional, and anxiety disorders in children, II: clinical characteristics. J Am Acad Child Adolesc Psychiatry 26:144–155, 1987

Regier DA, Kaelber CT, Rae DS, et al: Limitations of diagnostic criteria and assessment instruments for mental disorders: implications for research and policy. Arch Gen Psychiatry 55:109–115, 1998

Reich W: Diagnostic Interview for Children and Adolescents (DICA). J Am Acad Child Adolesc Psychiatry 39:59–66, 2000

Robins LN: Epidemiology: reflections on testing the validity of psychiatric interviews. Arch Gen Psychiatry 42:918–924, 1985

Robins LN, Cottler LB: Making a structured psychiatric diagnostic interview faithful to the nomenclature. Am J Epidemiol 160:808–813, 2004

Rutter M: Child psychiatric disorder: measures, causal mechanisms and interventions. Arch Gen Psychiatry 54:785–789, 1997

Shaffer D, Fisher P, Lucus CP, et al: NIMH Diagnostic Interview Schedule for Children, Version IV (NIMH DISC-IV): description, differences from previous versions and reliability of some common diagnoses. J Am Acad Child Adolesc Psychiatry 39:28–38, 2000

Sherrill JT, Kovacs M: Interview Schedule for Children and Adolescents (ISCA). J Am Acad Child Adolesc Psychiatry 39:67–75, 2000

Valla JP, Bergeron L, Berube H: The Dominic-R, a pictorial interview for 6- to 11-year-old children. J Am Acad Child Adolesc Psychiatry 39:85–93, 2000

Valla JP, Kovess V, Chan Chee C, et al: A French study of the Dominic Interactive. Soc Psychiatry Psychiatr Epidemiol 37:441–448, 2002

Weller EB, Weller RA, Svadjian H: Mood Disorders, in Child and Adolescent Psychiatry, A Comprehensive Textbook, 2nd Edition. Edited by Lewis M. Baltimore, MD, Williams & Wilkins, 1996, pp 650–665

Weller EB, Weller RA, Fristad M, et al: Children's Interview for Psychiatric Syndromes (ChIPS). J Am Acad Child Adolesc Psychiatry 39:76–84, 2000

Zarin DA, Earls F: Diagnostic decision making in psychiatry. Am J Psychiatry 150:197–206, 1993

Self-Assessment Questions

Select the single best response for each question.

6.1 According to Angold and Fisher (1999), clinician diagnoses are potentially fraught with numerous biases. All of the following are examples of such biases *except*

A. Making diagnoses before all relevant information is collected.

B. Collecting information selectively when confirming and/or ruling out a diagnosis.

C. Not systematically collecting and organizing information.

D. Not permitting one's special expertise to influence diagnostic assessment.

E. Assuming correlations in symptoms and illnesses that in reality are spurious or nonexistent.

6.2 *Construct validity* is defined as

A. How well a category as defined appears to describe a recognized illness.

B. Whether a category has meaning in terms of what it is designed to describe.

C. How well a category predicts a pertinent aspect of care.

D. How internally consistent a measure is.

E. How often different interviewers assign the same diagnosis.

6.3 Which of the statements concerning reliability is *false?*

A. Reliability includes how often different interviewers assign the same diagnosis.

B. Diagnostic tools need to be reliable in order to be useful.

C. Reliability ensures validity.

D. Reliability includes how internally consistent the measure is.

E. Reliability encompasses how consistently respondents report the same symptoms or diagnoses over time.

6.4 Which of the following statements concerning assessment of a diagnostic instrument's ability to detect cases is *true?*

A. *Sensitivity* is the percentage of individuals in a sample who have the disorder who are accurately identified by the interview.

B. *Predictive value positive* is the percentage of individuals in the defined sample positively identified by the interview who actually have the disorder.

C. *Specificity* is the percentage of individuals in a sample who do not have the disorder who are accurately identified by the interview as not having the disorder.

D. *Predictive value negative* is the percentage of individuals in the defined sample identified as not having the disorder by the interview who in fact do not have the disorder.

E. All of the above.

6.5   Although a number of structured diagnostic interviews are available for assessment of psychiatric illnesses in youth, these instruments have limitations. Examples of such limitations include all of the following *except*

    A.   Children may underreport new or unusual phenomena.
    B.   Children may lack the requisite attention span.
    C.   Children may lack the abstract awareness to understand the concepts.
    D.   Children may not be aware of the concept being described.
    E.   Children may lack the necessary verbal skills.

Rating Scales

Kathleen Myers, M.D., M.P.H.

Brent Collett, Ph.D.

This chapter discusses the use of rating scales in psychiatric assessment (Myers and Winters 2002a). The term *rating scale* refers to any instrument that permits rapid assessment of a behavior or psychological dimension by yielding a numerical score that is easily interpreted. The emphasis here is on scales that are routinely encountered in clinical practice. The text discusses general issues regarding the functioning and applications of rating scales, and the tables provide information regarding the availability of psychometric data supporting the functioning of these scales. All scales presented here have adequate functioning documented for their intended purposes.

Advantages and Disadvantages of Rating Scales

Rating scales are useful for community screening, monitoring at-risk youths, selecting homogeneous groups for treatment, and evaluating outcome. They provide systematic coverage and quantification of behaviors for comparison of an individ- ual with him- or herself and his or her peers over time, setting, and context.

Perhaps the greatest difficulty with rating scales is the user's unrealistic expectations (Myers and Winters 2002a; Piacentini 1993). Clinicians often inaccurately assume that an elevated score is equivalent to a diagnosis. Many scales used in youth were modified from adult measures and thus may not appropriately tap youths' experience. Finally, many popular scales do not have established technical adequacy, making it difficult to determine the appropriateness of a specific scale for a particular application.

Individual and situational factors can also affect a scale's performance. Youths who seek social acceptance may underreport symptoms ("denial" or "lying"), whereas those who feel overwhelmed may overreport symptoms ("faking"). Adult respondents' own characteristics may affect how they rate a youth, as is often seen in depressed mothers' tendency to overreport their children's behavioral problems. Poor agreement is noted among adults who rate a youth in different settings (e.g., teachers and parents), and only moderate agreement is achieved among adults in the same environment (e.g., mothers and fathers in the home). These disparities reflect both differences in reporters' perceptions and variations in youths' behavior as a function of context. Not surprisingly, there is also great disparity between youths' self-reports and adults' reports. These discrepancies highlight the need to collect information from multiple informants and the importance of viewing scales as a means of communication rather than as "the truth."

Psychometric Properties of Rating Scales

A scale's psychometric properties include estimates of reliability, validity, and the adequacy of normative data (Myers and Winters 2002a). *Reliability* refers to the consistency with which a scale's items measure the same construct, the stability of measurements over time, and the level of agreement across different raters. Lack of reliability is termed *random error*. *Validity* pertains to whether the scale accurately assesses what it was designed to assess. Lack of validity is referred to as *systematic error*. During scale development, normative data are collected to determine the range of scores in a population. Cutoff scores are then derived to determine thresholds for pathology versus typical variation. *Adequacy* of a scale for any given patient depends on how well the normative sample reflects that patient's background, given that normative values, cutoff scores, and even psychometric properties can vary by demographic, cultural, and clinical characteristics.

Broad-Band Rating Scales

Broad-band scales (Table 7–1) assess multiple dimensions of problematic and adaptive behavior (Myers and Collett 2004). Because these scales are not specific to a single diagnosis or construct, they are particularly useful for initial evaluation of a youth's problems and to focus further assessment. Because of the need for broad assessment, these scales tend to be lengthy, which often precludes their use for repeated administrations. Furthermore, they tend to include few items per subscale, sacrificing depth of assessment for breadth. Ideally, clinicians would supplement the information from these scales with diagnosis-specific scales, diagnostic interviews, and behavioral observations.

The Child Behavior Checklist (CBCL; Achenbach and Rescorla 2000, 2001) is the most popular broad-band scale used in research and clinical work and has been the gold standard among behavior rating scales since its development in the 1960s. In addition to the parent report form, the CBCL scales include the Teacher Report Form (TRF), the Youth Self-Report (YSR), and the Child Behavior Checklist 1½–5 (CBCL 1½–5) and Caregiver–Teacher Report Form (C-TRF) for preschoolers. These scales have recently been updated with new normative data and several modifications to item content and subscale structure. The age ranges for the CBCL and TRF have shifted slightly, as has the age range for the downward extension for toddlers and preschoolers. A new innovation for the CBCL 1½–5 is a language scale, intended to provide brief screening of this dimension given the frequent overlap between language delays and behavior problems among young children. Additionally, all of the scales can now be scored in accordance with DSM-IV-TR (American Psychiatric Association 2000) diagnoses.

Rating Scales Assessing Externalizing Behaviors

Rating scales are particularly useful for assessing externalizing behaviors, such as symptoms of attention-deficit/hyperactiv-

Table 7–1.   Psychometric properties of broad-band rating scales

Scale (ages for use)	Type of scale, number of items and subscales	Availability of normative data and reliability data	Availability of validity data
Child Behavior Checklist (CBCL)/ Teacher Report Form (TRF) (6–18 years): copyright held by Achenbach System of Empirically Based Assessment (ASEBA) (Achenbach and Rescorla 2001)	Parent–teacher report: 120 items; 8 problem subscales, 6 DSM-IV-TR subscales, 3 composite scales	Normative data available IC: yes (parent and teacher) TR: yes (parent and teacher) IR: yes (parent–parent; teacher–teacher; parent–teacher)	CONV: yes (parent & teacher with nonclinical) DIVG: NR DISC: yes (parent & teacher for clinical vs. nonclinical)
Child Behavior Checklist 1½–5 (CBCL 1½–5)/Caregiver–Teacher Report Form (C-TRF) (1½–5 years): copyright held by ASEBA (Achenbach and Rescorla 2000)	Parent, teacher, caregiver report: 102 problem items; 8 language items, 310 vocabulary words, 7 problem subscales, 5 DSM-IV-TR subscales, 2 language subscales, 3 composite scales	Normative data available IC: yes (parent and teacher) TR: yes (parent and teacher) IR: yes (parent–parent, teacher–teacher, parent–teacher)	CONV: yes (parent & teacher with various clinical & nonclinical) DIVG: NR DISC: yes (parent & teacher for clinical vs. nonclinical and for language—delayed vs. nondelayed)
Youth Self-Report (YSR) (11–18 years): copyright held by ASEBA (Achenbach and Rescorla 2000)	Self-report: 105 problem items; 8 problem subscales, 6 DSM-IV-TR subscales, 3 composite scales	Normative data available IC: yes TR: yes IR: yes (youth–parent & youth–teacher)	CONV: NR DIVG: NR DISC: yes (clinical vs. nonclinical)

Note.   CONV = convergent validity; DISC = discriminant validity; DIVG = divergent validity; IC = internal consistency reliability; IR = interrater reliability; TR = test–retest reliability; clinical = clinical samples; nonclinical = nonclinical samples; NR = not reported.

ity disorder (ADHD), oppositional defiant disorder (ODD), and conduct disorder (CD) (Collett et al. 2003a, 2003b). Such behaviors are publicly observable, and youths displaying these behaviors are referred because of problems they pose to parents and teachers in multiple situations. Youths tend to underestimate their misbehaviors, so adults are considered the optimal informants on narrow-band scales that focus on one specific externalizing construct, or behavior (Table 7–2). Ratings are generally obtained from multiple adults to describe youths' behaviors across various perspectives and settings. These scales are likely to demonstrate developmental relevance, or suitability, because they were developed for elementary-school children on the basis of their behaviors at home and school. Suitability of these scales for younger and older ages is less clear. Furthermore, research in this area has focused almost exclusively on externalizing behavior in boys, and less is known about the suitability of current assessment and conceptualization approaches for girls.

Several scales to assess ADHD are widely used in both research and clinical practice (Collett et al. 2003a). Among the most popular is the Conners Rating Scale—Revised (CRS-R; Conners 1997), an updated version of the original Conners Rating Scale (CRS). There are several abbreviated versions for parent, teacher, and youth self-report. In addition to multiple subscales assessing ADHD, the CRS-R also assesses common comorbidities. It has good technical adequacy for the assessment of ADHD but is less adequate for comorbid disorders. The full version is most useful for initial evaluation, while abbreviated versions facilitate ongoing monitoring. The CRS-R continues to be considered the primary ADHD rating scale.

Several researchers have developed ADHD scales by presenting symptom criteria from DSM-IV (American Psychiatric Association 1994) in a rating-scale format. Respondents rate the frequency with which a youth demonstrates each symptom. Scores are derived either by totaling the items or by using a symptom-count procedure in which items rated as occurring "often" or "very often" are considered present. Prominent examples include the Swanson, Nolan, and Pelham—IV Questionnaire (SNAP-IV; Swanson 1992) and the ADHD Rating Scale—IV (ADHD RS-IV; DuPaul et al. 1998). Although the SNAP-IV has been used in large-scale studies, data on its technical adequacy are lacking. By contrast, a great deal of psychometric and normative data support the technical adequacy of the ADHD RS-IV. Overall, these scales are especially useful for treatment monitoring because of their brevity, temporal stability, and low cost. The SNAP-IV is offered free online.

In contrast to the plethora of ADHD scales based on DSM-IV-TR, there are few diagnosis-based scales assessing other disruptive disorders, such as ODD and CD. However, several scales assess general externalizing behaviors without direct connection to DSM-IV-TR (Collett et al. 2003b). The Eyberg Child Behavior Inventory (ECBI; Eyberg and Pincus 1999) has a long history of extensive clinical and research use, particularly with young disruptive children. Although not specifically tied to DSM-IV, the ECBI assesses features of inattention, hyperactivity–impulsivity, and oppositionality. There is also a classroom version, the Sutter-Eyberg Student Behavior Inventory—Revised (SESBI-R; Eyberg and Pincus 1999). The psychometric properties of the ECBI and the SESBI-R are strong, and the normative data are adequate for most applications. Although the scales are normed through age 16 years, they are most appropriate for young children and may not adequately assess conduct problems seen in school-age children and adolescents.

Table 7–2. Psychometric properties of scales assessing externalizing behaviors

Scale (ages for use)	Type of scale, number of items	Availability of normative data and reliability data	Availability of validity data
ADHD Rating Scale—IV (ADHD RS-IV) (5–18 years): copyright held by Guilford Press (DuPaul et al. 1998)	Home (parent) & school (teacher) report: 18 items	Normative data available IC: yes (home & school [nonclinical]) TR: yes (home & school [nonclinical]) IR: yes (parent–teacher [nonclinical])	CONV: yes (nonclinical) DIVG: NR DISC: yes (ADHD vs. nonclinical; ADHD vs. clinical control; ADHD-I vs. ADHD-C) SENS and SPEC: yes (home & school versions)
Conners Rating Scale—Revised (CRS-R) (3–17 years): copyright held by Multi-Health Systems, Inc. (Conners 1997)	Parent, teacher, and adolescent reports: 80 items (parent), 59 items (teacher), 87 items (adolescent) Global index ADHD index DSM-IV-TR symptom subscales	Normative data available IC: yes (parent, teacher, adolescent [clinical & nonclinical]) TR: yes (parent, teacher, adolescent [clinical & nonclinical]) IR: yes (parent–teacher, parent–adolescent, teacher–adolescent [all for clinical & nonclinical])	CONV: NR DIVG: NR DISC: yes (ADHD vs. nonclinical) SENS and SPEC: yes (parent, teacher, adolescent versions)
Eyberg Child Behavior Inventory (ECBI) (2–16 years): copyright held by Psychological Assessment Resources (Eyberg and Pincus 1999)	Parent report: 36 items	Normative data available IC: yes (normative) TR: yes (3-week, 12-week, 10-month) IR: yes (mother–father)	CONV: yes DISC: yes (clinical vs. nonclinical; CD vs. nonclinical; LD vs. nonclinical; ADHD vs. ADHD/ ODD vs. ADHD/ODD/CD)
Home Situations Questionnaires (HSQ) (4–11 years): copyright held by Guilford Press (Barkley 1997)	Parent report: 16 items	Normative data available IC: yes (parent [nonclinical]) TR: yes (parent [nonclinical]) IR: yes (mother–father [nonclinical])	CONV: yes (nonclinical) DIVG: NR DISC: yes (ADHD vs. nonclinical)

Table 7–2. Psychometric properties of scales assessing externalizing behaviors *(continued)*

Scale (ages for use)	Type of scale, number of items	Availability of normative data and reliability data	Availability of validity data
School Situations Questionnaires (SSQ) (4–11 years): copyright held by Guilford Press (Barkley 1997)	Teacher report: 12 items	Normative data available IC: yes (teacher for nonclinical) TR: yes (teacher for clinical & nonclinical) IR: NR	CONV: yes (clinical & nonclinical) DIVG: NR DISC: yes (ADHD vs. nonclinical)
Sutter-Eyberg Student Behavior Inventory—Revised (SESBI-R) (2–17 years): copyright held by Psychological Assessment Resources (Eyberg and Pincus 1999)	Teacher report: 38 items	Normative data available IC: yes (normative) TR: yes (6-week; normative & clinical) IR: NR	CONV: yes DISC: yes (CD vs. nonclinical; SED vs. nonreferred) PRED: "supported"
Swanson, Nolan, and Pelham—IV questionnaire (SNAP-IV) (5–11 years): available online at http://www.adhd.net (Swanson 1992)	Parent–teacher report: 90 items, full version; 31 items, ADHD+ODD version	Limited normative data available IC: yes (teacher [clinical & nonclinical]) TR: NR IR: yes (parent–teacher [clinical & nonclinical])	No validity data available

Note. ADHD = attention-deficit/hyperactivity disorder; ADHD-I=ADHD, inattentive type; ADHD-C=ADHD, combined type; CD=conduct disorder; CONV=convergent validity; DISC=discriminant validity; DIVG=divergent validity; HSQ=Home Situations Questionnaire; IC=internal consistency reliability; IR=interrater reliability; LD=learning-disabled; ODD=oppositional defiant disorder; SED=seriously emotionally disturbed; SENS=sensitivity; SPEC=specificity; TR=test-retest reliability; clinical = clinical samples; nonclinical = nonclinical samples; NR=not reported.

The Home Situations Questionnaire (HSQ) and School Situations Questionnaire (SSQ) (Barkley 1997) are unique scales that focus on the environmental context in which deviant behaviors occur rather than the overall frequency of behavior problems. The scales include common household or classroom situations and ask respondents to indicate whether the behavior is problematic in that setting. For situations rated as problematic, respondents then rate their severity. These scales' utility lies in assessing effects of youths' behaviors on daily life, not in assessing any disorder. Thus, they are best used as adjuncts to diagnosis-based or construct-driven scales. The data they yield are used to prioritize targets for intervention, evaluate situational precipitants, and assess times of the day that may relate to interventions. These scales are sensitive to treatment gains achieved through medication and behavioral interventions. However, caution is warranted when interpreting an individual's scores with respect to the normative data, which are outmoded.

Rating Scales Assessing Internalizing Symptoms

Internalizing symptoms are not readily observable by others (Myers and Winters 2002b; Ohan et al. 2002; Winters et al. 2002). They represent youths' subjective distress and are best assessed by youths' self-report. Several aspects intrinsic to internalizing symptoms affect the functioning of these scales. Because youths' feelings of depression, anxiety, hopelessness, or suicidality wax and wane, a scale with good stability is needed to detect treatment effects. Additionally, internalizing symptoms overlap, so that depression rating scales also detect anxiety and suicidality, and vice versa. Thus, a scale with discriminant and divergent validity is especially valuable (Table 7–3).

■ Rating Scales Assessing Mood and Related Symptoms

Discriminating depressed youth is hampered by the high frequency of depressive symptoms in both clinical and community samples and by the laxity in the construct that these scales tap. Most depression rating scales measure distress rather than depression.

The Beck Depression Inventory (BDI; Beck 1993) is the most popular depression rating scale for adolescents, and its downward extension, the Children's Depression Inventory (CDI; Kovacs 1992), is the most popular scale for preadolescents. These scales assess cognitive and affective aspects of depression. A strength of the BDI for screening is its discrimination of depressed teens from those with anxiety and conduct disorders. The CDI has predictive validity. Both scales are sensitive to treatment effects, making them useful for monitoring. However, the CDI's poor sensitivity, specificity, and discriminant validity suggest that it predominantly measures distress.

The Center for Epidemiologic Studies Depression Scale (CES-D; Yonkers and Samson 2000a) similarly measures distress. Its popularity lies in its easy completion and availability in the public domain. The CES-D may be most useful for screening community samples or for monitoring the treatment of individual youth, but not for comparing different groups of youth.

The Reynolds Adolescent Depression Scale (RADS; Reynolds 1987a) and the Reynolds Child Depression Scale (RCDS; Reynolds 1989) offer the advantage of being the only depression rating scales that are based on a clear construct of depression, although this construct is somewhat outmoded. Another advantage is that the two versions used sequentially offer developmentally suitable assessment of youth over time.

Table 7–3.　Psychometric properties of scales assessing internalizing symptoms

Scale (ages for use)	Type of scale, number of items	Availability of normative data and reliability data	Availability of validity data
Beck Depression Inventory (BDI) (adolescents): copyright held by Psychological Corporation (Beck 1993)	Youth self-report: 21 items	No normative data available IC: yes (clinical & nonclinical) TR: yes (various clinical & nonclinical) IR: NR	CONV: yes (clinical & nonclinical) DISC: yes (clinical & nonclinical) DIVG: NR SENS & SPEC: yes (clinical)
Beck Hopelessness Scale (BHS) (adolescents): available at beckinst@gim.net (Beck 2005)	Self-report: 20 items	No normative data available IC: yes (clinical) TR: NR IR: NR	CONV: yes (clinical) DISC: yes (clinical) DIVG: NR
Center for Epidemiologic Studies Depression Scale (CES-D) (adolescents): public domain (Yonkers and Samson 2000a)	Youth self-report & parent report: 20 items	No normative data available IC: yes (clinical) TR: yes (clinical) IR: yes (clinical)	CONV: yes (clinical) CONV: yes (clinical) DISC: yes (clinical) DIVG: NR
Child Posttraumatic Stress Disorder—Reaction Index (CPTS-RI) (8–18 years): available from Robert Pynoos, M.D., at rpynoos@npih.medsch.ucla.edu (Pynoos 2005)	Clinician-administered or self-report: 20 items	No normative data available IC: yes (clinical [traumatized children]) TR: yes (clinical [traumatized teens]) IR: yes (clinical [traumatized teens])	CONV: yes (clinical [traumatized children]) DIVG: NR DISC: NR SENS: yes (clinical [traumatized children])
Children's Depression Inventory (CDI) (7–18 years): copyright held by Multi-Health Systems, Inc. (Kovacs 1992)	Youth self-report, parent report, teacher report: 27 items	Normative data available IC: yes (multiple) TR: yes (clinical & nonclinical) IR: yes (clinical)	CONV: yes (multiple) DIVG: NR DISC: yes (multiple) SENS & SPEC: yes (multiple)

Table 7–3. Psychometric properties of scales assessing internalizing symptoms *(continued)*

Scale (ages for use)	Type of scale, number of items	Availability of normative data and reliability data	Availability of validity data
Children's Depression Rating Scale— Revised (CDRS-R) (6–12 years): copyright held by Western Psychological Services (Poznanski and Mokros 1999)	Clinician-administered to child & parent: 17 items	No normative data available IC: yes (clinical) TR: yes (various clinical) IR: yes (various clinical)	CONC: yes (various clinical) CONV: yes (various clinical) DIVG: NR DISC: NR
Hopelessness Scale for Children (HSC) (children & adolescents): available from Alan Kazdin, Ph.D., at alan.kazdin@yale.edu (Kazdin 2005)	Self-report: 17 items	No normative data available IC: yes (clinical) TR: yes (clinical) IR: NR	CONV: yes (clinical) DISC: yes (clinical) DIVG: NR
Mania Rating Scale (MRS) (developed for adults): public domain (Yonkers and Samson 2000b)	Self-report: 11 items	No normative data available IC: yes (clinical) TR: NR IR: NR	CONC: yes (clinical) CONV: yes (clinical) DISC: yes (clinical) DIVG: yes (clinical) SENS & SPEC: yes (clinical)
Mania Rating Scale—Parent Form (MRS-P) (modification of MRS for children & adolescents): available from Eric Youngstrom, M.D., at eric.youngstrom@case.edu (Youngstrom et al. 2004)	Parent report: 11 items	No normative data available IC: yes (clinical) TR: NR IR: yes (clinical [parent–clinician])	CONC: NR CONV: NR DISC: yes (clinical) DIVG: NR SENS & SPEC: yes (clinical)

Table 7–3. Psychometric properties of scales assessing internalizing symptoms *(continued)*

Scale (ages for use)	Type of scale, number of items	Availability of normative data and reliability data	Availability of validity data
Multidimensional Anxiety Scale for Children (MASC) (children & adolescents): copyright held by Multi-Health Systems, Inc. (March 1997)	Youth self-report & parent report: 39 items	No normative data available IC: yes (clinical) TR: yes (clinical) IR: yes (clinical)	CONV: yes (clinical & nonclinical) DIVG: yes (clinical & nonclinical) DISC: yes (clinical)
Pediatric Anxiety Rating Scale (PARS) (5–15 years): available from Mark Riddle, M.D., at mriddle@jhmi.edu (Riddle 2005)	Clinician-administered to child & parent: 50 checklist items, 7 severity items	No normative data available IC: yes (clinical) TR: yes (clinical) IR: yes (clinical)	CONV: yes (clinical [clinician, parent, and child ratings]) DIVG: yes (clinical [clinician & parent ratings]) DISC: NR
Reynolds Adolescent Depression Scale (RADS) (adolescents) and Reynolds Children's Depression Scale (RCDS) (children): copyright held by Psychological Assessment Resources (Reynolds 1987a)	Youth self-report [RADS]; youth self-report & parent report [RCDS]: 30 items	Normative data available IC: yes (clinical & nonclinical) TR: yes (clinical & nonclinical) IR: NR	CONC: yes (clinical & nonclinical) CONV: yes (clinical & nonclinical) DISC: NR DIVG: NR
Reynold's Suicide Ideation Questionnaire for Adolescents (SIQ) (14–18 years) and Reynold's Suicide Ideation Questionnaire for Children (SIQ-Jr) (11–13 years): copyright held by Psychological Assessment Resources (Reynolds 1987b)	Youth self-report: 30 items	Normative data available IC: yes (school) TR: yes (school [SIQ, not SIQ-Jr] IR: NR	CONC: yes (school) CONV: yes (school & clinical) DIVG: NR DISC: yes (clinical)

Table 7–3. Psychometric properties of scales assessing internalizing symptoms *(continued)*

Scale (ages for use)	Type of scale, number of items	Availability of normative data and reliability data	Availability of validity data
Screen for Child Anxiety Related Emotional Disorders (SCARED) (9–19 years): available from Boris Birmaher, M.D., at birmaherb@msx.upmc.edu (Birmaher 2005)	Youth self-report & parent report: 41 items	No normative data available IC: yes (clinical) TR: yes (clinical) IR: yes (clinical)	CONV: yes (clinical) DIVG: NR DISC: yes (clinical) SENS & SPEC: yes (clinical)
Social Phobia Anxiety Inventory for Children (SPAI-C) (9–14 years): copyright held by Multi-Health Systems, Inc. (Beidel et al. 1988)	Self-report: 26 items	Normative data available IC: yes (clinical & nonclinical) TR: yes (clinical & nonclinical) IR: NR	CONV: yes (clinical & nonclinical) DIVG: yes (clinical & nonclinical) DISC: NR SENS & SPEC: yes (clinical & nonclinical)

Note. CONV = convergent validity; DISC = discriminant validity; DIVG = divergent validity; IC=internal consistency; IR = interrater reliability; SENS = sensitivity; SPEC = specificity; TR=test–retest reliability; clinical = clinical samples; nonclinical = nonclinical samples; NR = not reported.

The Children's Depression Rating Scale—Revised (CDRS-R; Poznanski and Mokros 1999) has a special niche in its clinician-rated format, thought to provide greater accuracy than self- or adult-report formats. The CDRS-R in combination with self-reports offers comprehensive yet efficient assessment that is sensitive to treatment.

The Reynolds Suicide Scales (Reynolds 1987b) include the Suicide Ideation Questionnaire for Adolescents (SIQ) for high school students and the Suicide Ideation Questionnaire for Children (SIQ-Jr) for middle school students. These popular scales measure the intensity and frequency of suicidal ideation. They perform well for screening, group discrimination, monitoring treatment, and following youth into high school.

The Beck Hopelessness Scale (BHS; Beck 2005) and its modification, the Hopelessness Scale for Children (HSC; Kazdin 2003), measure attributes about future expectations that correlate with suicidality. These popular scales function well in discriminating suicidal youth, in screening, in treatment monitoring, in longitudinal assessment, and in predicting suicide attempts.

The Mania Rating Scale (MRS; Yonkers and Samson 2000b), a clinician-administered scale used in youth diagnosed with bipolar disorder, has also been modified into a parent-report format (MRS-P; Youngstrom et al. 2004). Both the original MRS and the MRS-P are in early stages of evaluation with youth. There is some evidence of divergence and discrimination of bipolar disorder from ADHD and depression, as well as sensitivity to treatment. Much more work is needed. Nonetheless, because there are no established scales for early-onset bipolar disorder, this scale will increasingly be used. Prior to use, potential users should carefully examine the relevance of this scale for their application.

■ Rating Scales Assessing Anxiety Symptoms

In comparison with depression rating scales, anxiety rating scales show good construct validity, because they are based on established diagnostic criteria.

The Multidimensional Anxiety Scale for Children (MASC; March 1997; March et al. 1997) and the Screen for Child Anxiety Related Emotional Disorders (SCARED; Birmaher 2003; Birmaher et al. 1997, 1999) have subscales that correspond to various DSM-IV–defined anxiety disorders, such as social phobia (SocPh), separation anxiety disorder (SAD), and generalized anxiety disorder (GAD). These popular scales discriminate anxious youths from those with other disorders, including depression, a real strength. Both are sensitive to treatment. The SCARED offers the advantage of free online availability.

The Pediatric Anxiety Rating Scale (PARS; Research Unit on Pediatric Psychopharmacology Anxiety Study Group 2002; Riddle 2003) already has a niche as a result of the fact that it is clinician-administered. This scale rates frequency and severity of symptoms related to DSM-IV–defined GAD, SAD, and SocPh. It also measures impairment, a unique strength. The PARS was developed for drug trials and shows sensitivity to treatment effects. Its use with self-report scales allows comprehensive yet efficient assessment.

The Social Phobia and Anxiety Inventory for Children (SPAI-C; Beidel et al. 1988, 2000) measures a specific anxiety construct, social anxiety. It nicely discriminates social anxiety from other anxiety disorders. However, its sensitivity to treatment needs clarification. The Child Posttraumatic Stress Disorder—Reaction Index (CPTSD-RI; Pynoos 2003) is the most widely used measure of posttraumatic stress disorder (PTSD) symptoms in youth. It can be used as either a clinician-administered or a self-report scale, and it is sensitive to the effects of therapy. The CPTSD-RI functions well across cultures and types of trauma encompassing abuse, medical procedures, and war.

Rating Scales Assessing Impairment

The term *functional impairment* refers to deficits in role performance across various domains of functioning, including cognitive level, verbal abilities, academic achievement, social interactions, self-care, and use of leisure time. Functional impairment is a characteristic of the individual that indicates that individual's functioning across life's roles. By contrast, *severity of illness* is a characteristic of a disorder that indicates the seriousness or extent of the disorder. Severity does not identify the domains of life affected by illness. Thus, functional impairment defines "caseness." This is best evidenced by the inclusion of impairment (i.e., Axis V) in DSM-IV-TR. Caseness ultimately determines the services a youth receives (Winters et al. 2005).

Unidimensional, or global, scales synthesize functioning over many domains to describe overall impairment with a single score (Table 7–4). This score allows comparison of impairment across patients with different diagnoses and provides ease of measuring change over time. However, global scales do not disentangle functioning from symptomatology and do not consider which domains should be targeted for intervention. The Children's Global Assessment Scale (CGAS; Shaffer et al. 2000) is the most popular global scale. The clinician quickly rates the CGAS based on data obtained during the clinical assessment. The CGAS discriminates clinical from nonclinical groups. Scores below 61 define "caseness" and service utilization. The CGAS is appropriate for screening and for treatment monitoring. However, its sensitivity and specificity

have not been clearly established.

Multidimensional scales contain multiple independent subscales that describe the domains of functioning affected by illness (see Table 7–4). The Vineland Adaptive Behavior Scales, Survey Form (VABS; Sparrow et al. 1984) is the prototypical measure of impairment. The VABS is a semistructured interview with caregivers. There is also a Classroom Edition for teachers. The VABS addresses developmental skills in five domains: Daily Living Skills; Communication; Socialization; Motor Skills (for ages birth to 5 years), and a Maladaptive Behavior Domain (for ages 5 years and older). This instrument has representative normative data as well as norms for special populations (e.g., autistic youth). The VABS is appropriate for most clinical applications but is most commonly partnered with intelligence tests to determine service eligibility for developmentally impaired youths.

The Child and Adolescent Functional Assessment Scale (CAFAS; Hodges 2000) is a clinician-administered interview that covers a youth's functioning as well as caregiver needs. Specific behavioral descriptors are used to plan treatment. The CAFAS discriminates clinical severity and predicts service utilization, juvenile recidivism, legal involvement, and school attendance. An efficient screening tool, the CAFAS has shown sensitivity to treatment effects. A Web site provides updated information on the use of this scale in various state initiatives. The author offers training in the use of this popular scale.

Conclusion

The scales presented here do not substitute for diagnostic assessment and good clinical judgment. They augment diagnostic assessment and individualize assessment for specific applications. They offer the clinician a better understanding of

Table 7–4. Psychometric properties of scales assessing impairment

Scale (ages for use)	Type of scale, number of items	Availability of normative data and reliability data	Availability of validity data
Children's Global Assessment Scale (CGAS) (4–16 years): public domain (Shaffer et al. 2000)	Clinician-rated: 1 item w/100 points	No normative data available IC: NA TR: yes (clinical & nonclinical) IR: yes (clinical)	CONC: yes (clinical) CONV: yes (clinical) DISC: yes (clinical) DIVG: NR PRED: preliminary support (clinical)
Vineland Adaptive Behavior Scales (VABS), Survey Form (0–18 years): copyright held by American Guidance Service (Sparrow et al. 1984)	Clinician-administered to guardian: 297 items	Normative data available IC: yes (clinical & nonclinical) TR: yes (nonclinical) IR: yes (nonclinical)	CONC: yes (clinical & nonclinical) CONV: yes (clinical) DISC: yes (clinical & nonclinical) DIVG: NR PRED: NR
Child and Adolescent Functional Assessment Scale (CAFAS) (5–16 years): copyright held by Functional Assessment Systems (Hodges 2000)	Clinician rating or parent interview: 164 items	No normative data available IC: yes (clinical) TR: yes (clinical) IR: yes (clinical)	CONC: yes (clinical) CONV: yes (clinical) DISC: yes (clinical) DIVG: NR PRED: yes (clinical)

Note.   CONV = convergent validity; DISC = discriminant validity; DIVG = divergent validity; IC = internal consistency reliability; IR = interrater reliability; TR = test–retest reliability; clinical = clinical samples; nonclinical = nonclinical samples; NR = not reported.

youths' difficulties, quantify those difficulties in a manner that can be readily understood, and follow the response of those difficulties to treatment. Rating scales help to establish evidenced-based treatments that better ensure accountability in clinical practice and appropriate treatments for our young patients.

References

Achenbach TM, Rescorla LA: Manual for the ASEBA School-Age Forms & Profiles. Burlington, VT, University of Vermont, Research Center for Children, Youth, and Families, 2000. Available from the Achenbach System of Empirically Based Assessment (ASEBA), 1 South Prospect Street, Room 6436, Burlington, VT 05401-3456; phone: 802-656-8313 or 802-656-2608; Web site: http://www.aseba.org

Achenbach TM, Rescorla LA: Manual for the ASEBA Preschool Forms & Profiles. Burlington, VT, University of Vermont, Research Center for Children, Youth, and Families, 2001. Available from the Achenbach System of Empirically Based Assessment (ASEBA), 1 South Prospect Street, room 6436, Burlington, VT 05401-3456; phone: 802-656-8313 or 802-656-2608; Web site: http://www.aseba.org

American Psychiatric Association: Diagnostic and Statistical Manual of Mental Disorders, 4th Edition. Washington, DC, American Psychiatric Association, 1994

American Psychiatric Association: Diagnostic and Statistical Manual of Mental Disorders, 4th Edition, Text Revision. Washington, DC, American Psychiatric Association, 2000

Barkley RA: Defiant Children: A Clinician's Manual for Assessment and Parent Training, 2nd Edition. New York, Guilford, 1997. Available from the publisher's Web site: http://www.guilford.com

Beck AT: Beck Depression Inventory (BDI) Manual, 2nd Edition. San Antonio, TX, Psychological Corporation, 1993. Available from Psychological Corporation, 19500 Bulverde Road, San Antonio, TX 78259; phone: 800-872-1726; Web site: http://www.psychcorp.com

Beck AT: The Beck Hopelessness Scale (BHS), 2005. Available from the Beck Institute at beckinst@gim.net

Beidel DC, Turner SM, Morris TL: Social Phobia and Anxiety Inventory for Children (SPAI-C). North Tonawanda, NY, Multi-Health Systems, 1988. Available from Multi-Health Systems, Inc., 908 Niagara Falls Boulevard, North Tonawanda, NY 14120-2060; phone: 800-456-3003; Web site: http://www.mhs.com

Beidel DC, Turner SM, Hamlin K, et al: The Social Phobia and Anxiety Inventory for Children (SPAI-C): external and discriminative validity. Behav Ther 31:75–87, 2000

Birmaher B: Screen for Child Anxiety Related Emotional Disorders (SCARED), 2005. Available from the Division of Child Psychiatry, Western Psychiatric Institute and Clinic, 3811 O'Hara Street, Pittsburgh, PA 15213; e-mail: birmaherb@msx.upmc.edu

Birmaher B, Khetarpal S, Brent D, et al.: The Screen for Child Anxiety Related Emotional Disorders (SCARED): scale construction and psychometric characteristics. J Am Acad Child Adolesc Psychiatry 36:545–553, 1997

Birmaher B, Brent DA, Chiappetta L, et al: Psychometric properties of the Screen for Child Anxiety Related Emotional Disorders (SCARED): a replication study. J Am Acad Child Adolesc Psychiatry 38:1230–1236, 1999

Collett BR, Ohan JL, Myers KM: Ten-year review of rating scales, V: scales assessing attention-deficit/hyperactivity disorder. J Am Acad Child Adolesc Psychiatry 42:1015–1037, 2003a

Collett BR, Ohan JL, Myers KM: Ten-year review of rating scales, VI: scales assessing disruptive behavior disorders and externalizing behaviors. J Am Acad Child Adolesc Psychiatry 42:1143–1170, 2003b

Conners CK: Conners Rating Scale—Revised, Technical Manual. North Tonawanda, NY, Multi-Health Systems, 1997. Available from Multi-Health Systems, Inc., 908 Niagara Falls Boulevard, North Tonawanda, NY 14120-2060; phone: 800-456-3003; Web site: http://www.mhs.com

DuPaul GJ, Power TJ, Anastopoulos AD, et al: ADHD Rating Scale-IV: Checklist, Norms, and Clinical Interpretation. New York, Guilford, 1998. Available from the publisher's Web site: http://www.guilford.com

Eyberg SM, Pincus D: Eyberg Child Behavior Inventory and Sutter-Eyberg Student Behavior Inventory—Revised, Professional Manual. Odessa, FL, Psychological Assessment Resources, Inc., 1999. Available from Psychological Assessment Resources, Inc., 16204 N. Florida Avenue, Lutz, FL 33549; phone: 813-968-3003; Web site: http://www.parinc.com

Hodges K: Child and Adolescent Functional Assessment Scale, 2nd Revision. Ypsilanti, MI, Eastern Michigan University, Department of Psychology, 2000. Available from Kay Hodges, Ph.D., Functional Assessment Systems, LLC, 2140 Earhart Road, Ann Arbor, MI 48105; phone: 734-769-9725; fax: 734-769-1434; e-mail: hodges@provide.net; Web site: http://www.cafas.com

Kazdin AE: The Hopelessness Scale for Children (HSC), 2003. Available from Alan E. Kazdin, Ph.D., Yale University; e-mail: alan.kazdin@yale.edu

Kovacs M: Children's Depression Inventory Manual. North Tonawanda, NY, Multi-Health Systems, 1992. Available from Multi-Health Systems, Inc., 908 Niagara Falls Boulevard, North Tonawanda, NY 14120-2060; phone: 800-456-3003; Web site: http://www.mhs.com

March JS: Manual for the Multidimensional Anxiety Scale for Children (MASC). North Tonawanda, NY, Multi-Health Systems, 1997. Available from Multi-Health Systems, Inc., 908 Niagara Falls Boulevard, North Tonawanda, NY 14120-2060; phone: 800-456-3003; Web site: http://www.mhs.com

March JS, Parker JD, Sullivan K, et al: The Multidimensional Anxiety Scale for Children (MASC): factor structure, reliability, and validity. J Am Acad Child Adolesc Psychiatry 36:554–565, 1997

Myers KM, Collett BR: Rating scales in child and adolescent psychiatry, in The American Psychiatric Publishing Textbook of Child and Adolescent Psychiatry, 3rd Edition. Edited by Wiener JM, Dulcan MK. Arlington, VA, American Psychiatric Publishing, 2004, pp 149–163

Myers K, Winters NC: Ten-year review of rating scales, I: overview of scale functioning, psychometric properties, and selection. J Am Acad Child Adolesc Psychiatry 41:114–122, 2002a

Myers K, Winters NC: Ten-year review of rating scales, II: scales for internalizing disorders. J Am Acad Child Adolesc Psychiatry 41:634–659, 2002b

Ohan JL, Myers K, Collett BR: Ten-year review of rating scales, IV: scales assessing trauma and its effects. J Am Acad Child Adolesc Psychiatry 41:1401–1422, 2002

Piacentini J: Checklists and ratings scales, in Handbook of Child and Adolescent Assessment, Vol 167. Edited by Ollendick TH. Boston, MA, Allyn & Bacon, 1993, pp 82–97

Poznanski EO, Mokros HB: Children's Depression Rating Scale—Revised (CDRS-R). Los Angeles, CA, Western Psychological Services, 1999. Available from Western Psychological Services, 12031 Wilshire Boulevard 90025-1251; phone: 800-648-8857; Web site: http://www.wpspublish.com

Pynoos RS: The Child Posttraumatic Stress Disorder—Reaction Index (CPTSD-RI), 2005. Available from Robert Pynoos, M.D., Trauma Psychiatry Service, University of California, Los Angeles, 300 UCLA Medical Plaza, Los Angeles, CA 90024-6968; e-mail: rpynoos@npih.medsch.ucla.edu

Research Unit on Pediatric Psychopharmacology Anxiety Study Group: The Pediatric Anxiety Scale (PARS): development and psychometric properties. J Am Acad Child Adolesc Psychiatry 41:1061–1069, 2002

Reynolds WM: Reynolds Adolescent Depression Scale (RADS) and Reynolds Children's Depression Scale (RCDS). Odessa, FL, Psychological Assessment Resources, Inc., 1987a. Available from Psychological Assessment Resources, Inc., 16204 N. Florida Avenue, Lutz, FL 33549; phone: 813-968-3003; Web site: http://www.parinc.com

Reynolds WM: Suicide Ideation Questionnaire (SIQ): Professional Manual. Odessa, FL, Psychological Assessment Resources, Inc., 1987b. Available from Psychological Assessment Resources, Inc., 16204 N. Florida Avenue, Lutz, FL 33549; phone: 813-968-3003; Web site: http://www.parinc.com

Riddle M: The Pediatric Anxiety Rating Scale (PARS), 2005. Available from Mark A. Riddle, M.D., Division of Child and Adolescent Psychiatry, Johns Hopkins Medical Institutions, Children's Center, Suite 346, 600 North Wolfe Street, Baltimore, MD 21287-3325; e-mail: mriddle@jhmi.edu

Shaffer D, Gould MS, Bird H, et al: Children's Global Assessment Scale (CGAS), in Handbook of Psychiatric Measures. Edited by American Psychiatric Association Task Force for the Handbook of Psychiatric Measures. Washington, DC, American Psychiatric Association, 2000, pp 363–365

Sparrow SS, Balla DA, Cicchetti DV: Interview Edition Survey Form Manual: Vineland Adaptive Behavior Scales (VABS). Circle Pines, MN, American Guidance Service, 1984. Available from AGS Publishing, 4201 Woodland Road, Circle Pines, MN 55014-1796; phone: 800-328-2560; fax: 800-471-8457; e-mail: customerservice@agsnet.com; Web site: http://www.agsnet.com

Swanson J: School-Based Assessments and Interventions for ADD Students. Irvine, CA, KC Publishing, 1992

Swanson J, Schuck S, Mann M, et al: Categorical and dimensional definitions and evaluations of symptoms of ADHD: the SNAP and SWAN rating scales, 2001. Available at: http://www.adhd.net

Winters NC, Myers K, Proud L: Ten-year review of rating scales, III: scales for suicidality, cognitive style, and self-esteem. J Am Acad Child Adolesc Psychiatry 41:1050–1181, 2002

Winters NC, Collett BR, Myers KM: Ten-year review of rating scales, VII: scales assessing functional impairment. J Am Acad Child Adolesc Psychiatry 44:309–338, 2005

Yonkers KA, Samson J: Center for Epidemiologic Studies Depression Scale (CES-D), in Handbook of Psychiatric Measures. Edited by American Psychiatric Association Task Force for the Handbook of Psychiatric Measures. Washington, DC, American Psychiatric Association, 2000a, pp 523–526

Yonkers KA, Samson J: Young Mania Rating Scale (YMRS), in Handbook of Psychiatric Measures. Edited by American Psychiatric Association Task Force for the Handbook of Psychiatric Measures. Washington, DC, American Psychiatric Association, 2000b, pp 540–542

Youngstrom EA, Findling RL, Calabrese JR, et al.: Comparing the diagnostic accuracy of six potential screening instruments for bipolar disorder in youth aged 5 to 17 years. J Am Acad Child Adolesc Psychiatry 43:847–858, 2004. Available from Eric A. Youngstrom, Ph.D., Case Western Reserve University; e-mail: eric.youngstrom@case.edu

Self-Assessment Questions

Select the single best response for each question.

7.1   The *reliability* of a rating instrument

     A. Is equivalent to random error.

     B. Refers to the consistency with which an instrument measures a construct in the same way every time.

     C. Pertains to whether the instrument accurately assesses what it was designed to measure.

     D. Is inversely proportional to the validity of the instrument.

     E. Is reduced when the measured construct changes over time.

7.2   Which of the following is the best example of a broad-band rating scale?

     A. Conners Rating Scale—Revised.

     B. Children's Depression Inventory.

     C. Hopelessness Scale for Children.

     D. Child Behavior Checklist.

     E. ADHD Rating Scale—IV.

7.3   All of the following statements pertaining to broad-band rating scales are correct *except*

     A. They include measurements of both internalizing and externalizing behaviors.

     B. They assess a variety of clinical problems.

     C. They may be lengthy and cumbersome to complete.

     D. They assess for both breadth and depth of pathology in all clinical domains.

     E. They are best used to identify problems that will require further evaluation.

7.4   The Conners Rating Scale—Revised

     A. Includes parent, teacher, and youth self-report versions.

     B. Mostly assesses internalizing behaviors.

     C. Includes some abbreviated versions, but only for youth self-report.

     D. Has no mechanism for assessing common comorbid conditions.

     E. Is most useful for initial assessment in its abbreviated version.

7.5   Which of the following scales measuring internalizing symptoms is clinician-administered rather than self-reported?

     A. Beck Depression Inventory.

     B. Children's Depression Inventory.

     C. Children's Depression Rating Scale.

     D. Beck Hopelessness Scale.

     E. Hopelessness Scale for Children.

Laboratory and Diagnostic Testing

Robert L. Hendren, D.O.

XiaoYan He, M.D.

Systematic assessment and objective measurement are essential in psychiatric evaluation. A thorough review of the history and a clinical interview are cornerstones in the evaluation and management of behavioral and emotional disturbances in children. In addition, careful medical evaluation and laboratory testing are important for three reasons: 1) to identify an unrecognized medical condition that may be causing the psychiatric symptoms, 2) to determine baseline values of physiological parameters that may be affected by psychotropic medications, and 3) to identify any medical condition that may be complicated by medication treatment. With a rapidly growing number of tests and technical instruments available to physicians treating psychiatric disorders in both the hospital setting and outpatient practice, learning about and effectively using laboratory and diagnostic tests is challenging yet crucial. Decisions about testing must be made for individual circumstances because clear guidelines are rarely available. This chapter focuses on the utility of the more commonly considered laboratory tests and neuroimaging studies in both initial assessment and clinical management.

Laboratory Testing in Initial Assessment

■ Baseline Laboratory Tests

The potential value of a laboratory test depends on its sensitivity in detecting a specific disorder and the prevalence of the disorder in the relevant population. In the child or adolescent with negative medical history and physical examination findings for whom the expected risk for a specific medical disorder is low, the likelihood that a laboratory test will identify a true positive finding is minimal. However, when there is a positive medical history or physical findings suggesting a medical illness, specific laboratory tests should be used as clinically necessary. Some experts recommend the following laboratory tests as part of a comprehensive examination and/or premedication workup: 1) complete blood count (CBC), differential, and hematocrit; 2) urinalysis; 3) blood urea nitrogen (BUN) level; 4) serum electrolytes for sodium, potassium, chloride, calcium, phosphate, and carbon dioxide content; 5) liver function tests for aspartate aminotransferase (AST), alanine aminotransferase (ALT), alkaline phosphatase, and bilirubin; and 6) lead level in children younger than age 7 years when risk factors are present and in older children when indicated (Green 2001). However, the utility of routine laboratory tests is not clear. Sheline and Kehr (1990) studied 252 psychiatric inpatients to evaluate how often screening test findings revealed important clinical information. Although 49% of the patients had a coexisting medical illness, in only 6% did laboratory test findings lead to changes in clinical management. Anfinson and Kathol (1992) noted that whereas screening tests frequently generate abnormal results, in only 0.8%–4.0% are findings clinically significant. In their review, no specific laboratory tests were recommended on a routine basis.

Given this background, certain laboratory tests can provide valuable information to confirm or validate diagnoses. Careful consideration should be given to obtaining the following tests for individuals at increased risk for particular medical problems.

Hematological Measures

It is suggested that a CBC should always be a part of a routine screen (Green 2001). The CBC is sensitive to a wide range of medical problems that can cause, compli-cate, or mimic psychiatric conditions. Selective screening should be considered for individuals at increased risk for anemia, such as cow's milk–fed infants, toddlers, adolescent girls, pregnant teens, and recent immigrants from developing countries. Iron deficiency and iron deficiency anemia are still relatively common in toddlers, adolescent girls, and women of childbearing age (Ania et al. 1994). Anemia can be associated with a wide range of mental status changes, including asthenia, depression, and psychosis. Obtaining follow-up hematocrit and hemoglobin values is recommended if the screening red blood cell (RBC) count is abnormal. The white blood cell (WBC) count should be considered in the baseline screening before initiating certain psychotropic medications, such as clozapine, lithium, and carbamazepine, as well as in treatment monitoring. A WBC differential is recommended if clinical manifestations of infectious diseases or leukemia are present. Additional discussion of hematological measures can be found in Rosse et al. (1989) and Speicher (1998).

Biochemical Measures

Serum electrolytes.   Neuropsychiatric complications may be the cause or result of serum electrolyte abnormalities. For instance, hyponatremia may be the result of the syndrome of inappropriate secretion of antidiuretic hormone (SIADH), psychogenic polydipsia, or carbamazepine use. Clinicians should consider the resulting hyponatremia as a possible cause of anorexia, depression, irritability, lethargy, or confusion. Another example is hypokalemia, which can be associated with significant weakness and electrocardiographic changes. When an adolescent girl presents with binge-purge behavior, self-induced vomiting, or laxative abuse, testing potassium level and treating hypokalemia can be lifesaving.

Renal Function Tests

Abnormal BUN levels may be associated with various mental status changes. For patients who are taking lithium, tests for BUN levels, creatinine clearance, and 24-hour urine protein levels are frequently used in pretreatment and follow-up evaluation. Urinalysis is important in the evaluation of certain organic mental disorders secondary to disorders such as diabetes, SIADH, and hepatobiliary disease.

Liver Function Tests

Abnormal liver enzyme values may be associated with certain psychiatric conditions. In patients with bulimia, testing for serum amylase levels has been proposed as a method to help monitor binge-purge activities. Baseline serum amylase levels for patients who engage in severe bingeing are reportedly higher than for control subjects without eating disorders or those with nonbulimic anorexia (Green 2001).

Baseline liver function should be assessed prior to initiating anticonvulsant treatment, especially valproate and carbamazepine therapy. Liver function should be monitored more often during the first several weeks of therapy and every 6–12 months afterward (Janicak et al. 2001). Although routine monitoring is not recommended for atomoxetine, very rare reports of altered liver function in patients receiving this agent suggest that monitoring of liver function should be considered in patients with the potential for compromised liver function.

Neuroendocrine Tests

The association of the "metabolic syndrome" with atypical antipsychotics has led the U.S. Food and Drug Administration (FDA) to order the manufacturers of all six second-generation antipsychotics to include warning language about hyperglycemia and diabetes mellitus. The FDA recommends monitoring of blood glucose and lipids in patients taking atypical antipsychotics (see section titled "Selective Serotonin Reuptake Inhibitors, Monoamine Oxidase Inhibitors, Neuroleptics, and Stimulants," later in this chapter).

Thyroid hormone is responsible for normal growth and development. Abnormalities in the concentration of thyroid hormones can result in psychiatric symptoms, including anxiety, depression, panic, restlessness, mental retardation, and psychosis. Laboratory tests to detect thyroid dysfunction include serum thyroxine (T_4), triiodothyronine (T_3), resin uptake, thyroid-stimulating hormone (TSH), and serum T_3 levels. Significant differences in basal thyroid hormone and T_4 elevations are reported in adolescents with depression and those with mania compared with control subjects (Sokolov et al. 1994). However, most studies report normal thyroid function (TSH) in depression in both adolescents (Khan 1987; Kutcher et al. 1991) and prepubertal children (Garcia et al. 1991).

Kutcher (1997) suggested that there is no evidence to support the use of basal neuroendocrine laboratory testing for either screening or diagnostic purposes in child and adolescent psychiatric patients. He further suggested that special stimulation tests, such as the dexamethasone suppression test (DST), the thyrotropin-releasing hormone (TRH) test, and the corticotropin-releasing hormone (CRH) test, have not demonstrated diagnostic validity for any child and adolescent psychiatric disorder. However, if family and clinical history or physical examination findings indicate a possible thyroid disorder, a screening test for T_4 and T_3 resin uptake are recommended (Leo et al. 1997).

Abnormal thyroid function can result in behavior that may resemble attention-deficit/hyperactivity disorder (ADHD) (Weiss and Stein 1999). Three thyroid disorders have been reported to be associated with ADHD-like symptoms: hyperthyroidism, hypothyroidism, and the syndrome of resistance to thyroid hormone (Pear et al. 2001). Several studies have concluded that routine TSH screening in children with nonfamilial ADHD is not indicated (Elia et al. 1994; Toren et al. 1997; Valentine et al. 1997). However, it is indicated for children with a family history of thyroid disorder or physical signs of goiter, low birth weight, growth retardation, and speech and hearing impairment (Zametkin et al. 1998).

Other neuroendocrine tests, including those for plasma cortisol and catecholamines, amylase and lipase, antidiuretic hormone (ADH), growth hormone, prolactin, and testosterone and estrogen, are used for evaluation of a variety of endocrine disorders that may manifest as psychiatric symptoms.

Baseline Drug Screening

Serum toxicology and urine toxicology are commonly used to determine whether a patient is using one or more psychoactive substances. Drug screening is limited by the time needed to obtain results and the risk of false-positive and false-negative results. Positive results may not prove substance abuse or dependence but do indicate substance use. Negative results are not sufficient to rule out substance use. A positive result on an immunoassay screen test should be followed by confirmation by a more sensitive method (Bukstein 1997). A drug screen should be requested for adolescents who present with new-onset psychosis, behavioral changes, or severe anxiety, and when substance abuse is suspected.

Baseline Electrocardiogram

Various medical conditions and psychotropic medications predispose patients to cardiac risks. Baseline electrocardiography

(ECG) should be considered when elements of risk are present. For instance, a pretreatment electrocardiogram should be obtained for patients with known cardiac disease or at high cardiac risk (e.g., family history of sudden death or cardiac arrhythmia, hypertension, or cardiac diseases) when psychotropic medication with cardiac effects is being considered. Some antipsychotics, especially thioridazine, are known to cause QTc interval prolongation. Ziprasidone is a newer atypical antipsychotic medication that prolongs the QT interval more than do haloperidol, olanzapine, quetiapine, and risperidone but less than do mesoridazine and thioridazine (FDA 2000). Data on the effect of ziprasidone on ECG indicate an approximately 20-ms increase in the QT interval but no cases of mortality from overdose, torsade de pointes, or excess in sudden death and unexpected deaths (Goodnick 2001). However, it is important to ask apparently healthy patients if they have had syncope, a family history of sudden death, or long QT syndrome. If any of these are present, a pretreatment electrocardiogram should be obtained (Glassman and Bigger 2001). Tricyclic antidepressants (TCAs) can cause cardiac arrhythmia, so ECG should be considered to monitor possible adverse effects on cardiac function with these medications.

Cardiac monitoring with α-adrenergic agents such as clonidine is controversial. The American Heart Association guidelines (Gutgesell et al. 1999) do not recommend baseline or monitoring ECG.

■ Special Populations

Suicide Attempters

Clinicians should order blood toxicology workups for patients who have overdosed on prescribed or abused drugs. The severity of specific organ involvement can be assessed by the appropriate tests. An electrocardiogram should be obtained for patients who have overdosed with a TCA. Liver function tests are important for assessing patients who have overdosed with acetaminophen, and serum electrolyte values are needed to assess anion gap in cases of aspirin overdose. Radiological assessment may help evaluate damage caused by a self-inflicted injury.

Children With Unexplained Weight Loss

Children and adolescents with a history of starvation, bingeing, and/or purging who are being evaluated for symptoms of weight loss, depression, or anxiety need a medical and laboratory assessment to determine the degree of weight loss and to identify a potential medical emergency, especially for those with a history of anorexia nervosa and/or bulimia nervosa.

Hypercarotenemia is a common finding in patients with anorexia nervosa, especially in those in the restrictor subtype. Measuring serum beta-carotene value in patients with restricting or purging anorexia provides supporting evidence for the diagnosis, especially in atypical presentations (Boland et al. 2001). However, the significance of elevated beta-carotene levels for prognosis and treatment of anorexia nervosa is unproven. Recent research implicates an association of disturbed neuropeptide Y release and pathological behavior in patients with bulimia nervosa. Significantly higher levels of plasma leptin and neuropeptide Y in patients with bulimia and significantly lower levels in patients with anorexia than in control subjects have also been reported (Baranowska et al. 2001). Nevertheless, measurement of neuropeptide Y in children and adolescents with eating disorders is not recommended for diagnosis or treatment. Increased serum cholesterol and decreased free T_4 levels are found in patients with bulimia nervosa; however, the mechanism and consequences of the abnormality are uncertain (Pauporte and Walsh 2001).

Patients with anorexia nervosa often have functional cardiac abnormalities secondary to their nutritional depletion, including decreased left ventricular mass and varying degrees of left ventricular systolic dysfunction. A study measuring myocardial performance index (MPI) for global ventricular function in patients with anorexia nervosa (Eidem et al. 2001) found a significantly elevated left ventricular MPI, which indicated a subclinical degree of ventricular impairment. The study suggested the potential clinical utility of MPI in the early identification of subclinical left-ventricular dysfunction in patients with anorexia nervosa.

Serum and urine electrolyte tests should be used routinely in assessment of children and adolescents with weight loss. Laboratory screening for serum hypokalemia and hypochloremia should be considered for individuals with bulimia nervosa (Wolfe et al. 2001). The ratio of urine sodium to chloride has been reported to predict bulimic behavior (Crow et al. 2001) better than do traditional screening tests such as that for serum hypokalemia.

For patients with eating disorders, a CBC with differential count should be obtained to monitor anemia and leukopenia, as should findings for serum electrolyte (especially potassium and BUN) and amylase levels and urinalysis (Rosse et al. 1989). Additional tests, including ECG and TSH and those for other pituitary hormones, may be useful to assess effects of starvation, laxative abuse, dehydration, and abnormal electrolyte levels.

An enlarged parotid gland associated with an elevated amylase level is commonly observed in patients who binge and vomit. The serum amylase level is an excellent way to monitor vomiting in patients with bulimia who deny purging (Halmi 1999).

Profound osteopenia is a serious complication of anorexia nervosa. Patients with anorexia nervosa are at high risk for fracture (Espallargues et al. 2001) and osteoporosis (Zipfel et al. 2001). The clinician who treats adolescents with eating disorders should educate them regarding the danger of bone fragility and the risk of fracture and should consider X-ray examination to determine the reduction of bone density and size if the patient's history and condition indicate.

Children With Neurodevelopmental Disorders

The benefits of genetic diagnosis in children with neurodevelopmental disorders include 1) recognition of recurrent risk, which is useful in genetic counseling; 2) prediction of prognosis; 3) elimination of unnecessary laboratory tests; 4) establishment of guidelines for disorder management; and 5) family support (i.e., cooperation with family's request to identify etiological factors) (Carey and McMahon 1999).

In fragile X syndrome, a fragile site on the X chromosome is usually detected by cytogenetic testing in individuals with mental retardation but not in individuals with only emotional or learning problems. With the discovery of the *FMR1* gene, DNA testing can identify not only individuals affected by fragile X syndrome but also all carriers of the syndrome. Routine screening for fragile X syndrome has been suggested for schoolchildren with learning disabilities (Slaney et al. 1995), and a saliva DNA test as an alternative to the blood DNA test for such a screening program has been evaluated (Hagerman et al. 1994). The use of subtelomeric fluorescence in situ hybridization (FISH) analysis with specific DNA probes for chromosome 15q duplications or deletions in children with autism, for chromosome 22q13 deletions (Havens et al. 2004) in children with developmental delay, and for specific alterations known to be associated with other disorders may yield useful informa-

tion regarding etiology (Hansen and Hagerman 2003).

Examination of karyotype (morphology and number of chromosomes) is important in the evaluation of possible sex chromosomal abnormality. Girls with an abnormal number of X chromosomes have psychosocial, educational, and behavioral problems. In Turner syndrome (45, XO), deficits in nonverbal abilities, visuospatial processing, visual memory, and visual construction are clear and consistent findings. These individuals have lower self-esteem, poor peer relationships and social skills, and short attention span. Boys with Klinefelter syndrome (47, XXY) have cognitive deficits in verbal ability and language processing.

Prader-Willi syndrome is caused by absence of the normally active paternal inherited gene at chromosome 15 (q11–q13 region) or by deletion. Prader-Willi syndrome can be diagnosed most efficiently by a molecular diagnostic test using southern hybridization and methylation-sensitive probes, fluorescent in situ hybridization, and polymerase chain reaction technique (Dykins and Cassidy 1999). Establishing the diagnosis of Williams syndrome is another example of the clinical benefit of molecular genetics in child and adolescent psychiatry (Morris and Mervis 1999).

Wilson's disease is an autosomal-recessive inherited disorder of abnormal copper metabolism, which results in decreased intellectual functioning, inappropriate behavior, anxiety, depression, psychosis, and movement disorder. However, it is not diagnosed by genetic tests. Serum ceruloplasmin, serum, and urine copper tests are usually used to evaluate patients for Wilson's disease. It is critical for clinicians to consider Wilson's disease in the differential diagnosis of psychotic young adults with a movement disorder, because the disease is treatable.

Neuroimaging and Electroencephalographic Evaluation

Neuroimaging technology, including structural magnetic resonance imaging (MRI), magnetic resonance spectroscopy (MRS), functional MRI, positron emission tomography (PET), and single-photon emission computed tomography (SPECT), holds great promise for neurodevelopmental diagnosis and treatment. Recent research studies demonstrate improved specificity of neuroimaging findings for ADHD (Schulz et al. 2004), bipolar disorder (Blumberg et al. 2004), autism (Brambilla et al. 2004), first-episode psychosis (Wood et al. 2003), and other developmental disorders (Greicius 2003). However, the conclusion that neuroimaging evaluations are not yet valid diagnostic tests in child and adolescent psychiatry (Hendren et al. 2000) continues to hold. Although each of these modalities has particular advantages in biomedical research, magnetic resonance technology is the most suited to assessment and research in child and adolescent psychiatry (Pine 2001). In clinical practice, use of MRI should be seriously considered in all cases involving rapid onset of severe psychopathology, significant abnormal findings on neurological examination, seizures, or the presence of certain genetic syndromes (Hoon and Melhem 2000).

Structural MRI creates images of brain structures that can be measured to determine volumes in a region of interest (Frank and Pavlakis 2001). MRS is a measure of metabolism and reflects changes that occur over weeks and months (Stoll et al. 2000). Functional MRI measures oxygen consumption in brain regions of interest and reflects changes that occur over minutes or hours on the basis of a task-response paradigm (O'Tuama et al. 1999).

PET has limited use in children because of the expense and risk associated with the isotopes necessary for the procedure and the paucity of children without a disorder who have been studied as normal control subjects (O'Tuama et al. 1999). SPECT uses less radioactive isotope and is therefore less expensive and has less perceived risk in children, but it does not have the spatial resolution of PET. Although some authors promote the use of SPECT in diagnosis and treatment matching (Amen 2001), there are no analyses in the scientific peer-reviewed literature of the validity of SPECT for this purpose.

Electroencephalography (EEG) is indicated when a seizure disorder is a possibility and may identify relationships to decreased cognitive function (Ballaban-Gil and Tuchman 2000). Minor, nonspecific abnormalities occur in up to 30% of children and do not require treatment.

Laboratory Tests in Treatment Management

One of the goals of initial laboratory testing is to obtain baseline information for patients who are likely to receive psychotropic medications. Following are guidelines for monitoring several commonly used psychotropic medications.

■ Tricyclic Antidepressants

TCAs are commonly associated with adverse effects on blood pressure and heart rate (Walsh et al. 1999). Pretreatment baseline measurement and regular monitoring of blood pressure, pulse, and ECG are therefore essential. Biederman et al. (1995) reported desipramine-associated sudden death in children between ages 4 and 14 years, which has led to a careful examination of the potential cardiac effects of tricyclics in children. Several subsequent reports of sudden death associated with imipramine and desipramine (Varley and McClellan 1997) have further increased interest in investigation of TCAs' cardiac effects in children and adolescents.

Johnson et al. (1996) found no consistent pattern of electrocardiographic interval changes related to dosage, age, treatment duration, or plasma levels of desipramine and imipramine in children. Although some argue that ECG should not be routinely used until the dose is above 2.5–3.5 mg/kg, it is recommended currently that routine ECG be done before initiating TCA treatment and that follow-up ECG be done when clinically indicated (Zametkin et al. 1998).

The American Psychiatric Association Task Force on the Use of Laboratory Tests in Psychiatry (1985) concluded that blood-level measurements of TCAs are unequivocally useful. TCA blood levels might be ordered for the following: 1) patients who have questionable compliance, 2) patients who have a poor response to a "typical" dose, 3) patients who experience side effects at a very low dose, 4) patients who are potentially very sensitive to side effects, and 5) patients for whom treatment is urgent and who require a potentially therapeutic medication level in as short a time as possible. Therapeutic blood levels of TCA are described by the Task Force as follows: Total imipramine and its metabolite, desmethylimipramine, should exceed 150 ng/mL; for nortriptyline, a therapeutic range is between 50 and 150 ng/mL; for desipramine, the therapeutic level should be above 125 ng/mL. TCA blood levels are generally obtained 9–12 hours after the last dose, and blood for determining medication levels should be drawn when TCA dosage is at a steady state (at least 5 days after initiation of or change in medication dosage).

■ Selective Serotonin Reuptake Inhibitors, Monoamine Oxidase Inhibitors, Neuroleptics, and Stimulants

Currently, no baseline laboratory tests are indicated before the initiation of selective serotonin reuptake inhibitors or monoamine oxidase inhibitors if findings from the review of systems are negative for medical disorders. A urine pregnancy test should be ordered for sexually active female adolescents. For patients who are about to begin treatment with a neuroleptic, especially pimozide or clozapine, a CBC, liver function test, and electrocardiogram are necessary for monitoring potential adverse effects. The American Diabetes Association recommends measurement of fasting blood sugar at baseline, at 12 weeks, and then at least annually when treatment is initiated in adults without diabetes and when dosages are increased in adults with diabetes (American Diabetes Association et al. 2004). They also recommend monitoring of lipids and triglycerides at baseline, 12 weeks, and annually along with regular weight monitoring. Although the FDA does not recommend routine monitoring of prolactin levels with risperidone treatment, hyperprolactinemia-associated symptoms have led some researchers to advocate regular monitoring (Toren et al. 2004). No laboratory tests are indicated for methylphenidate or amphetamine. Questions have been raised regarding an association of Adderall XR with sudden death, but causality and need for cardiac monitoring have not been established. However, with evidence linking pemoline to liver failure (Marotta and Roberts 1998; Safer et al. 2001), a baseline liver function test should be obtained, and liver function should be closely monitored, in patients receiving treatment with that agent; parents and patients should be educated about the risks and the signs and symptoms of liver toxicity (Adcock et al. 1998).

Lithium

Lithium can have significant adverse effects on the thyroid, kidney, heart, and developing fetus and may cause a benign elevation of the CBC. It is recommended that pretreatment evaluation include a CBC, serum electrolytes test, BUN test, serum creatinine test, thyroid function tests, urinalysis, and an electrocardiogram (Morihisa et al. 1999). For sexually active female patients, a urine pregnancy test should be ordered.

For acute mania, a therapeutic lithium level is suggested for adults, from a lower range of 0.8–1.0 mEq/L to an upper range of 1.4–1.5 mEq/L (Carroll et al. 1987), but no therapeutic range is established for children and adolescents. A steady-state lithium level is generally obtained 4 or 5 days after the last dosage change. The lithium blood level should be checked every 5 days until an adequate therapeutic concentration is achieved or adverse effects preclude further increases (Janicak et al. 2001). For maintenance therapy, lower lithium levels of 0.6–1.0 mEq/L are recommended (Gelenberg et al. 1989).

The optimal frequency of follow-up laboratory tests has not been established. However, laboratory work is warranted if adverse effects increase or the patient's health status changes.

Anticonvulsants

Carbamazepine has been implicated in aplastic anemia, leukopenia, thrombocytopenia, and anemia as well as slow atrioventricular conduction. Pretreatment laboratory work should include liver function tests, an electrocardiogram, and hematological measures, including CBC and platelet count, serum iron assay, and reticulocyte count. Hematological measures should be repeated weekly for the first 3 months of treatment because of the risk of carbamazepine-related aplastic anemia, agranulocytosis, leukopenia, and thrombocytopenia (Zametkin et al. 1998). A urine pregnancy test should be obtained for sexually active teenagers. A CBC should be immediately obtained if there are any signs or symptoms of bone marrow suppression such as fever, malaise, sore throat, and petechiae. A therapeutic carbamazepine level for psychiatric disorders has not been established, but a laboratory level of 8–12 ng/mL is used when treating partial complex seizures. Carbamazepine level monitoring, especially in the first several weeks of therapy, is crucial because of the phenomenon of autometabolism and potential drug interactions.

For patients taking valproic acid, baseline liver function tests are recommended because of potential hepatotoxicity. An elevated incidence of birth defects in children whose mothers took valproic acid prior to or during their pregnancy suggests that a urine pregnancy test should always be obtained before initiation of treatment. A therapeutic level of 50–125 µg/mL for the treatment of mania has been suggested (Bowden et al. 1996). Measuring the serum level of valproic acid is important for predicting adverse effects and monitoring compliance.

References

Adcock KG, MacElroy DE, Wolford ET, et al: Pemoline therapy resulting in liver transplantation. Ann Pharmacother 32:422–425, 1998

Amen DG: Why don't psychiatrists look at the brain? NeuroPsychiatry Reviews 2:1,19–21, 2001

American Diabetes Association, American Psychiatric Association, American Association of Clinical Endocrinologists, North American Association for the Study of Obesity: Consensus development conference on antipsychotic drugs and obesity and diabetes. Diabetes Care 27:596–601, 2004

American Psychiatric Association Task Force on the Use of Laboratory Tests in Psychiatry: Tricyclic antidepressants blood level measurements and clinical outcome: an APA Task Force report. Am J Psychiatry 142:155–162, 1985

Anfinson TJ, Kathol RG: Screening laboratory evaluation in psychiatric patients: a review. Gen Hosp Psychiatry 14:248–257, 1992

Ania BJ, Suman VJ, Fairbanks VF, et al: Prevalence of anemia in medical practice: community versus referral patients. Mayo Clin Proc 69:730–733, 1994

Ballaban-Gil K, Tuchman R: Epilepsy and epileptiform EEG: association with autism and language disorders. Ment Retard Dev Disabil Res Rev 6:300–308, 2000

Baranowska B, Wolinska-Witort E, Wasilewska-Dziubinska E, et al: Plasma leptin, neuropeptide Y (NPY) and galanin concentrations in bulimia nervosa and in anorexia nervosa. Neuroendocrinol Lett 22:365–358, 2001

Biederman J, Thisted RA, Greenhill LL, et al: Estimation of the association between desipramine and the risk for sudden death in 5- to 14-year-old children. J Clin Psychiatry 56:87–93, 1995

Blumberg HP, Kaufman J, Martin A, et al: Significance of adolescent neurodevelopment for the neural circuitry of bipolar disorder. Ann N Y Acad Sci 1021:376–383, 2004

Boland BB, Beguin C, Zech F, et al: Serum beta-carotene in anorexia nervosa patients: a case-control study. Int J Eat Disord 30:299–305, 2001

Bowden CL, Janicak PG, Orsulak P, et al: Relationship of serum valproate concentration to response in mania. Am J Psychiatry 153:765–770, 1996

Brambilla P, Hardan AY, di Nemi SU, et al: The functional neuroanatomy of autism. Funct Neurol 19:9–17, 2004

Bukstein O: Practice parameters for the assessment and treatment of children and adolescents with substance use disorders. J Am Acad Child Adolesc Psychiatry 36 (10 suppl): 140S–156S, 1997

Carey JC, McMahon WM: Neurobehavioral disorders and medical genetics, in Handbook of Neurodevelopmental and Genetic Disorders in Children. Edited by Goldstein S, Reynolds CR. New York, Guilford, 1999, pp 38–60

Carroll JA, Jefferson JW, Greist JH: Psychiatric uses of lithium for children and adolescents. Hosp Community Psychiatry 38:927–928, 1987

Crow SJ, Rosenberg ME, Mitchell JE, et al: Urine electrolytes as markers of bulimia nervosa. Int J Eat Disord 30:279–287, 2001

Dykins EM, Cassidy SB: Prader-Willi syndrome, in Handbook of Neurodevelopmental and Genetic Disorders in Children. Edited by Goldstein S, Reynolds CR. New York, Guilford, 1999, pp 525–554

Eidem BW, Cetta F, Webb JL, et al: Early detection of cardiac dysfunction: use of the myocardial performance index in patients with anorexia nervosa. J Adolesc Health 29:267–270, 2001

Elia J, Gulotta C, Rose SR, et al: Thyroid function and attention-deficit/hyperactivity disorder. J Am Acad Child Adolesc Psychiatry 33:169–172, 1994

Espallargues M, Sampietro-Colom L, Estrada MD, et al: Identify bone mass–related risk factors for fracture to guide bone densitometry measurements: a systematic review of the literature. Osteoporos Int 2:811–822, 2001

FDA Briefing Document for Zeldox Capsules (Ziprasidone). New York, Pfizer Inc, July 18, 2000, p 116

Frank Y, Pavlakis SG: Brain imaging in neurobehavioral disorders. Pediatr Neurol 25:278–287, 2001

Garcia MR, Ryan ND, Rabinovitch H, et al: Thyroid stimulating hormone response to thyrotropin in prepubertal depression. J Am Acad Child Adolesc Psychiatry 30:398–406, 1991

Gelenberg AJ, Kane JM, Keller MB, et al: Comparison of standard and low levels of lithium for maintenance treatment of bipolar disorder. N Engl J Med 321:1489–1493, 1989

Glassman AH, Bigger TJ Jr: Antipsychotic drugs: prolonged QTc interval, torsade de pointes, and sudden death. Am J Psychiatry 158:1774–1782, 2001

Goodnick PJ:. Ziprasidone: profile on safety. Expert Opin Pharmacother 2:1655–1662, 2001

Green WH: Child and Adolescent Clinical Psychopharmacology, 3rd Edition. Philadelphia, PA, Lippincott Williams & Wilkins, 2001, pp 22–26

Greicius MD: Neuroimaging in developmental disorders. Curr Opin Neurol 16:143–146, 2003

Gutgesell H, Atkins D, Barst R, et al: AHA Scientific Statement: cardiovascular monitoring of children and adolescents receiving psychotropic drugs. J Am Acad Child Adolesc Psychiatry 38:1047–1050, 1999

Hagerman RJ, Wilson P, Staney LW, et al: Evaluation of school children at high risk for fragile X syndrome utilizing buccal cell FMR-1 testing. Am J Med Genet 51:474–481, 1994

Halmi KA: Eating disorders: anorexia nervosa, bulimia nervosa, and obesity, in Textbook of Psychiatry, 3rd Edition. Edited by Hales RE, Yudofsky SC, Talbott JA. Washington, DC, American Psychiatric Press, 1999, pp 983–1002

Hansen RL, Hagerman RJ: Contributions of pediatrics, in Autism Spectrum Disorders: A Research Review for Practitioners. Edited by Ozonoff S, Rogers SJ, Hendren RL. Washington, DC, American Psychiatric Publishing, 2003, pp 87–110

Havens JM, Visootsak J, Phelan MC, et al: 22q13 deletion syndrome: an update and review for the primary pediatrician. Clin Pediatr (Phila) 43:43–53, 2004

Hendren RL, DeBacker I, Pandina G: Review of neuroimaging studies of child and adolescent psychiatric disorders from the past ten years. J Am Acad Child Adolesc Psychiatry 39:815–828, 2000

Hoon AH, Melhem ER: Neuroimaging: applications in disorders of early brain development. J Dev Behav Pediatr 21: 291–302, 2000

Janicak PG, Davis JM, Preskorn SH, et al: Principles and Practice of Psychopharmacotherapy, 3rd Edition. Philadelphia, PA, Lippincott Williams & Wilkins, 2001

Johnson A, Guiffre RM, O'Malley K: ECG changes in pediatric patients on tricyclic antidepressants, desipramine, and imipramine. Can J Psychiatry 41:102–106, 1996

Khan AU: Biochemical profile of depressed adolescents. J Am Acad Child Adolesc Psychiatry 26:873–878, 1987

Kutcher SP: Child and Adolescent Psychopharmacology. Philadelphia, PA, WB Saunders, 1997

Kutcher S, Malkin D, Silverberg J, et al: Nocturnal cortisol, thyroid stimulating hormone, and growth hormone secretory profiles in depressed adolescents. J Am Acad Child Adolesc Psychiatry 30:407–414, 1991

Leo RJ, Batterman-Faunce JM, Pickhardt D, et al: Utility of thyroid screening in adolescent psychiatric inpatients. J Am Acad Child Psychiatry 36:103–111, 1997

Marotta PJ, Roberts EA: Pemoline hepatotoxicity in children. J Pediatr 132:894–897, 1998

Morihisa JM, Rosse RB, Cross CD, et al: Laboratory and other diagnostic tests in psychiatry, in Textbook of Psychiatry, 3rd Edition. Edited by Hales RE, Yudofsky SC, Talbott JA. Washington DC, American Psychiatric Press, 1999, pp 281–316

Morris CA, Mervis CB: Williams syndrome, in Handbook of Neurodevelopmental and Genetic Disorders in Children. Edited by Goldstein S, Reynolds CR. New York, Guilford, 1999, pp 555–590

O'Tuama LA, Dickstein DP, Neeper R, et al: Functional brain imaging in neuropsychiatric disorders of childhood. Child Neurol 14:207–221, 1999

Pauporte J, Walsh BT: Serum cholesterol in bulimia nervosa. Int J Eat Disord 30:294–298, 2001

Pear PL, Weiss RE, Stein MA: Medical mimics: medical and neurological conditions simulating ADHD. Ann N Y Acad Sci 931:97–112, 2001

Pine DS: Functional magnetic resonance imaging in children and adolescents, in Advances in Brain Imaging. Edited by Morihisa JM (Review of Psychiatry Series, Vol 20, No 4; Oldham JM, Riba MB, series eds). Washington, DC, American Psychiatric Publishing, 2001, pp 53–82

Rosse RB, Giese AA, Deutsch SI, et al: A Concise Guide to Laboratory and Diagnostic Testing in Psychiatry. Washington, DC, American Psychiatric Association, 1989

Safer DJ, Zito JM, Gardner JE: Pemoline hepatotoxicity and postmarketing surveillance. J Am Acad Child Adolesc Psychiatry 40:622–629, 2001

Schulz KP, Fan J, Tang CY, et al: Response inhibition in adolescents diagnosed with attention deficit hyperactivity disorder during childhood: an event-related FMRI study. Am J Psychiatry 161:1650–1657, 2004

Sheline Y, Kehr C: Cost and utility of routine admission laboratory testing for psychiatric inpatients. Gen Hosp Psychiatry 12:329–334, 1990

Slaney SF, Wilkie AOM, Hirst MC, et al: DNA testing for fragile X syndrome in schools for learning difficulties. Arch Dis Child 72:33–37, 1995

Sokolov S, Kutcher S, Joffe R: Basal thyroid indices in adolescent depression and bipolar disorder. J Am Acad Child Adolesc Psychiatry 33:469–475, 1994

Speicher CE: The Right Test: A Physician's Guide to Laboratory Medicine, 3rd Edition. Philadelphia, PA, WB Saunders, 1998

Stoll AL, Renshaw PF, Yurgelunn-Todd DA, et al: Neuroimaging in bipolar disorder: what have we learned? Biol Psychiatry 48:505–517, 2000

Toren P, Karasik A, Eldar S, et al: Thyroid function in attention deficit hyperactivity disorder. J Psychiatr Res 31:359–363, 1997

Toren P, Ratner S, Laor N, et al: Benefit–risk assessment of atypical antipsychotics in the treatment of schizophrenia and comorbid disorders in children and adolescents. Drug Saf 27:1135–1156, 2004

Valentine J, Rossi E, O'Leary P, et al: Thyroid function in a population of children with attention deficit hyperactivity disorder. J Paediatr Child Health 33:117–120, 1997

Varley CK, McClellan J: Case study: two additional sudden deaths with tricyclic antidepressants. J Am Acad Child Adolesc Psychiatry 36:390–394, 1997

Walsh BT, Greenhill LL, Giardina EG, et al: Effects of desipramine on autonomic input of the heart. J Am Acad Child Adolesc Psychiatry 38:1186–1192, 1999

Weiss RE, Stein MA: Thyroid function and attention deficit hyperactivity disorder, in Attention Deficit Disorders and Hyperactivity in Children and Adults. Edited by Accardo PJ, Blondis TA, Whitman BY, et al. New York, Marcel Dekker, 1999, pp 419–430

Wolfe BE, Metger ED, Levine JM, et al: Laboratory screening for electrolyte abnormalities and anemia in bulimia nervosa: a controlled study. Int J Eat Disord 30:288–293, 2001

Wood SJ, Berger G, Velakoulis D, et al: Proton magnetic resonance spectroscopy in first episode psychosis and ultra high-risk individuals. Schizophr Bull 29:831–843, 2003

Zametkin AJ, Ernst M, Silver R: Laboratory and diagnostic testing in child and adolescent psychiatry. J Am Acad Child Adolesc Psychiatry 37:464–472, 1998

Zipfel S, Seibel MJ, Lowe B, et al: Osteoporosis in eating disorders: a follow-up study of patients with anorexia and bulimia nervosa. J Clin Endocrinol Metab 86:5227–5233, 2001

Self-Assessment Questions

Select the single best response for each question.

8.1 In a study conducted by Sheline and Kehr (1990), the use of screening tests in psychiatric inpatients led to changes in clinical management in what percentage of cases?

  A. 1%.
  B. 6%.
  C. 10%.
  D. 14%.
  E. None of the above.

8.2 Laboratory tests recommended as part of a comprehensive examination or pre-medication workup include all of the following *except*

  A. Complete blood count (CBC).
  B. Urinalysis.
  C. Thyroid panel.
  D. Liver function tests.
  E. Blood urea nitrogen (BUN).

8.3 Which of the following thyroid disorders has been reported to be associated with attention-deficit/hyperactivity disorder (ADHD)–like symptoms?

  A. Hyperthyroidism.
  B. Syndrome of resistance to thyroid hormone.
  C. Hypothyroidism.
  D. All of the above.
  E. None of the above.

8.4 For patients who attempt suicide by drug overdose, recommended medical/laboratory tests depend on the specific substance taken. Which of the following recommendations is *incorrect?*

  A. Blood toxicology workup for overdose on illegal substances.
  B. Liver function test for acetaminophen overdose.
  C. Serum electrolytes for aspirin overdose.
  D. Electrocardiogram (ECG) for selective serotonin reuptake inhibitor (SSRI) overdose.
  E. None of the above.

8.5 Peer-reviewed articles support the use of single-photon emission computed tomography (SPECT) to rule out which of the following disorders in children?

  A. ADHD.
  B. Wilson's disease.
  C. Seizure disorder.
  D. Prader-Willi syndrome.
  E. None of the above.

Presentation of Findings and Recommendations

Héctor R. Bird, M.D.

The postassessment (or "informing") interview is a crucial aspect of the diagnostic process in child and adolescent psychiatry (Group for the Advancement of Psychiatry 1957). Its main purposes are to share the clinician's observations with the child's parents, to elaborate further on parental feelings and perceptions, and to discuss the clinician's recommendations so as to arrive collaboratively at a plan that will be helpful to both the child and his or her family. It is generally the parents who have brought the child to treatment, and it is they who will need to implement the clinician's recommendations. If treatment is indicated, the parents must work out the practical arrangements to enable their child to see the clinician and to subsidize the cost of treatment.

Parents generally approach this interview with a great deal of anxiety. Guilt is the underlying emotion generating their anxiety, and parents bring this guilt with them into the office. Quite often, guilt is externalized as anger toward their child and often toward the clinician. Parents view their child as their product (not entirely inaccurately), but this leads them to see their child's failings and difficulties as their own failure and to view their child's pathology as an affront to the adequacy of their parenting abilities. For many parents, the postassessment interview is the day of reckoning on which the "guilty" verdict will be passed by the all-knowing professional—the moment when all their parental flaws and all their mistakes and faulty child-rearing practices will be exposed. The parents generally arrive at the office on the defensive, anticipating an accusatory finger pointed at them, with a view of the clinician as their adversary. Thus, the clinician's first task is to provide these anxious parents with reassurance and support (Cox 1994).

One important way to provide support and reassurance to the parents is by conveying that regardless of the developmental, behavioral, or emotional difficulties, their child is basically a good person. Although the parents may believe that they have "failed" in bringing up their child (and in some respects, this may indeed be true), it is important to make them feel that there are equally many things that they have done "right." This first step in the information-sharing process must heavily emphasize the child's observed assets: "Johnny is a very nice kid. He's engaging…sensitive…good at relating to others…witty…affectionate…has a great sense of humor…. There's a lot about him to be proud of." At this stage, one must be cautious to maintain a balance between the positive and the negative. To deny any kind of parental influence on the child's difficulties and to attribute everything to genetics or to temperament can be as detrimental as pointing the accusatory finger at the parents and placing the blame entirely on the way they have brought up their child. The parents must be brought to the realization that they have as much to do with what are perceived as their child's positive characteristics as they may have to do with what are seen as their child's liabilities. If this balance of positive and negative is achieved, the parents will be more receptive to the information shared with them.

The informing interview should not be a lecture in which the clinician does all the talking. The next step is to move into the problem areas and to summarize what has happened since the onset of the consultation process: "When you first came to see me three weeks ago, your major concerns seemed to be that Johnny's work in school had gone downhill and that his teachers complained that he does not pay attention in class….I wonder what your thoughts about this have been since we last met." In this interview it is important to share what has happened since the parents were last seen during the diagnostic process. How has their child reacted to the diagnostic interviews? What has his or her behavior been like? Has he or she given the parents any feedback about the meetings with the clinician? Have there

been any observable changes in the child's behavior or emotional state?

It is also important that the parents understand that what is "wrong" with their child is not simply the maladaptive behavior that is manifested but that these behaviors are closely linked to the child's emotions and cognitions. This understanding is often facilitated by an elaboration of those insights about their child, about themselves, and about family interactions that may have been gained during the diagnostic process. It is thus crucial to de-emphasize how the child behaves and to emphasize how the child feels and sees the world. Many parents require more than one session to explore their motivations, to relieve their guilt about having failed or their anger at their child, and, when treatment is indicated, to overcome their resistance to treatment.

Another important factor that serves to reassure the parents and to gain their confidence and alliance is for the clinician to be perceived as a reliable and competent professional whose observations and recommendations can be trusted. From their brief contact during the diagnostic process, the parents may have developed fantasies about the clinician, some of which may already be transference reactions. When a recommendation for treatment is being made, it is pertinent to explain to parents, "I have a feeling that I can be helpful to your child, but I have known your child for only a few days, and you have known your child all his or her life. From what you have observed about me, do you think I am the kind of person whom he or she will find helpful?" Although this is in many ways a leading question, given that most parents would find it difficult to reply "No, you are not," this line of questioning opens up a dialogue and communicates to parents that the clinician is not an all-powerful, all-knowing expert who will rescue their child. Rather, it conveys that the clinician sees possible limitations to his or her capacities, as well as the need to have a good fit between patient and therapist.

To enhance communication with the parents, the clinician should avoid technical jargon and should provide observations and comments in lay terms. Even with highly educated parents, technical terms may not necessarily have the same meaning as they have for a trained professional. Greenspan (1981) recommended that information about the child be addressed in a developmental context. It is easier for parents to accept a statement such as "Your child relates to others more like a 2-year-old would" than "There is a disturbance in the way your child relates to other children," or "Your child is extremely immature in the way that he or she relates to others."

The clinician should limit the content of the interview with the parents to those areas that will help the patient and should limit the extent to which either parent may discuss individual problems to the exclusion of the identified patient.

The postdiagnostic interview with parents whose child's prognosis is poor, such as an autistic child or a child with mental retardation, is particularly sensitive. Regardless of the diagnosis or prognosis that can be anticipated, it is obviously impossible for any clinician to predict the future unequivocally for an individual patient. It behooves the clinician to be well versed in the literature and in recent findings about the disorder at hand so that a realistic appraisal of what or what not to expect can be communicated. The clinician should not feed into the parents' denial mechanisms by minimizing the severity of the psychopathology, but by the same token, the parents should not be allowed to leave the clinician's office in hopelessness and despair. Follow-up sessions are indicated with such parents to help them shape their expectations. Prognosis is poor only when the real

outcome is much worse than the anticipated outcome. Outcome must be dissected into its component parts. If the child is intellectually dull and the family expects him or her to have a brilliant career, then prognosis is extremely poor. If the parents can tone down their level of expectation and can see their child as a productive member of society in a more modest role, then the prognostic statement can be more favorable.

Confidentiality

Clearly, a child's family, particularly the parents, constitutes the child's most important source of social support. Often the clinician is hesitant to use this source of support to its fullest because of restricted conceptions of confidentiality that preclude discussion of the child's problems with the parents. This barrier often impairs the clinician's ability to find the most effective approach to helping the patient (Barth 1986).

The child clinician's task is complicated because the therapeutic alliance is twofold: the therapeutic contract must be negotiated with the child and with both parents. Particularly for a child whom one expects to have in treatment, a goal of the informing interview is to ensure that there is an alliance with the parents as well as the child. The alliance with the parents will serve to maintain the child in treatment when resistance surfaces. In an intact family, the clinician must share the results of the evaluation with both parents and must accommodate both parents in setting up appointments. When there is a marital separation, the quality of the relationship between the parents dictates whether separate appointments are needed. Even under those circumstances, it is desirable that both parents share the session with the clinician. An observation of their interaction can provide the clinician with a firsthand view of circumstances that the child faces on a daily basis.

From the very first contact with the patient, the clinician should inform the patient of the process that will be followed. Both the child and the family should know that the child will be interviewed individually, that there may be a family interview, and that after a number of sessions the clinician will meet with the parents to convey results of the evaluation and recommendations. The child should be made aware that the purpose of this informing interview is to share information so that his or her parents can be more helpful and that the interview is not a forum to manipulate the parents or to chide them on the patient's behalf.

The clinician can promise confidentiality within certain limits, and the child must know these limits from the outset. As a general rule, the clinician can promise confidentiality to a child with the proviso that information which, in the clinician's judgment, is potentially self-destructive or destructive to others will be shared with those who can protect the child. In those instances, the clinician specifically breaches confidentiality to protect the child and those around him or her. The rubrics "self-destructive" and "destructive to others" include issues such as suicidality, antisocial behaviors, sexual promiscuity, and use of drugs or alcohol. To most children and adolescents, these limitations to confidentiality are reassuring and promote a sense of safety as well as confidence rather than mistrust in the clinician. Before meeting with the parents, the clinician should ask the patient about information that the patient wants to keep confidential, and this information should be kept confidential as long as the aforementioned proviso is upheld. The clinician also should inquire whether the patient would like the clinician to emphasize a particular topic while meeting with the parents. This inquiry often pro-

motes, from an early stage, a view of the clinician as a helping agent (Adams 1982; Simmons 1969).

Confidentiality is qualitatively different for younger children than for adolescents. Younger children find it difficult to conceive of events or circumstances that their parents either do not know or should not know. It usually is not necessary to include younger children in the postdiagnostic interview, and most children accept that the clinician must meet with parents privately.

Adolescence, however, is the second stage of separation-individuation, and regardless of whether it is acknowledged by the adolescent, the issues of privacy and confidentiality are of paramount importance, possibly of greater importance than they are for adult patients (Bird 1995). Any real or imagined breach of the adolescent's confidence may irreversibly block the patient's capacity to ever trust a particular clinician. As a general rule, the adolescent should be given the option to be present at meetings with the parents for the purpose of presenting findings and making recommendations. Some adolescents choose to be present; others presumably do not care. However, the choice should be theirs, and parents should be advised at the outset that their children are allowed to make this decision. Regardless of an adolescent's choice, before the informing interview, the clinician should specifically discuss with the adolescent what the parents will be told at the meeting. The adolescent then can provide the clinician with specific feedback and can discuss details that will be shared with the parents. This discussion with the adolescent also has therapeutic purpose in that it conveys to the adolescent the clinician's impressions and recommendations, as well as the clinician's opinion that the adolescent is the central person in the entire process. This approach places the clinician and the patient on the same team.

Therapeutic Alliance

The therapeutic alliance that the clinician hopes to establish with the patient must be preceded by a therapeutic alliance with the patient's parents. Either parent, as a senior member of the family and one who controls the family resources, is in a position to sabotage the clinician's efforts and to act out any resistance to treatment. For this reason, parents' collaboration is essential. Several factors are relevant to a family's remaining in therapy, including the therapist's activity and directiveness, the congruence between family expectations and the therapist's response, and the family's ability to influence the consultation. Parents, and patients in general, seem to prefer active and directive clinicians. This is particularly true of families who attend low-cost clinics, but this preference probably applies to families at all socioeconomic and educational levels. Studies of adults have shown that when therapists provided feedback that the patients' communications had been perceived, these patients were more likely to continue in therapy after the initial consultation (Roter 1989). The experience in child psychiatry is similar to what is generally experienced in medicine: patient compliance and satisfaction are strongly related to the physician's providing adequate feedback and information. It appears that sharing information in this way enhances patients' sense of empowerment and their conviction that they will be active participants in the therapeutic process.

The way that findings and recommendations are discussed with the family can have therapeutic and prognostic implications. The informing interview is a critical aspect of the diagnostic process. If this interview is handled poorly, it can lead to premature closure of a process that is potentially beneficial and therapeutic to the child and family. When done thoughtfully and sensitively, the informing interview can relieve parental anxiety and guilt, provide alternative ways for parents to view and deal with their children's difficulties, and establish an alliance between the clinician and family (Duehn and Proctor 1977; Stevenson 1971).

References

Adams PL: A Primer of Child Psychotherapy, 2nd Edition. Boston, MA, Little, Brown, 1982

Barth RP: Social and Cognitive Treatment of Children and Adolescents. San Francisco, CA, Jossey-Bass, 1986

Bird H: Psychiatric treatment of adolescents, in Kaplan and Sadock's Comprehensive Textbook of Psychiatry, 6th Edition. Edited by Kaplan HI, Sadock BJ. Baltimore, MD, Williams & Wilkins, 1995, pp 2439–2446

Cox AD: Interviews with parents, in Child and Adolescent Psychiatry: Modern Approaches. Edited by Rutter M, Taylor E, Hersov L. Oxford, UK, Blackwell Scientific, 1994, pp 34–50

Duehn WD, Proctor EK: Initial clinical interaction and premature discontinuance in treatment. Am J Orthopsychiatry 47:284–290, 1977

Greenspan SI: The Clinical Interview of the Child. New York, McGraw-Hill, 1981

Group for the Advancement of Psychiatry (GAP): The Diagnostic Process in Child Psychiatry (Report No 38). New York, Group for the Advancement of Psychiatry, 1957

Roter D: Which facets of communication have strong effects on outcome: a meta-analysis, in Communicating With Medical Patients. Edited by Stewart M, Roter D. London, Sage, 1989, pp 183–196

Simmons JE: Psychiatric Examination of Children. Philadelphia, PA, Lea & Febiger, 1969

Stevenson I: The Diagnostic Interview, 2nd Edition. New York, Harper & Row, 1971

Self-Assessment Questions

Select the single best response for each question.

9.1   The main purposes of the postassessment or "informing" interview in regard to a child or adolescent patient include which of the following?

   A. Sharing the clinician's observation with the child's parents.
   B. Elaborating further on parental feelings and perceptions.
   C. Discussing the clinician's recommendations.
   D. Arriving at a plan that will be helpful to the child and the family.
   E. All of the above.

9.2   Which of the following statements concerning confidentiality in children and adolescents is *false?*

   A. Confidentiality is qualitatively different for younger children than for adolescents.
   B. The clinician can promise confidentiality to a child with the proviso that information that is potentially self-destructive or destructive to others will be shared with those who may protect the child.
   C. It is usually necessary to include younger children in the postdiagnostic interview.
   D. The issues of confidentiality are of greater importance to adolescent patients than they are for adult patients.
   E. None of the above.

9.3   Factors that are relevant to a family's remaining in therapy include all of the following *except*

   A. The therapist's activity and directiveness.
   B. The family's ability to influence the consultation.
   C. The congruence between the family's expectations and the therapist's response.
   D. The severity of the child's psychiatric disorder.
   E. The family's perception that they are active participants in the therapeutic process.

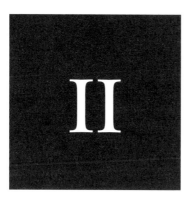

Developmental Disorders

Mental Retardation

Ludwik S. Szymanski, M.D.

Lawrence C. Kaplan, M.D.

Mental Retardation as a Psychosocial Phenomenon

■ Definitions of Mental Retardation

The 2002 Definition of the American Association on Mental Retardation

In 2002, the American Association on Mental Retardation (AAMR) published *Mental Retardation: Definition, Classification, and Systems of Supports,* 10th Edition, with the following definition:

> Mental retardation is a disability characterized by significant limitations both in intellectual functioning and in adaptive behavior as expressed in conceptual, social, and practical adaptive skills. This disability originates before age 18. (p. 8)

"Significant limitations" are defined as an IQ standard score at least 2 SD below the mean of an individually administered assessment instrument. The standard error of measurement for the instrument, usually between 3 and 5 points, has to be taken into account. Three general types of adaptive behavior are listed (instead of 10 specific adaptive skills as in DSM-IV-TR

[American Psychiatric Association 2000]). For the diagnosis of mental retardation to apply, the performance on a standardized instrument measuring adaptive behavior should be at least 2 SD below the mean in one of these types of adaptive behavior or in an overall score. The importance of clinical judgment is highlighted, not as a substitute for the use of an appropriate measurement but for assessment of the results, drawing conclusions, and planning for treatment and needed supports. Thus, a person can be diagnosed as having mental retardation of higher or lower severity than that which the IQ score alone would indicate, depending on the level of adaptive skills.

This definition refers to the current level of functioning, regardless of etiology; therefore, mental retardation is not necessarily viewed as a lifelong condition. It is required that the limitations be seen in the context of person's environment, culture, language diversity, and coexisting limitations, such as physical, sensory, and behavioral. The definition uses a "multidimensional" (essentially biopsychosocial) approach to mental retardation that includes five dimensions:

1. Intellectual abilities
2. Adaptive behavior
3. Participation, interactions, and social roles
4. Health (physical and mental)
5. Context (including environment and culture)

Thus, this definition stresses the importance of comorbidity of mental disorders with mental retardation in determining the person's functioning. It also stresses that the functioning of the individual with mental retardation results from interaction of the individual's capabilities, the environment, and available supports. Thus, even if there is a defined etiology, such as Down syndrome due to trisomy 21, the actual level of associated mental retardation will be influenced by factors such as presence of associated disabilities (e.g., sensory impairments), educational and other opportunities, attitudes of caregivers, and level of stimulation.

The DSM-IV-TR Definition

The DSM-IV-TR definition of mental retardation (Table 10–1) uses an IQ cutoff of 70, retains the subdivision into four levels of severity (mild, moderate, severe, and profound) based on the IQ score, and lists 10 types of adaptive behaviors. No general diagnosis of mental retardation is available. Separate diagnostic codes are used for each of the severity levels. Mental retardation is coded on Axis II.

Related Terms

Developmental disability.   This term is not synonymous with *mental retardation*. It is defined by the Developmental Disabilities Assistance and Bill of Rights Act of 2000 (Public Law 106–402) as follows:

> The term "developmental disability" means a severe, chronic disability of an individual that

> i. is attributable to a mental or physical impairment or combination of mental and physical impairments.
> ii. is manifested before the individual attains age 22 years.
> iii. is likely to continue indefinitely.
> iv. results in substantial functional limitations in three or more of the following areas of major life activity: self-care. receptive and expressive language, learning, mobility, self-direction, capacity for independent living, economic self-sufficiency.
> v. reflects the individual's need for a combination and sequence of special, interdisciplinary, or generic services, individualized supports, or other forms of assistance that are of lifelong or extended duration and are individually planned and coordinated.

A child from birth to age 9 who has a substantial developmental delay may be considered to have a developmental disability without meeting 3 or more of the above criteria without services and supports, has a high probability of meeting those criteria later in life.

Dual diagnosis.   This term has been used to denote people with mental retardation and a comorbid mental disorder. However, most mental health professionals use it to refer to comorbidity of mental illness and substance abuse disorder.

Intellectual disability.   This term, as well as the term *cognitive disability,* is being proposed to replace *mental retardation,* which is considered offensive by many. *Intellectual disability* is now in common use in the United Kingdom and many other English-speaking countries.

■ Initial Clinical Presentation

Mental retardation is usually diagnosed in one of the following circumstances:

- When a syndrome with a characteristic physical phenotype known to be asso-

Table 10–1.   DSM-IV-TR diagnostic criteria for mental retardation

A.   Significantly subaverage intellectual functioning: an IQ of approximately 70 or below on an individually administered IQ test (for infants, a clinical judgment of significantly subaverage intellectual functioning).

B.   Concurrent deficits or impairments in present adaptive functioning (i.e., the person's effectiveness in meeting the standards expected for his or her age by his or her cultural group) in at least two of the following areas: communication, self-care, home living, social/interpersonal skills, use of community resources, self-direction, functional academic skills, work, leisure, health, and safety.

C.   The onset is before age 18 years.

  Code based on degree of severity reflecting level of intellectual impairment:

317	**Mild Mental Retardation:**	IQ level 50–55 to approximately 70
318.0	**Moderate Mental Retardation:**	IQ level 35–40 to 50–55
318.1	**Severe Mental Retardation:**	IQ level 20–25 to 35–40
318.2	**Profound Mental Retardation:**	IQ level below 20 or 25
319	**Mental Retardation, Severity Unspecified:**	when there is strong presumption of mental retardation but the person's intelligence is untestable by standard tests

Source.   Reprinted from the *Diagnostic and Statistical Manual of Mental Disorders*, 4th Edition, Text Revision. Washington, DC, American Psychiatric Association, 2000. Copyright 2000, American Psychiatric Association. Used with permission.

ciated with mental retardation (e.g., Down syndrome) is diagnosed.

• In the course of diagnostic assessment for a disorder of the central nervous system (CNS) (e.g., seizures) that may be comorbid with mental retardation.

• When a child is referred for assessment of developmental delay (e.g., in language or motor development) or school failure. The more severe the mental retardation, the more frequently it is associated with diagnosable medical/neurological disorders and the earlier it is diagnosed. On the other hand, mild mental retardation is usually diagnosed later, such as during early school years, when academic failure becomes obvious. Even then, the initial concern might be about other manifestations, such as disruptive behavior, until detailed psychological assessment discloses the intellectual impairment. It is important to remember that, by definition, mental retardation is not necessarily a lifelong disorder. Some individ-

uals may meet the criteria for mild mental retardation during school years because of failure in academic learning, but with proper services and training, they can acquire adaptive and independence skills to the level that these criteria are no longer met.

■ Differential Diagnosis

In *learning disorders* and *communication disorders,* the impairments are usually more circumscribed and limited to a specific domain, unlike the generalized impairments that characterize mental retardation. *Pervasive developmental disorders* are characterized by qualitative impairments in social interaction and communication, whereas children with otherwise uncomplicated mental retardation do relate to others, even if in a manner immature for their age. *Dementia* is diagnosed if specific multiple cognitive impairments, including memory impairment, are present and represent decline from the previous level of functioning. Dementia may be diagnosed at any age, whereas criteria for mental retardation require an age at onset before 18 years. Theoretically, both dementia and mental retardation might be diagnosed if the insult to the brain was postnatal, but because of difficulty in establishing premorbid level of functioning, such double diagnosis is not recommended before age 4–6 years, or in cases in which the condition is sufficiently described by the diagnosis of mental retardation alone.

■ **Epidemiology**

The estimates of the prevalence of mental retardation have varied, depending on the definition and the methodology used. Under the current definition (based on an IQ cutoff at about 2 SDs and the presence of impairments in adaptive behavior), the prevalence is estimated to be about 1% of the general population. The prevalence of mild mental retardation is thought to be 0.37%–0.59%, and of moderate, severe, and profound mental retardation combined, 0.3%–0.4% (McLaren and Bryson 1987). Data from the National Health Interview Survey for 1994–1995 indicate that the combined prevalence of mental retardation and developmental disabilities in the United States is 1.58% of the population (excluding people living in residential settings of four or more people). The prevalence of mental retardation alone was estimated to be 0.78% (University of Minnesota 2000).

The prevalence of mental retardation is highest among school-age children, because they are faced with academic learning tasks that require cognitive abilities. The prevalence declines in the adult age group, when good adaptive skills, particularly for work, assume more importance. Mental retardation is also more prevalent in males than in females (1.6:1)

People with mental retardation often have associated medical, neurological, and sensory disorders. Seizure disorders are estimated to occur in 15%–30%, motor handicaps (including cerebral palsy) in 20%–30%, and sensory impairments in 10%–20% of this population (McLaren and Bryson 1987). The prevalence of these associated disorders is higher when the retardation is more severe.

Mental Retardation as a Biomedical Phenomenon

■ **Pathoetiology**

It is helpful to consider mental retardation as a developmental and behavioral manifestation of variations in the form, function, and adaptation of the CNS (Leroy 1992). The health professional also must consider the contribution of other organ systems, as well as the important effect of the environment on human beings, each of whom has unique responses to the various stresses and challenges of life.

With rapid advances in the prenatal and early postnatal detection of certain conditions, and with improvements in medical and educational supports, a number of clinical conditions traditionally associated with particular patterns of mental retardation appear to be quite different from their earlier descriptions (Curry et al. 1997; Mayes et al. 1985). This underscores the importance of understanding mental retardation as a reflection of embryonic, perinatal, and postnatal influences, with the balance among these characterizing the individual's actual clinical status (Kaplan 1985).

Three basic etiological categories can assist the clinician in formulating diagnoses, as outlined in Table 10–2:

1. Prenatal errors in morphogenesis of the CNS and/or other systems severe enough to alter normal development.

2. Alterations in the intrinsic biological environment of an individual such that the function of the CNS is also altered (such alterations may be established prenatally but can evolve postnatally).

3. Extraordinary extrinsic influences, resulting in a drastic change in mental function.

Errors in Morphogenesis

In this group of conditions, embryonic development and fetal development are altered (Jones 1997). Approximately 4% of live-born infants are found, in the first year of life, to have major errors of morphogenesis, 20% of which involve CNS effects that may cause mental retardation.

Errors in morphogenesis may be due to malformations (failure of tissue to form normally from the time of conception), deformations (alteration of normally forming tissues by abnormal mechanical forces), and disruptions (in utero injury or toxicity to tissues) (Hudgins and Cassidy 1999).

Malformations are usually sporadic or multifactorial (Wuu et al. 1991). Examples of multiple malformation syndromes include Brachmann–de Lange syndrome, Prader-Willi syndrome (Ben-Asher and Lancet 2004; Butler et al. 2004; Kaplan et al. 1987; Zipf 2004), Pena-Shokeir syndrome (an autosomal-recessive disorder involving severe mental retardation and upper motor neuron disease), and Down syndrome (Hall 1986; Pueschel and Pueschel 1992). Implied in all of these examples is the concept that some signal or operator, such as an identified gene or chromosome or an unidentified stimulus, promotes a cascade of abnormal CNS growth and development.

Deformations are changes in the form or growth of tissues and organ systems that have been influenced by unusual me-

Table 10–2. Etiological categories of mental retardation

Errors in morphogenesis of the CNS
Malformation and malformation syndromes
Disruption (injury) to developing central
  nervous system

Alterations in the intrinsic biological environment affecting the CNS
Inborn errors in metabolism
Non-inborn changes in metabolism

Extraordinary extrinsic influences or events in the CNS
Hypoxia
Trauma
Poisoning

Note.   CNS = central nervous system.

chanical forces (Graham 1988; Samlaska et al. 1989). These deformations may be due to an abnormally shaped uterus compressing the developing calvarial bones and resulting in simple cosmetic changes in the shape of the head (plagiocephaly) or to abnormal fetal movement that may result in fixed contractures at birth, hip dislocation, or clubfoot (Dunn and Clarren 1986; Graham 1988). Rarely do deformations themselves cause mental retardation, but identifying them is helpful because they may point to underlying congenital neurological conditions that are associated with mental retardation.

Disruptions involve catastrophic gestational damage of formed or forming tissues and organ systems of the embryo or fetus. This category includes effects of the large and growing group of teratogens, chemicals, and toxins that can disrupt normal morphogenesis. These include well-known substances such as alcohol, the largest cause of preventable mental retardation in the United States today; the anticoagulant sodium warfarin (Coumadin); and cocaine, a substance whose long-term effects, though incompletely understood, appear to be significant, even in the absence of distinct physical findings at birth (Astley et al. 2000; Bony et al. 2002; Hoyme et al. 2005; Koren et al. 1992). Also included in the group of disruptions are certain viruses, particularly toxoplasmosis, rubella, and cytomegalovirus, and, less commonly, the effects of maternal hyperthermia and intrauterine vascular accidents involving either placenta or fetal cerebral blood vessels (Hoyme et al. 1990).

For all of the mechanisms of abnormal morphogenesis outlined, the effect on the developing CNS may follow an identifiable pattern or may be variable and depend on the extent, duration, and intensity of the abnormal genetic, environmental, and/or physical influences. These general categories require careful consideration of family history and of drug and toxin exposure during the pregnancy. In these categories the clinician also is likely to see patterns among children based on their physical appearance and possibly on their developmental outcome. An example of this concept can be seen in males with fragile X syndrome in whom the sex-linked mode of inheritance often can be identified when taking a family history but also in whom specific phenotypic features can be identified. In this example of a malformation syndrome, mutations of the *FMR1* gene on the X chromosome supports the idea of inheritance of a gene for mental retardation through the maternal X chromosome (Pozdnyakova et al. 2005). A similar gene–chromosome behavioral–developmental association may also hold for Angelman's syndrome, which involves abnormalities in the molecular structure of chromosome 15 (Kaplan et al. 1987; Kishino et al. 1997; C. Williams 2005).

The identification of these general groups also permits the clinician to understand which conditions involving mental retardation may be preventable. Examples include fetal alcohol syndrome, in which abstinence from alcohol is the prevention, and fetal rubella syndrome, in which maternal immunity against the rubella virus is preventive (Hanshaw and Dudgeon 1978; Hoyme et al. 2005; Katz et al. 1998; Rittler et al. 2004).

Alterations in the Intrinsic Biological Environment

There are several circumstances under which changes in the brain's biochemical environment lead to mental retardation. These include genetically determined enzyme deficiencies (Leroy 1992), such as phenylalanine hydroxylase deficiency, resulting in the preventable mental retardation of phenylketonuria (Levy et al. 2003; Scriver and Clow 1980; Weglage et al. 2001). Precise diagnosis is important in these conditions because of the possibility of prevention or arrest of the mental retardation (Guttler et al. 1999; Nichols 1988). Another cause of mental retardation in an otherwise normal CNS is the injury to cortical tissue encountered in profound hypoglycemia.

Although the mechanisms of certain conditions are not fully understood, the natural history of children with certain clinical diagnoses is nonetheless useful in the selection of a strategy to evaluate them. For example, Rett's disorder presents the challenge of a female with loss of milestones within the first 2 years of life progressing to dementia and with autismlike behavior, for which a biochemical marker has now been identified (Einspieler et al. 2005; Holm 1985; Ravn et al. 2005). Nonetheless, the abnormal movements seen in these children and their slow clinical deterioration suggest that the nature of this condition is neurodegenerative rather than, for example, related to a congenital, structural CNS abnormality.

Effects of Extraordinary Extrinsic Influences

A number of accidental and environmental factors may contribute to the pathogenesis of mental retardation. Obvious examples include perinatal asphyxia, neonatal airway obstruction with profound hypoxemia, anesthesia complications, near drownings, poisonings, and head trauma (Kuban and Leviton 1994). Although few data precisely correlate specific clinical and historical factors with the degree of CNS and behavioral impairment, developmental prognosis can be built in part on the sense one has of both the duration of injury and the effectiveness of interventions.

Frequently, a child or an adult with mental retardation secondary to a catastrophic event presents with obvious upper motor neuron disease, especially secondary to profound hypoxia. One must not conclude, however, that mental retardation invariably co-occurs with the motor impairment that characterizes cerebral palsy. Numerous individuals with cerebral palsy are delayed in certain developmental domains but do not have mental retardation.

Finally, although insults to an otherwise normal brain are usually static in nature and occur in the context of a single accident, the so-called plasticity of the human CNS contributes to the wide variability seen in the outcome of specific types of injury and should be taken into consideration in the evaluation process. This might explain, for example, why the child commencing a course of rehabilitation after head trauma may later recover some skills.

■ Medical Evaluation of the Child With the Question of Mental Retardation

The algorithm in Figure 10–1 illustrates the importance of a systematic approach in the identification and evaluation of mental retardation (Kaplan 1989).

Family and Gestational Histories

Maternal obstetrical history should include attention to miscarriages or infertility, drug and chemical exposure, and fetal movement in particular. Additional history of fetal distress or premature labor can also be helpful. Parents usually can accurately report diminished fetal activity or problems in the size of the fetus, and this should alert the clinician to review or request further prenatal obstetrical data. A family history of mental retardation may provide very helpful information, especially in males (fragile X syndrome). In obtaining a drug or alcohol history, it is useful to ask about both the amount and the frequency of exposure.

General Physical Examination

The finding of three or more minor anomalies (phenotypic features that are obvious but not medically consequential) should alert the examiner to the possibility of a syndrome of abnormal morphogenesis. A finding of microcephaly in the newborn tells the examiner that brain growth and development were prenatally abnormal, raising the possibility of a malformation syndrome or of gestational disruption to the CNS. This finding should lead the clinician to obtain a head ultrasound and cranial computed tomography (CT) scan or a magnetic resonance imaging (MRI) scan if these are available. Abnormal scalp hair patterns are also often helpful in predicting cerebral dysgenesis because these patterns reflect the growth of the brain and resultant stretching of the scalp (Samlaska et al. 1989). Their abnormal appearance often implies problems of brain growth as early as the eighteenth week of gestation.

Midface asymmetry, especially undergrowth and abnormalities of the facial midline, may point to an underlying CNS malformation resulting in mental retar-

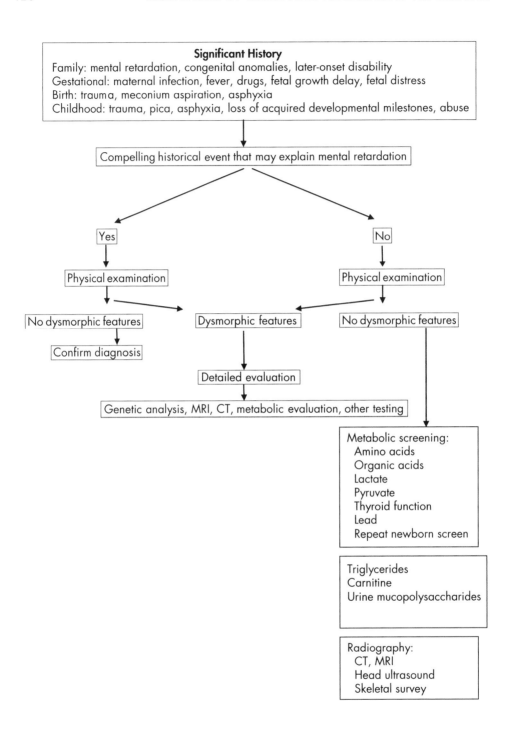

Figure 10–1.   Diagnostic approach to mental retardation for all ages.

dation. Close-set eyes (hypotelorbitism) often are encountered when a problem of the midline axis of the brain is present (Jones 1997; Tessier 1976). However, none of these findings is pathognomonic for the diagnosis of mental retardation. Rather, such features represent clues that mental retardation may occur, and its likelihood is greater when the dysgenesis is severe.

The neurological examination or neurodevelopmental evaluation should include careful attention to the symmetry of movements, the pitch of the infant's or child's cry, and response to stimuli (e.g., a bell or hand clapping). Often a high-pitched cry suggests long-standing prenatal insults. The child with irregular movements, extreme irritability, or hyperactive startle response may also be at risk for developmental disabilities. It should be pointed out, however, that although failure to respond to sounds or visual stimuli may signal that the child is deaf or blind, neither diagnosis implies mental retardation.

Laboratory Investigations

A number of screening studies are available. The urine amino acid screen plays an important role in the identification of conditions that may be treated through diet (e.g., phenylketonuria) (Levy et al. 2003; Wilcken et al. 1980).

Serum levels of lactate, pyruvate, bicarbonate, and venous pH recently have become recognized as being helpful in identifying any inborn errors of metabolism, especially if the individual has been acidotic.

When pica or significant lead exposure is suspected in the child with mental retardation, determining the blood level of lead can be critical. Anemia also may be significant (Needleman et al. 1990).

MRI is particularly helpful in assessing gray and white matter differentiation, posterior fossa anatomy, and myelination patterns. The CT scan has become the standard for the evaluation of ventricular enlargement and, when interpreted by an experienced specialist, defines much of what MRI can provide.

■ Relation of Specific Mental Retardation Conditions to Cytogenetic and Molecular Genetic Analysis

Since the 1990s, advances in molecular genetics and refinements in cytogenetic technology have increased the accuracy of diagnosis for a number of syndromes associated with mental retardation (Delach et al. 1995; Tantravahi et al. 2003). These techniques include fluorescence in situ hybridization (FISH), other specific DNA marker methods, and the application of quantitatively calibrated DNA probes to differentiate among clinical entities that share abnormal microscopic features on standard karyotype analysis.

Unlike high-resolution banding, these newer molecular techniques define abnormal regions of the human genome—DNA molecules that correlate with certain clinical features. Furthermore, these molecular variations allow geneticists to search for similar patterns in parents and other relatives, thereby enhancing their ability to provide genetic counseling regarding the possibility of recurrence.

Prader-Willi syndrome represents an example of a condition in whose diagnosis specific DNA markers have replaced extended prophase (high-resolution) banding techniques. This syndrome is characterized by hypotonia, obesity, developmental and behavioral problems (including mental retardation), hyperphagia (typically after the first year of life), hypogonadism in males, and dysmorphic features, including a narrow-appearing forehead, downslanting palpebral fissures, small-appearing hands and feet, and downturning of the corners of the mouth. Children often present in the neonatal period with low muscle tone and failure to thrive, a feature seen in a number of conditions (Kaplan et al. 1987). Before DNA probes were available for the q11–q12 region of chromosome 15, banding procedures identified micro-deletions in this region in approximately 50% of children with clinical features of Prader-Willi syndrome. DNA analysis now enables molecular confirmation of the diagnosis in most cases (Varela et al. 2005).

Angelman's syndrome also frequently presents with hypotonia and failure to thrive in infancy but evolves gradually to include ataxia, spasticity and other movement disorders, and mental retardation (Knoll et al. 1990). Phenotypically, children with Angelman's syndrome have prognathism. Historically, a tendency in some of these children toward excitability and uncontrolled laughter prompted the unfortunate eponym *happy puppet syndrome.*

Before a chromosome 15 deletion similar to that found in children with Prader-Willi syndrome was identified, Angelman's syndrome was diagnosed in children solely on the basis of clinical features. FISH studies now accurately identify subtle molecular differences in the q11–q12 region of chromosome 15 between these two entities (Delach et al. 1994). The molecular analysis has shown that in Prader-Willi syndrome, the deletion is of the chromosome of paternal origin, and in Angelman's syndrome, the deletion is of the chromosome of maternal origin.

The fragile X syndrome of X-linked mental retardation was initially identified by a constriction at the end of the long arm of the X chromosome (site Xq27.3), resulting in the appearance of a fragment being broken off, or "fragile." This cyto-

genetic finding is thought to occur in 1 of 250 males and in 1 of 2,500 females (Pozdnyakova and Regan 2005). Fragile X syndrome is the most common inherited form of mental retardation. In the past few years, analysis with DNA probes has identified the *FMR1* gene, with an unstable DNA sequence of CGG. In individuals without fragile X syndrome, this sequence has up to 54 repeats; in carriers, 52–230 (premutation); and in affected individuals, more than 230 (full mutation). The premutation inherited by a daughter from her mother tends to increase in length (expansion) and may result in full mutation in the next generation. The expansion does not occur in father-to-daughter transmission. The clinical features in affected prepubertal males include mental retardation, language impairment, gaze aversion, self-stimulatory behaviors, and a presentation similar to that of attention-deficit/hyperactivity disorder (ADHD). Initially, this clinical presentation suggested that many of these individuals had autistic disorder, but review of later studies did not support this association (Pozdnyakova and Regan 2005).

In carrier females, learning disabilities and/or mild mental retardation are seen. Physical phenotype, most obvious in postpubertal males, includes large testes, midfacial underdevelopment (resulting in long, narrow face), and large ears. Currently, the DNA studies are used for definite diagnosis, and they are extremely useful in determining carrier state in maternal relatives as well as in females with developmental difficulties and a family history of mental retardation. Some of the clinical features of fragile X syndrome seen in adults may not be noted in young children, particularly macroorchidism. Thus, a family history of mental retardation and speech and language disorder/autism further justifies obtaining the DNA study. It is important, however, to remember that routine karyotype analysis still has utility, because a number of aneuploidy and polyploidy chromosome anomalies are not diagnosable by molecular studies. Examples of these include XXY syndrome and XYY syndrome.

The support and treatment of children and adults with conditions such as Prader-Willi syndrome, Angelman's syndrome, and fragile X syndrome are most effective as a multidisciplinary effort. The input from geneticists, nutritionists, developmental psychologists, and physical, occupational, and speech therapists is as essential as the contribution of the developmental pediatrician and child psychiatrist. Nutritional management requires collaboration between these and other professionals. This collaboration is particularly important in helping parents understand the sensitive relationship between potential compulsive eating patterns and the child's self-image and response to educational strategies.

Other conditions that are diagnosed by molecular studies include Williams syndrome and a variety of conditions involving deletions (e.g., cri du chat syndrome) for which DNA probes now exist. Rett's disorder, although not associated with any known molecular abnormality, may represent another example of a unique clinical entity, similar in presentation among unrelated individuals, for which a molecular marker eventually will be found. Like the conditions described, it is characterized by discrete clinical features (loss of developmental milestones, which accelerates in the second decade of life; atypical hand movements; progressive dementia) with similar natural history in affected individuals. No biochemical marker has yet been identified; however, the fact that this condition occurs only in females suggests that the X chromosome is involved (Kerr 1991).

Psychiatry of Mental Retardation

An important cause of maladaptation in a person with mental retardation is inappropriate behavior (rather than the severity of the disability). As described later in this section, people with mental retardation are at increased risk for mental disorders. Thus, all efforts should be taken to ensure early recognition and treatment of mental/behavioral disorders.

■ Personality Development and Developmental Crises

A common misconception about people with mental retardation is that they are a homogeneous group with similar characteristics, behaviors, and personality patterns, such as lack of inhibitions and moral sense, rigidity, and attention seeking (Reiss 1994). In fact, all kinds of personality and behavior problems are encountered among persons with mental retardation, just as in the population at large. A personality feature frequently found in children with mental retardation (but not unique to them) is negative self-concept, probably related to experiences of failure or to messages of disappointment and rejection received from significant people and society (Reiss 1994; Szymanski and Crocker 1985). These children often expect failure, especially when faced with new tasks.

Recent research in molecular genetics has also led to increased interest in genetic determinants of behavior in mental retardation–associated syndromes. This is discussed in detail below, in the section "Genetics and Behavior: Behavioral Phenotypes."

Behavioral and developmental problems commonly encountered at various ages are summarized in Table 10–3.

Table 10–3.   Common behavioral and developmental problems leading to psychiatric referral in individuals with mental retardation

Age group	Behavioral problems	Developmental problems	Other	Comments
Early childhood	Reduced or exaggerated attachment behaviors, over/under activity level, irritability, passivity, eating/sleeping problems	Delay in motor development, language, play skills, social interaction skills	Differential diagnosis with pervasive developmental disorder; advice concerning educational plan, second opinion	Presentation may be related to behavioral phenotype.
School age	Impulsivity, inattention, overactivity, disruptive/aggressive behavior, withdrawal	Social interaction problems: indiscriminate, age inappropriate, poor social skills	Academic failure, advice concerning educational plan, second opinion	Presentation may be related to behavioral phenotype. Behavioral problems may be a reaction to inappropriate school placement.
Adolescence	Depression, withdrawal, noncompliance, aggression	Social interaction problems: isolated, sometimes exploited, poor social skills	Sexually inappropriate behaviors or sexual exploitation by others; planning for the future	Less disabled individuals may have more problems in realizing their delays.

■ Issues Related to Sexuality

In regard to the sexuality of persons with mental retardation, misconceptions and myths abound—for example, that people with mental retardation are uninhibited, are unable to learn social mores, or are not interested in sexuality. For most adolescents with mental retardation, pubertal development is normal but emotional development is lagging. Unfortunately, these youngsters, in their quest for social acceptance, may become victims of sexual and other exploitation by their peers who do not have mental retardation.

The best intervention here is prevention through early sexuality education, starting with helping the adolescent to develop a positive self-image and progressing to teaching social interaction skills and, finally, to teaching about sexuality, which should include principles of appropriate relevant social behaviors. In the past, many states' statutes permitted sterilization of people with mental retardation, either involuntarily or by legal guardian's permission. At present, no sterilization of minors or legally incompetent adults is permitted, except for rare cases in which court permission is obtained.

■ Parental Reactions and Adaptation to Mental Retardation in a Child

Children whose retardation is diagnosed at birth or in early infancy usually have severe retardation and an associated physical syndrome or impairment. The child's health problems may be overwhelming, and often the diagnosis is unexpected. The manner in which the parents are told about the child's condition is crucial (Lynch and Staloch 1988). In particular, the physician should take adequate time for this informing conference, listen to the parents' concerns, express empathy and compassion but not pity or personal value judgments, and provide detailed and helpful information about available services and what the parents can do to promote the child's development.

Parental sadness should not be confused with a pathological depression. Some parents may have various intermixed reactions, whereas others may have generally negative initial reactions, followed by denial, and ending with constructive adjustment (Mary 1990).

Mild retardation unassociated with physical abnormalities is usually diagnosed later in life. Some parents who believe the child's developmental delay is caused by emotional problems may have sought psychiatric consultation. Some families may deny the child's developmental problems and subject the child to continuous tests and consultations, looking for a diagnosis more acceptable than mental retardation.

Family adaptation will be influenced by the balance between the innate strengths of the family, the available supports and services, and child-related factors such as severity of the handicap, communication skills, the need for medical care, and behavioral and emotional problems. Parents need adequate explanations for the child's condition and concrete help in finding the needed services. Peer support by other families can be very helpful.

The role of brothers and sisters (especially older ones) is most important, as role models and often as protectors. Many, as adults, report that the experience of having a handicapped sibling made them more empathetic and better people. Many also choose careers in helping professions, such as speech therapy or social work. However, their adjustment may be compromised if they are subjected to undue pressure from the parents to assume responsibility for the care of the disabled sibling.

■ Epidemiology of Mental Disorders in Mental Retardation

Available reports of prevalence studies note quite diverse results because of methodological problems such as biased selection of study cohorts, use of different definitions of mental retardation, use of different diagnostic criteria for various mental disorders, and diagnostic techniques that varied from retrospective reviews of charts to detailed psychiatric interviews with patients and multiple informants (review: Dykens 2000; Kerker et al. 2004). Yet, most studies have agreed that the prevalence of mental disorders in this population is much higher than in children without mental retardation. In recent, population-based studies, between 32% and 37% of children with mental retardation had another psychiatric diagnosis (Linna et al. 2004; Stromme and Diseth 2000). Virtually all major diagnostic categories were represented. A number of factors contribute to this high prevalence (Dykens 2000): lowered ability to solve problems and deal with stresses due to reduced cognitive skills; poor language skills, leading to use of behavior, especially disruptive, as means of communication; repeated experiences of failure, leading to poor self-image and learned helplessness, which might be associated with depression (Dagnan and Sandhu 1999); poor pragmatic skills and social skills; and the neuropathology underlying the mental retardation and associated disabilities, which might also contribute to certain aberrant behaviors. Symptoms of mental disorders in this population may be persistent over time (Tonge and Einfeld 2000).

■ Genetics and Behavior: Behavioral Phenotypes

Historically, there had been a tendency to see certain behavioral patterns as typical for people with mental retardation. Usually these were inappropriate behaviors, sometimes even contradictory, such as passive and aggressive, asexual and sexually disinhibited. People with Down syndrome were described as charmers, attention-seeking, "Prince Charming." At their extreme, these views led to the belief that maladaptive behavior in people with mental retardation was genetically determined and contributed to the eugenic movement in the early part of the twentieth century, with its resulting involuntary sterilization of people with mental retardation. In the later backlash, these views were seen as stereotyping, and behaviors of these people as due only to the attitudes of other people in their environment. At present, it seems that there has been a partial return to the earlier views. No one denies that environment exerts a powerful influence in shaping a person's behavior, but as there have been developments in molecular genetics, increasing attention has been paid to genetic factors. The concept of behavioral phenotypes has become increasingly popular. It has been defined by Dykens (1995) as "the heightened probability or likelihood that people with a given syndrome will exhibit certain behavioral and developmental sequelae relative to those without the syndrome" (p. 523). Most of these behaviors are not unique to the particular syndrome (such as hyperactivity), but some might be, such as extreme overeating in people with Prader-Willi syndrome or extreme self-biting of hands and mouth in Lesch-Nyhan syndrome (Dykens 2000). Some of these behaviors (or at least their frequency and intensity) may be associated with the type of the genetic abnormality. For example, maladaptive behaviors are more frequent or intense in people with Prader-Willi syndrome due to paternal deletion on chromosome 15 than in those with maternal uniparental disomy (Dykens 2000). Thus, these patients offer a unique opportunity to study the genetic underpinnings of behavior.

■ Psychiatric Clinical Assessment

Comprehensive Context

Psychiatric clinical assessment of persons with mental retardation has two interrelated aspects: assessment of the mental retardation and assessment of comorbid mental disorder. Considering the multiplicity of cognitive and other deficiencies most of these individuals have, the assessment should be done within a framework of comprehensive understanding of the patient's biomedical and psychosocial problems. The principles of psychiatric assessment are summarized in Table 10–4.

Table 10–4. Principles of psychiatric assessment of persons with mental retardation

Comprehensive, biopsychosocial context—Review/update/obtain:

Etiological/medical workup
Cognitive profile (not just overall IQ)
Communication skills
Environment (family, supports, services)
Current and past psychiatric history
Individual's strengths

Utilize multiple informants

Patient interview/observation:

Allow sufficient time
If possible, see patient in natural
  environment

Referral

Children and adolescents with mental retardation are referred for psychiatric evaluation for a variety of reasons, overt and covert, just like those without mental retardation (AACAP 1999). Not infrequently the referral is initiated by several people, for different and sometimes contradictory reasons. For example, a teacher might expect a diagnosis of mental disorder and a prescription for medication "for aggression," whereas a parent might want a recommendation for a transfer to a better school. Common reasons for referral are summarized in Table 10–5.

Table 10–5. Common reasons for referral to a psychiatrist

Disturbed behavior (especially disruptive)
Search for diagnosis (often of mental
  disorder rather than of retardation)
Poor developmental progress
Help in educational planning

Patient's History

A detailed and comprehensive history from multiple informants (e.g., parents, sitters, teachers, therapists, classroom aides) is essential (AACAP 1999). Components of a comprehensive history are summarized in Table 10–6.

Interviewing Techniques

Interviewing techniques have been described elsewhere in detail (AACAP 1999; Reiss 1994; Szymanski 1977, 1980b).

The interviewer must assess the patient's communication skills and adapt to them, if necessary using the caregivers as "interpreters." Leading questions—those requiring "yes" or "no" answers—must be avoided. The interviewer must make sure that the each question is understood and use concrete examples, if needed. Nonverbal techniques such as play, drawing, and various activities are helpful if appropriate to the child's chronological age. People with mental retardation are sensitive to being treated as eternal children or as "stupid" and might be insulted if an age-inappropriate activity is suggested or very simple questions are asked of them.

Table 10–6.   Patient's history

Presenting symptoms

Concrete behavioral description; examples

Variability in time, place, with different caregivers

Symptom change over time

Correlation with environmental events

Antecedents and consequences for patient's behavior

Past history and personality patterns, strengths and weaknesses

Adaptive skills, learning, self-care, leisure/recreation

Attention span, activity level, socialization, communication skills

Unusual behaviors (e.g., stereotypies, rituals, self-injury)

Psychiatric history

Evaluations, diagnoses, hospitalizations, treatment, medications

Alternative treatments (diets, supplements, manipulations)

Educational/work history

Detailed program description, patient's response

Attitudes of teachers/peers

Family/environmental history

Understanding of and reaction to child's disabilities

Attitudes toward child's growth (dependence vs. independence)

Long-term expectations

Family's cultural context

For this reason it might be better, with more verbal people, to avoid standard questions of a "formal" mental status examination and disguise them instead within a casual conversation. The patient's knowledge, understanding, and feelings about the disability should be explored; the best time to do so is after first asking about strengths and abilities. General behavior—social communication, attention, activity level, any unusual behaviors, and mood—must be observed.

Often, an unobtrusive initial observation in the waiting room will provide valuable information.

Assessment of Clinical Data

The data obtained during diagnostic evaluation must be viewed in the context of the child's total clinical presentation (behavioral, psychological, and physical), developmental and communication level, associated disabilities (especially sensory and neurological), environmental and cultural factors and events, education, and experience. For example, a boy who is withdrawn and talks to himself may be hallucinating, may be rejected by his peers and feel depressed and lonely, may be trying to attract his teacher's attention, or may be talking to an imaginary friend appropriate to his developmental age. The diagnostic statement should integrate these data and include, in addition to a formal diagnostic label, a review of the patient's strengths, liabilities, and needs for support in all applicable domains; factors initiating and maintaining the problem; and a comprehensive treatment plan. The possibility of an underlying general medical disorder must always be considered. Individuals with mental retardation might not be able to report on their signs and symptoms; some disorders with psychiatric manifestations are more common in certain conditions (e.g., thyroid disorders in Down syndrome); a physical discomfort in a nonverbal person might be communicated via overt behaviors; and, as a group, these individuals frequently receive medications that have behavioral side effects.

The Use of DSM-IV-TR Terminology

The categorical diagnosis is not sufficient to describe the patient adequately; a brief but comprehensive statement enumerating the reasons for making the formal diagnosis as well as the environmental, psychological, and biomedical issues and the person's needs for support is also necessary. This could follow the five dimensions outlined in the AAMR diagnostic manual (American Association on Mental Retardation 2002). The standard diagnostic criteria—DSM-IV-TR (American Psychiatric Association 2000)—should be used. In most people with mild mental retardation, there are sufficient communicative skills to permit making the diagnosis and using the criteria in the same manner as in people who do not have mental retardation. If the person's communicative language is significantly impaired, the diagnosis must be based primarily on history and observations of behavior. A useful publication (Royal College of Psychiatrists 2001) describes how the expression of mental disorders in adults may be influenced by mental retardation.

The descriptive term "behavior disorder" is neither defined nor recognized by DSM-IV-TR, although it is listed in ICD-10 (*International Classification of Diseases and Related Health Problems,* 10th Revision; World Health Organization 1992). Presumably, this term might be used to describe behavioral problems that occur solely in certain situations (e.g., aggression that manifests only at school in an overcrowded classroom) and that are not symptomatic of a diagnosable mental disorder.

■ Diagnosis of Specific Mental Disorders

Disorders Usually First Diagnosed in Infancy, Childhood, or Adolescence

Pervasive developmental disorders. A common differential diagnostic question is whether the patient has mental retardation or autism. However, the diagnoses of retardation and autism frequently coexist. In particular, diagnostic confusion commonly arises if the child has self-stimulatory behaviors and significant delay in language development. This constellation is frequently seen in children with mental retardation who do not have autistic disorder. They usually do not show the core symptoms of autistic disorder: qualitative impairments in reciprocal social relationships and social communication. They usually relate well, especially to familiar people, albeit more appropriately to their developmental rather than chronological age. Some patients, especially those with poor language skills, may avoid contact with people whom they do not understand. Such avoidance is sometimes mistaken for social withdrawal, but careful observation of the child on several occasions in nondemanding situations and detailed developmental history will usually lead to the correct diagnosis.

Attention-deficit/hyperactivity disorder and disruptive disorders. Overactivity and poor attention span are frequent reasons for psychiatric referral of children with mental retardation. It is thought that the prevalence of ADHD is similar among people with mental retardation and those without it, ranging from 4% to 11% (Feinstein and Reiss 1996). Most of the DSM-IV-TR criteria for ADHD are based on observable behaviors and therefore generally can be applied to people with mental retardation. The symptoms should be evaluated in the context of the person's developmental level. Care should be exercised to recognize situation-specific inattentiveness occurring only in one setting, usually in reaction to environmental factors such as lack of structure or a boring or difficult activity. ADHD-like symptoms may be also a part of some behavioral phenotypes, such as fragile X, or a side effect of medications, such as barbiturates, and may be confused with akathisia due to neuroleptics.

Conduct disorders occur frequently. Disobedience and noncompliance are common reasons for referral. As with ADHD, the diagnostic assessment should consider the child's developmental level, the child's understanding of the rules, and the appropriateness of the educational program (if the problems happen primarily in the school).

Feeding and eating disorders.　Pica and rumination disorder, not uncommon in people with severe and profound mental retardation, are separate diagnostic categories in DSM-IV-TR. In the presence of mental retardation, these disorders are diagnosed if the problem is severe enough to be the focus of clinical attention. Care should be exercised to assess for the presence of an underlying physiological disorder, such as gastroesophageal reflux and peptic ulcers caused by *Helicobacter pylori* (the latter disorder having been reported quite frequently in institutional populations). Some cases of pica were reported in which a zinc or iron deficiency was present, and the symptoms abated with dietary supplementation (Lofts et al. 1990).

Mental Disorders Due to a General Medical Condition

This category replaced the various categories of "organic" mental disorders, which previously had been used indiscriminately in mental retardation. DSM-IV-TR diagnostic criteria require that neuropathology be present and that its causative relation to the behavioral manifestations be proven. A diagnosis of this type might be inferred from the nature of the clinical symptoms (e.g., if they are typical for a temporal lobe pathology, which has been demonstrated) and whether a chronological correlation between the onset of behavioral and neurological manifestations is found. Related to this might be behavioral adverse effects of medications.

Schizophrenia and Other Psychotic Disorders

Schizophrenia and mental retardation were often confused in the past, and individuals with severe mental retardation were sometimes thought to have psychosis because of their bizarre, self-stimulatory behaviors. Current estimates of the prevalence of schizophrenia in people with mental retardation range from about 1%, as accepted for the general population (Reiss 1994), to about 2%–3% (Bregman 1991; Fraser and Nolan 1994). Children with a psychotic disorder may be first referred to a psychiatrist owing to a suspicion of mental retardation because psychosis may be associated with cognitive deficiencies (Russell and Tanguay 1981). Persons with certain mental retardation syndromes, especially velocardiofacial syndrome and Prader-Willi syndrome (Dykens 2000), have been reported to be at increased risk for psychotic disorders.

In people with mild mental retardation who are verbal, the diagnosis of comorbid psychotic disorder usually can be made in the same manner as in people without mental retardation, and the diagnosis of subtypes of schizophrenia is also possible. However, documenting delusions and hallucinations is difficult if not impossible in people with severe mental retardation, especially if they are nonverbal (Reid 1993). In some people without sufficient language to report delusions or hallucinations, the presence of grossly disorganized behavior coexisting with negative symptoms might be sufficient evidence for the diagnosis of schizophrenia (although not of its specific subtype) or of psychotic disorder not otherwise specified.

Depressive Disorders

Although mood disorders among people with mental retardation are about as frequent as mood disorders in the general population, they often remain undiagnosed (Feinstein and Reiss 1996; Gillberg et al. 1986; Reiss 1994; Sovner and Hurley 1983), especially if the individual's behavior is not disturbing to others. Suicide can also occur among children, adolescents, and adults with mental retardation (Patja et al. 2001; Walters et al. 1995).

The diagnosis is more difficult if the person lacks language skills to express the traditional symptoms of depression (e.g., poor self-image and hopelessness). However, most of the DSM-IV-TR criteria for a major depressive episode can be satisfied on the basis of observation and history, even if the patient is not verbal: depressed or irritable mood, diminished interest in activities, significant weight loss or gain, insomnia or hypersomnia, psychomotor agitation or retardation, fatigue, and diminished ability to concentrate. The mood changes may be reported by the patient or by others. Children and adolescents with mild mental retardation and good language skills usually can describe the same symptoms as those without mental retardation. They may, however, use simple and concrete statements; for example, they may say that they feel sick and weak, rather than depressed, or complain that no one likes them, rather than say that they feel worthless (AACAP 1999). Depression in this population also has been found to be strongly associated with aggressive behavior (Reiss and Rojahn 1993). Such behaviors could be a method of affective expression in people with limited language or even a form of self-defense against caregivers' expectations and pressure to perform and comply. Depression has been also reported in people with Down syndrome (Szymanski and Biederman 1984).

The differential diagnosis of depression versus dementia often emerges in people with mental retardation—especially in people with Down syndrome, because of its association with Alzheimer's disease. Clinical dementia in individuals with Down syndrome does not occur before the fourth or even fifth decade of life and is associated with loss of skills and memory. This contrasts with depression, in which there is diminished interest and productivity but no actual loss of skills. Another important differential diagnosis is with thyroid disorders, to which people with Down syndrome are prone. Depressive symptoms may be also a side effect of certain beta-blockers, such as propranolol, sometimes used in the treatment of aggressive behavior.

Bipolar Disorder

Manic symptoms may be noticed more readily than depression because they are usually disturbing to caregivers. Otherwise, problems with the diagnosis are similar to those noted for depressive disorders. The symptoms must be evaluated in the context of developmental level—for example, a nonverbal adolescent with significant mental retardation would not exhibit grandiosity, pressured speech, flight of ideas, and buying sprees, but there may be noticeable insomnia, hyperactivity, screaming, increased masturbation, distractibility, and irritability. Inappropriately elevated mood may be expressed through yelling, laughter, and dancing. Caregivers familiar with the individual will notice a mood change. In some children and adolescents with severe mental retardation, the mood changes are rapid-cycling, as often as every few days (Jan et al. 1994). Periodic disruptive behaviors may be related to an undiagnosed bipolar disorder, but more often they represent a reaction to usual life stresses that occur periodically, such as staff and school changes.

Anxiety Disorders

Generalized anxiety disorder, phobias, and panic disorder occur in this population but are often misdiagnosed as a nonspecific "behavior disorder." The diagnosis can be usually made though interview with the patient (if sufficiently verbal) and caregivers (Feinstein and Reiss 1996; Masi et al. 2000).

Obsessive-Compulsive Disorder

The diagnosis of obsessive-compulsive disorder requires that the compulsions be a response to the obsessions and thus that the anxiety and distress associated with the obsessions be identified. This can usually be done for people with mild mental retardation and sufficient language skills. In persons with autistic disorder, and in those with significant mental retardation and poor or no language, the diagnosis is often inferred from the person's repetitive, ritualistic behaviors. However, it is not clear whether such behaviors represent an actual obsessive-compulsive disorder. In such individuals, the diagnosis of stereotypic movement disorder may be used.

Posttraumatic Stress Disorder

This diagnosis, often related to sexual abuse, is often missed (Ryan (1994). The individual may not be able to report abuse, but it might be suspected if symptoms such as excessive masturbation, loss of toilet training, sleep disorder, avoidance of places or people possibly associated with the abuse, heightened arousal, and vigilance appear. People with mental retardation may subjectively perceive the traumatic event as threatening, even if it would not be perceived as such by a person of similar age without mental retardation. Children and adolescents with mental retardation are at a particular risk for sexual abuse. They are considered "safe" victims because they may have problems in reporting the abuse, and if they do, they may not be believed. Mentally retarded victims may even cooperate with the perpetrator, because of their tendency to trust others and the belief that by cooperating they will make a friend.

Self-Injurious Behaviors and Stereotypic Behaviors

A variety of repetitive and seemingly nonfunctional behaviors may occur in individuals with mental retardation and/or autism, such as body rocking, head banging, and hand shaking. Because this is a very heterogeneous group, there is no single treatment approach, and accurate differential diagnosis is essential (Gualtieri 1989). If association with another mental disorder can be ruled out and the behavior is the focus of treatment, the DSM-IV-TR category of stereotypic movement disorder can be used. If there is tissue damage that requires medical treatment, the specifier "with self-injurious behavior" is added. The self-injurious behaviors (SIBs) may lead to serious damage (e.g., retinal detachment and blindness due to head banging, or self-biting that may lead to virtual limb amputation). It is important to rule out an underlying physical discomfort due to a medical problem; for example, head banging might be due to migraine headache or earache from otitis. SIBs also are associated with disorders such as autism, blindness, and certain behavioral phenotypes, such as Lesch-Nyhan and fragile X syndromes. An excellent review is provided by Harris (1995).

Aggression

Aggressive behavior is one of the most common reasons for psychiatric referral in people of all ages who have mental retardation; the term encompasses behaviors as diverse as swearing (verbal aggression) and life-threatening violence. There is no discrete disorder called *aggression;* aggressive behavior can be associated with psychopathology, such as psychosis, ADHD, paranoid traits, personality and conduct disorders, and affective disorders (Connor and Steingard 1996; Reiss 1994). It can represent a learned behavior related to exposure to aggressive role models, to certain antecedents, or to consequences such as reactions of the caregivers that will reinforce the aggressive behavior. It can be related to neuropathology, such as head injury, and to certain seizure disorders. Thus, comprehensive diagnostic assessment, biomedical, psychiatric, and psychosocial, is a precondition to treatment (Connor and Steingard 1996; Harris 1995, p. 478).

■ Treatment of Mental Disorders in People With Mental Retardation

Developing a Treatment Plan

The following guidelines are important to the success of the treatment:

- A comprehensive diagnostic psychiatric assessment is a prerequisite to any treatment plan. It should result in a comprehensive understanding of the person's strengths, disabilities, maladaptive behaviors, and needs in all domains. Biomedical, psychological, and environmental factors that could have initiated and/or maintained the problem—such as inappropriate school or residential placement, lack of appropriate supports, or inconsistent management by caregivers—should be explored.
- Clear goals of treatment should be established, regularly reviewed, and updated as necessary. The ultimate goal is not only removal of inappropriate behaviors or other symptoms but also achievement of an optimally feasible quality of life for the individual, as measured by objective criteria and individual's subjective satisfaction (Schalock and Begab 1990; Szymanski 2000). Facilitation of a sense of self-worth, leading to a positive self-image, which may prevent development of learned helplessness, passivity, or maladaptive defenses, is important, as is learning self-care and independence-related skills.
- The treatment should be comprehensive; all of the patient's needs, not just the disruptive behaviors, should be addressed. These needs may include medical problems, self-care skills, communication skills, interpersonal relating, education and/or work, and recreation.
- Collaboration of the psychiatrist with all members of the treatment team responsible for each of those aspects is essential. All involved caregivers should agree on the treatment goals and approaches.
- Choice of psychiatric interventions should be guided by the best risk–benefit ratio. They should be integrated with the patient's total treatment program, including medical, educational, behavioral, and habilitative interventions. The least intrusive approaches should be chosen first.
- Behaviors and skills that will be an index of progress should be identified, and means of monitoring them should be established. Adverse treatment effects should be monitored regularly, because the patient may not be able to report them.
- Human rights and legal requirements (such as obtaining legal informed consent for use of medications) should be respected.

Psychotherapies

There have been few controlled studies on the efficacy of psychotherapies in people with mental retardation but many reports on individual cases and smaller, uncontrolled groups (for a review, see Beail 2003). Cognitive-behavioral approaches have been found useful in teaching skills of self-management, and psychodynamic psychotherapy has shown utility in reducing emotional distress and improving self-image and social functioning.

The following guidelines for individual and group therapy have been described (Hollins 2001; Reiss 1994; Sigman 1985; Stavrakaki and Klein 1985; Szymanski 1980a):

The available literature agrees on the following guidelines as essential to the success of both individual and group therapy:

- The therapist should be willing, trained, flexible, supportive, eclectic, and able to serve as a role model for the patient.
- The patient should have basic skills of verbal or nonverbal communication.
- The therapy often must be directive, concrete, repetitious, and structured but permit spontaneous expression.
- Nonverbal communication (e.g., play activities for modeling real-life situations and learning ways of handling them) may be very helpful.
- An eclectic approach is needed, using reality-oriented cognitive techniques, behavior modification, role modeling, and family supports.
- The therapy should be a part of a comprehensive treatment program, with all involved working as a team and regularly communicating.
- In the course of therapy, the patient should acquire a constructive understanding of his or her disabilities, balanced by an appreciation of his or her strengths, leading to development of a positive self-image.

Behavior Modification

Essentially the same techniques are used as for people without mental retardation, with allowances to accommodate patients' developmental level and communication skills. For example, nonverbal, severely handicapped individuals may need a reward immediately after the desired behavior occurs in order to recognize the connection between reward and behavior. The focus should be not only on eliminating objectionable behaviors (Reiss 1994) but also on teaching appropriate replacement behaviors. Ignoring inappropriate behaviors works only if sufficient social and other rewards are given for appropriate ones. The treatment should be generalized to all settings and caregivers, such as through training parents to apply the same techniques at home that are used at school.

Aversive techniques (punishment) are rarely used, and then only very briefly in exceptional circumstances limited to dangerous SIBs and aggression that do not respond to thorough application of other treatments.

Family-Directed Interventions

All families of people with mental retardation should be provided with comprehensive support and information about the nature of child's problems, genetics, appropriate expectations, behavioral management techniques, entitlements for education and other services, and resources and support groups. Some families may need support in alleviating guilt feelings, if these are present, or modifying overprotective or overdemanding attitudes toward the child. Optimally, families should be able to integrate the child into family life and expect him or her to do chores, even if minimal, to let the child feel like a valued family member. Psychiatrists may be particularly effective in helping the parents to recognize the child's strengths and to learn to derive gratification regardless of the level of disability.

Pharmacotherapy

Common mistakes in the use of psychotropic drugs in people with mental retardation include treating single nonspecific symptoms, without prior diagnostic understanding; continuing the treatment without evidence of effectiveness; using medications alone, without other interventions; and using medications as a substitute for education and training (Matson et al. 2000).

Research on the use of these agents in children and adolescents with mental retardation has been limited (Aman et al. 2000). However, there is no evidence that the presence of low IQ changes the mechanism of drug action and its effectiveness, although this might vary in different syndromes associated with mental retardation. The frequency of side effects in this population might not be the same as that in populations without mental retardation (AACAP 1999). People with Down syndrome may be sensitive to anticholinergic drugs, which may lead to cognitive impairment and delirium. Lithium might also lead to cognitive dulling; because of irregular fluid intake, there is higher risk of toxicity. Sedative-hypnotic drugs may have the paradoxical effect of behavioral disinhibition.

The Centers for Medicare and Medicaid Services (formerly the Health Care Financing Administration) have issued helpful guidelines for the use of psychotropics in people with mental retardation. The main points of these guidelines are

- Comprehensive diagnostic evaluation *prior* to drug initiation (and not afterward, to justify drug use)
- Baseline behavioral data
- Prior trial of less intrusive treatments if applicable; medication to be used only as part of a comprehensive treatment/habilitation program; use of the lowest effective dose

- Avoidance of reducing patient's functioning as a result of the medication
- Careful monitoring of side effects
- Continuation of the drug only if it is clearly proven effective and safe

For an excellent review of current knowledge of psychopharmacology in the field of mental retardation, see Reiss and Aman (1998).

Antipsychotics. In people with mental retardation, antipsychotic drugs have a long history of use for virtually any behavioral symptoms rather than for their principal indications (e.g., psychosis). At present, atypical antipsychotics, because of their effectiveness and more favorable side-effect profile, are the drugs of choice. People with mental retardation may be more at risk for weight gain and metabolic syndrome, as well as tardive akathisia and dyskinesia; when antipsychotics are abruptly discontinued, behavioral symptoms, such as irritability, insomnia, and weight loss, may emerge (Gualtieri et al. 1986). Most published studies are anecdotal, but controlled ones are starting to appear. There are case reports of the effectiveness of risperidone in children and adolescents with psychosis, SIB, and aggression (Dosen 2001). These drugs may be effective in psychotic disorders, bipolar disorder, Tourette's disorder, and possibly severe conduct disorders associated with mental retardation (Cheng-Shannon et al. 2004). However, adverse effects of weight gain and development of metabolic syndrome are major risks that can be overlooked by caregivers, who may feel that these effects are preferable to the aggressive/disruptive behavior. In one study, ziprasidone was reported to reduce maladaptive behaviors without leading to weight gain, and even to normalize weight and metabolic indices that had been substantially increased from previous treatment with another medication (Cohen et al. 2003).

Antidepressants. Newer antidepressants, chiefly the selective serotonin reuptake inhibitors (SSRIs), are used as first-line agents for the treatment of depression and obsessive-compulsive symptoms and, recently, for ADHD and anxiety disorders, in children and adolescents with mental retardation (Dosen 2001; Sovner et al. 2001). However, use of these agents may be now markedly curtailed due to concerns about emergence of suicidal ideation. SSRIs have been found in preliminary studies to be helpful, at least temporarily, for SIBs in some individuals. The choice of the particular SSRI largely depends on the side-effect profile.

Lithium. At present, because of side effects, lithium has been largely replaced by anticonvulsants as the first-line treatment. In people with mental retardation, lithium has been found to be useful occasionally in the treatment of aggressive behaviors (Langee 1990; McCracken and Diamond 1988). As with other drugs, side effects must be closely monitored, because the patient may not be able to report them.

Anticonvulsants. Other than their most common use in treatment of seizure disorders, anticonvulsants have been increasingly used in the general population, as well as in people with mental retardation, as mood stabilizers, and they have been reported as useful in controlling aggressive behavior (Glue 1989; Langee 1989; Sovner 1991). Hyponatremia and water intoxication are important side effects of carbamazepine that are sometimes overlooked. It also appears that phenobarbital, although helpful in controlling seizures, might result in hyperactivity and behavior problems (Alvarez 1998).

Anxiolytics. Anxiolytics have been used periodically in people with mental retardation for long-term treatment of aggressive behavior. However, there is no clear evidence of their effectiveness. People with mental retardation who receive benzodiazepines are described as being at risk for cognitive and memory impairments. Paradoxical reactions, such as behavioral disinhibition and an increase in stereotypic behaviors and SIBs, might occur. Behavioral side effects, including aggression, irritability, agitation, and worsening of preexisting maladaptive behaviors, have been reported to occur at a rate of 13%. For these reasons, it has been suggested that benzodiazepines should be prescribed only at low dosages and for limited durations (Kalachnik et al. 2002). Some studies have found buspirone to be effective, with few side effects. SSRIs are also tried occasionally as anxiolytics (review; AACAP 1999).

Stimulants. In persons with ADHD comorbid with mental retardation, stimulant drugs, in conjunction with behavioral intervention, may lead to an improvement in attention and hyperactivity. However, there is concern about side effects, particularly tics, especially in people who already exhibit stereotypic behaviors. Clonidine has been used for the treatment of ADHD in this population, and it may be effective in reducing overactivity. It is available in patch form, which may be important with people unwilling to take oral medication. However, blood pressure and pulse rate monitoring requires some cooperation.

Beta-blockers. Since the appearance of reports on the effectiveness of propranolol in the treatment of rage episodes after brain damage (D.T. Williams et al. 1982), beta-blockers have been used quite extensively for the treatment of "generic" aggression in people with mental retardation. The results have been mixed, most likely because of the heterogeneity of the aggressive behavior. Because depression is a potential side effect of these agents, they may reduce not only the patient's disruptive behavior but also his or her global level of functioning.

Other agents.   Naltrexone, an opiate receptor antagonist, has been studied in the treatment of SIBs in adults with severe mental retardation, on the basis of the hypothesis that the endogenous opioid system has a role in their pathogenesis. The results have been mixed; with some persons showing improvement and others experiencing exacerbation of the SIB.

Nonestablished treatments.   Some families have tried treating their children's mental retardation with various diets and regimens of vitamins, minerals, and other nutritional supplement combinations, such as megavitamin treatment; vitamin B_6 with magnesium; and gluten-free, yeast-free, and casein-free diets. However, there are no empirical studies supporting these treatments' effectiveness, and results of initial reports have not been subsequently reproduced. With some supplements, there is a danger of side effects, such as with very high doses of fat-soluble vitamins. It is important that clinicians specifically ask families about use of such agents.

■ Education and Habilitation of Persons With Mental Retardation

Children and adolescents with mental retardation and other disabilities are now expected to attend public schools, live at home, and participate in age-appropriate community activities. The goal of education and habilitation of persons with mental retardation is to help them achieve the highest possible quality of life (Schalock and Begab 1990). Our current approach is based on the "normalization principle," which refers to providing peo-

ple with mental retardation "patterns and conditions of everyday life which are as close as possible to the norms and patterns of the mainstream of society" (Nirje 1969, p. 181; Wolfensberger 1995).

Public Law 94–142 of 1975, with its subsequent amendments (now codified as IDEA [Individuals with Disabilities Education Act]), made appropriate public education available to all who needed it. The current standard is *inclusion,* which refers to placing a child in an age-appropriate regular classroom and providing in that classroom all services necessary because of the child's limitations. There should be collaboration between special-education and regular teachers, synchronization of the topics being taught to disabled and nondisabled students, employment of nondisabled peers as teaching buddies, provision of an individual teaching aide, and provision of appropriate special therapies.

In addition to federal laws, there are state laws pertaining to services for persons with disabilities. Clinicians should be aware of the current laws and regulations in their jurisdictions, in order to inform the families of children with disabilities whom they see about their right to services and to advocate for them. The local chapter of The ARC of the United States (formerly the Association for Retarded Citizens of the United States; 101 Wayne Avenue, Suite 650, Silver Spring, MD 20910; 301-565-3842) can provide valuable assistance in this regard. The ARC's Web site (http://www.thearc.org) offers a great deal of information on mental retardation and other developmental disabilities as well as links to various resources and organizations, including ones for families of persons with specific disorders (e.g., Down syndrome, Prader-Willi syndrome). Another very helpful Web site is that of the Federation for Children With Special Needs (http://www.fcsn.org).

References

Alvarez N: Barbiturates in the treatment of epilepsy in people with intellectual disability. J Intellect Disabil Res 42 (suppl 1):16–23, 1998

Aman MG, Collier-Crespin A, Lindsay RL: Pharmacotherapy of disorders in mental retardation. Eur Child Adolesc Psychiatry 9 (suppl 1): I98–I107, 2000

American Academy of Child and Adolescent Psychiatry [AACAP]: Practice parameters for the assessment and treatment of children, adolescents, and adults with mental retardation and comorbid mental disorders. J Am Acad Child Adolesc Psychiatry 38 (12, suppl):5S–31S, 1999

American Association on Mental Retardation: Mental Retardation: Definition, Classification, and Systems of Supports, 10th Edition. Washington, DC, American Association on Mental Retardation, 2002

American Psychiatric Association: Diagnostic and Statistical Manual of Mental Disorders, 4th Edition, Text Revision. Washington, DC, American Psychiatric Association, 2000

Astley SJ, Bailey D, Talbot C, et al: Fetal alcohol syndrome (FAS) primary prevention through FAS diagnosis, II: a comprehensive profile of 80 birth mothers of children with FAS. Alcohol 35:509–519, 2000

Beail N: What works for people with mental retardation? Critical commentary on cognitive-behavioral and psychodynamic psychotherapy research. Ment Retard 41:468–472, 2003

Ben-Asher E, Lancet D: NIPBL gene responsible for Cornelia de Lange syndrome, a severe developmental disorder. Isr Med Assoc J 6:571–572, 2004

Bony C, Zyka F, Tiran-Rajaofera I, et al: Warfarin fetopathy. Arch Pediatr 9:705–708, 2002

Bregman J: Current developments in the understanding of mental retardation, part II: psychopathology. J Am Acad Child Adolesc Psychiatry 30:861–872, 1991

Butler MG, Bitytel DC, Kibiryeva N, et al: Behavioral differences among subjects with Prader-Willi syndrome and type I or type II deletion and maternal disomy. Pediatrics 113 (3 pt 1): 565–573, 2004

Cheng-Shannon J, McGough JJ, Pataki C, et al: Second-generation antipsychotic medications in children and adolescents. J Child Adolesc Psychopharmacol 14:372–394, 2004

Clarren SK, Smith DW, Hansen JW: Helmet treatment for plagiocephaly and congenital muscular torticollis. J Pediatr 94:43–46, 1979

Cohen S, Fitzgerald B, Okos A, et al: Weight, lipids, glucose, and behavioral measures with ziprasidone treatment in a population with mental retardation. J Clin Psychiatry 64:60–62, 2003

Connor DF, Steingard RJ: A clinical approach to the pharmacotherapy of aggression in children and adolescents. Ann N Y Acad Sci 794:290–307, 1996

Curry C, Stevenson R, Aughton D: Evaluation of mental retardation: recommendations of a consensus conference. Am J Med Genet 72:468–477, 1997

Dagnan D, Sandhu S: Social comparison, self-esteem and depression in people with intellectual disability. J Intellect Disabil Res 43:372–379, 1999

Delach J, Rosengren S, Kaplan L, et al: Comparison of high resolution chromosome banding and fluorescence in situ hybridization (FISH) for the diagnosis of Prader-Willi syndrome and Angelman syndrome. Genetics 52:85–91, 1995

Dosen A: Pharmacotherapy in mentally retarded children, in Treating Mental Illness and Behavior Disorders in Children and Adults With Mental Retardation. Edited by Dosen A, Day K. Washington, DC: American Psychiatric Publishing, 2001, pp 429–450

Dunn KB, Clarren SK: The origin of prenatal and postnatal postural deformities. Pediatr Clin North Am 33:1277–1297, 1986

Dykens EM: Measuring behavioral phenotypes: provocations from the "new genetics." Am J Ment Retard 99:522–532, 1995

Dykens EM: Annotation: psychopathology in children with intellectual disability. J Child Psychol Psychiatry 41:407–417, 2000

Einspieler C, Kerr AM, Prechtl HF: Is the early development of girls with Rett disorder really normal? Pediatr Res 57(5 pt 1):696–700, 2005

Feinstein C, Reiss AL: Psychiatric disorder in mentally retarded children and adolescents: the challenges of meaningful diagnosis. Child Adolesc Psychiatr Clin N Am 5:827–852, 1996

Gillberg C, Persson E, Grufman M, et al: Psychiatric disorders in mildly and severely mentally retarded urban children and adolescents: epidemiological aspects. Br J Psychiatry 149:68–74, 1986

Glue P: Rapid cycling affective disorder in the mentally retarded. Biol Psychiatry 26:250–256, 1989

Graham JM Jr: Smith's Recognizable Patterns of Human Deformation. Philadelphia, PA, WB Saunders, 1988

Gualtieri CT: The differential diagnosis of self-injurious behavior in mentally retarded people. Psychopharmacol Bull 25:358–363, 1989

Gualtieri CT, Schroeder SR, Hicks RE, et al: Tardive dyskinesia in young mentally retarded individuals. Arch Gen Psychiatry 43:335–340, 1986

Guttler F, Azen C, Guldberg P, et al: Relationship among genotype, biochemical phenotype, and cognitive performance in females with phenylalanine hydroxylase deficiency: report from the Maternal Phenylketonuria Collaborative Study. Pediatrics 104:258–262, 1999

Hoyme HE, May PA, Kalberg WO, et al: A practical approach to diagnosis of fetal alcohol spectrum disorders: clarification of the 1996 Institute of Medicine criteria. Pediatrics 115:39–47, 2005

Hagerman RJ, Silverman AC (eds): Fragile X Syndrome: Diagnosis, Treatment, and Research. Baltimore, MD, Johns Hopkins University Press, 1996

Hall JG: Invited editorial comment: analysis of Pena-Shokeir phenotype. Am J Med Genet 25:99, 1986

Hanshaw GB: Developmental abnormalities associated with congenital CMV infection. Advances in Teratology 4:64–93, 1970

Harris JC: Developmental Neuropsychiatry. Oxford, UK, Oxford University Press, 1995

Hollins S: Psychotherapeutic methods, in Treating Mental Illness and Behavior Disorders in Children and Adults With Mental Retardation. Edited by Dosen A, Day K. Washington, DC, American Psychiatric Publishing, 2001, pp 27–44

Holm VA: Rett's syndrome: a progressive developmental disability in girls. J Dev Behav Pediatr 6:32–36, 1985

Holmes LB: Congenital malformations, in Manual of Neonatal Care. Edited by Doherty JP, Stark AR. Boston, MA, Little, Brown, 1980, pp 91–96

Hoyme EH, Higginbottom MC, Jones KL: Vascular etiology of disruptive structural defects in monozygotic twins. Pediatrics 67:288–291, 1981

Hoyme HE, May PA, Kalberg WO, et al: A practical approach to diagnosis of fetal alcohol spectrum disorders: clarification of the 1996 Institute of Medicine criteria. Pediatrics 115:39–47, 2005

Hudgins L, Cassidy S: Congenital anomalies, in Developmental Behavioral Pediatrics, 3rd Edition. Edited by Levine MD, Carey WB, Crocker AC. Philadelphia, PA, WB Saunders, 1999, pp 249–262

Jan JE, Abroms IF, Freeman RD, et al: Rapid cycling in severely multidisabled children: a form of bipolar affective disorder? Pediatr Neurol 10:34–39, 1994

Jones KL: Smith's Recognizable Patterns of Human Malformation, 5th Edition. Philadelphia, PA, WB Saunders, 1997

Kalachnik JE, Hanzel TE, Sevenich R, et al: Benzodiazepine behavioral side effects: review and implications for individuals with mental retardation. Am J Ment Retard 107:376–410, 2002

Kaplan LC: Assessment and management of infants and children with multiple congenital anomalies, in Developmental Disabilities: Delivery of Medical Care for Children and Adults. Edited by Rubin IL, Crocker AC. Philadelphia, PA, Lea & Febiger, 1989, pp 97–116

Kaplan LC: Neural tube defects, in Manual of Neonatal Care. Edited by Cloherty JP, Start AR. Boston, MA, Little, Brown, 1998

Kaplan LC, Wharton R, Elias E, et al: Clinical heterogeneity associated with deletions in the long arm of chromosome 15: report of three new cases and their possible genetic significance. Am J Med Genet 28:45–53, 1987

Katz SL, Gershon AA, Hotez PJ, et al (eds): Krugman's Infectious Diseases of Children, 10th Edition. St. Louis, MO, Mosby, 1998

Kerker BD, Owens PL, Zigler E, et al: Mental health disorders among individuals with mental retardation: challenges to accurate prevalence estimates. Public Health Rep 119:409–417, 2004

Kerr AM: Rett syndrome: British longitudinal study, in Mental Retardation and Medical Care. Edited by Roosendaal JJ. Proceedings of the European Congress on Mental Retardation and Medical Care, Zeist, Uitgeverij Kerokebosch, April 21–24, 1991

Kishino T, Lalande M, Watstaff J: *UBE3A/E6-AP* mutations cause Angelman syndrome. Nat Genet 15:70, 1997

Knoll JH, Nichols RD, Magenis RE, et al: Angelman syndrome: three molecular classes identified with chromosome 15q11q13 specific DNA markers. Am J Hum Genet 47:149–155, 1990

Koren G, Gladstone D, Robeson C, et al: The perception of teratogenic risk of cocaine. Teratology 46:567–571, 1992

Kuban KCK, Leviton A: Cerebral palsy. N Engl J Med 330: 188–195, 1994

Laird CD: Proposed mechanism of inheritance and expression of the human fragile X syndrome of mental retardation. Genetics 117:587–590, 1987

Langee HR: A retrospective study of mentally retarded patients with behavioral disorders who were treated with carbamazepine. Am J Ment Retard 93:640–643, 1989

Langee HR: Retrospective study of lithium use for institutionalized mentally retarded individuals with behavior disorders. Am J Ment Retard 94:448–452, 1990

Leroy JG: Heredity, development and behavior, in Developmental-Behavioral Pediatrics, 2nd Edition. Edited by Levine MD, Carey WB, Crocker AC. Philadelphia, PA, WB Saunders, 1992, pp 193–212

Levy HL, Waisbren SE, Flemming G, et al: Pregnancy experiences in the woman with mild hyperphenylalaninemia. Pediatrics 112:1548–1552, 2003

Linna SL, Moilanen I, Ebeling H, et al: Psychiatric symptoms in children with intellectual disability. Eur Child Adolesc Psychiatry 8 (suppl 4):77–82, 1999

Lofts RH, Schroeder SR, Maier RH: Effects of serum zinc supplementation on pica behavior of persons with mental retardation. Am J Ment Retard 95:103–109, 1990

Lynch EC, Staloch NH: Parental perceptions of physicians' communication in the informing process. Ment Retard 26:77–81, 1988

Mary NL: Reactions of black, Hispanic, and white mothers to having a child with handicaps. Ment Retard 28:1–5, 1990

Masi G, Favilla L, Mucci M: Generalized anxiety disorder in adolescents and young adults with mild mental retardation. Psychiatry 63:54–64, 2000

Matson JL, Bamburg JW, Mayville EA, et al: Psychopharmacology and mental retardation: a 10 year review (1990–1999). Res Dev Disabil 21:263–296, 2000

Mayes LC, Kirk V, Haywood N, et al: Changing cognitive outcome in preterm infants with hyaline membrane disease. Am J Dis Child 139:20–24, 1985

McCracken JT, Diamond RP: Bipolar disorder in mildly retarded adolescents. J Am Acad Child Adolesc Psychiatry 27:494–499, 1988

McLaren J, Bryson SE: Review of recent epidemiological studies of mental retardation: prevalence, associated disorders, and etiology. Am J Ment Retard 92:243–254, 1987

Needleman HL, Schell A, Bellinger D, et al: The long-term effects of exposure to low doses of lead in childhood. An 11-year follow-up report. N Engl J Med 322:83–88, 1990

Nichols EK: Human Gene Therapy. Cambridge, MA, Harvard University Press, 1988

Nirje B: The normalization principle and its human management applications, in Changing Patterns in Residential Services for the Mentally Retarded. Edited by Kugel R, Wolfensberger W. Washington, DC, President's Committee on Mental Retardation, 1969, p 181

Patja K, Iivanainen M, Raitasuo S, et al: Suicide mortality in mental retardation: a 35-year follow-up study. Acta Psychiatr Scand 103:307–311, 2001

Pozdnyakova I, Regan L: New insights into fragile X syndrome. Relating genotype to phenotype at the molecular level. FEBS J 272:872–878, 2005

Pueschel SM, Pueschel JK (eds): Biomedical Concerns in Persons With Down Syndrome. Baltimore, MD, Paul H Brookes, 1992

Ravn K, Nielsen JB, Skjeldal OH, et al: Large genomic rearrangements in MECP2. Hum Mutat 25:324, 2005

Reid AH: Schizophrenic and paranoid syndromes in persons with mental retardation: assessment and diagnosis, in Mental Health Aspects of Mental Retardation. Edited by Fletcher RJ, Dosen A. New York, Lexington Books, 1993, pp 98–110

Reiss S: Handbook of Challenging Behavior: Mental Health Aspects of Mental Retardation. Worthington, OH, IDS Publishing, 1994

Reiss S, Aman M: Psychotropic Medication & Developmental Disabilities: The International Consensus Handbook. Columbus, OH, Ohio State University, 1998

Reiss S, Rojahn J: Joint occurrence of depression and aggression in children and adults with mental retardation. J Intellect Disabil Res 37:287–294, 1993

Rittler M, Lopez-Camelo J, Castilla EE: Monitoring congenital rubella embryopathy. Birth Defects Res A Clin Mol Teratol 70:939–943, 2004

Royal College of Psychiatrists: DC-LD (Diagnostic Criteria for Psychiatric Disorders for Use With Adults With Learning Disabilities/Mental Retardation). London, Gaskell, 2001

Russell AT, Tanguay PE: Mental illness and mental retardation: cause or coincidence? Am J Ment Defic 85:570–574, 1981

Ryan R: Posttraumatic stress disorder in persons with developmental disabilities. Community Ment Health J 30:45–54, 1994

Samlaska CP, James WD, Sperling LC: Scalp whorls. J Am Acad Dermatol 21(3 pt 1):553–556, 1989

Schalock RL, Begab MJ (eds): Quality of Life: Perspectives and Issues. Washington, DC, American Association on Mental Retardation, 1990

Scriver CL, Clow CL: Phenylketonuria: epitome of human biochemical genetics (2 parts). N Engl J Med 303:1336–1394, 1980

Seshia SS, Johnston R, Kasian G: Non-traumatic coma in childhood: clinical variables in prediction of outcome. Dev Med Child Neurol 25:493–501, 1983

Sigman M: Individual and group psychotherapy with mentally retarded adolescents, in Children With Emotional Disorders and Developmental Disabilities. Edited by Sigman M. Orlando, FL, Grune & Stratton, 1985, pp 259–276

Sovner R: Use of anticonvulsant agents for treatment of neuropsychiatric disorders in the developmentally disabled, in Mental Retardation: Developing Pharmacotherapies. Edited by Ratey JJ. Washington, DC, American Psychiatric Publishing, 1991, pp 83–106

Sovner R, Hurley AD: Do the mentally retarded suffer from affective illness? Arch Gen Psychiatry 40:61–67, 1983

Sovner R, Pary R, Dosen A, et al: Antidepressant drugs, in Treating Mental Illness and Behavior Disorders in Children and Adults with Mental Retardation. Edited by Dosen A, Day K. Washington, DC, American Psychiatric Publishing, 2001, pp 179–200

Stavrakaki C, Klein C: Psychotherapies with the mentally retarded. Psychiatr Clin North Am 9:733–743, 1985

Stromme P, Diseth TH: Prevalence of psychiatric diagnoses in children with mental retardation: data from a population-based study. Dev Med Child Neurol 42:266–270, 2000

Szymanski LS: Psychiatric diagnostic evaluation of mentally retarded individuals. J Am Acad Child Psychiatry 16:67–87, 1977

Szymanski LS: Happiness as a goal of treatment. Journal of the American Association on Mental Retardation 105:352–362, 2000

Szymanski LS, Biederman J: Depression and anorexia nervosa of persons with Down syndrome. Am J Ment Defic 89:246–251, 1984

Szymanski LS, Crocker AC: Mental retardation, in Comprehensive Textbook of Psychiatry, 4th Edition. Edited by Kaplan HI, Sadock BJ. Baltimore, MD, Williams & Wilkins, 1985, pp 1635–1671

Szymanski LS: Individual psychotherapy with retarded persons, in Emotional Disorders of Mentally Retarded Persons. Edited by Szymanski LS, Tanguay PE. Baltimore, MD, University Park Press, 1980a, pp 131–148

Szymanski LS: Psychiatric diagnosis of retarded persons, in Emotional Disorders of Mentally Retarded Persons. Edited by Szymanski LS, Tanguay PE. Baltimore, MD, University Park Press, 1980b, pp 61–81

Tantravahi U, Nicholls RD, Stroh H, et al: Quantitative calibration and use of DNA probes for investigating chromosome abnormalities in the Prader-Willi syndrome. Am J Med Genet 33:78–87, 1989

Tantravahi U, Wheeler P: Molecular testing for prenatal diagnosis. Clin Lab Med 23:481–502, 2003

Tessier P: Anatomical classification of facial, cranio-facial, and latero-facial clefts. J Maxillofac Surg 4:69–92, 1976

Tonge B, Einfeld S: The trajectory of psychiatric disorders in young people with intellectual disabilities. Aust N Z J Psychiatry 34:80–84, 2000

University of Minnesota, the College of Education and Human Development: MR/DD Data Brief, Vol 2, No. 1, p 5, 2000. Available at: http://rtc.umn.edu/nhis/databrief2/index.html. Accessed July 2003

Varela MC, Kok F, Setian N, et al: Impact of molecular mechanisms, including deletion size, on Prader-Willi syndrome phenotype: study of 75 patients. Clin Genet 67:47–52, 2005

Walters AS, Barrett RP, Knapp LG, et al: Suicidal behavior in children and adolescents with mental retardation. Res Dev Disabil 16:85–96, 1995

Weglage J, Pietsch M, Feldmann R, et al: Normal clinical outcome in untreated subjects with mild hyperphenylalaninemia. Pediatr Res 49:532–536, 2001

Wilcken B, Smith A, Brown DA: Urine screening for aminoacidopathies: is it beneficial? Results of a long-term follow-up of cases detected by screening one million babies. J Pediatr 97:492–496, 1980

Williams CA: Neurological aspects of the Angelman syndrome. Brain Dev 27:88–94, 2005

Williams DT, Mehl R, Yudofsky S, et al: The effects of propranolol on uncontrolled rage outbursts in children and adolescents with organic brain dysfunction. J Am Acad Child Psychiatry 21:129–135, 1982

Wolfensberger W: The Principle of Normalization in Human Services. Toronto, Ontario, Canada, National Institute on Mental Retardation, 1972

World Health Organization: International Classification of Diseases and Related Health Problems, 10th Revision. Geneva, World Health Organization, 1992

Wuu KD, Chiu PC, Li Sy, et al: Chromosomal and biochemical screening on mentally retarded school children in Taiwan. Jpn J Human Genet 36:267–274, 1991

Zipf WB: Prader-Willi syndrome: the care and treatment of infants, children, and adults. Adv Pediatr 51:409–434, 2004

Self-Assessment Questions

Select the single best response for each question.

10.1 DSM-IV-TR (American Psychiatric Association 2000) criteria require an IQ score in which of the following ranges for a diagnosis of "severe mental retardation"?

  A. Below 20–25.
  B. Between 20–25 and 35–40.
  C. Between 35–40 and 50–55.
  D. Between 50–55 and 70.
  E. None of the above.

10.2 Data from the National Health Interview Survey for 1994–1995 (University of Minnesota 2000) indicate that the combined prevalence of mental retardation and developmental disabilities in the United States during that period was approximately what percentage of the population?

  A. 1.5%.
  B. 3%.
  C. 5%.
  D. 7%.
  E. 9%.

10.3 Prader-Willi syndrome in children is characterized by all of the following *except*

  A. Obesity.
  B. Hypogonadism in males.
  C. Spasticity.
  D. Dysmorphic features.
  E. Hyperphagia.

10.4 DNA probes and molecular biology analyses have identified the q11–q12 region of chromosome 15 as the abnormal region of the human genome responsible for which of the following syndromes?

  A. Prader-Willi syndrome and Angelman's syndrome.
  B. Angelman's syndrome and fragile X syndrome.
  C. Prader-Willi syndrome and fragile X syndrome.
  D. Prader-Willi syndrome and Williams syndrome.
  E. Fragile X syndrome and Rett's disorder.

10.5 The most common inherited form of mental retardation is

  A. Angelman's syndrome.
  B. Rett's disorder.
  C. Williams syndrome.
  D. Prader-Willi syndrome.
  E. Fragile X syndrome.

10.6 Current estimates of the prevalence of schizophrenia in individuals with mental retardation are in the range of

  A. 1%–3%.
  B. 3%–5%.
  C. 5%–8%.
  D. 8%–10%.
  E. 10%–12%.

Autistic Disorders

Luke Y. Tsai, M.D.

Definition and Diagnostic Criteria

■ Historical Background

In 1943, Kanner described a group of 11 children with a previously unrecognized disorder. He noted a number of characteristic features in these children, such as an inability to develop relationships with people, extreme aloofness, a delay in speech development, and noncommunicative use of speech. Other features included repeated simple patterns of play activities and islets of ability. He described these children as having "come into the world with innate inability to form the usual, biologically provided affective contact with people" (Kanner 1943, p. 250). Despite the variety of individual differences that appeared in the case descriptions, Kanner believed that only two features were of diagnostic significance: autistic aloneness and obsessive insistence on sameness. He adopted the term *early infantile autism* to describe this disorder and called attention to the fact that its symptoms were already evident in infancy.

However, controversy continued over the definition of the disorder because the name *autism* was ill chosen. It led to confusion with Bleuler's (1911/1950) use of the same term to describe schizophrenia in adults. This confusion led many clinicians to use terms such as *childhood schizophrenia, borderline psychosis, symbiotic psychosis,* and *infantile psychosis* as interchangeable diagnoses. Each label had its definition and roots in a particular view of the nature and causation of autism.

In an attempt to clarify the confusion, Eisenberg and Kanner (1956) reduced the essential symptoms to two: extreme self-isolation and preoccupation with the preservation of sameness. The peculiar abnormality of language was considered to be secondary to the disturbance of human relatedness and, hence, not essential. They also expanded the age at onset to the first 2 years of life.

Rutter (1968) critically analyzed the existing empirical evidence and proposed four essential characteristics of infantile autism: 1) a lack of social interest and responsiveness; 2) impaired language, ranging from absence of speech to peculiar speech patterns; 3) bizarre motor behavior, ranging from rigid and limited play patterns to more complex ritualistic and compulsive behavior; and 4) early onset, before age 30 months. These features were present in nearly all children with autism. There were many other specific features, but they were unevenly distributed. The definitions of Kanner (1943) and Rutter (1968) paved the way for two sets of criteria that were widely used by clinicians all over the world: ICD-9-CM (*International Classification of Diseases and Related Health Problems,* 9th Revision, Clinical Modification) (U.S. Department of Health and Human Services 1980) and DSM-III (American Psychiatric Association 1980).

■ Diagnostic Concepts

Although ICD-9-CM and DSM-III had similar definitions and diagnostic criteria for infantile autism, differences in the concept of autism were apparent. In ICD-9-CM, infantile autism was classified as a subtype of "psychoses with origin specific to childhood," whereas in DSM-III and DSM-III-R (American Psychiatric Association 1987), infantile autism was viewed as a type of pervasive developmental disorder (PDD), defined as a group of severe, early developmental disorders characterized by delays and distortions in the development of social skills, cognition, and communication.

In 1994, the American Psychiatric Association published DSM-IV (with its Text Revision, DSM-IV-TR, published in 2000), which continues to adopt the diagnostic term *pervasive developmental disorders.* In DSM-IV and DSM-IV-TR, these disorders included 1) autistic disorder; 2) Rett's disorder; 3) childhood disintegrative disorder; 4) Asperger's disorder; and 5) pervasive developmental disorder not otherwise specified (PDDNOS), including atypical autism. These texts also offer operational diagnostic criteria for all of the subtypes of PDDs except PDDNOS. It is obvious that the concept of PDDs in DSM-IV and DSM-IV-TR is a

"splitters" approach. This approach supports the taxonomic validity of each subtype and aims to facilitate research in the subclassification of these disorders. Although the DSM-IV and DSM-IV-TR diagnostic criteria for PDDs are based on a field study (Volkmar et al. 1994), it is expected that these criteria will not satisfy everyone and will be revised when improved understanding and further knowledge are gained. Nonetheless, it is hoped that refinement of the criteria would not only ensure more reliable diagnosis but also provide further support for the taxonomic validity of the various subtypes of PDDs.

Although the concept of PDDs was retained in DSM-III-R, the diagnostic criteria for autistic disorder were revised considerably. The DSM-III criteria were descriptive, whereas the menu-like scheme of DSM-III-R criteria required the presence of a minimum number of criteria in each of the three cardinal areas of deficits. The revised criteria were much more concrete, observable, and operational than those in DSM-III. The revised criteria did not require raters to determine subjectively whether a "pervasive impairment" or a "gross deficit" was present; hence, clinicians no longer hesitated to use the diagnosis of autistic disorder in older and higher-functioning autistic individuals. DSM-III-R broadened the diagnostic concept of autism from that in DSM-III, allowing for the gradation of behavior seen in autistic individuals. In the DSM-IV and DSM-IV-TR diagnostic criteria for autistic disorder, the total number of diagnostic criteria has been reduced to 12, and the required minimum number for a diagnosis of autistic disorder has been reduced to 6 (Table 20–1). These changes were made to facilitate the use of the criteria by clinicians while the diagnostic validity and reliability are maintained at a high level.

Table 11–1.   DSM-IV-TR diagnostic criteria for autistic disorder

A.   A total of six (or more) items from (1), (2), and (3), with at least two from (1), and one each
     from (2) and (3):
     (1)   qualitative impairment in social interaction, as manifested by at least two of the
           following:
           (a) marked impairment in the use of multiple nonverbal behaviors such as eye-to-eye
               gaze, facial expression, body postures, and gestures to regulate social interaction
           (b) failure to develop peer relationships appropriate to developmental level
           (c) a lack of spontaneous seeking to share enjoyment, interests, or achievements with
               other people (e.g., by a lack of showing, bringing, or pointing out objects of
               interest)
           (d) lack of social or emotional reciprocity
     (2)   qualitative impairments in communication as manifested by at least one of the
           following:
           (a) delay in, or total lack of, the development of spoken language (not accompanied
               by an attempt to compensate through alternative modes of communication such as
               gesture or mime)
           (b) in individuals with adequate speech, marked impairment in the ability to initiate or
               sustain a conversation with others
           (c) stereotyped and repetitive use of language or idiosyncratic language
           (d) lack of varied, spontaneous make-believe play or social imitative play appropriate
               to developmental level
     (3)   restricted repetitive and stereotyped patterns of behavior, interests, and activities, as
           manifested by at least one of the following:
           (a) encompassing preoccupation with one or more stereotyped and restricted patterns
               of interest that is abnormal either in intensity or focus
           (b) apparently inflexible adherence to specific, nonfunctional routines or rituals
           (c) stereotyped and repetitive motor mannerisms (e.g., hand or finger flapping or
               twisting, or complex whole-body movements)
           (d) persistent preoccupation with parts of objects

B.   Delays or abnormal functioning in at least one of the following areas, with onset prior
     to age 3 years: (1) social interaction, (2) language as used in social communication, or
     (3) symbolic or imaginative play.

C.   The disturbance is not better accounted for by Rett's disorder or childhood disintegrative
     disorder.

Source.   Reprinted from the *Diagnostic and Statistical Manual of Mental Disorders,* 4th Edition, Text
Revision. Washington, DC, American Psychiatric Association, 2000. Copyright 2000, American Psychiatric Association. Used with permission.

Diagnostic Rating Scales

Several commonly used diagnostic rating
scales have been developed for clinicians
and investigators to screen individuals
for suspected autistic disorder and to
diagnose the disorder: the Autism Behavior Checklist (ABC), Autism Diagnostic Interview—Revised (ADI-R), Autism Diagnostic Observation Schedule
(ADOS), Pre-Linguistic Autism Diagnostic Observation Schedule (PL-ADOS),
Autism Screening Questionnaire (ASQ),
Autism Spectrum Disorder Screening
Questionnaire (ASDSQ), Checklist for
Autism in Toddlers (CHAT), and Child-

hood Autism Rating Scales (CARS). All of these scales have been tested for their validity and reliability.

Clinical Features

■ Age at Onset

Several studies have demonstrated that children younger than 3 years can be reliably identified as potentially having PDDs (Baird et al. 2000; Lord 1995; Stone et al. 1999).

Kanner (1943) described autism as beginning shortly after birth. In a study of parental recognition of developmental abnormalities in a sample of 82 consecutive referrals, De Giacomo and Fombonne (1998) found that the mean age of children was 19.1 months when the parents first became concerned and that the first professional advice was sought when children were 24.1 months old.

Other investigators, however, have observed that in perhaps one-third of the autistic children, parents reported a clinical picture indistinguishable from that of Kanner's original autism, which arose after a period of seemingly normal development (up to age 2 years). Whether early development in these children had been truly normal in all aspects is difficult to determine. Subtle signs occurring during the first 2 years of life may have been forgotten, overlooked, or denied by the parents because of difficulty in recall, anxiety, or lack of knowledge of normal child development. Nonetheless, a few investigators had reported the onset of typically autistic behavior in the third to fifth year of life.

Davidovitch et al. (2000) interviewed 39 mothers of autistic children and found that 19 (47.5%) of the autistic children regressed in verbal and nonverbal communication and social abilities but not in motor abilities. Mean age of regression was 24

months, with 11 children who regressed before that age and 8 who regressed after that age. There was little difference between those children who regressed and those who did not in maternal perceptions and reports of development, family, and medical history. Kobayashi and Murata (1998) studied setback phenomenon (regression) in 179 children for whom precise records about infancy were available. They found a significantly higher rate of epilepsy and a significantly lower level of language development on entering elementary school among the setback group compared with the non-setback group.

■ Deficits in Social Behavior

Social deficits were considered by Kanner (1943) to be central to the pathogenesis of autism. Autistic infants tend to avoid eye contact and to show little conventional interest in the human voice. They do not assume an anticipatory posture or put up their arms to be picked up in the way that children do who are not autistic. They are indifferent to affection and seldom show facial responsiveness. As a result, parents often suspect that the child is deaf. In more intelligent autistic individuals, lack of social responsiveness may not be obvious until well into the second year of life.

In early childhood, autistic children continue to show deviation in eye contact, but they may enjoy a tickle or may passively accept physical contact, such as lap sitting. They do not develop a bonding relationship with their parents. They generally do not follow their parents around the house. They tend to lack social referencing and to not look toward an adult in the presence of an ambiguous and unfamiliar stimulus. Most autistic children do not show normal separation or stranger anxiety. Adults usually are treated as interchangeable, so that these children may approach a stranger almost as readily as they do their parents. They generally are not interested in being with or playing with other children, or they may even actively avoid other children.

In middle childhood, greater awareness of the attachment to parents and other familiar adults may develop. However, serious social difficulties continue. These children show a lack of interest in playing group games, and they are unable to form peer relationships. Some of the least disabled may become passively involved in other children's games or physical play. However, this apparent sociability is usually superficial.

As autistic children grow older, they may become affectionate and friendly with their parents and siblings. However, they seldom initiate social contacts and they show an apparent lack of positive interest in people. Some of the less severely impaired autistic individuals may desire friends. However, a lack of response to other people's interests and emotions as well as a lack of appreciation of humor often result in the autistic youngster's saying or doing socially inappropriate things that usually prevent the development of friendships.

■ Problems in Communication

Impairment in Nonverbal Communication

Autistic infants show their needs through crying and screaming. In early childhood, they may develop the concrete gesture of pulling adults by the hand to the object that is desired or wanted. This is often done without a socially appropriate facial expression. Nodding and shaking of the head are seldom seen either as a substitute for or as an accompaniment of speech. They generally do not participate in imitative games. These children are less likely than other children to copy or follow their parents' activities.

In middle and late childhood, they use gestures infrequently, even when they understand other people's gestures fairly well. A small number of autistic children do develop imitative play skills, but these tend to be stereotyped repetitive actions based on their own experience.

Generally speaking, autistic children are able to show their emotions of joy, fear, or anger, but they tend to show only the extreme of emotions. Facial expressions that ordinarily reinforce meaning are usually absent. Some autistic people appear wooden and expressionless much of the time.

Impairment in Understanding of Speech

Comprehension of speech is impaired to various degrees. Severely retarded autistic people may never develop any awareness of the meaning of speech. Children who are less severely impaired may follow simple instructions given in an immediate present context or with the aid of gestures. When impairment is mild, only the comprehension of subtle or abstract meanings may be affected. Humor and idiomatic expressions can be confusing for even the brightest autistic person.

Impairment in Speech Development

Many autistic people have an impaired amount or pattern of babble in their first year. About one-half of autistic patients remain mute for their entire lives (Ricks and Wing 1976). When speech has developed, it usually reveals many abnormalities. Meaningless immediate or delayed echolalia may be the only kind of speech acquired in some autistic individuals. However, although the echolalic speech may be produced quite accurately, the child often has little or no comprehension of its meaning. When echolalia is extreme, distorted syntax and fragmented speech patterns result. Other autistic people may develop appropriate use of phrases copied from others. This is often accompanied by pronoun reversal in the early stages of language development.

Often the mechanical production of speech is impaired. The speech may be like that of a robot, characterized by a monotonous, flat delivery with little lability, change of emphasis, or emotional expression. Some children may use speech primarily for self-stimulatory purposes. Such speech tends to be repetitive in nature, with words, phrases, or sounds being produced over and over without any apparent relation to the environment or ongoing activity. Problems of pronunciation are common in young autistic children, but these tend to diminish with increasing age. There may be a marked contrast between clearly enunciated echolalic speech and poorly pronounced spontaneous speech. There may be chanting or singsong speech, with odd prolongation of sounds, syllables, and words. A question-like intonation may be used for propositional statements. Odd respiratory rhythms may produce staccato speech in some autistic individuals.

Immature and abnormal grammatical constructions are often present in the spontaneous speech of autistic people. Words and phrases may be used idiosyncratically, or phrases may be telegraphic and distorted. Words of similar sound or related meaning may be muddled. Autistic people may label objects by their use or else coin words of their own. Prepositions, conjunctions, and pronouns often are dropped from phrases or are used incorrectly.

When functional speech develops, it tends not to be used in the usual way for social communication. Usually autistic people rely on stereotyped phrases and repetition when they talk. Their speech almost always fails to convey imagination, abstraction, or subtle emotion. Their language skills are generally poor in talking about anything outside the immediate

context. They tend to talk about their special interests, and the same information tends to recur whenever the same subject is raised. The most advanced autistic people may be able to exchange concrete pieces of information that interest them, but once the conversation departs from this level, they become lost and may withdraw from social contact. In general, the ordinary to-and-fro chatter of a reciprocal interaction is lacking. Thus, they give the impression of talking *to* someone rather than *with* someone.

■ Unusual Patterns of Behavior

Autistic children's unusual responses to their environment may take several forms. All of the items of behavior mentioned here are common in autistic children, but a single child seldom shows all the features at one time.

Resistance to Change

Autistic children are disturbed by changes in the familiar environment, and tantrums may follow even a minor change in everyday routine. Many autistic children line up toys or objects and become very distressed if these are disturbed. The behavior is twice as common in retarded autistic children as in autistic youngsters with normal intelligence (Bartak and Rutter 1976). Almost all autistic children resist learning or practicing a new activity.

Ritualistic or Compulsive Behaviors

Ritualistic or compulsive behaviors usually involve rigid routines (e.g., insistence on eating particular foods) or stereotyped, repetitive motor acts, such as hand clapping or finger mannerisms (e.g., twisting, flicking movements carried out near the face). Some children develop preoccupations, such as spending a great deal of time memorizing weather information, state capitals, or birth dates of family members. In adolescence, some of these behaviors may develop into obsessional symptoms (e.g., repeatedly asking the same question, which must be answered in a specific manner) and compulsive behaviors (e.g., compulsive touching of certain objects). Ritualistic or compulsive behaviors are more often displayed by nonretarded people with autism than by retarded people with autism (Bartak and Rutter 1976).

Abnormal Attachments

Many autistic children develop intense attachments to odd objects (e.g., pipe cleaners, small plastic toys). The child may carry the object at all times and protest or throw tantrums if it is removed; if the object is not eventually returned to the child, he or she frequently chooses a new object.

Unusual Responses to Sensory Experiences

Children with autism may have a fascination with lights, patterns, sounds, spinning objects, and tactile sensations. Objects often are manipulated without regard for their usual functions. Young autistic children may perseveringly line up, stack, or twirl objects. They may repetitively flush toilets or turn on and off light switches. They may have a continuing preoccupation with certain features of objects, such as their texture, taste, smell, color, or shape. These children are often either underresponsive or overresponsive to sensory stimuli. Thus, they may be suspected of being deaf, nearsighted, or blind. Autistic children may actively avoid gentle physical contact but react with intense pleasure to rough games. Some autistic children may follow extreme food fads.

■ Disturbance of Motility

The typical motor milestones may be delayed, but they are often within normal range. Young autistic children usually have difficulties with motor imitation, especially when they have to learn by watching and when the movements have to be reversed in direction. Many young autistic children are markedly overactive, but they may become underactive in adolescence. The autistic child often displays grimacing, hand flapping or twisting, toe walking, lunging, jumping, darting or pacing, body rocking and swaying, and head rolling or banging. Some of these movements appear to be involuntary. In some cases, they may appear intermittently, whereas in other cases, they are continuously present. They are usually interrupted by episodes of immobility and odd posturing, with head bowed and arms flexed at the elbow. Many children with autism exhibit body-tensing movements when they are excited about or absorbed in some sensory experience, such as watching a spinning toy.

■ Intelligence and Cognitive Deficits

Most autistic children are mentally retarded (Rutter 1978). About 40%–60% of autistic children have an IQ below 50; only 20%–30% have an IQ of 70 or more. Follow-up studies have shown that retardation present at the time of initial diagnosis tends to persist (Freeman et al. 1985).

A Wechsler Adult Intelligence Scale (WAIS) profile characterized by a verbal IQ lower than performance IQ (VIQ < PIQ) with the lowest subtest score on comprehension and highest on block design had been associated with autistic disorder. However, a study of 81 high-functioning subjects with autistic order by Siegel et al. (1996) found that autistic individuals could demonstrate a wide range of ability levels and patterns on the Wechsler scales, without a single characteristic prototype.

Although autistic children with low IQ and those with high IQ are similar in terms of the main symptoms associated with autism, those with a low IQ show a more severely impaired social development and are more likely to display deviant social responses, such as touching or smelling people, stereotypies, and self-injury (Bartak and Rutter 1976). One-third of mentally retarded autistic youngsters develop seizure disorders; this condition is less prevalent in those who are not retarded (Rutter 1978). The prognosis is both worse and different for autistic people with low IQ (Rutter 1970). Because the difference in outcome according to IQ is so marked, it is essential to obtain an accurate assessment of intelligence during the initial evaluation of every autistic child.

Kanner (1943) noted the excellent rote memories of autistic children. The most common areas of special skills tend to be musical, mechanical, and mathematical abilities. Rutter and Lockyer (1967) noted that in contrast to a clinic control group matched for IQ, autistic children generally had a superior performance on the subtests requiring manipulative or visuospatial skills or immediate memory, whereas they did poorly on tasks demanding symbolic or abstract thought and sequential logic. Other studies have shown that cognition in autistic children is impaired, particularly in capacity for imitation, comprehension of spoken words and gestures, flexibility, inventiveness, rule formation and application, and information use.

■ Associated Features

The affective expression of autistic people may be flattened, excessive, or inappropriate to the situation. Their mood often is labile. Sobbing, crying, or screaming may be unexplained or inconsolable. Inappropriate laughing and giggling may occur for no obvious reason. Real dangers, such as moving vehicles or heights, may not be appreciated by a young autistic child, but the same child may be terrified of harmless objects or situations, such as a stuffed animal or visiting a relative's house. Peculiar habits, such as hair pulling or biting parts of the body, are sometimes present, particularly in mentally retarded autistic children. Lack of dizziness after spinning has often been observed, and some autistic children love to spin themselves for long periods.

At some stage during childhood, particularly before 8 years of age, the majority of autistic children studied have been reported to have sleep problems, including one or more of the following: extreme sleep latencies (difficulty falling asleep), lengthy periods of night waking, shortened night sleep, and early waking (Elia et al. 2000b; Patzold et al. 1998; Taira et al. 1998). Other investigators, however, raised the question of parental oversensitivity to sleep disturbance of their autistic children (Schreck and Mulick 2000; Tsai 1997).

Comorbid Psychiatric Disorders

Many investigators have found that in addition to the core autistic symptomatologies (i.e., impairment in social interaction; impairment in communication; and restricted repetitive and stereotyped patterns of behavior, interests, and activities), many autistic individuals develop other behavioral and/or psychiatric symptoms that may be considered clinical manifestations of comorbid psychiatric disorders. In summary, 64% of autistic individuals had poor attention and concentration; 36%–48% were hyperactive; 43%–88% had morbid or unusual preoccupation; 37% had obsessive phenomena; 16%–86% engaged in compulsions or rituals; 50%–89% had stereotyped utterance; 68%–74% had stereotyped mannerism; 17%–74% had anxiety or fears; 9%–44% showed depressive mood, irritability, agitation, and inappropriate affect; 11% had sleep problems; 24%–43% had a history of self-injury; and 8% presented with tics (for a review, see Tsai 2004). These investigators, however, did not specifically examine the incidence of diagnosable psychiatric disorders in their samples.

On the basis of the observations as described above, the DSM-III, DSM-III-R, and DSM-IV/DSM-IV-TR diagnostic classification systems consider some of these behavioral and/or psychiatric symptoms (e.g., abnormalities of posture and motor behavior, odd responses to sensory input or fascination with some sensations, self-injurious behavior, excessive fearfulness in response to harmless objects or events, generalized anxiety and tension, abnormalities of mood, abnormalities in sleeping) to be "associated features" of autistic disorder. On the other hand, the DSM classifications considered the symptoms of motor stereotypies (e.g., hand clapping; peculiar hand movements; and rocking, dipping, and swaying movements of the whole body) and verbal stereotypies (e.g., repetition of words or phrases) to be diagnostic criteria for autistic disorder (under the categories of markedly restricted repertoire of activities and interests and of qualitative impairments in communication, respectively). However, these motor and verbal stereotypies are frequently noted in individuals with Tourette's disorder and have been considered as diagnostic features of Tourette's disorder.

Research on the specific relationship between these associated features and autistic symptoms is sparse or nonexistent. It is not clear whether these emergent behavioral and psychiatric symptoms are developmentally related symptoms and behaviors of autistic disorder or whether they should really be considered symptoms of comorbid psychiatric disorders.

Because of difficulties in communicating with other people, as well as in showing appropriate affect, autistic individuals do not appear to resist their compulsions, to complain about the compulsive acts, or to manifest distress. This increases the possibility that clinicians may hesitate to diagnose additional psychiatric disorders in people with autistic disorder. Nevertheless, some case reports have described other specific types of psychiatric disorders occurring in autistic individuals. These include reports of unipolar and bipolar affective disorders, anxiety disorder, anorexia nervosa, obsessive-compulsive disorder, schizophrenia, and Tourette's disorder (for a review, see Tsai 2004). Given the relatively high frequencies of the associated features and the increasing number of case reports of autism associated with other major psychiatric disorders, a significant number of individuals with autistic disorder may also have coexisting major psychiatric disorders (Tsai 1996).

To allow effective treatment of people with autistic disorder who may also have one or more comorbid psychiatric disorders, the current diagnostic criteria of certain psychiatric disorders and assessment techniques must be modified and refined. For example, the diagnosis of obsessive-compulsive disorder may be considered in lower-functioning autistic individuals even in the absence of clear ego dystonicity, or the diagnosis of major depression may be considered in nonverbal and/or lower-functioning autistic people even in the absence of subjectively reported depressed mood, worry, guilty feeling, and suicidal ideation.

Yet some of the additional behavioral and/or psychiatric symptoms in autistic people as described above have been viewed as results of these individuals' inability to cope with environmental demands and physical discomfort. Thus, these symptoms have been viewed as "maladaptive behaviors" of autistic disorder and have been treated mainly with behavior modification techniques. However, if these associated behavioral and/or psychiatric symptoms are considered as symptoms of various comorbid psychiatric disorders, pharmacotherapy can be a safe and efficacious treatment for these symptoms in autistic people (Tsai 2001).

Medical Disorders

Some medical disorders have been observed to have an increased rate of co-occurrence with autistic disorder:

- Epilepsy has been noted in 4%–42% of autistic people (Giovanardi et al. 2000). Several reports have suggested that many autistic individuals first develop seizures in adolescence (Deykin and MacMahon 1979; Rutter 1984). Volkmar and Nelson (1990) reported that the risk that autistic people will develop seizures is highest during early childhood. A prospective study of epilepsy in children with autistic spectrum disorder found that about 5% of those with an autistic condition had epilepsy. Most had onset of seizures before age 1 year (Wong 1993). In a retrospective study of 60 patients (mean age 17 years 2 months), the prevalence of electroencephalographic paroxysmal abnormalities without epilepsy was 6.7% (4 patients); seizure onset was after age 12 years in 40 patients (66.7%). The most common type of epilepsy was partial in 45% (Rossi et al. 1995) to 65.2% (Giovanardi et al. 2000) of subjects. Rossi et al.

(1995) noted that electroencephalographic paroxysmal abnormalities were mostly focal and multifocal. Females with autism seemed to be more frequently affected by seizures than were males (Elia et al. 1995).

- Among patients with tuberous sclerosis (TSC), 20%–25% also met criteria for autistic disorder (Baker et al. 1998; Smalley 1998).

- In a sample of 25 Swedish patients with Mobius syndrome, a condition characterized by involvement of the sixth and seventh cranial nerves, six patients also met criteria for autism (Miller et al. 1998).

- About 7% of individuals with Down syndrome also had autistic disorder (Kent et al. 1999).

- In a study of 17 congenitally blind children, four had definite or likely autism, based on the Autism Behavior Checklist completed by the parents and teachers (Goodman and Minne 1995).

- A population-based study found the prevalence of Angelman's syndrome to be 4 in 49,000 Swedish children. All 4 children in the study with Angelman's syndrome also met full criteria for the diagnosis of autistic disorder (Steffenburg et al. 1996).

Differential Diagnosis

Autism should be distinguished from the following conditions.

■ Asperger's Disorder

Asperger's disorder is a syndrome described by Asperger (1944/1991) as an abnormal personality trait that is not evident until the third year of life. The main features are a lack of social intuition, leading to naive and tactless behavior and difficulty with social relationships; normal intelligence but with poor coordination and visuospatial perception; and obsessive preoccupation or circumscribed interest patterns. Wing (1981) reported that the picture described by Asperger could be seen in some adults who clearly had classic autism as children but who had made progress in language and other skills. This finding suggested that Asperger's disorder be considered as a mild form of autism. DSM-IV and DSM-IV-TR, however, classify Asperger's disorder as distinct from autism. If additional features described by Asperger (1944/1991) and other clinicians (e.g., extremely argumentative with a condescending attitude, verbally abusing other children, hitting other children, and lashing out and knocking objects over, interested in violence) (Gillberg 2000) but not included in DSM-IV-TR would also be considered as diagnostic features of Asperger's disorder, autistic disorder could be much more easily differentiated from Asperger's disorder.

■ Rett's Disorder

Children with Rett's disorder develop "autistic features" during the rapid developmental regression stage (usually appears at age 1–2 years). The features include lack of sustained interest in people or objects; stereotypic responses to environmental stimuli; absent or very limited interpersonal contact; manifestation of great anxiety and apparent fear when confronted with an unfamiliar situation, or even without evident stimulation; loss of already acquired elements of language; stereotypic hand movements, such as hand-washing movements in front of the mouth or chest and rubbing motions of the hands; and repetitive blows on the teeth, grabbing of the tongue, and other movements (Hagberg et al. 1983). However, the clinical course is quite different from that of autism, with Rett's disorder progressing from relatively normal devel-

opment up to about age 6 months to various forms of progressive neurological impairment, a progression not seen in autism. Furthermore, a methyl-CpG-binding protein 2 mutation can be found in almost every patient with classical Rett's disorder but not in patients with autistic disorder.

■ Childhood Disintegrative Disorder

In childhood disintegrative disorder, development usually appears normal or near normal up to age 3 or 4 years, at which time profound regression and behavioral disintegration take place. Children with childhood disintegrative disorder have loss of speech and language, loss of social skills, and loss of interest in objects. These children have impaired interpersonal relationships and develop stereotypies and mannerisms. Sometimes these disorders develop after some clear-cut organic brain disease. More often, no clinical signs of neurological damage are apparent, but the subsequent course and postmortem studies often reveal some kind of organic cortical degeneration (Rutter 1977). The patterns of symptomatology differ in crucial aspects from those of autism.

■ Mental Retardation

People with mental retardation often have behavioral abnormalities similar to those seen in people with autism. In mental retardation, generalized delays in development occur across many areas. Some children, especially those with Down syndrome, are quite sociable and can communicate in gesture and mime.

■ Developmental Language Disorder

Children with a developmental language disorder may show some autistic behavior, especially before age 5 years. They may develop disturbances in relating and social responses, but they do not manifest the perceptual disturbances (e.g., sensory hyperreactivity or hyporeactivity) that are characteristic of autistic children (Ornitz and Ritvo 1976). However, children with language disorder are much more likely to be able to relate to others by nonverbal gestures and expressions. When they do acquire speech, they also demonstrate communicative intent and emotion, characteristics that are not present in verbal autistic children. Furthermore, children with a language disorder have some imaginative play, which is markedly deficient in autistic children (Bartak et al. 1975). Cantwell et al. (1989) reported an interim follow-up study of a group of "higher-functioning" boys with autism and a control group of boys with severe receptive developmental language disorder. They noted that in middle childhood very few of the autistic boys had good language skills at follow-up evaluation, whereas nearly one-half of the group with language disorder was communicating well, a striking difference in view of the initial general similarity.

■ Obsessive-Compulsive Disorder

Bartak and Rutter (1976) noted that about 68% of the 14 nonretarded autistic children in their study had shown rituals. About 80% of these children also had "quasi-obsessive" behaviors. Difficult adaptation to new situations was found in about 74% of these children. Rumsey et al. (1985b) reported that stereotyped, repetitive movements were highly prevalent (78%) and were directly observable among the nine higher-functioning autistic men they studied. The movement most frequently observed involved the hands or arms with individual finger movement, rotating movements or whole-body rocking, and pacing.

Some of these obsessive and/or compulsive symptoms have obvious similarities to those seen in obsessive-compulsive disorder. However, in a case-controlled study, McDougle et al. (1995) found that the autistic subjects, as compared with the obsessive-compulsive subjects, were significantly less likely to experience thoughts with aggressive, contamination, sexual, religious, symmetric, and somatic content and were less likely to engage in cleaning, checking, and counting behaviors. Repetitive behaviors in the form of ordering, hoarding, telling or asking, touching, tapping, and rubbing occurred significantly more frequently in the autistic patients compared with the patients with obsessive-compulsive disorder.

■ Tourette's Disorder

Compulsive and ritualistic behaviors (e.g., keeping objects neatly arranged and routines unchanged; compulsive touching of people and things nearby; compulsive shouting and swearing; echoing of words, sounds, and actions) that can occur in Giles de la Tourette syndrome (or the syndrome of chronic multiple tics) resemble some phenomena that occur in autism. Sometimes separating symptoms of Tourette's disorder from the symptoms of autism can be difficult. However, the examination of the total behavior pattern and developmental history should make the diagnosis clear. Individuals with Tourette's disorder are aware of their disorder. They are frightened and distressed because they do not feel that they can control it. They usually do not have significantly delayed and deviant language and speech development, and their tics often have a waxing and waning pattern.

■ Schizophrenia

One well-established finding is that autistic children almost never develop a thought disorder with delusions and hallucinations. Children with childhood-onset schizophrenia can be differentiated from children with autistic disorder on the basis of age at onset, developmental history, family history, and clinical features. For almost all autistic children and adolescents, the age of disorder onset is before 5 years, whereas the onset of schizophrenia in childhood is most often during preadolescence or adolescence.

■ Selective Mutism

In selective mutism, the child refuses to speak in almost all social situations, despite the ability to comprehend spoken language and to speak. The child may communicate by gestures, nodding or shaking the head, or, in some cases, by monosyllabic or short, monotone utterances. The same child may talk normally at home with family members. Autistic children retain their characteristic language abnormalities in all situations. In any case, the whole pattern of behavior is markedly different in the two conditions.

■ Landau-Kleffner Syndrome

Landau-Kleffner syndrome (LKS) is a neurological syndrome in which children's development is normal until, usually, age 3–5 years, and then, without evident cause, the children have an abrupt or gradual loss of language ability. The regression of language development involves a profound impairment in both language comprehension and expression and may first manifest as deafness or inattentiveness to sound, sometimes called auditory agnosia. In many children with LKS, the regression of language development is closely preceded, accompanied, or followed by the onset of seizure disorders and/or electroencephalographic abnormalities (Hirsch et al. 1990; Landau and Kleffner 1957; Stefanatos et al. 1995). The syndrome is also called *acquired aphasia with convulsive disorder in children, acquired epileptiform aphasia of child-*

hood, and *acquired epileptica aphasia.*

In about 25% of autistic individuals, difficulties are not apparent until after the second birthday (Short and Schopler 1988). Some of these children may have actual regression in language development and have electroencephalographic abnormalities or a seizure disorder. Although some investigators argue that for such patients the disorder diagnosis should be LKS instead of autistic disorder or PDDNOS (Stefanatos et al. 1995), other researchers disagree with this point of view (Volkmar et al. 1996).

Available published data indicate that nonverbal skills and social interaction skills tend to be preserved in LKS. The behavioral problems with restricted repetitive and stereotyped patterns of behavior, interests, and activities are not as prominent in LKS as in autistic disorder. In many subjects with LKS, characteristic multifocal spikes and spike-and-wave discharges with marked activation of these discharges occur during sleep (Hirsch et al. 1990; Stefanatos et al. 1995), an electroencephalographic pattern rarely presented in autistic disorder.

The age at onset of LKS is usually much later than that of autistic disorder. Children with autistic disorder usually have delayed language development, whereas children with LKS have normal language development before the onset of LKS. The available data indicate that subjects with LKS most likely would not qualify for a diagnosis of autistic disorder. However, some subjects with LKS may qualify for a diagnosis of PDDNOS as defined by DSM-IV-TR.

■ Fragile X Syndrome

Fragile X syndrome has been recognized as a cause of nonspecific mental retardation. Some studies reported that individuals with fragile X syndrome were described as autistic or having autistic features that were most apparent in childhood. Hagerman

(1992) reported that 15% of individuals with fragile X syndrome also had autistic disorder. Bailey et al. (1998) reported that 14 of 57 boys (approximately 25%) with fragile X syndrome scored above the cutoff for autism on the Childhood Autism Rating Scale.

However, the prevalence of the fragile X anomaly among autistic people has been reported to be between 0% and 20% (Piven et al. 1991b), with a general consensus that the actual prevalence is 2%–5% (Hallmayer et al. 1994). A question had been raised regarding the differential diagnosis between fragile X syndrome and autistic disorder. A carefully designed study of 58 mentally retarded men with fragile X syndrome matched for age, cognitive level, living conditions, and length of institutionalization with 58 mentally retarded men without fragile X syndrome (Maes et al. 1993) reported that the core features of autism, namely social indifference and severely disturbed social relations, generally were not found in the fragile X group. The adults with fragile X syndrome had average interpersonal and communicative skills. They were more sensitive to social contact and attention from others and approached not only new physical environments but also other people with great openness and interest (Maes et al. 1993). It appears that individuals with a nonautistic fragile X syndrome have clinical features that are clearly distinguishable from those of autistic disorder. In subjects with fragile X syndrome and autistic features, the possibility of fragile X syndrome with a comorbid condition of autistic disorder or PDDNOS should be considered.

Epidemiology

■ Prevalence

DSM-IV-TR suggests the prevalence of autistic disorder to be 2–5 cases per 10,000 children in the United States (American Psychiatric Association 2000). Epidemiological studies in North America, Europe, Japan, and Israel have estimated the prevalence of autism to be between 0.15 and 34 per 10,000 children (for a review, see Tsai 2004). The trend is for more recent studies to report a higher frequency.

In an extensive review of the prevalence of autism, Fombonne (1999) noted a median prevalence of 5.2 per 10,000 children worldwide. The prevalence significantly increased with publication year. The median rate was 7.2 per 10,000 children for 11 surveys carried out worldwide since 1989, suggesting changes in case definition and improved recognition as the reasons for higher rates. It is not clear whether prevalence rates of autism in cities differ from those in rural districts.

The prevalence of autistic disorder in children with mental retardation is reported to be 8.9%–11.7% (Nordin and Gillberg 1996).

■ Sex Ratio

All studies of autism have shown a predominance of boys over girls. Ratios of 3 or 4 boys to 1 girl have consistently been reported (Tsai 1986). In addition, several studies have found that autistic girls tend to have a greater degree of morbidity—that is, more often, a greater proportion of autistic females than autistic males are severely impaired (Tsai 1986). Females with autism seemed to be more frequently affected by seizures than were males (Elia et al. 1995). Boutin et al. (1997) noted that females with autism and patients with low IQ and autism had more first-degree relatives with cognitive disability. Volkmar et al. (1993) reported that the sex differences were primarily confined to IQ, and the other matrices of severity of autism were not prominent. However, in a study of 21 males and 21 females with autism who were higher functioning, McLennan et al. (1993) found that the autistic males were rated to be more severely autistic than the females on several measures of early social development but not in any other areas.

These findings indicate that there may be significant sex differences in the occurrence and the severity of autism, and they warrant further study.

■ Socioeconomic Class

Kanner (1943) originally observed that families of his patients were predominantly of an upper socioeconomic status. However, later population studies (Tsai et al. 1982; Wing 1980) did not support Kanner's idea. As pointed out by Tsai et al. (1982), most of the studies showing high socioeconomic class bias were conducted before 1970, and those showing no bias were carried out after that date. When the possible effects of parental educational and occupational achievements and patterns of referral were controlled, autistic people were found in all socioeconomic classes.

Etiology

■ Known Medical Conditions

There is general agreement that autistic disorder has an organic basis, but there is less agreement on the frequency with which it is associated with known medical conditions. After a review of the literature, Rutter et al. (1994) concluded that the rate of known medical conditions in autism is probably about 10%, and that the rate is higher in autistic disorder associated with profound mental retardation and in atypical autism. In a French epidemiological survey, Fombonne and colleagues (1997) concluded that known

medical disorders (excluding epilepsy and sensory impairments) were associated with less than 10% of the cases of autism. Gillberg and Coleman (1996) reported a higher rate of 24.4% having known comorbid medical conditions but found a similar trend for higher rates of medical disorders among autistic individuals with severe mental retardation. Barton and Volkmar (1998) retrospectively reviewed medical records of 211 subjects with autism and found that the prevalence of medical conditions suspected to have an association with autism varied between 10% and 15% and, with a less strict definition of *medical condition*, between 25% and 37%. Nonetheless, these medical conditions or disorders were not considered to be causes of autistic disorder.

■ Congenital Factors

Results of numerous studies show that many autistic children have organic brain disorders. A wide variety of neurological disorders have been reported: cerebral palsy, congenital rubella, toxoplasmosis, TSC, cytomegalovirus infection, lead encephalopathy, meningitis, encephalitis, severe brain hemorrhage, many types of epilepsy, and others. Many of these neurological or congenital disorders derive from prenatal, perinatal, and neonatal complications. Several investigators have reported that such complications (reduced optimality) appear with increased frequency in the histories of autistic patients. These factors include increased maternal age, firstborn children and those born fourth or later, bleeding after the first trimester, maternal use of medication, and meconium in amniotic fluid (Tsai 1987). Juul-Dam et al. (2001) also reported an association of unfavorable events in pregnancy, delivery, and the neonatal phase and autism. Burd and colleagues (1999) identified five variables (decreased birth weight, low maternal education, later start of prenatal care, having a previous termination of pregnancy, and increasing father's age) associated with increased risk of autism.

On the other hand, Lord et al. (1991) proposed that pre- and perinatal factors play less of a role in autism in higher-functioning individuals. Piven et al. (1993) found that the reported association between optimality and autism in autistic probands and their siblings might be the result of failure to control for birth order. Bolton et al. (1997) noted that the optimality score was significantly elevated in both autistic probands and those with Down syndrome and concluded that obstetric adversities associated with autism either represented an epiphenomenona of the condition or derived from some shared risk factor(s). Other investigators reported no significant obstetric adversity in mothers of autistic subjects (Cryan et al. 1996; Deb et al. 1997).

Because of the lack of uniformity in applying diagnostic criteria to autism as well as to the selection of obstetric complications, the findings on the association between optimality and autism should be accepted cautiously. Also, the data reviewed here do not indicate a unifying pathological process in autism.

■ Genetic Factors

Research since the 1980s has convincingly indicated that autism is a genetic disorder. This conclusion is based mainly on data from family studies, twin studies, and chromosome studies. Autism has been reported to be associated with various chromosomal abnormalities (for a review, see Tsai 2004). Autism is likely genetically heterogeneous, with variability of clinical features.

Some genetic syndromes are associated with autism, including phenylketonuria (Knoblock and Pasamanick 1975),

fragile X syndrome, and TSC. Some investigators have found a high prevalence of fragile X syndrome in people with autism (Bloomquist et al. 1985), but others have been unable to replicate this finding (Payton et al. 1989). About 20%–25% of patients with TSC also meet criteria for autistic disorder (Baker et al. 1998; Smalley 1998). The mechanism underlying the association of autism and TSC is unclear. It is speculated that autism may arise if TSC gene mutations occur at critical stages of neural development in the brain (Smalley 1998).

As mentioned earlier, one study found 4 of 49,000 Swedish children to have Angelman's syndrome. All 4 children also met full criteria for the diagnosis of autistic disorder (Steffenburg et al. 1996). Maternal truncation mutation in the *UBE3A/E6-AP* gene in chromosome 15q11–13 has been known to cause Angelman's syndrome. This finding suggests that the possible gene for autism may be identified in the 15q11–13 region (Herzing et al. 2001).

Several studies have shown that between 2% and 7% of the siblings of children with autism have the same condition (Bolton et al. 1994; Chudley et al. 1998; Ritvo et al. 1989; Smalley 1991; Tsai et al. 1981). When this estimated incidence is compared with the risk for autism in the general population, the rate of autism in siblings is 50 times higher.

Ritvo et al. (1985) reported a study involving 281 families enrolled in the University of California, Los Angeles Registry for Genetic Studies in Autism. They included (by parental report) 22 sets of monozygotic twins concordant for autism; 18 sets of dizygotic twins, of whom 2 sets were concordant for autism; and 46 sets of nontwin siblings concordant for autism. Twenty-one pairs (11 monozygotic and 10 dizygotic) of twins and 1 set of identical triplets were identified in the

Nordic countries (Denmark, Finland, Iceland, Norway, and Sweden) (Steffenburg et al. 1989). The concordance for autism by pair was 91% in the monozygotic and 0% in the dizygotic pairs. In most of the pairs discordant for autism, the autistic twin had been under more perinatal stress. It was concluded that the results supported the hypothesis that autism had a hereditary component and that perinatal complication was a contributory factor in some cases.

Folstein and Rutter (1977) studied 21 same-sex autistic twin pairs and found that 4 of 11 monozygotic twin pairs (36%) were concordant for autism, as compared with 0 of 10 (0%) dizygotic twins. Discordance was usually associated with definite or suggestive evidence of organic brain dysfunction in the affected twin. This first British twin sample was reexamined along with a second total-population British sample of autistic twins and triplets. In the combined sample of 44 sets of twins and triplets, 60% of monozygotic pairs were concordant for autism, compared with no dizygotic pairs. When a broader spectrum of related cognitive or social abnormalities was applied to the sample, 92% of the monozygotic pairs were concordant for the spectrum, compared with 10% of the dizygotic pairs. The findings indicate that autism is under a high degree of genetic control and suggest that multiple genetic loci are involved (Bailey et al. 1995). The findings also suggest that autism might develop because of a combination of genetic predisposition and biological impairment.

On the basis of the findings from their twin study, Folstein and Rutter (1977) suggested that autism is one manifestation of an underlying genetic liability to cognitive dysfunction; that is, a cognitive disorder may present in its mildest form as learning disabilities and in its most severe form as autism. To date, family studies of autism seem to provide some support for such a hypothesis. The sibling data show that between 6% and 24% of the siblings of autistic probands have cognitive disorders (including autism, mental retardation, and learning disability) and/or speech-language disorders (August et al. 1981; Bolton et al. 1994; Freeman et al. 1986; Piven et al. 1990).

Szatmari and colleagues (1995) reported that rates of cognitive impairments and psychiatric symptoms were not found more frequently in parents or relatives of probands with PDD compared with relatives of control subjects. Other investigators have reported that parents of autistic children had increased rates of anxiety disorder (Piven et al. 1991a), major depressive disorder (Bolton et al. 1998; R. DeLong and Nohria 1994; Piven and Palmer 1999; Smalley et al. 1995), social phobia (Piven and Palmer 1999; Smalley et al. 1995), motor tics and obsessive-compulsive disorder (Bolton et al. 1998), and higher rates of particular characteristics (rigidity, aloofness, hypersensitivity to criticism, and anxiousness), speech and pragmatic language deficits, and limited friendships (Piven et al. 1997). Murphy and colleagues (2000) noted significantly increased expression of anxiety, impulsiveness, aloofness, shyness, oversensitivity, irritability, and eccentricity among relatives of subjects with autism. Gillberg et al. (1992) reported that mothers of autistic subjects tended to have schizoaffective disorder and that Asperger's disorder was more common among first-degree relatives of children with autism compared with control subjects. Plumet et al. (1995) reported that the brothers of a group of autistic females had a lower verbal performance. Folstein et al. (1999) found that parents of autistic children scored slightly but significantly lower on the WAIS-R Full Scale and Performance IQ and on the Word Attack Test from the Woodcock-Johnson battery compared with parents of control subjects. These findings suggest some association between autism and other major psychiatric disorders and verbal performance, but more study is needed to define the genetic implications.

With the recent advancement of molecular genetic techniques, a number of whole-genome screenings for linkage have been carried out in several samples of autistic subjects.

Two chromosomes have received the most attention: 7q and 15q. Several studies focused on chromosome 7q in autistic subjects have identified chromosome band 7q31–33 as the likely susceptibility locus (Ashley-Koch et al. 1999; Barrett et al. 1999; Gong et al. 2004; International Molecular Genetic Study of Autism Consortium 2001; Warburton et al. 2000; Wassink et al. 2001). Several other studies have found evidence in support of linkage to the 15q11–13 region (Bass et al. 2000; Cook et al. 1998; Craddock and Lendon 1999; Maddox et al. 1999; Martin et al. 2000; McCauley et al. 2004; Repetto et al. 1998; Rineer et al. 1998; Wolpert et al. 2000) and 15q22–23 region (M. Smith et al. 2000). Furthermore, the duplication of 15q11–13 was found to be maternally inherited (Cook et al. 1997b; Martinsson et al. 1996). Salmon et al. (1999), however, believed that the role of 15q11–13 is minor, at best, in the majority of individuals with autism. Lauritsen et al. (1999) proposed some candidate regions on chromosomes 7q21 and 10q21.2.

Several genes have been proposed as candidates for association with autism. Cook et al. (1997a) provided evidence of linkage and association between the serotonin transporter gene (*HTT*) in the 15q11–13 region and autism. Yirmiya et al. (2001) and Conroy et al. (2004) also

showed evidence for an association between the polymorphism of the serotonin transporter region and autism. Other investigators, however, were not able to replicate this finding (Klauck et al. 1997; Maestrini et al. 1999; Persico et al. 2000; Zhong et al. 1999). Tordjman et al. (2001) noted that transmission of *HTT* promoter alleles did not differ between probands with autism and their unaffected siblings. However, allelic transmission in probands depended on severity of impairment in the social and communication domains. It was concluded that *HTT* promoter alleles by themselves do not convey risk for autism but rather modify the severity of autism in the social and communication domains. Careful replication studies are necessary before it can be determined that the proposed markers and candidate genes have a role in the development of autism.

The data available show reasonable evidence that genetic factors play a major contributory role in a subgroup of autistic individuals. However, several genome-wide screens for susceptibility genes have been performed with limited concordance of linked loci. These data seem to indicate that there are numerous genes of weak effect involved in the development of autistic disorder and/or that autistic disorder is genetically heterogeneous. Nonetheless, at present the most interesting chromosome regions being studied for possible links to autistic disorder are chromosomes 7q31–35, 15q11–13, and 16p13.3 (Lauritsen and Ewald 2001).

■ Immunological Factors

Several studies have suggested the possibility of an immune defect in autistic disorder. Chess (1977) reported an increased frequency of autism in individuals with congenital rubella. Deykin and Mac-Mahon (1979) found that autism was associated with prenatal rubella or influenza infection in about 5% of patients.

In a further study of the activity of the natural killer cell (a large granular lymphocyte and a likely part of basic defense mechanism against virus-infected cells and malignancy), 12 (39%) of the autistic subjects were found to have significantly reduced natural killer cell activity (Warren et al. 1987).

Gupta et al. (1998) examined Th1-like and Th2-like cytokines in CD4+ and CD8+ T cells in children with autism and found an imbalance of cytokines. They speculated that such an imbalance is a cause of autism.

Denney et al. (1996) reported that children with autism had a lower percentage of helper-inducer cells and a lower helper:suppressor ratio, with both measures inversely related to the severity of autistic symptoms.

Scifo et al. (1996) proposed that the mechanisms underlying opioid–immune interactions are altered and may play a role in the development of autism.

Weizman et al. (1982) investigated the cell-mediated immune response to human myelin basic protein (a component of myelin) by using the macrophage migration inhibition factor test. The results were interpreted as suggesting that a cell-mediated autoimmune response to brain antigen exists in some autistic individuals. This hypothesis was supported by a report that described 19 of 33 autistic subjects (58%) as testing positive for antibodies to myelin basic protein—a rate more than six times higher than in nondisabled and retarded control subjects (Singh et al. 1993). In a further study, Singh et al. (1997) found a significant increase in incidence of autoantibodies to neuron-axon filament protein and autoantibodies to glial fibrillary acidic protein in autistic subjects. It was speculated that these autoantibodies might be related to autoim-

mune pathology of autism. Singh et al. (1998) further reported an association between virus serology and brain autoantibody in autistic subjects and proposed a hypothesis that virus-induced autoimmune response might play a causal role in autism. Connolly et al. (1999) found immunoglobulin G (IgG) antibrain autoantibodies in 27% of sera and immunoglobulin M (IgM) autoantibodies in 36% of sera from children with autistic spectrum disorder. The findings were speculated to mean that autoimmunity might play a role in the pathogenesis of language and social development abnormalities in a subset of children with autism.

Monoclonal antibody D8/17–positive cells were found in 14 of 18 patients (78%) with autism. As severity of repetitive behaviors significantly correlated with D8/17 expression, Hollander et al. (1999) suggested that D8/17 expression could serve as a marker for compulsion severity within autism.

Todd and Ciaranello (1985) reported that about one-third of the autistic children in their study had an unusual antibody circulating in their blood and spinal fluid. This antibody appeared to attack the receptor for serotonin (5-hydroxytryptamine [5-HT]). In a further study, Todd et al. (1988, p. 647) concluded that "if an antibody-mediated autoantigen recognition is important in, or related to, established infantile autism, only a few antigens are involved."

All these findings seem to suggest that depressed immune function, autoimmune mechanism, or faulty immune regulation (deficiency in some components of immune system and excesses in others) may be associated with the etiology of autism. However, interpretation of the data is hampered by conceptual and methodological differences between studies. Both the clinical significance of the immune changes and the causal connection between immune changes and autistic symptoms remain to be elucidated by more extensive studies.

■ Neurological Factors

Neurological abnormalities have been reported in 30%–50% of autistic patients (Tsai et al. 1981), including hypotonia or hypertonia, disturbance of body schema, clumsiness, choreiform movements, pathological reflexes, myoclonic jerking, drooling, abnormal posture and gait, dystonic posturing of hands and fingers, tremor, ankle clonus, emotional facial paralysis, and strabismus. These are all signs of dysfunction in the basal ganglia, particularly the neostriatum, and closely related structures of the medial aspects of the frontal lobe or limbic system.

Several investigators have reported that some individuals with autism (between 12% and 46%) had macrocephaly (head circumference in the 97th percentile or higher) (Fidler et al. 2000; Lainhart et al. 1997). Fidler et al. (2000) also noted that the first-degree relatives of these patients also had a higher rate of macrocephaly when compared against a published normative sample. However, Courchesne et al. (1999) reported that the brain weight was normal in most postmortem studies of autistic subjects. Rare cases of microcephaly have also been observed. Other investigators questioned the specificity of macrocephaly to autism (Ghaziuddin et al. 1999).

■ Neuroanatomical Factors

Computed Tomography Scan Studies

Findings of computed tomography (CT) studies have been inconsistent.

Magnetic Resonance Imaging Studies

Magnetic resonance imaging (MRI) studies have reported cerebellar hypoplasia and/or a small brain stem, including the midbrain, pons, and medulla oblongata;

smaller amygdala; reduced size of corpus callosum; smaller area dentate within the limbic system; reduced volume of hippocampus; smaller right anterior cingulate gyrus; significantly increased total brain, total tissue, and total lateral ventricle volumes; increased volume of the caudate nuclei; and increased total volume of cerebellum and cerebellar hemispheres (for a review, see Tsai 2004). Other studies, however, have not found any abnormalities in the posterior fossa structures of the brain, particularly the cerebellum (for a review, see Tsai 2004) or the hippocampus (Piven et al. 1998).

In a study of 22 boys with low-functioning autism, Elia et al. (2000a) reported a significant negative correlation between the midsagittal area of the cerebrum and age and a positive correlation between the midsagittal area of the midbrain and some subscales of the Psychoeducational Profile—Revised.

Howard et al. (2000) found that individuals with high-functioning autism had neuropsychological profiles characteristic of effects of amygdala damage, and that the same individuals also had abnormalities of medial temporal lobe brain structure, notably bilateral enlarged amygdala volumes.

On the other hand, Ciesielski and Knight (1994) found that the abnormal MRI cerebellar morphology was similar for both the high-functioning autistic subjects and those who had had childhood leukemia and had been treated with radiotherapy and intrathecal chemotherapy. The abnormal MRI macromorphology of the vermis may be nonspecific to autism. Nonetheless, the finding of cerebellar abnormalities is consistent with microscopic postmortem findings. Although the link between the cerebellar abnormalities and autism has yet to be determined, MRI technology has provided an exciting new avenue for future in vivo studies of the brain.

Differences in MRI study results may have been due to subjects' ages, subjects' cognitive functioning level, the number of subjects, and the area measurement method used.

Functional Magnetic Resonance Imaging Studies

Using functional magnetic resonance imaging (fMRI), Baron-Cohen et al. (1999) found that attempting to judge from the expression of another person's eyes what that other person might be thinking or feeling activated the frontotemporal regions but not the amygdala of autistic subjects. These results seemed to provide support for the social brain theory of normal function and the amygdala theory of autism (Baron-Cohen et al. 2000).

Ring et al. (1999) employed the Embedded Figures Task and fMRI in a study of autistic patients' brain activation patterns. Although the developmentally normal control subjects showed activated prefrontal areas, the autistic subjects showed greater activation of ventral occipitotemporal regions. The findings suggest that the healthy control subjects invoked a greater contribution from the working memory system, while the autistic subjects depended to an abnormally large extent on visual systems for object feature analysis.

Using fMRI as subjects performed visually paced finger movement, Muller et al. (2001) found that in general, the autistic group had less pronounced activation compared with control subjects. The control subjects showed greater activation in perirolandic and supplementary motor areas, whereas the autistic subjects had greater activation in posterior and prefrontal cortices.

Magnetic Resonance Spectroscopy Studies

Minshew et al. (1993) used magnetic resonance spectroscopy (MRS) to study 11 high-functioning autistic individuals. The pilot study found that the autistic group had decreased levels of phosphocreatine and esterified ends. As neuropsychological and language test performance of these subjects declined, levels of the most labile energy phosphate compound and of membrane building blocks decreased and levels of membrane breakdown products increased. These results indicate alterations in brain energy and phospholipid metabolism in autism that correlate with neuropsychological and language deficits. Otsuka et al. (1999) used MRS to examine the right hippocampus–amygdala region and left cerebellar hemisphere of 27 autistic patients between ages 2 and 18 years. The N-acetylaspartate (NAA) concentration was significantly decreased. It was speculated that the decreased NAA concentration might be due to neuronal hypofunction or immature neurons. Chugani et al. (1999) reported that autistic children had lower levels of NAA in the cerebellum. The significance of these findings is unclear, but this research approach merits further exploration.

Positron Emission Tomography Studies

Rumsey et al. (1985a), using positron emission tomography (PET), reported substantially elevated use of glucose throughout many parts of the brain in 10 autistic men compared with control subjects. Heh et al. (1989) reported no significant differences in mean cerebellar glucose metabolism between 7 adult patients with autism and 8 age-matched control subjects, although all mean glucose rates for the autistic patients were either equal to or greater than those of the control subjects. Zilbovicius et al. (2000) reported that autistic patients tended to have highly significant hypoperfusion in both temporal lobes centered in the associative auditory and adjacent multimodal cortex. Haznedar et al. (2000)

noted significant glucose metabolic reductions in both the anterior and posterior cingulate gyri.

Using PET to study five high-functioning autistic adults, Muller et al. (1998) found that the activation in the right dentate nucleus and in the left frontal area 46 was reduced during verbal, auditory, and expressive language and enhanced during motor speech. This finding may indicate impairment of the dentatothalamocortical pathway. Muller et al. (1999) also reported a reversed hemispheric dominance during verbal auditory stimulation; a trend toward reduced activation of the auditory cortex during acoustic stimulation; and reduced cerebellar activation during use of nonverbal auditory perception and possibly expressive language. These findings were considered as compatible with previous findings of cerebellar anomalies.

Siegel and colleagues (1992) used [^{18}F]fluoro-2-deoxyglucose PET to assess regional cerebral glucose metabolic rate (GMR) in 16 high-functioning autistic adults and 26 nonautistic control subjects. Autistic subjects had an abnormal anterior rectal gyrus asymmetry, in which the left side was larger than the right, which is the reverse of the normal asymmetry in that region. The autistic group also showed a low GMR in the left posterior putamen and a high GMR in the right posterior calcarine cortex. Brain regions with GMRs greater than 3 standard deviations from the normal mean were more prevalent in the autistic group than in the control group.

In a study of serotonin synthesis in the dentatothalamocortical pathway in seven boys and one girl with autism, Chugani et al. (1997) found asymmetries of serotonin synthesis in the frontal cortex, thalamus, and dentate nucleus of the cerebellum in all seven boys but not in the one girl. Decreased serotonin synthesis

was found in the frontal cortex and thalamus in five of the seven boys (71%) and in the right frontal cortex and thalamus in the two remaining boys (29%). In all seven boys, elevated serotonin synthesis in the contralateral dentate nucleus was observed. These serotonergic abnormalities in a brain pathway were considered as one mechanism underlying the pathophysiology of autism.

Zilbovicius et al. (1992) measured regional cerebral blood flow with single photon emission computed tomography (SPECT) in 21 autistic children; no cortical regional abnormalities were found. In another study of five autistic children, Zilbovicius et al. (1995) used SPECT twice during the children's development: at age 3–4 years and 3 years later. A transient frontal hypoperfusion was found in the autistic children at age 3–4 years. However, by age 6–7 years, these children's frontal perfusion had attained normal values. These results indicate delayed frontal maturation in childhood autism.

Chiron and colleagues (1995) used [^{133}Xe]SPECT to study 18 autistic children between the ages of 4 and 17 years. The regional cerebral blood flow (rCBF) in autistic subjects was decreased in the left hemisphere, particularly in the region of the sensorimotor and language-related cortex.

Starkstein et al. (2000) measured rCBF using [^{99m}Tc]HMPAO SPECT in 30 autistic patients and noted significantly low perfusion in the right temporal lobe (basal and inferior areas), occipital lobes, thalami, and left basal ganglia.

Hashimoto et al. (2000) performed SPECT in 22 autistic patients and reported lower rCBF in both laterotemporal and dorsomediolateral areas. The rCBF was significantly higher in the right temporal and right parietal lobes than that in the left ones. Inversely, the rCBF in the frontal and occipital lobes was significantly higher on the left side than on the right side. A positive correlation between rCBF and IQ was observed in the left laterotemporal and both dorsomediolateral frontal areas, and a negative one was noted in the cerebellar vermis area.

Ohnishi et al. (2000) assessed the relationship between rCBF and symptom profiles in 23 autistic children and found decreased rCBF in the bilateral insula, superior temporal gyri, and left prefrontal cortices. Impairments in communication and social interaction were thought to be related to the altered perfusion in the medial prefrontal cortex and anterior cingulate gyrus, and the obsessive desires for sameness were associated with altered perfusion in the right mediotemporal lobe.

■ Biochemical Factors

The results obtained from neuropathology and brain imaging studies strongly suggest that the cerebral defect in autism is microscopic or functional, without major gross neuroanatomical pathology. Thus, the neurochemical correlates in autism must be examined.

Serotonin Studies

Many studies consistently have reported that about one-third of autistic individuals have hyperserotonemia (Anderson et al. 1987). There are three possible explanations for this condition: 1) enhanced platelet uptake, storage, or volume; 2) increased synthesis; and 3) decreased catabolism.

Marazziti et al. (2000) investigated the 5-HT transporter by means of the specific binding of [^{3}H]paroxetine in 20 autistic children and adolescents. The results showed a significantly higher density of [^{3}H]paroxetine binding sites in autistic subjects than in healthy control

subjects, suggesting the presence of serotonergic dysfunction in autism.

Although some previous studies found that the platelets' handling of 5-HT appeared to be normal in autistic individuals (Anderson et al. 1985), other studies indicated that the role of the platelets might need to be reexamined (Katsui et al. 1986). Furthermore, the autistic probands and their first-degree relatives had strong familial resemblance. There was positive correlation of both platelet-rich plasma 5-HT and platelet-poor (free) plasma 5-HT between autistic probands and their first-degree relatives (Kuperman et al. 1985; Leboyer et al. 1999). The platelet-rich plasma 5-HT levels of autistic subjects with affected siblings (i.e., with either autistic disorder or PDDNOS) were significantly higher than those of the autistic subjects without affected siblings, and autistic subjects without affected siblings had 5-HT levels significantly higher than those of control subjects. The results suggest that 5-HT levels in autistic subjects may be associated with genetic liability to autism (Piven et al. 1991c).

The studies of 5-HT synthesis in autism have been conflicting. Several studies have not found any difference between autistic and nonautistic subjects (Minderaa et al. 1987). The ratio of serum tryptophan to large neutral amino acids is considered a reliable marker of tryptophan availability for brain serotonin synthesis. D'Eufemia et al. (1995) found a significantly lower serum ratio in the autistic subjects compared with the nonautistic control subjects.

The occurrence of hyperserotonemia in autistic people does not appear to be the result of decreased catabolism of 5-HT. No consistent correlations have been found between blood levels of 5-HT and any autistic behaviors or symptoms. Moreover, hyperserotonemia has also been found in some children with severe retardation. The mechanism and importance of hyperserotonemia in autism are unclear.

Dopamine Studies

Campbell (1977) reported that neuroleptics, which are dopamine receptor–blocking agents, modulated several symptoms involving the motor system (e.g., hyperactivity, stereotypies, aggression, and self-injury) and made autistic children more compliant and receptive to special-education procedures. On the other hand, dopamine agonists, such as stimulants, may worsen preexisting stereotypies, aggression, and hyperactivity in autistic children.

Studies of dopamine in autism have focused on the measurement of homovanillic acid (HVA), the main metabolite of dopamine. Findings of studies have been inconsistent. HVA concentrations have not been shown to correlate with any autistic behaviors or symptoms.

Epinephrine and Norepinephrine Studies

Plasma norepinephrine level has been reported to be elevated in autistic subjects (Lake et al. 1977), but in platelets, both epinephrine and norepinephrine levels were significantly lower in the autistic group compared with the control group (Launay et al. 1987).

No difference in cerebrospinal fluid levels, plasma levels, and urinary excretion of MHPG (3-methoxy-4-hydroxyphenylglycol), as well as urinary excretion rates of epinephrine, norepinephrine, and vanillylmandelic acid, has been found between autistic subjects and control subjects (Minderaa et al. 1994).

Other Monoamine Studies

Martineau et al. (1992) reported that the urinary levels of dopamine and its derivatives HVA, 3,4-dihydroxyphenylacetic acid (DOPAC), 3-methoxytyramine (3MT), epinephrine, norepinephrine, and 5-HT and its metabolite 5-hydroxyindoleacetic acid (5-HIAA) in autistic children between ages 2 and 12.5 years decreased significantly with age. The results suggest a maturation defect of the monoaminergic system in autism.

■ Vaccinations

The hypothesis that measles, mumps, and rubella (MMR) vaccines cause autism was first raised by reports of cases in which developmental regression occurred soon after MMR vaccination. However, several major epidemiological studies failed to find any evidence to support a causal association between MMR vaccine and autism (Farrington et al. 2001; Kaye et al. 2001; Taylor et al. 1999). Concern has also been raised about possible association between MMR vaccine–induced mercury (thimerosal) exposure and autism (Bernard et al. 2001). The evidence, however, does not support such a hypothesis (Chez et al. 2004; Halsey et al. 2001; Parker et al. 2004).

■ Other Biological Factors

Gastrointestinal Abnormalities

Horvath et al. (1999) reported high rates of reflux esophagitis, chronic gastritis, and chronic duodenitis in 36 children with autism. Unrecognized gastrointestinal disorders were considered to be a contributing factor to the behavioral problems of nonverbal autistic subjects.

Abnormal Intestinal Permeability

An altered intestinal permeability was found in 9 of 21 autistic subjects (43%) (D'Eufemia et al. 1996). It was speculated that an altered intestinal permeability could represent a possible mechanism for the increased passage through the gut mucosa of peptides derived from food, with subsequent behavioral abnormalities in these patients.

Summary of Other Biological Factors

Although hypotheses are intriguing, they have been based on findings from studies with very small samples; thus, more studies are needed.

■ Neuropsychological Factors

Several studies suggest that autistic people may have a diminished or altered capacity for selectively channeling information for further internal attention and processing, as well as differential hemispheric involvement in attentional deficits (Courchesne 1987; Dawson et al. 1988). Courchesne et al. (1994) reviewed autopsy, MRI, and neurophysiological findings and proposed that in autism, cerebellar maldevelopment may contribute to an inability to execute rapid attention shifts, which undermines social and cognitive development.

Investigators have found that autistic individuals had deficits of face recognition (Boucher et al. 1998; Celani et al. 1999), voice recognition (Boucher et al. 1998), and emotion recognition (Bormann-Kischkel et al. 1995; Celani et al. 1999). Based on results of tasks used in studies of amygdala dysfunction in autism, Adolphs et al. (2001) suggested that such dysfunction might contribute to an impaired ability to link visual perception of socially relevant stimuli with retrieval of social knowledge and with elicitation of social behavior. However, Loveland et al. (1997) reported that people with autism could use affective information from multiple sources to recognize emotions in much the same ways as people of comparable developmental level without autism.

A deficit in theory of mind ability (i.e., the ability to make inferences about others' mental states) has been described as the core deficit in autism (Jolliffe and Baron-Cohen 1999; Ozonoff et al. 1991). However, other investigators reported that autism did not involve a specific impairment in theory of mind ability (Yirmiya and Shulman 1996) and that theory of mind deficits are not unique to autism (Buitelaar et al. 1999; Yirmiya et al. 1998). Further, Rieffe et al. (2000) studied the understanding of atypical emotions in 23 high-functioning children with autism spectrum disorders (mean age, 9 years 3 months) and concluded that the theory of mind ability of such children might be intact.

There is growing interest in the studying of the precursors to the ability of conceiving other people's minds. Investigators have found that autistic individuals have deficits in two candidate precursors, imitation and joint attention (Charman et al. 1997; Roeyers et al. 1998).

Many studies have shown that autistic individuals perform at a much lower level than control subjects on tests of executive functioning, defined as tasks requiring subjects to hold information in mind while suppressing a prepotent response (Bennetto et al. 1996; Ozonoff et al. 1991). A significant proportion of parents and siblings of autistic children have been observed to also have impaired executive functioning (Hughes et al. 1999). However, other investigators reported that executive functioning in autistic children was not impaired (Griffith et al. 1999; Russell et al. 1999) or impairment was not universally presented (Liss et al. 2001).

■ Birth Season

A proposed higher risk of autism in certain birth months has not been consistently replicated.

■ Summary of Etiology

As yet, no specific causes of autistic disorder have been identified. Neurobiological
investigations in autism have found various
abnormalities. However, no single measure
of the abnormalities has been found consistently, and the etiological implications of
the findings are far from clear, possibly
because autistic disorder is a behavior-
defined syndrome that includes several
distinct conditions. It is anticipated that future studies will determine a range of biological etiologies for the subgroups consti-
tuting autistic disorder.

Treatment

There is no cure for autism, because its etiology is unknown. However, comprehensive intervention, including parental counseling, behavior modification, special
education in a highly structured environment, sensory integration training, speech
therapy, social skills training, and medications, has demonstrated significant treatment effects in many autistic individuals
(American Academy of Child and Adolescent Psychiatry 1999; Tsai 2001).

■ Special-Education
    Intervention

Emphasis is placed on promoting the autistic child's more normal social and linguistic developments and on minimizing
the child's maladaptive behaviors (e.g.,
hyperactivity, stereotypies, self-injury, aggressiveness), which interfere with or are
incompatible with the child's adaptive
functioning and learning. There has been
an increasing focus on early identification
and treatment of preschool autistic children through special-education programs
in highly structured environments and on
working closely with the family members
of autistic children to help them cope better with the problems faced at home and

to increase positive interaction (Jocelyn et
al. 1998; Koegel et al. 1996; Ozonoff and
Cathcart 1998).

There has been an increasing focus on
providing education services/interven-
tions through "regular education programs" (i.e., inclusion education) with
strong special-education support. Some
general student peers have demonstrated
their usefulness and effectiveness in helping their autistic classmates to increase
reading fluency, make correct responses to
reading comprehension questions and
social interactions, and decrease inappropriate behaviors (Goldstein et al. 1992;
Laushey and Heflin 2000; Pierce and
Schreibman 1997).

Educational treatment should be intensive and sustained and should emphasize acquisition of self-care, social,
and job skills. It is critical that each student's educational intervention plan be
truly individualized and take into consideration both the student's weaknesses/
deficits and strengths/talents.

■ Computer-Based Treatment

A computer-based intervention with a
motivating multimedia program has been
demonstrated to increase reading and
communication skills in children with
autism (Heimann et al. 1995) and to
increase their ability to construct correct
sentences and to use more appropriate
vocal responses (Yamamoto and Miya
1999). Some investigators have attempted
to use virtual reality technologies to teach
autistic children new coping skills that
may then be generalized in their everyday
lives (Max and Burke 1997; Strickland
1997).

■ Behavior Therapy

Extensive research in behavior therapy
since the 1960s has shown that many autistic children can be taught special skills in

social adaptation and cognitive and motor skills. Their maladaptive behavior can also be ameliorated significantly. Lovaas et al. (1976) reviewed the principles involved in behavior therapy with autistic children. A few points are emphasized here: First, behavior therapy programs should be designed for individual children because autistic children vary greatly in their disabilities and family circumstances. Treatment approaches that work for certain patients may not work for others. Second, autistic children have an impaired ability to generalize from one situation to another, so the skills they have learned in a hospital or school tend not to transfer to the home or other settings. It is crucial in treatment to plan the approach specifically to ensure that the changes in the child's clinical state are being carefully monitored, that the problems in each setting are dealt with, and that steps are taken to encourage generalization of behavior changes. Third, because one of the treatment goals is to promote the child's social development, long-term residential treatment is not usually appropriate.

Intensive behavior therapy in early childhood is critical, and preliminary data seemed to show long-lasting positive effects (McEachin et al. 1993; Sheinkopf and Siegel 1998; T. Smith et al. 2000). A home-based approach, which trains parents, siblings, and local special-education teachers to carry out behavior therapies, has been important (Knott et al. 1995). It may be difficult for some parents and siblings of autistic patients to carry out such therapies. Some studies reported that parents and siblings of autistic individuals had significant personality adjustment difficulties, with a high degree of anxiety (Weiss 1991), and they tended to have higher scores on depression and stress ratings than did control subjects (Gold 1993; Koegel et al. 1992). Several factors have been identified as significantly influenc-

ing adjustment of families with an autistic child: the severity of the child's disorder, mother's social support, mother's perceived locus of control, and family service agency affiliation (Henderson and Vandenberg 1992).

■ Speech and Language Therapies

Licensed speech and language therapists have developed treatments aimed at stimulating the individual's natural ability for and interest in learning language. The treatments customarily take place in one-to-one sessions held 2 or 3 hours per week. However, no scientific studies have evaluated whether any form of speech and language therapy helps individuals with autism. Speech and language therapy sessions should also include peers, siblings, and parents so that the therapist can assess the learning effect on the autistic child (i.e., whether the child applies the newly learned skills in other settings with other people).

■ Social Skills Training

Both individual and group social skills training may be helpful to older and higher-functioning individuals with autism. Some autistic individuals enjoy meeting with other people who have similar difficulties. The therapist working with these individuals should facilitate such social contacts within the context of an activity- or special interest–oriented group. However, the therapist should also create or facilitate opportunities for these individuals to meet with nonautistic friends or peers so that they have opportunities to learn or to practice appropriate social skills. Autistic individuals tend not to learn social skills naturally. They have to be taught to recognize social cues and how to react to them. They need to be told how to monitor and modify their own inappropriate social behaviors.

These skills can be taught through role modeling, role playing, social stories, cartooning, and video recordings, using rules, visual cues, and positive behavioral reinforcement. To ensure success, the first step is to identify specific measurable target behaviors that must be learned. It is important to teach one skill at a time and then build a repertoire. Each new skill to be learned should be broken into smaller components or steps. The new skill should be taught using multiple methods and building in ways that would ensure generalizing such a skill in many different situations or settings.

Group social skills training sessions must be structured with very specific rules. At the outset, carefully scripted rules that specify appropriate responses should be taught and discussed. The students would then be taught to know when they are being unintentionally insulting, tactless, or inappropriate. Alternative and appropriate skills should be taught and practiced with positive reinforcement strategies (i.e., rewards) to increase use of the newly learned social skills. Autistic individuals usually do not possess a sense of humor, tell jokes, or use metaphors. They tend to interpret words and phrases literally. It is important to teach how to appreciate humor, jokes, metaphors, and irony, as well as to practice discerning when to appropriately use them.

Cognitive Therapy

Individual cognitive psychotherapy may be helpful to higher-functioning autistic individuals. The focus of therapy is to help them understand the social behavior of other people and to see how their own behavior can be viewed as unusual. Additional therapeutic group experiences can provide these individuals with more insight into their disabilities, helping them to accept their limitations in some areas and to discover their strengths and potentials in others. Thus, cognitive therapy can also prevent depression in these individuals.

Sensorimotor Therapies

One of the oldest and most popular notions about children with developmental delays, including those with autism, is that they have difficulty processing sensory input from the environment and/or translating such input into effective action.

Sensory Integration Therapy

In sensory integration therapy (SIT), a therapist stimulates an individual's skin and vestibular systems. This stimulation consists of activities such as swinging in a hammock suspended from the ceiling, spinning in circles on specially constructed chairs, brushing parts of the individual's body, and engaging in physical activities that require balance. There is no information on the treatment length that is required to yield significantly positive results, if any. Nonetheless, because SIT resembles play and most children with autism enjoy it, SIT can be used as a reward or positive reinforcer to enhance speech/communication and social skills training. Furthermore, SIT may offer enjoyable and healthy physical activity, which is as important for autistic patients as for typically developing children.

Auditory Integration Training

In auditory integration training (AIT), various compact discs are selected containing music determined to be the best for the person receiving the therapy. The music is then played on a standard compact disc player and fed through an electronic device. The person listens to the music through standard headphones.

The treatment consists of 20 half-hour sessions at a rate of 2 per day over a period of 10 days.

However, in 1998, the American Academy of Pediatrics stated that there was not enough information to support the claims that AIT improved communication skills in autistic children.

■ Music Therapy

The implementation of music therapy involves interactions of the therapist, client, and music that initiate and sustain musical and nonmusical change processes. As the musical elements of rhythm, melody, and harmony are elaborated across time, the therapist and client can develop a relationship that may improve the quality of life. Music therapy may include singing, movement to music, and playing instruments.

Music therapy can be carried out in a private setting, but it can also be incorporated into school. An interested parent could also learn techniques for using music as a teaching tool at home. Music therapy has been used for many years to treat autistic individuals. It does seem to improve the quality of life of some autistic people.

■ Pharmacotherapy

Aman et al. (1995) surveyed the prevalence and pattern of medication therapy among autistic individuals in North Carolina. In all, 33.8% of the survey sample (taken from the caseloads of 838 care providers) was taking some psychotropic drug or vitamin for autism or associated behavior/psychiatric problems. More than 50% of the sample was taking some psychotropic, antiepileptic, vitamin, or "medical" agent. Martin et al. (1999b) reviewed the rates and pattern of psychotropic drug use in 109 high-functioning children, adolescents, and adults with PDD enrolled in the Yale Child Study Center's Project on Social Learning Disabilities. In all, 55% of the sample was taking psychotropics, with 29.3% taking two or more medications simultaneously. Antidepressants were the most commonly used drugs (32.1%), followed by stimulants (20.2%) and neuroleptics (16.5%).

Pharmacotherapy does not alter the natural history or course of autistic disorder. It can be helpful, however, in controlling specific symptoms such as hyperactivity, withdrawal, stereotypies, self-injury, aggressiveness, and sleep disorders. This subject has been reviewed by Tsai (2001).

Neuroleptics

Low-potency typical neuroleptics, such as chlorpromazine, have little or no therapeutic effect because they cause excessive sedation, even at low doses. On the other hand, haloperidol, a high-potency neuroleptic, has demonstrated both short- and long-term efficacy in young autistic children (ages 2.6–7.2 years) (Campbell et al. 1983). Haloperidol was significantly superior to placebo in reducing symptoms of withdrawal and stereotypies in these children. The combination of haloperidol and contingent reinforcement was found to be most effective in facilitating the acquisition of imitative speech. A long-term study of haloperidol by Campbell et al. (1983) reported that the effect lasts for 6 months to 2.5 years. At optimal doses, no adverse effects were noted. When above-optimal doses were given, excessive sedation was most common, followed by acute dystonic reaction. However, since the introduction of newer atypical neuroleptics, the role of haloperidol in autistic disorder has decreased and has been limited mostly to the treatment of tic disorders. When it is used, patients must be very carefully monitored for side effects.

Agonists, Antagonists, and Blockers

Fenfluramine, an antiserotonergic anorectic, was initially reported as showing positive effects, but subsequent data from a multicenter study (Campbell et al. 1988b) and an independent study failed to confirm any positive effects (Leventhal et al. 1993).

Naltrexone, an opiate antagonist, has been reported to have positive effects on hyperactivity, social relatedness, and self-injury (Campbell et al. 1993; Kolmen et al. 1997). However, other investigators did not find such effects (Gillberg 1995; Willemsen-Swinkels et al. 1996). Naltrexone treatment did not lead to improvement in communication skills (Feldman et al. 1999). Willemsen-Swinkels et al. (1995) reported increased incidence of stereotyped behavior with naltrexone treatment.

Clomipramine, a 5-HT reuptake blocker with unique anti-obsessional properties, has been shown to be effective in reducing compulsive and ritualistic behaviors, stereotypies, and aggressive and impulsive behaviors and in improving social relatedness (Gordon et al. 1993; McDougle et al. 1992). However, Sanchez et al. (1996) reported that clomipramine was not therapeutic and was associated with serious side effects.

Fluoxetine, a 5-HT reuptake blocker, likewise has been reported to reduce overall autistic symptoms (Buchsbaum et al. 2001; Cook et al. 1992; G.R. DeLong et al. 1998; Fatemi et al. 1998) but also to induce significant side effects, including restlessness, hyperactivity, agitation, vivid dreams, decreased appetite, and insomnia (Cook et al. 1992; Fatemi et al. 1998).

Fluvoxamine, a 5-HT reuptake blocker, was reported to be more effective than placebo in short-term treatment of symptoms of autism (i.e., social relatedness, repetitive thoughts and behavior, maladaptive behav-

ior, and aggression) in 15 adults (McDougle et al. 1996).

Sertraline, a 5-HT reuptake blocker, was reported as effective in reducing self-injury and aggression in mentally retarded autistic patients (Hellings et al. 1996) and in transition-associated anxiety and agitation in autistic children (Steingard et al. 1997).

A low dosage of venlafaxine, a potent inhibitor of neuronal serotonin and norepinephrine reuptake, was reported as effective in six subjects with autism. Improvement was noted in repetitive behaviors and restricted interests, social deficits, communication and language function, inattention, and hyperactivity (Hollander et al. 2000).

Clonidine, an α_2-adrenergic receptor agonist, showed effectiveness in reducing several hyperarousal behaviors and in improving social relationships in some autistic patients. However, clonidine also caused significant drowsiness and decreased activity levels (Fankhauser et al. 1992).

Risperidone, a potent 5-HT$_{2A}$-dopamine D$_2$ antagonist with additional dopamine antagonistic properties, seemed to reduce repetitive behavior, aggression, anxiety or nervousness, depression, irritability, self-injury, and overall behavioral symptoms (Findling et al. 1997b; Horrigan and Barnhill 1997; McDougle et al. 1998; Zuddas et al. 2000). However, weight gain is common (Findling et al. 1997b; Horrigan and Barnhill 1997; Zuddas et al. 2000). The rate of increase lessened over a period of time, and after drug withdrawal, considerable weight loss was observed in the patients who had previously shown the most significant weight increase (Zuddas et al. 2000).

Quetiapine fumarate is an antagonist at multiple neurotransmitter receptors in the brain: serotonin 5-HT$_{1A}$, 5-HT$_2$, dopamine D$_1$ and D$_2$, histamine H$_1$, and α_1-

adrenergic and α_2-adrenergic receptors. In an open-label quentiapine treatment in six autistic children, Martin et al. (1999a) reported that there was no significant improvement as rated on the Clinical Global Impression Scale and that quetiapine was poorly tolerated and associated with serious side effects.

Olanzapine is a selective monoaminergic antagonist to the following receptors: serotonin 5-HT$_{2A/2C}$, dopamine D$_1$ through dopamine D$_4$, muscarinic M$_1$ through muscarinic M$_5$, histamine H$_1$, and adrenergic. Five of six children treated with olanzapine showed improved scores on the Clinical Global Impression Scale (Malone et al. 2001). Weight gain is common with olanzapine treatment.

Stimulants

The use of stimulants in autism has not received extensive evaluation. Quintana et al. (1995) reported modest but statistically significant improvement with the use of methylphenidate in 10 autistic children. Handen et al. (2000) reported that 8 of 13 autistic children (62%) showed a positive response to methylphenidate, based on a minimum 50% decrease on the Conners Hyperactivity Index. Stimulants are frequently reported to exacerbate irritability, insomnia, and aggression in clinical populations (Posey and McDougle 2000).

Anticonvulsants

Anticonvulsants have been used to treat autistic symptoms. Hollander and colleagues (2001) reported that 10 of 14 autistic patients (71%) taking divalproex sodium were rated as having sustained response to treatment. It appeared that the responders were those who had associated features of affective instability, impulsivity, and aggression as well as those with a history of electroencephalographic abnormalities or seizures.

Natural and Synthetic Hormones

Secretin is a peptide hormone that stimulates pancreatic secretion. After the initial report of positive effect of secretin treatment of three autistic subjects (Horvath et al. 1998), many children with autism have received secretin treatment. However, several large-sample controlled studies have failed to demonstrate any significant positive treatment effect for autism (Chez et al. 2000; Coniglio et al. 2001; Dunn-Geier et al. 2000; Roberts et al. 2001), and a worsening in autistic symptoms during secretin treatment was noted by Robinson (2001).

The effects of neuropeptide ORG 2766, a synthetic analogue of adrenocorticotropic hormone, were studied in 34 autistic children. ORG 2766 was reported to increase the amount and quality of social interaction (Buitelaar et al. 1992). However, in a later study of 50 children with autism between ages 7 and 15 years and with a Performance IQ above 60, ORG 2766 failed to improve social and communicative behavior at the group level. Future studies should examine whether ORG 2766 differentially affects various subtypes of autism (Buitelaar et al. 1996).

Other Medications and Supplements

Niaprazine is a histamine H$_1$-receptor antagonist with marked sedative properties. Niaprazine was administered at 1 mg/kg/day for 60 days in 25 subjects with autism. A positive effect was noted in 13 patients (52%), particularly for hyperkinesias, unstable attention, resistance to change and frustration, mild anxiety, aggression, and sleep problems (Rossi et al. 1999).

R-THBP (6R-L-$erythro$-5,6,7,8-tetra-hydrobiopterin), a cofactor for tyrosine hydroxylase in the biosynthetic pathway of catecholamines and serotonin, was reported as effective in improving autistic children's social functioning—mainly eye contact and desire to interact and in the number of words or sounds that the children used (Fernell et al. 1997; Komori et al. 1995).

The efficacy of pyridoxine (vitamin B_6) plus magnesium has been controversial. Some short-term (2-week to 30-day) studies reported positive results (Pfeiffer et al. 1995; Tsai 1992). However, interpretation of these findings must be tempered because of methodological problems inherent in many of the studies (Pfeiffer et al. 1995). Other investigators could not confirm such findings (Findling et al. 1997a; Tolbert et al. 1993).

N,N-dimethylglycine (DMG), a dietary supplement, has been reported, in nonmedical literature, to be beneficial in children with autism. Two studies failed to find any significant difference between groups given DMG and those given placebo (Bolman and Richmond 1999; Kern et al. 2001).

Summary of Drug Efficacy Studies

Placebo-controlled trials of larger samples and long-term studies are needed before conclusions about the efficacy of any of these drugs can be drawn.

■ Pharmacotherapy for Clinical Conditions

Some clinical conditions in autistic disorder and associated psychiatric disorders are potentially drug responsive. For some conditions, the administration of certain drugs has been based on well-documented research, but for others, further research is required. I base these suggestions on my limited clinical and empirical experiences and those of a few other investigators because little research has been done in this field.

In unusual behaviors such as resistance to change, stereotypies, ritualistic and compulsive behaviors, and abnormal attachments, haloperidol, clomipramine, or selective serotonin reuptake inhibitors may be considered (Gordon et al. 1993; Tsai 2001).

In patients with severe hyperactivity, attention-deficit/hyperactivity disorder and impulsivity, clonidine (Ghaziuddin et al. 1992), guanfacine, or imipramine may be considered in low- or midlevel-functioning autistic individuals with or without other neurological disorders, such as seizure disorders and Tourette's disorder. Haloperidol may be considered for patients who do not respond to clonidine, guanfacine, or imipramine. In high-functioning individuals without other neurological disorders, stimulants may be tried first. Guanfacine, clonidine, and imipramine may be considered in patients who do not respond to stimulants or in those who have other neurological disorders (Tsai 2001).

In autistic patients with tic-like symptoms, haloperidol and pimozide should be tried first because they are more potent than clonidine. Risperidone and fluoxetine have been reported to be effective in the treatment of tic disorders. In some cases, the combination of haloperidol or pimozide with fluoxetine may be needed (Tsai 2001).

For treatment of social withdrawal in people with autistic disorder, naltrexone and fluoxetine may be considered (Tsai 2001).

In depressed individuals with autism and a strong family history of unipolar affective illness, tricyclic antidepressants, such as desipramine, or other 5-HT reuptake blockers may be considered (Ghaziuddin and Tsai 1991). Close monitoring of the drug response is critical in these patients, because clinicians have noted that the depressive episode became a hypomanic episode in some patients. Lithium may be the drug of choice in patients with a family history of bipolar affective illness and symptoms of mania.

Some autistic individuals may become aggressive and physically attack other people. Some of the aggressive behaviors may be related to frustrations. Most of the aggressive behaviors, however, do not seem to have any clear cause. They are of great concern because of their devastating effects. For individuals who demonstrate frequent aggressive behaviors and who do not respond to behavioral interventions, risperidone or olanzapine may be the drug of choice. Trazodone, carbamazepine, lithium, and propranolol may be considered in patients who do not respond to risperidone or olanzapine treatment (Tsai 2001).

Self-injurious behavior such as head banging, finger, hand, or wrist biting, and scratching of face or extremities may occur in lower-functioning autistic individuals. A selective serotonin reuptake inhibitor or naltrexone may be the drug of first choice (Campbell et al. 1988a; Tsai 2001). Haloperidol or trazodone may be considered for individuals who do not respond to naltrexone treatment.

Unusual sleeping patterns are common in autistic children. Some children develop complete reversed sleep pattern; that is, they sleep during the day and wake during the night. The key to solve such a problem is to reverse the sleep cycle through a well-planned regimen. Some autistic children seem to need a much longer time to settle down for sleep (i.e., have initial insomnia) and/or need less sleep than most nonautistic children. Children with these sleep disturbances tend to keep the entire family awake every night. Melatonin may be the drug of first choice (Jan et al. 1994; Tsai 2001). Some autistic children may respond to antihistamines, such as diphen-

hydramine and hydroxyzine, or to clonidine. In other, more severe cases, tricyclic antidepressants, such as imipramine or trazodone (Gualtieri 1991; Tsai 2001), may be considered.

In autistic individuals who develop clear delusions, hallucinations, and bizarre behaviors, including catatonia, an atypical neuroleptic (e.g., risperidone, olanzapine, quetiapine) may be the drug of first choice (Tsai 2001). Other antipsychotic medications, such as haloperidol, thiothixene, and loxapine, are the second-line drugs of choice.

Because the above information was developed mainly from experience with small samples of autistic children treated with psychotropic medications, a great deal of work remains to be done to verify these medications' efficacy in adolescents and adults with autistic disorder.

■ Summary of Treatment

As yet, no single treatment modality can alter the course of autism. Achieving significant treatment goals for autistic children requires comprehensive treatment programs, which include behavior modification and special education in a highly structured environment. Pharmacotherapy may be useful to control symptoms and behaviors that are not responsive to behavior modification or special-education techniques.

Clinical Course and Prognosis

Autism is a disorder with a chronic course. Although social, conceptual, linguistic, and obsessive difficulties frequently persist, they do so in forms that are rather different from those shown in early years. In a 12-year prospective study of 53 autistic children, 68% achieved scores within their original IQ group, 23% moved into higher IQ groups, and 9% moved down to lower

IQ groups. The Vineland Adaptive Behavior Scores (VABS) were consistently lower than cognitive scores, and maladaptive behaviors were found to occur with equal frequency in the high-, medium-, and low-IQ groups (Freeman et al. 1991). In a further study, Freeman et al. (1999) observed that autistic subjects improved with age in all domains of VABS. The rate of growth in communication and daily living skills was related to initial IQ, whereas rate of growth in social skills was not. In a group of preschool autistic children reevaluated at a mean age of 10–13 years, Sigman et al. (1999) found little change in the diagnosis of autism but sizable improvements in intellectual and language abilities. Harris and Handleman (2000) reexamined the educational placement of 27 preschool autistic children 4 to 6 years later. It was found that having a higher IQ at intake and being of younger age were both predictive of being in a regular education class after discharge from an intensive treatment program, whereas having a lower IQ and being older at intake were closely related to placement in a special-education classroom.

A small group of autistic children— 22% in Gillberg's (1991) study—showed a progressive deterioration during adolescence, characterized by a general intellectual decline. Between 7% and 28% of autistic children who had shown no clinical evidence of neurological disorder in early childhood first developed seizures in adolescence or early adulthood. The seizures were usually major but tended to occur infrequently (Rutter 1977). During adolescence, hyperactivity is often replaced by marked underactivity and lack of initiative and drive. Some autistic people may have increased anxiety and tension. They may have sexual curiosity (Konstantareas and Lunsky 1997) that may lead to socially embarrassing behavior, such as masturbation in public or self-exposure (Van

Bourgondien et al. 1997). A Japanese follow-up study of 201 young adults reported that about 31.5% had some marked deterioration during adolescence but that 43.2% had shown marked improvement during that period (Kobayashi et al. 1992). On the basis of data from the California developmental disabilities registry, Shavelle and Strauss (1998) reported that people with autism have an increased mortality risk that increases with age. The mortality ratio for females was strikingly higher than for males.

In a Swedish sample, Gillberg (1991) found that a minority of people with autism had a productive, self-supporting adult life. However, even those with good adjustment generally continued to have difficulties in relationships and some oddities of behavior. Gillberg (1991) also reported that about two-thirds of the individuals with autism remained dependent on others throughout life. Ballaban-Gil et al. (1996), in a study of 54 adolescents and 45 adults, reported that behavior difficulties continued to be a problem in 69% of the subjects; 90% of both adolescents and adults had persisting social deficits; only 35% achieved normal or near-normal fluency; and only 29% had achieved normal or near-normal comprehension of oral language. Piven et al. (1996) reported significant change over time in autistic behaviors, generally in the direction of improvement, particularly in communication and social behaviors. Mawhood et al. (2000) found that at about age 23 or 24 years, autistic subjects showed significant improvement in verbal IQ and receptive language scores. However, about 74% had severe social difficulties (Howlin et al. 2000).

The University of North Carolina program Treatment and Education of Autistic and Related Communication Handicapped Children (Division TEACCH) has found that when community services are available and provide adequate educational and vocational training, only a minority (i.e., 8%) of autistic individuals are placed in institutions (Schopler et al. 1982). Ballaban-Gil et al. (1996) noted that 53% of 45 autistic adults lived in residential placement; only 11% of adults were employed on the open market, all in menial jobs, an additional 16% were employed in sheltered workshops. Howlin et al. (2000) reported that by age 23 or 24 years, many autistic adults still lived with their parents, few had close friends or permanent jobs, and ratings of social interaction indicated abnormalities in a number of different areas.

Three factors were consistently related to outcome: 1) IQ, 2) the presence or absence of speech, and 3) the severity of the disorder. IQ alone best predicts only those with poor outcome. A high nonverbal score with no subsequent language development is of no predictive value, whereas if language subsequently develops, the nonverbal score is a useful guide to later general IQ scores (Rutter 1970). One additional factor, work/school status, was found to be the best predictor of work or academic performance at follow-up (DeMyer et al. 1973). Other variables have been reported to be significantly associated with outcome (although the correlations are less strong than for the previous three variables): 1) amount of time spent in school, 2) rating of social maturity, 3) rating of social behavior, 4) developmental milestones, and 5) comorbid neuropsychiatric disorders.

Conflicting findings have been reported for several variables in relation to outcome: sex, brain dysfunction or damage, and the category "untestable child." Factors that were unrelated to outcome included birth weight, perinatal complications, age at onset, history of a period of normal development before onset, late development of seizures, socioeconomic class, broken home, family history of mental illness, and type of treatment.

Research Issues

A range of neurobiological abnormalities associated with autistic disorder has been found, although the replicability of specific findings has not been high. The inconsistent findings may be the result of a number of factors, including the use of different diagnostic criteria for patient selection; failure to control for developmental factors (i.e., many studies included both children and adults); lack of suitable control groups (i.e., most studies used nonretarded rather than mentally retarded control subjects and hence failed to control for concomitant mental retardation found in most of the autistic subjects); failure to control for concomitant medical disorders (particularly central nervous system pathologies); and use of medications that may significantly affect a subject's neurochemical or neurophysiological responses. Nevertheless, the lack of consistent and specific findings can also be viewed as supporting evidence for the existence of many different subgroups within autistic disorder.

Future neurobiological research should 1) focus on the question of specificity and selectivity within each of the subgroups; 2) avoid combining high-functioning autistic subjects with those who have Asperger's disorder, as many studies did in the past; 3) integrate many levels of inquiry for neurobiological information associated with autism; 4) put more emphasis on developing agreeable, reliable, and valid diagnostic instruments to identify comorbid psychiatric disorders in autistic individuals; and 5) involve collaboration between multiple research centers from various countries to study various races and ethnic groups.

The amount of research into pharmacotherapy for autistic disorder has steadily increased since the 1980s. However, studies have been complicated by various factors, including a tremendous range of syndrome expression, uncommunicative subjects, treatment with multiple medications combined with nonpharmacological interventions, failure to include behavioral measures, and absence of long-term outcome measures.

Future psychopharmacological research should emphasize the use of randomized, double-blind, placebo-controlled, crossover designs; the involvement of multicenters with extensive cross-site training; and the use of uniform diagnostic criteria to study medication treatment in autistic children and adolescents. Communication problems may be solvable by several strategies, including careful questioning of care providers; specially adapted and sensitive rating scales with good clinician reliability; laboratory tests; and physical examinations. The broad heterogeneity of subjects will require that outcome measures be sensitive to individual change over a wide spectrum of treatment response and side effects.

Future psychopharmacological investigations should focus on the efficacy of combined treatments such as pharmacotherapy with behavior therapy or group therapy, because it is highly unlikely that curative medications for autism will be developed in the near future.

References

Adolphs R, Sears L, Piven J: Abnormal processing of social information from faces in autism. J Cogn Neurosci 13:232–240, 2001

Aman MG, Van Bourgondien ME, Wolford PL, et al: Psychotropic and anticonvulsant drugs in subjects with autism: prevalence and patterns of use. J Am Acad Child Adolesc Psychiatry 34:1672–1681, 1995

American Academy of Child and Adolescent Psychiatry: Practice parameters for the assessment and treatment of children, adolescents, and adults with autism and other pervasive developmental disorders. J Am Acad Child Adolesc Psychiatry 38 (12, suppl):32S–54S, 1999

American Psychiatric Association: Diagnostic and Statistical Manual of Mental Disorders, 3rd Edition. Washington, DC, American Psychiatric Association, 1980

American Psychiatric Association: Diagnostic and Statistical Manual of Mental Disorders, 3rd Edition, Revised. Washington, DC, American Psychiatric Association, 1987

American Psychiatric Association: Diagnostic and Statistical Manual of Mental Disorders, 4th Edition. Washington, DC, American Psychiatric Association, 1994

American Psychiatric Association: Diagnostic and Statistical Manual of Mental Disorders, 4th Edition, Text Revision. Washington, DC, American Psychiatric Association, 2000

Anderson GM, Schlicht KR, Cohen DJ: Two-dimensional high-performance liquid chromatographic determination of 5-hydroxyindoleacetic acid and homovanillic acid in urine. Anal Biochem 144:27–31, 1985

Anderson GM, Freedman DX, Cohen DJ, et al: Whole blood serotonin in autistic and normal subjects. J Child Psychol Psychiatry 28:885–900, 1987

Ashley-Koch A, Wolpert CM, Menold MM, et al: Genetic studies of autistic disorder and chromosome 7. Genomics 61:227–236, 1999

Asperger H: Die autistischen psychopathen im kindesalter (1944), in Autism and Asperger Syndrome. Translated by Frith U. Cambridge, UK, Cambridge University Press, 1991, pp 37–92

August GJ, Stewart MA, Tsai L: The incidence of cognitive disabilities in the siblings of autistic children. Br J Psychiatry 138:416–422, 1981

Bailey A, Le Couteur A, Gottesman I, et al: Autism as a strong genetic disorder: evidence from a British twin study. Psychol Med 25:63–77, 1995

Bailey DB Jr, Mesibov GB, Hatton DD, et al: Autistic behavior in young boys with fragile X syndrome. J Autism Dev Disord 28:499–508, 1998

Baird G, Charman T, Baron-Cohen S, et al: A screening instrument for autism at 18 months of age: a 6-year follow-up study. J Am Acad Child Adolesc Psychiatry 39:694–702, 2000

Baker P, Piven J, Sato Y: Autism and tuberous sclerosis complex: prevalence and clinical features. J Autism Dev Disord 28:279–285, 1998

Ballaban-Gil K, Rapin I, Tuchman R, et al: Longitudinal examination of the behavioral, language, and social changes in a population of adolescents and young adults with autistic disorder. Pediatr Neurol 15:217–223, 1996

Baron-Cohen S, Ring HA, Wheelwright, et al: Social intelligence in the normal and autistic brain: an fMRI study. Eur J Neurosci 11:1891–1898, 1999

Baron-Cohen S, Ring HA, Bullmore ET, et al: The amygdala theory of autism. Neurosci Biobehav Rev 24:355–364, 2000

Barrett S, Beck JC, Bernier R, et al: Autosomal genomic screen for autism: collaborative linkage study of autism. Am J Med Genet 88:609–615, 1999

Bartak L, Rutter M: Differences between mentally retarded and normally intelligent autistic children. J Autism Child Schizophr 6:109–120, 1976

Bartak L, Rutter M, Cox A: A comparative study of infantile autism and specific developmental receptive language disorder, I: the children. Br J Psychiatry 126:127–145, 1975

Barton M, Volkmar F: How commonly are known medical conditions associated with autism? J Autism Dev Disord 28:273–278, 1998

Bass MP, Menold MM, Wolpert, et al: Genetic studies in autistic disorder and chromosome 15. Neurogenetics 2:219–226, 2000

Bennetto L, Pennington BF, Rogers SJ: Intact and impaired memory functions in autism. Child Dev 67:1816–1835, 1996

Bernard S, Enayati A, Redwood L, et al: Autism: a novel form of mercury poisoning. Med Hypotheses 56:462–471, 2001

Bleuler E: Dementia Praecox oder Gruppe der Schizophrenien (1911). Translated by Zinkin J. New York, International Universities Press, 1950

Bloomquist HK, Bohman M, Edvinsson SO, et al: Frequency of fragile X syndrome in infantile autism: a Swedish multicenter study. Clin Genet 27:113–117, 1985

Bolman WM, Richmond JA: A double-blind, placebo-controlled, crossover pilot trial of low dose dimethylglycine in patients with autistic disorder. J Autism Dev Disord 29:191–194, 1999

Bolton P, Macdonald H, Pickles A, et al: A case-control family history study of autism. J Child Psychol Psychiatry 35:877–900, 1994

Bolton PF, Murphy M, Macdonald H, et al: Obstetric complication in autism: consequences or causes of the condition? J Am Acad Child Adolesc Psychiatry 36:272–281, 1997

Bolton PF, Pickles A, Murphy M, et al: Autism, affective and other psychiatric disorders: patterns of familial aggregation. Psychol Med 28:385–395, 1998

Bormann-Kischkel C, Vilsmeier M, Baude B: The development of emotional concepts in autism. J Child Psychol Psychiatry 36:1243–1259, 1995

Boucher J, Lewis V, Collis G: Familiar face and voice matching and recognition in children with autism. J Child Psychol Psychiatry 39:171–181, 1998

Boutin P, Maziade M, Merette C, et al: Family history of cognitive disabilities in first-degree relatives of autistic and mentally retarded children. J Autism Dev Disord 27:165–176, 1997

Buchsbaum MS, Hollander E, Hazenedar MM, et al: Effect of fluoxetine on regional cerebral metabolism in autistic spectrum disorder: a pilot study. Int J Neuropsychopharmacol 4:119–125, 2001

Buitelaar JK, Van Engeland H, de Kogel KH, et al: The adrenocorticotrophic hormone (4–9) analog ORG 2766 benefits autistic children: report on a second controlled clinical trial. J Am Acad Child Adolesc Psychiatry 31:1149–1156, 1992

Buitelaar JK, Dekker ME, van Ree JM, et al: A controlled trial with ORG 2766, an ACTH-(4–9) analog, in 50 relatively able children with autism. Euro Neuropsychopharmacol 6:13–19, 1996

Buitelaar JK, van der Wees M, Swaab-Barneveld H, et al: Theory of mind and emotion-recognition functioning in autistic spectrum disorders and in psychiatric control and normal children. Dev Psychopathol 11:39–58, 1999

Burd L, Severud R, Kerbeshian J, et al: Prenatal and perinatal risk factors for autism. J Perinat Med 27:441–450, 1999

Campbell M: Treatment of childhood and adolescent schizophrenia, in Psychopharmacology in Childhood and Adolescence. Edited by Wiener JM. New York, Basic Books, 1977, pp 101–118

Campbell M, Perry R, Bennett WG, et al: Long-term therapeutic efficacy and drug-related abnormal movements: a prospective study of haloperidol in autistic children. Psychopharmacol Bull 19:80–83, 1983

Campbell M, Adams P, Perry R, et al: Naltrexone in infantile autism. Psychopharmacol Bull 24:135–139, 1988a

Campbell M, Adams P, Small AM, et al: Efficacy and safety of fenfluramine in autistic children. J Am Acad Child Adolesc Psychiatry 4:434–439, 1988b

Campbell M, Anderson LT, Small AM, et al: Naltrexone in autistic children: behavioral symptoms and attentional learning. J Am Acad Child Adolesc Psychiatry 32:1283–1291, 1993

Cantwell DP, Baker L, Rutter M, et al: Infantile autism and developmental dysphasia: a comparative follow-up into middle childhood. J Autism Dev Disord 19:19–31, 1989

Celani G, Battacchi MW, Arcidacono L: The understanding of the emotional meaning of facial expressions in people with autism. J Autism Dev Disord 29:57–66, 1999

Charman T, Sweettenham J, Baron-Cohen S, et al: Infants with autism: an investigation of empathy, pretend play, joint attention, and imitation. Dev Psychol 33:781–789, 1997

Chess S: Follow-up report on autism in congenital rubella. J Autism Dev Disord 7:69–81, 1977

Chez MG, Buchanan CP, Bagan BT, et al: Secretin and autism: a two-part clinical investigation. J Autism Dev Disord 30:87–94, 2000

Chez MG, Chin K, Hung PC: Immunizations, immunology, and autism. Semin Pediatr Neurol 11:214–217, 2004

Chiron C, Leboyer M, Leon F, et al: SPECT of the brain in childhood autism: evidence for a lack of normal hemispheric asymmetry. Dev Med Child Neurol 37:849–860, 1995

Chudley AE, Gutierrez E, Joycelyn LJ, et al: Outcomes of genetic evaluation in children with pervasive developmental disorder. J Dev Behav Pediatr 19:321–325, 1998

Chugani DC, Muzik O, Rothermel R, et al: Altered serotonin synthesis in the dentatothalamocortical pathway in autistic boys. Ann Neurol 42:666–669, 1997

Chugani DC, Sundram BS, Behen M, et al: Evidence of altered energy metabolism in autistic children. Prog Neuropsychopharmacol Biol Psychiatry 23:635–641, 1999

Ciesielski KT, Knight JE: Cerebellar abnormality in autism: a nonspecific effect of early brain damage? Acta Neurobiol Exp (Warsz) 54:151–154, 1994

Coniglio SJ, Lewis JD, Lang C, et al: A randomized, double-blind, placebo-controlled trial of single-dose intravenous secretin as treatment for children with autism. J Pediatr 138:649–655, 2001

Connolly AM, Chez MG, Pestronk A, et al: Serum autoantibodies to brain in Landau-Kleffner variant, autism, and other neurologic disorders. J Pediatr 134:607–613, 1999

Conroy J, Meally E, Kearney G, et al: Serotonin transporter gene and autism: a haplotype analysis in an Irish autistic population. Mol Psychiatry 9:587–593, 2004

Cook EH Jr, Rowlett R, Jaselskis C, et al: Fluoxetine treatment of children and adults with autistic disorder and mental retardation. J Am Acad Child Adolesc Psychiatry 31:739–745, 1992

Cook EH Jr, Courchesne RY, Lord C, et al: Evidence of linkage between the serotonin transporter and autistic disorder. Mol Psychiatr 2:247–250, 1997a

Cook EH Jr, Lindgren V, Leventhal BL, et al: Autism or atypical autism in maternally but not paternally derived proximal 15q duplication. Am J Hum Genet 60:928–934, 1997b

Cook EH Jr, Courchesne RY, Cox NJ, et al: Linkage-disequilibrium mapping of autistic disorder. Am J Hum Genet 62:1077–1083, 1998

Courchesne E: A neurophysiological view of autism, in Neurobiological Issues in Autism. Edited by Schopler E, Mesibov GB. New York, Plenum, 1987, pp 285–324

Courchesne E, Townsend J, Akshoomoff NA, et al: Impairment in shifting attention in autistic and cerebellar patients. Behav Neurosci 108:848–865, 1994

Courchesne E, Muller RA, Saitoh O: Brain weight in autism: normal in the majority of cases, megalencephalic in rare cases. Neurology 52:1057–1059, 1999

Craddock N, Lendon C: Chromosome Workshop: chromosomes 11, 14, and 15. Am J Med Genet 88:244–254, 1999

Cryan E, Byrne M, O'Donovan A, et al: A case-control study of obstetric complications and later autistic disorder. J Autism Dev Disord 26:453–460, 1996

Davidovitch M, Glick L, Holtzman G, et al: Developmental regression in autism: maternal perception. J Autism Dev Disord 30:113–119, 2000

Dawson G, Finley C, Phillips S, et al: Reduced P3 amplitude of the event-related brain potential: relationship to language ability in autism. J Autism Dev Disord 18:493–504, 1988

Deb S, Prasad KB, Seth H, et al: A comparison of obstetric and neonatal complications between children with autistic disorder and their siblings. J Intellect Disabil Res 41(pt 1): 81–86, 1997

De Giacomo A, Fombonne E: Parental recognition of developmental abnormalities in autism. Eur Child Adolesc Psychiatry 7:131–136, 1998

DeLong GR, Teague LA, McSwain Kamran M: Effects of fluoxetine treatment in young children with idiopathic autism. Dev Med Child Neurol 40:551–562, 1998

DeLong R, Nohria C: Psychiatric family history and neurological disease in autistic spectrum disorders. Dev Med Child Neurol 36:441–448, 1994

DeMyer M, Barton S, DeMyer W, et al: Prognosis in autism: a follow-up study. J Autism Child Schizophr 3:199–246, 1973

Denney DR, Frei BW, Gaffney G: Lymphocyte subsets and interleukin-2 receptors in autistic children. J Autism Dev Disord 26:87–97, 1996

D'Eufemia P, Finocchiaro R, Celli M, et al: Low serum tryptophan to large neutral amino acids ratio in idiopathic infantile autism. Biomed Pharmacother 49:288–292, 1995

D'Eufemia P, Celli M, Finocchiaro R, et al: Abnormal intestinal permeability in children with autism. Acta Paediatr 85:1076–1079, 1996

Deykin E, MacMahon B: The incidence of seizures among children with autistic symptoms. Am J Psychiatry 126: 1310–1312, 1979

Dunn-Geier J, Ho HH, Auersperg E, et al: Effect of secretin on children with autism: a randomized controlled trial. Dev Med Child Neurol 42:796–802, 2000

Eisenberg L, Kanner L: Early infantile autism 1943–55. Am J Orthopsychiatry 26:556–566, 1956

Elia M, Musumeci SA, Ferri R, et al: Clinical and neurophysiological aspects of epilepsy in subjects with autism and mental retardation. Am J Ment Retard 100:6–16, 1995

Elia M, Ferri R, Musumeci SA, et al: Clinical correlates of brain morphometric features of subjects with low-functioning autistic disorder. J Child Neurol 15:504–508, 2000a

Elia M, Ferri R, Musumeci SA, et al: Sleep in subjects with autistic disorder: a neurophysiological and psychological study. Brain Dev 22:88–92, 2000b

Fankhauser MP, Karumanchi VC, German ML, et al: A double-blind, placebo-controlled study of the efficacy of transdermal clonidine in autism. J Clin Psychiatry 53:77–82, 1992

Farrington CP, Miller E, Taylor B: MMR and autism: further evidence against a causal association. Vaccine 19:3632–3635, 2001

Fatemi SH, Realmuto GM, Khan L, et al: Fluoxetine in treatment of adolescent patients
with autism: a longitudinal open trial. J Autism Dev Disord 28:303–307, 1998

Feldman HM, Kolmen BK, Gonzaga AM: Naltrexone and communication skills in
young children with autism. J Am Acad
Child Adolesc Psychiatry 38:587–593, 1999

Fernell E, Watanabe Y, Adolfsson Y, et al: Possible effects of tetrahydrobiopterin treatment
in six children with autism: clinical and
positron emission tomography data—a pilot study. Dev Med Child Neurol 39:313–
318, 1997

Fidler DJ, Bailey JN, Smalley SL: Macrocephaly
in autism and other pervasive developmental
disorders. Dev Med Child Neurol 42:737–
740, 2000

Findling RL, Maxwell K, Scotese-Wojtila L, et al:
High-dose pyridoxine and magnesium administration in children with autistic disorder: an absence of salutary effects in a double-blind, placebo-controlled study. J Autism
Dev Disord 27:467–478, 1997a

Findling RL, Maxwell K, Wiznitzer M: An open
clinical trial of risperidone monotherapy in
young children with autistic disorder. Psychopharmacol Bull 33:155–159, 1997b

Folstein S, Rutter M: Infantile autism: a genetic study of 21 twin pairs. J Child Psychol
Psychiatry 18:297–321, 1977

Folstein S, Santangelo SL, Gilman SE, et al: Predictors of cognitive test patterns in autism
families. J Child Psychol Psychiatry 40:1117–
1128, 1999

Fombonne E: The epidemiology of autism: a
review. Psychol Med 29:769–786, 1999

Fombonne E, du Mazaubrun C, Cans C, et al:
Autism and associated medical disorders in
a French epidemiological survey. J Am Acad
Child Adolesc Psychiatry 36:1561–1569,
1997

Freeman BJ, Ritvo ER, Needleman R, et al:
The stability of cognitive and linguistic parameters in autism: a five-year prospective
study. J Am Acad Child Psychiatry 24:459–
464, 1985

Freeman BJ, Ritvo ER, Yokota A, et al: Autism,
forme fruste: psychometric assessments of
first-degree relatives, in Biological Psychiatry. Edited by Shagass E, Perris C, Struwe G,
et al. New York, Elsevier Science, 1986, pp
1487–1488

Freeman BJ, Rahbar B, Ritvo ER, et al: The stability of cognitive and behavioral parameters in autism: a twelve-year prospective
study. J Am Acad Child Adolesc Psychiatry
30:479–482, 1991

Freeman BJ, Del'Homme M, Guthrie D, et al:
Vineland Adaptive Behavior Scale scores as
a function of age and IQ in 210 autistic children. J Autism Dev Disord 29:379–384, 1999

Ghaziuddin M, Tsai L: Depression in autistic
disorder. Br J Psychiatry 159:721–723, 1991

Ghaziuddin M, Tsai L, Ghaziuddin N: Clonidine for autism. J Child Adolesc Psychopharmacol 2:1–2, 1992

Ghaziuddin M, Zaccagnini J, Tsai L, et al: Is
megalencephaly specific to autism? J Intellect Disabil Res 43(pt 4):279–282, 1999

Gillberg C: Outcome in autism and autistic-
like conditions. J Am Acad Child Adolesc
Psychiatry 30:375–382, 1991

Gillberg C: Endogenous opioid and opiate antagonists in autism: brief review of empirical findings and implications for clinicians.
Dev Med Child Neurol 37:239–245, 1995

Gillberg C: Autism and Asperger Syndrome.
Cambridge, UK, Cambridge University
Press, 2000

Gillberg C, Coleman M: Autism and medical
disorders: a review of the literature. Dev
Med Child Neurol 38:191–202, 1996

Gillberg C, Gillberg IC, Steffenburg S: Siblings and parents of children with autism:
a controlled population-based study. Dev
Med Child Neurol 34:389–398, 1992

Giovanardi Rossi P, Posar A, Parmeggiani A:
Epilepsy in adolescents and young adults
with autistic disorder. Brain Dev 22:102–
106, 2000

Gold N: Depression and social adjustment in
siblings of boys with autism. J Autism Dev
Disord 23:147–163, 1993

Goldstein H, Kaczmarek L, Pennington R, et al: Peer-mediated intervention: attending to, commenting on, and acknowledging the behavior of preschoolers with autism. J Appl Behav Anal 25:289–305, 1992

Gong X, Jia M, Ruan Y, et al: Association between the FOXP2 gene and autistic disorder in Chinese population. Am J Med Genet B Neuropsychiatr Genet 127:113–116, 2004

Goodman R, Minne C: Questionnaire screening for comorbid pervasive developmental disorders in congenitally blind children: a pilot study. J Autism Dev Disord 25:195–203, 1995

Gordon CT, State RC, Nelson JE, et al: A double-blind comparison of clomipramine, desipramine, and placebo in the treatment of autistic disorder. Arch Gen Psychiatry 50:441–447, 1993

Griffith EM, Pennington BF, Wehner EA, et al: Executive functions in young children with autism. Child Dev 70:817–832, 1999

Gualtieri CT: Neuropsychiatry and Behavioral Pharmacology. New York, Springer-Verlag, 1991

Gupta S, Aggarwal S, Rashanravan B, et al: Th1- and Th2-like cytokines in CD4+ and CD8+ T cells in autism. J Neuroimmunol 85:106–109, 1998

Hagberg BA, Aicardi J, Dias K, et al: A progressive syndrome of autism, dementia, ataxia, and loss of purposeful hand use in girls: Rett's syndrome—report of 35 cases. Ann Neurol 14:471–479, 1983

Hagerman R: Medical aspects of the fragile X syndrome, in The Fragile X Child. Edited by Schopmeyer BB, Lowe F. San Diego, CA, Singular Publishing Group, 1992, pp 19–29

Hallmayer J, Pintado E, Lotspeich L, et al: Molecular analysis and test of linkage between the FMR-1 gene and infantile autism in multiplex families. Am J Hum Genet 55:951–959, 1994

Halsey NA, Hyman SL, Conference Writing Panel: Measles-mumps-rubella vaccine and autistic spectrum disorder: report from the New Challenges in Childhood Immunizations Conference convened in Oak Brook, IL, June 12–13, 2000. Pediatrics 107:E84, 2001

Handen BL, Johnson CR, Lubetsky M: Efficacy of methylphenidate among children with autism and symptoms of attention-deficit hyperactivity disorder. J Autism Dev Disord 30:245–255, 2000

Harris SL, Handleman JS: Age and IQ at intake as predictors of placement for young children with autism: a four- to six-year follow-up. J Autism Dev Disord 30:137–142, 2000

Hashimoto T, Sasaki M, Fukumizu M, et al: Single-photon emission computed tomography of the brain in autism: effect of the developmental level. Pediatr Neurol 23:416–420, 2000

Haznedar MM, Buchsbaum MS, Wei TC, et al: Limbic circuitry in patients with autism spectrum disorder studied with positron emission tomography and magnetic resonance imaging. Am J Psychiatry 157:1994–2001, 2000

Heh CWC, Smith R, Wu J, et al: Positron emission tomography of the cerebellum in autism. Am J Psychiatry 146:242–245, 1989

Heimann M, Nelson KE, Tjus T, et al: Increasing reading and communication skills in children with autism through an interactive multimedia computer program. J Autism Dev Disord 25:459–480, 1995

Hellings JA, Kelley LA, Gabrielli WF, et al: Sertraline response in adults with mental retardation and autistic disorder. J Clin Psychiatry 57:333–336, 1996

Henderson D, Vandenberg B: Factors influencing adjustment in the families of autistic children. Psychol Rep 71:167–171, 1992

Herzing LB, Kim SJ, Cook EH Jr, et al: The human aminophospholipid-transporting ATPase gene *ATP10C* maps adjacent to *UBE3A* and exhibits similar imprinted expression. Am J Hum Genet 68:1501–1505, 2001

Hirsch E, Marescaux C, Maquet P, et al: Landau-Kleffner syndrome: a clinical and EEG study of five cases. Epilepsia 31:756–767, 1990

Hollander E, DelGiudice-Asch G, Simon L, et al: B lymphocyte antigen D8/17 and repetitive behaviors in autism. Am J Psychiatry 156:317–320, 1999

Hollander E, Kaplan A, Cartwright C, et al: Venlafaxine in children, adolescents, and young adults with autism spectrum disorders: an open retrospective clinical report. J Child Neurol 15:132–135, 2000

Hollander E, Dolgoff-Kaspar R, Cartwright C, et al: An open trial of divalproex sodium in autism spectrum disorders. J Clin Psychiatry 62:530–534, 2001

Horrigan JP, Barnhill LJ: Risperidone and explosive aggressive autism. J Autism Dev Disord 27:313–323, 1997

Horvath K, Stefanatos G, Sokolski KN, et al: Improved social and language skills after secretin administration in patients with autistic spectrum disorders. J Assoc Acad Minor Phys 9:9–15, 1998

Horvath K, Papadimitriou JC, Rabsztyn A, et al: Gastrointestinal abnormalities in children with autistic disorder. J Pediatr 135:533–535, 1999

Howard MA, Cowell MA, Boucher J, et al: Convergent neuroanatomical and behavioural evidence of an amygdala hypothesis of autism. Neuroreport 11:2931–2935, 2000

Howlin P, Mawhood L, Rutter M: Autism and developmental receptive language disorder—a follow-up comparison in early adult life, II: social, behavioural, and psychiatric outcomes. J Child Psychol Psychiatry 41:561–578, 2000

Hughes C, Plumet MH, Leboyer M: Towards a cognitive phenotype for autism: increased prevalence of executive dysfunction and superior spatial span amongst siblings of children with autism. J Child Psychol Psychiatry 40:705–718, 1999

International Molecular Genetics Study of Autism Consortium (IMGSAC): Further characterization of autism susceptibility locus *AUTS1* on chromosome 7q. Hum Mol Genet 10:973–982, 2001

Jan JE, Espezel H, Appleton RE: The treatment of sleep disorders with melatonin. Dev Med Child Neurol 36:97–107, 1994

Jocelyn LJ, Casiro OG, Beattie D, et al: Treatment of children with autism: a randomized controlled trial to evaluate a caregiver-based intervention program in community day-care centers. J Dev Behav Pediatr 19:326–334, 1998

Jolliffe T, Baron-Cohen S: The Strange Stories Test: a replication with high-functioning adults with autism or Asperger syndrome. J Autism Dev Disord 29:395–406, 1999

Juul-Dam N, Townsend J, Courchesne E: Prenatal, perinatal, and neonatal factors in autism, pervasive developmental disorder–not otherwise specified, and the general population. Pediatrics 107:E63, 2001

Kanner L: Autistic disturbances of affective contact. Nervous Child 2:217–250, 1943

Katsui T, Okuda M, Usuda S, et al: Kinetics of H-serotonin uptake by platelets in infantile autism and developmental language disorder (including five pairs of twins). J Autism Dev Disord 16:69–76, 1986

Kaye JA, del Mar Melero-Montes M, et al: Mumps, measles, and rubella vaccine and the incidence of autism recorded by general practitioners: a time trend analysis. BMJ 322:460–463, 2001

Kent L, Evans J, Paul M, et al: Comorbidity of autistic spectrum disorders in children with Down syndrome. Dev Med Child Neurol 41:153–158, 1999

Kern JK, Miller VS, Cauller PL, et al: Effectiveness of *N,N*-dimethylglycine in autism and pervasive developmental disorder. J Child Neurol 16:169–173, 2001

Klauck SM, Pouska F, Benner A, et al: Serotonin transporter (*5-HTT*) gene variants associated with autism? Hum Mol Genet 6:2233–2238, 1997

Knoblock H, Pasamanick B: Some etiologic and prognostic factors in early infantile autism and psychosis. Pediatrics 55:182–191, 1975

Knott F, Lewis C, Williams T: Sibling interaction of children with learning disabilities: a comparison of autism and Down's syndrome. J Child Psychol Psychiatry 36:965–976, 1995

Kobayashi R, Murata T: Setback phenomenon in autism and long-term prognosis. Acta Psychiatr Scand 98:296–303, 1998

Kobayashi R, Murata T, Yoshinaga K: A follow-up study of 201 children with autism in Kyushu and Yamaguchi areas, Japan. J Autism Dev Disord 22:395–411, 1992

Koegel RL, Schreibman L, Loos LM, et al: Consistent stress profiles in mothers of children with autism. J Autism Dev Disord 22:205–216, 1992

Koegel RL, Bimbela A, Schreibman L: Collateral effects of parent training on family interactions. J Autism Dev Disord 26:347–359, 1996

Kolmen BK, Feldman HM, Handen BL, et al: Naltrexone in young autistic children: replication study and learning measures. J Am Acad Child Adolesc Psychiatry 36:800–802, 1997

Komori H, Matsuishi T, Yamada S, et al: Cerebrospinal fluid biopterin and biogenic amine metabolites during oral R-THBP therapy for infantile autism. J Autism Dev Disord 25:183–193, 1995

Konstantareas MM, Lunsky YJ: Sociosexual knowledge, experience, attitude, and interests of individuals with autistic disorder and developmental delay. J Autism Dev Disord 27:397–413, 1997

Kuperman S, Beeghly JH, Burns TL, et al: Serotonin relationships of autistic probands and their first-degree relatives. J Am Acad Child Psychiatry 24:189–190, 1985

Lainhart JE, Piven J, Wzorek M, et al: Macrocephaly in children and adults with autism. J Am Acad Child Adolesc Psychiatry 36:282–290, 1997

Lake CR, Ziegler MG, Murphy DL: Increased norepinephrine levels and decreased dopamine-beta-hydroxylase activity in primary autism. Arch Gen Psychiatry 34:553–556, 1977

Landau WM, Kleffner FR: Syndrome of acquired aphasia with convulsive disorder in children. Neurology 7:523–530, 1957

Launay JM, Bursztejn C, Ferrari P, et al: Catecholamine metabolism in infantile autism: a controlled study of 22 autistic children. J Autism Dev Disord 17:333–347, 1987

Lauritsen M, Ewald H: The genetics of autism. Acta Psychiatr Scand 103:411–427, 2001

Lauritsen M, Mors O, Mortensen PB, et al: Infantile autism and associated autosomal chromosome abnormalities: a register-based study and a literature survey. J Child Psychol Psychiatry 40:335–345, 1999

Laushey KM, Heflin LJ: Enhancing social skills of kindergarten children with autism through the training of multiple peers as tutors. J Autism Dev Disord 30:183–193, 2000

Leboyer M, Philipppe A, Bouvard M, et al: Whole blood and plasma beta-endorphin in autistic probands and their first-degree relatives. Biol Psychiatry 45:158–163, 1999

Leventhal BL, Cook EH, Morford M, et al: Clinical and neurochemical effects of fenfluramine in children with autism. J Neuropsychiatry Clin Neurosci 5:307–315, 1993

Liss M, Fein D, Allen D, et al: Executive functioning in high-functioning children with autism. J Child Psychol Psychiatry 42:261–270, 2001

Lord C: Follow-up of two-year-olds referred for possible autism. J Child Psychol Psychiatry 36:1365–1382, 1995

Lord C, Mulloy C, Wendelboe M, et al: Pre- and perinatal factors in high-functioning females and males with autism. J Autism Dev Disord 21:197–209, 1991

Lovaas OI, Schreibman L, Koegel RL: A behavior modification approach to the treatment of autistic children, in Psychopathology and Child Development. Edited by Schopler E, Reichler RJ. New York, Plenum, 1976, pp 291–310

Loveland KA, Tunali-Kotoski B, Chen YR, et al: Emotion cognition in autism: verbal and nonverbal information. Dev Psychopathol 9:579–593, 1997

Maddox LO, Menold MM, Bass MP, et al: Autistic disorder and chromosomes 15q11-q13: construction and analysis of a BAC/PAC contig. Genomics 62:325–331, 1999

Maes B, Fryns JP, Van Walleghem M, et al: Fragile-X syndrome and autism: a prevalent association or a misinterpreted connection? Genet Couns 4:245–263, 1993

Maestrini E, Lai C, Marlow A, et al: Serotonin transporter (5-HTT) and gamma-aminobutyric acid receptor subunit beta3 (GABR3) gene polymorphisms are not associated with autism in the IMGSA families. The International Molecular Genetic Study of Autism Concertium. Am J Med Genet 88:492–496, 1999

Malone RP, Cater J, Sheikh RM, et al: Olanza-pine versus haloperidol in children with autistic disorder: an open pilot study. J Am Acad Child Adolesc Psychiatry 40:887–894, 2001

Marazziti D, Muratori F, Cesari A, et al: Increased density of the platelet serotonin transporter in autism. Pharmacopsychiatry 33:165–168, 2000

Martin A, Koenig K, Scahill L, et al: Open-label quetiapine in the treatment of children and adolescents with autistic disorder. J Child Adolesc Psychopharmacol 9:99–107, 1999a

Martin A, Scahill, Klin A, et al: Higher-functioning pervasive developmental disorders: rates and pattern of psychotropic drug use. J Am Acad Child Adolesc Psychiatry 38:923–931, 1999b

Martin ER, Menold MM, Wolpert CM, et al: Analysis of linkage disequilibrium in gamma-aminobutyric acid receptor subunit genes in autistic disorder. Am J Med Genet 96:43–48, 2000

Martineau J, Barthelemy C, Jouve J, et al: Monoamines (serotonin and catecholamines) and their derivatives in infantile autism: age-related changes and drug effects. Dev Med Child Neurol 34:593–603, 1992

Martinsson T, Johannesson T, Vujic M, et al: Maternal origin of the dup (15) chromosome in infantile autism. Eur Child Adolesc Psychiatry 5:185–192, 1996

Mawhood L, Howlin P, Rutter M: Autism and developmental receptive language disorder: a comparative follow-up in early adult life, I: cognitive and language outcomes. J Child Psychol Psychiatry 41:547–559, 2000

Max ML, Burke JC: Virtual reality for autism communication and education, with lessons for medical training simulators. Stud Health Technol Inform 39:46–53, 1997

McCauley JL, Olson LM, Delahanty R, et al: A linkage disequilibrium map of the 1-Mb 15q12 GABA(A) receptor subunit cluster and association to autism. Am J Med Genet B Neuropsychiatr Genet 131:51–59, 2004

McDougle CJ, Price LH, Volkmar FR, et al: Clomipramine in autism: preliminary evidence of efficacy. J Am Acad Child Adolesc Psychiatry 31:746–750, 1992

McDougle CJ, Kresch LE, Goodman WK, et al: A case-controlled study of repetitive thoughts and behavior in adults with autistic disorder and obsessive-compulsive disorder. Am J Psychiatry 152:772–777, 1995

McDougle CJ, Naylor ST, Cohen DJ, et al: A double-blind, placebo-controlled study of fluvoxamine in adults with autistic disorder. Arch Gen Psychiatry 53:1001–1008, 1996

McDougle CJ, Holmes JP, Carlson DC, et al: A double-blind, placebo-controlled study of risperidone in adults with autistic disorder and other pervasive developmental disorders. Arch Gen Psychiatry 55:633–641, 1998

McEachin JJ, Smith T, Lovaas OI: Long-term outcome for children with autism who received early intensive behavioral treatment. Am J Ment Retard 97:359–372, 1993

McLennan JD, Lord C, Schopler E: Sex differences in higher functioning people with autism. J Autism Dev Disord 23:217–227, 1993

Miller MT, Stromland K, Gillberg C, et al: The puzzle of autism: an ophthalmologic contribution. Trans Am Ophthalmol Soc 96:369–385, 1998

Minderaa RB, Anderson GM, Volkmar FR, et al: Urinary 5-hydroxyindoleacetic acid and whole blood serotonin and tryptophan in autistic and normal subjects. Biol Psychiatry 22:933–940, 1987

Minderaa RB, Anderson GM, Volkmar FR, et al: Noradrenergic and adrenergic functioning in autism. Biol Psychiatry 36:237–241, 1994

Minshew NJ, Goldstein G, Dombrowski SM, et al: A preliminary MRS study of autism: evidence for undersynthesis and increased degradation of brain membranes. Biol Psychiatry 33:762–773, 1993

Muller RA, Chugani DC, Behen ME, et al: Impairment of dentate-thalamo-cortical pathway in autistic men: language activation data from positron emission tomography. Neurosci Lett 245:1–4, 1998

Muller RA, Behen ME, Rothermel RD, et al: Brain mapping of language and auditory perception in high-functioning autistic adults: a PET study. J Autism Dev Disord 29:19–31, 1999

Muller RA, Pierce K, Ambrose JB, et al: Atypical patterns of cerebral motor activation in autism: a functional magnetic resonance study. Biol Psychiatry 49:665–676, 2001

Murphy M, Bolton PF, Pickles A, et al: Personality traits of the relatives of autistic probands. Psychol Med 30:1411–1424, 2000

Nordin V, Gillberg C: Autism spectrum disorder in children with physical or mental disability or both, I: clinical and epidemiological aspects. Dev Med Child Neurol 38:297–313, 1996

Ohnishi T, Matsuda H, Hashimoto T, et al: Abnormal regional cerebral blood flow in childhood autism. Brain 123(pt 9): 1838–1844, 2000

Ornitz EM, Ritvo ER: The syndrome of autism: a critical review. Am J Psychiatry 133:609–621, 1976

Otsuka H, Harada M, Mori K, et al: Brain metabolites in the hippocampus-amygdala region and cerebellum in autism: an 1H-MR spectroscopy study. Neuroradiol 41:517–519, 1999

Ozonoff S, Cathcart K: Effectiveness of home program intervention for young children with autism. J Autism Dev Disord 28:25–32, 1998

Ozonoff S, Pennington BF, Rogers SJ: Executive function deficits in higher-functioning autistic individuals: relationship to theory of mind. J Child Psychol Psychiatry 32:1081–1105, 1991

Parker SK, Schwartz B, Todd J, et al: Thimerosal-containing vaccines and autistic spectrum disorder: a critical review of published original data. Pediatrics 114:793-804, 2004; erratum in Pediatrics 115:200, 2005

Patzold LM, Richdale AL, Tonge BJ: An investigation into sleep characteristics of children with autism and Asperger's disorder. J Paediatr Child Health 34:528–533, 1998

Payton JB, Steele MW, Wenger SL, et al: The fragile X marker and autism in perspective. J Am Acad Child Adolesc Psychiatry 28:417–421, 1989

Persico AM, Militerni R, Bravaccio C, et al: Lack of association between serotonin transporter gene promotor variants and autistic disorder in two ethnically distinct samples. Am J Med Genet 96:123–127, 2000

Pfeiffer SI, Norton J, Nelson L, et al: Efficacy of vitamin B_6 and magnesium in the treatment of autism: a methodology review and summary of outcomes. J Autism Dev Disord 25:481–493, 1995

Pierce K, Schreibman L: Multiple peer use of pivotal response training to increase social behaviors of classmates with autism: results from trained and untrained peers. J Appl Behav Anal 30:157–160, 1997

Piven J, Palmer P: Psychiatric disorder and the broad autism phenotype: evidence from a family study of multiple-incidence autism families. Am J Psychiatry 156:557–563, 1999

Piven J, Gayle J, Chase G, et al: A family history of neuropsychiatric disorders in adult siblings of autistic individuals. J Am Acad Child Adolesc Psychiatry 29:177–183, 1990

Piven J, Chase GA, Landa R, et al: Psychiatric disorders in the parents of autistic individuals. J Am Acad Child Adolesc Psychiatry 30:471–478, 1991a

Piven J, Gayle J, Landa R, et al: The prevalence of fragile X in a sample of autistic individuals diagnosed using a standardized interview. J Am Acad Child Adolesc Psychiatry 30:825–830, 1991b

Piven J, Tsai GC, Nehme E, et al: Platelet serotonin, a possible marker for familial autism. J Autism Dev Disord 21:51–59, 1991c

Piven J, Simon J, Chase GA, et al: The etiology of autism: pre-, peri- and neonatal factors. J Am Acad Child Adolesc Psychiatry 32: 1256–1263, 1993

Piven J, Harper J, Palmer P, et al: Course of behavioral change in autism: a retrospective study of high-IQ adolescents and adults. J Am Acad Child Adolesc Psychiatry 35:523–529, 1996

Piven J, Palmer P, Landa R, et al: Personality and language characteristics in parents from multiple-incidence autism families. Am J Med Gene 74:398–411, 1997

Piven J, Bailey J, Ranson BJ, et al: No difference in hippocampus volume detected on magnetic resonance imaging in autistic individuals. J Autism Dev Disord 28:105–110, 1998

Plumet MH, Goldblum MC, Leboyer M: Verbal skill in relatives of autistic females. Cortex 31:723–733, 1995

Posey DJ, McDougle CJ: The pharmacotherapy of target symptoms associated with autistic disorder and other pervasive developmental disorders. Harv Rev Psychiatry 8:45–63, 2000

Quintana H, Brimaher B, Stedge D, et al: Use of methylphenidate in the treatment of children with autistic disorder. J Autism Dev Disord 25:283–294, 1995

Repetto GM, White LM, Bader PJ, et al: Interstitial duplications of chromosome region 15q11q13: clinical and molecular characterization. Am J Med Genet 79:82–89, 1998

Ricks DM, Wing L: Language, communication and the use of symbols, in Early Childhood Autism. Edited by Wing L. Oxford, UK, Pergamon, 1976, pp 93–134

Rieffe C, Meerum Terwogt M, Stockmann L: Understanding atypical emotions among children with autism. J Autism Dev Disord 30:195–203, 2000

Rineer S, Finucane B, Simon EW: Symptoms among children and young adults with isodicentric chromosome 15. Am J Med Genet 81:428–433, 1998

Ring HA, Baron-Cohen S, Wheelwright S, et al: Cerebral correlates of preserved cognitive skills in autism: a functional study of embedded figures task performance. Brain 122:1305–1315, 1999

Ritvo ER, Freeman BJ, Mason-Brothers A, et al: Concordance for the syndrome of autism in 40 pairs of afflicted twins. Am J Psychiatry 142:74–77, 1985

Ritvo ER, Jorde LB, Mason-Brothers A, et al: The UCLA–University of Utah epidemiologic survey of autism: recurrence risk estimate and genetic counseling. Am J Psychiatry 146:1032–1036, 1989

Roberts W, Weaver L, Brian J, et al: Repeated doses of porcine secretin in the treatment of autism: a randomized, placebo-controlled trial. Pediatrics 107:E71, 2001

Robinson TW: Homeopathic secretin in autism: a clinical pilot study. Br Homeopath J 90:86–91, 2001

Roeyers H, Van Oost P, Bothuyne S: Immediate imitation and joint attention in young children with autism. Dev Psychopathol 10:441–450, 1998

Rossi PG, Parmeggiani A, Bach V, et al: EEG features and epilepsy in patients with autism. Brain Dev 17:169–174, 1995

Rossi PG, Posar A, Parmeggiani A, et al: Niaprazine in the treatment of autistic disorder. J Child Neurol 14:547–550, 1999

Rumsey JM, Duara R, Grady C, et al: Brain metabolism in autism: resting cerebral glucose utilization rates measured with positron emission tomography. Arch Gen Psychiatry 42:448–455, 1985a

Rumsey JM, Rapoport JL, Sceery WR: Autistic children as adults: psychiatric, social and behavioral outcomes. J Am Acad Child Psychiatry 24:465–473, 1985b

Russell J, Jarrold C, Hood B: Two intact executive capacities in children with autism: implications for the core executive dysfunction in the disorder. J Autism Dev Disord 29:103–112, 1999

Rutter M: Concepts of autism: a review of research. J Child Psychol Psychiatry 9:1–25, 1968

Rutter M: Autistic children: infancy to adulthood. Semin Psychiatry 2:435–450, 1970

Rutter M: Infantile autism and other child psychoses, in Child Psychiatry: Modern Approaches. Edited by Rutter M, Hersov L. Oxford, UK, Blackwell Scientific, 1977, pp 717–747

Rutter M: Diagnosis and definition, in Autism: A Reappraisal of Concepts and Treatment. Edited by Rutter M, Schopler E. New York, Plenum, 1978, pp 1–25

Rutter M: Autistic children growing up. Dev Med Child Neurol 26:122–129, 1984

Rutter M, Lockyer L: A five to fifteen year followup study of infantile psychosis, I: description of sample. Br J Psychiatry 113:1169–1182, 1967

Rutter M, Bailey A, Bolton P, et al: Autism and known medical conditions: myth and substance. J Child Psychol Psychiatry 35:311–322, 1994

Salmon B, Hallmayer J, Rogers T, et al: Absence of linkage and linkage disequilibrium to 15q11–q13 markers in 139 multiplex families with autism. Am J Med Genet 88:551–556, 1999

Sanchez LE, Campbell M, Small AM, et al: A pilot study of clomipramine in young autistic children. J Am Acad Child Adolesc Psychiatry 35:537–544, 1996

Schopler E, Mesibov GB, Baker A: Evaluation of treatment for autistic children and their parents. J Am Acad Adolesc Child Psychiatry 21:262–267, 1982

Schreck KA, Mulick JA: Parental report of sleep problems in children with autism. J Autism Dev Disord 30:127–135, 2000

Scifo R, Cioni M, Nicolosi A, et al: Opioid–immune interaction in autism: behavioural and immunological assessment during a double-blind treatment with naltrexone. Ann Ist Super Sanita 32:351–359, 1996

Shavelle RM, Strauss D: Comparative mortality of person with autism in California, 1980–1996. J Insur Med 30:220–225, 1998

Sheinkopf SJ, Siegel B: Home-based behavioral treatment of young children with autism. J Autism Dev Disord 28:15–23, 1998

Short AB, Schopler E: Factors relating to age of onset. J Autism Dev Disord 18:207–216, 1988

Siegel BV Jr, Asarnow R, Tanguay P, et al: Regional cerebral glucose metabolism and attention in adults with a history of childhood autism. J Neuropsychiatry Clin Neurosci 4:406–414, 1992

Siegel DJ, Minshew NJ, Goldstein G: Wechsler IQ profiles in diagnosis of high-functioning autism. J Autism Dev Disord 26:389–406, 1996

Sigman M, Ruskin E, Arbeile S, et al: Continuity and change in the social competence of children with autism, Down syndrome, and developmental delays. Monogr Soc Res Child Dev 64:1–114, 1999

Singh VK, Warren RP, Odell JD, et al: Antibodies to myelin basic protein in children with autistic behavior. Brain Behav Immun 7:97–103, 1993

Singh VK, Warren R, Averett R, et al: Circulating autoantibodies to neuronal and glial filament proteins in autism. Pediatr Neurol 17:88–90, 1997

Singh VK, Lin SX, Yang VC: Serological association of measles virus and human herpesvirus-6 with brain autoantibodies in autism. Clin Immunol Immunopathol 89:105–108, 1998

Smalley SL: Genetic influences in autism. Psychiatr Clin North Am 14:125–139, 1991

Smalley SL: Autism and tuberous sclerosis. J Autism Dev Disord 28:407–414, 1998

Smalley SL, McCracken J, Tanguay P: Autism, affective disorder, and social phobia. Am J Med Genet 60:19–26, 1995

Smith M, Filipek PA, Wu C, et al: Analysis of a 1-megabase deletion in 15q22-q23 in an autistic patient: identification of candidate gene for autism and of homologous DNA segments in 15q22-q23 and 15q11-q13. Am J Med Genet 96:765–770, 2000

Smith T, Groen AD, Wynn JW: Randomized trial of intensive early intervention for children with pervasive developmental disorder. Am J Ment Retard 105:269–285, 2000

Starkstein SE, Vazquez S, Vrancic D, et al: SPECT findings in mentally retarded autistic individuals. J Neuropsychiatr Clin Neurosci 12:370–375, 2000

Stefanatos GA, Grover W, Geller E: Case study: corticosteroid treatment of language regression in pervasive developmental disorder. J Am Acad Child Adolesc Psychiatry 34:1107–1111, 1995

Steffenburg S, Gillberg C, Hellgren L, et al: A twin study of autism in Denmark, Finland, Iceland, Norway and Sweden. J Child Psychol Psychiatry 30:405–416, 1989

Steffenburg S, Gillberg C, Steffenburg U, et al: Autism in Angelman syndrome: a population-based study. Pediatr Neurol 14:131–136, 1996

Steingard R, Zimnitzky B, DeMaso DR, et al: Sertraline treatment of transition-associated anxiety and agitation in children with autistic disorder. J Child Adolesc Psychopharmacol 7:9–15, 1997

Stone WL, Lee EB, Ashford L, et al: Can autism be diagnosed accurately under 3 years? J Child Psychol Psychiatry 40: 219–226, 1999

Strickland D: Virtual reality for the treatment of autism. Stud Health Technol Inform 44:81–86, 1997

Szatmari P, Jones MB, Fisman S, et al: Parents and collateral relatives of children with pervasive developmental disorders: a family history study. Am J Med Genet 60:282–289, 1995

Taira M, Takase M, Sasaki H: Sleep disorder in children with autism. Psychiatr Clin Neurosci 52:182–183, 1998

Taylor B, Miller E, Farrington CP, et al: Autism and measles, mumps, and rubella vaccine: no epidemiological evidence for a causal association. Lancet 353:2026–2029, 1999

Todd RD, Ciaranello RD: Demonstration of inter- and intraspecies differences in serotonin binding sites by antibodies from an autistic child. Proc Natl Acad Sci U S A 82:612–616, 1985

Todd RD, Hickok IM, Anderson GM, et al: Antibrain antibodies in infantile autism. Biol Psychiatry 23:644–647, 1988

Tolbert L, Haigler T, Waits MM, et al: Brief report: lack of response in an autistic population to a low dose clinical trial of pyridoxine plus magnesium. J Autism Dev Disord 23:193–199, 1993

Tordjman S, Gutknecht L, Carlier M, et al: Role of the serotonin transporter gene in behavioral expression of autism. Mol Psychiatry 6:434–439, 2001

Tsai LY: Infantile autism and schizophrenia in childhood, in The Medical Basis of Psychiatry. Edited by Winokur G, Clayton P. Philadelphia, PA, WB Saunders, 1986, pp 331–351

Tsai LY: Pre-, peri-, and neonatal factors in autism, in Neurobiological Issues in Autism. Edited by Schopler E, Mesibov GB. New York, Plenum, 1987, pp 179–189

Tsai LY: Medical treatment in autism, in Autism: Identification, Education, and Treatment. Edited by Berkell DE. Hillsdale, NJ, Lawrence Erlbaum, 1992, pp 151–184

Tsai LY: Brief report: comorbid psychiatric disorders of autistic disorder. J Autism Dev Disord 26:159–163, 1996

Tsai LY: Sleep problems and effective treatment in children with autism. Proceedings of the Autism Society of America National Conference, pp 183–184, 1997

Tsai LY: Taking the Mystery Out of Medication in Autism/Asperger Syndromes. Arlington, TX, Future Horizons Inc., 2001

Tsai LY: Autistic disorder, in The American Psychiatric Publishing Textbook of Child and Adolescent Psychiatry, 3rd Edition. Edited by Wiener JM, Dulcan MK. Washington, DC, American Psychiatric Publishing, 2004, pp 261–315

Tsai LY, Stewart MA, August G: Implication of sex differences in the familial transmission of infantile autism. J Autism Dev Disord 11:165–173, 1981

Tsai Ly, Stewart MA, Faust M, et al: Social class distribution of fathers and children enrolled in the Iowa autism program. J Autism Dev Disord 12:211–222, 1982

U.S. Department of Health and Human Services: International Classification of Diseases, 9th Revision, Clinical Modification. Washington, DC, U.S. Department of Health and Human Services, 1980

Van Bourgondien ME, Reichle NC, Palmer A: Sexual behavior in adults with autism. J Autism Dev Disord 27:113–125, 1997

Vincent JB, Kolozsvari D, Roberts WS, et al: Mutation screening of X-chromosomal neuroligin genes: no mutations in 196 autism probands. Am J Med Genet B Neuropsychiatr Genet 129:82–84, 2004

Volkmar FR, Nelson DS: Seizure disorders in autism. J Am Acad Child Adolesc Psychiatry 29:127–129, 1990

Volkmar FR, Szatmari P, Sparrow SS: Sex difference in pervasive developmental disorders. J Autism Dev Disord 23:579–591, 1993

Volkmar FR, Kline A, Siegel B, et al: Field trial for autistic disorder in DSM-IV. Am J Psychiatry 151:1361–1367, 1994

Volkmar FR, Cook EH Jr, Lord C, et al: Autism and related conditions (letter). J Am Acad Child Adolesc Psychiatry 35:401–402, 1996

Warburton P, Baird G, Chen W, et al: Support for linkage of autism and specific language impairment to 7q3 from two chromosome rearrangement involving 7q31. Am J Med Genet 96:228–234, 2000

Warren RP, Foster A, Margaretten NC: Reduced natural killer cell activity in autism. J Am Acad Child Adolesc Psychiatry 26:333–335, 1987

Wassink TH, Piven J, Vieland VJ, et al: Evidence supporting *WNT2* as an autism susceptibility gene. Am J Med Genet 105:406–413, 2001

Weiss SJ: Personality adjustment and social support of parents who care for children with pervasive developmental disorders. Arch Psychiatr Nurs 5:25–30, 1991

Weizman A, Weizman R, Szekely GA, et al: Abnormal immune response to brain tissue antigen in the syndrome of autism. Am J Psychiatry 139:1462–1465, 1982

Willemsen-Swinkels SH, Buitelaar JK, Nijhof GJ, et al: Failure of naltrexone hydrochloride to reduce self-injurious and autistic behavior in mentally retarded adults: double-blind placebo-controlled studies. Arch Gen Psychiatry 52:766–773, 1995

Willemsen-Swinkels SH, Buitelaar JK, van Engeland H: The effect of chronic naltrexone treatment in young autistic children: a double-blind placebo-controlled crossover study. Biol Psychiatry 39:1023–1031, 1996

Wing L: Childhood autism and social class: a question of selection. Br J Psychiatry 137:410–417, 1980

Wing L: Asperger's syndrome: a clinical account. Psychol Med 11:115–129, 1981

Wolpert CM, Menold MM, Bass MP, et al: Three probands with autistic disorder and isodicentric chromosome 15. Am J Med Genet 96:365–372, 2000

Wong V: Epilepsy in children with autistic spectrum disorder. J Child Neurol 8:316–322, 1993

Yamamoto J, Miya T: Acquisition and transfer of sentence construction in autistic students: analysis by computer-based teaching. Res Dev Disabil 20:355–377, 1999

Yirmiya N, Shulman C: Seriation, conservation, and theory of mind abilities in individuals with autism, individuals with mental retardation, and normally developing children. Child Dev 67:2045–2059, 1996

Yirmiya N, Erel O, Shaked M, et al: Meta-analyses comparing theory of mind abilities of individuals with autism, individuals with mental retardation, and normally developing individuals. Psychol Bull 124:283–307, 1998

Yirmiya N, Pilowsky T, Nemanov L, et al: Evidence for an association with serotonin transporter region polymorphism and autism. Am J Med Genet 105:381–386, 2001

Zhong N, Ye L, Ju W, et al: *5-HTTLPR* variants not associated with autistic spectrum disorders. Neurogenetics 2:129–131, 1999

Zilbovicius M, Garreau B, Tzourio N, et al: Regional cerebral blood flow in childhood autism: a SPECT study. Am J Psychiatry 149:924–930, 1992

Zilbovicius M, Garreau B, Samson Y, et al: Delayed maturation of the frontal cortex in childhood autism. Am J Psychiatry 152:248–252, 1995

Zilbovicius M, Boddaert N, Belin P, et al: Temporal lobe dysfunction in childhood autism: a PET study. Am J Psychiatry 157:1988–1993, 2000

Zuddas A, Di Martino A, Muglia P, et al: Long-term risperidone for pervasive developmental disorder: efficacy, tolerability, and discontinuation. J Child Adolesc Psychopharmacol 10:79–90, 2000

Self-Assessment Questions

Select the single best response for each question.

11.1 Which of the following is an essential characteristic of infantile autism, as proposed by Rutter (1968)?

A. Onset before age 30 months.
B. Bizarre motor behavior.
C. Impaired language.
D. Lack of social interest and responsiveness.
E. All of the above.

11.2 All of the following are pervasive developmental disorders *except*

A. Autistic disorder.
B. Mental retardation.
C. Rett's disorder.
D. Childhood disintegrative disorder.
E. Asperger's disorder.

11.3 A common comorbid medical condition noted in patients with autism is epilepsy. Which of the following statements is *true?*

A. The risk of epilepsy in patients with autism is highest during late adolescence.
B. A prospective study of epilepsy in children with autistic spectrum disorders found a rate of 5%.
C. The most common type of epilepsy is generalized or grand mal seizures.
D. Males with autism have seizures more frequently than do females with autism.
E. None of the above.

11.4 All of the following psychopharmacological agents have been reported to decrease autistic symptoms *except*

A. Fluoxetine.
B. Fluvoxamine.
C. Quetiapine.
D. Venlafaxine.
E. Sertraline.

11.5 Which of the following factors has consistently been shown to be related to outcome in autistic patients?

A. Age at onset.
B. Family history of mental illness.
C. IQ.
D. Perinatal complications.
E. Birth weight.

12

Developmental Disorders of Communication, Motor Skills, and Learning

Carl Feinstein, M.D.

Jennifer M. Phillips, Ph.D.

Developmental disorders of communication, motor skills, and learning are common conditions with significant implications for both children's mental health and their ability to function successfully at school and in other psychosocial contexts. The relationship of these disorders to other DSM disorders is complex. Although they are included under Axis I clinical disorders in DSM-IV-TR (American Psychiatric Association 2000), they stand apart from the other Axis I disorders of childhood, which describe emotional or behavioral abnormalities. However, they are very common as comorbid conditions in children with psychiatric disorders. Unfortunately, many children with learning, language, and

motor disorders have significant psychiatric disorders but are never referred for treatment of their mental health problems.

Many of these disorders are overlapping in occurrence and etiologically intertwined. Communication disorders and motor skills disorders often co-occur with learning disorders. Developmental reading disorder (dyslexia) is closely associated with and related to developmental language disorder (American Speech-Language-Hearing Association 2002; Hummel and Feinstein 1997). Many children who have language disorders develop learning disorders during the school-age years (American Academy of Child and Adolescent Psychiatry 1998;

Schoenbrodt et al. 1997). There is also a reported higher rate of occurrence of developmental coordination disorder with both communication and learning disorders (American Psychiatric Association 2000).

The high prevalence and multiple adverse consequences of these disorders constitute a major public health and public policy concern. Estimates of the prevalence of learning disorders in students in the United States have ranged from 1% to 10%. Up to 15% of children have a language disorder (American Academy of Child and Adolescent Psychiatry 1998; American Psychiatric Association 2000; Castrogiovanni 2002; U.S. Department of Education 1995). In total, about 10%–20% of children and adolescents have communication and/or learning disorders. About 50% of these children have a comorbid psychiatric disorder (American Academy of Child and Adolescent Psychiatry 1998; Beitchman and Young 1997). In addition to being at risk for psychiatric disorders, these children are also at risk for delinquency, early school dropout, and poor academic achievement (American Academy of Child and Adolescent Psychiatry 1998; Beitchman et al. 1986; Cantwell and Baker 1991).

The child and adolescent psychiatrist plays a critical role in the assessment and treatment of children with communication, motor skills, and learning disorders. Effective treatment of children with these issues, as well as secondary prevention of psychiatric disorders, requires a coordinated multidisciplinary intervention (Silver and Hagin 1989). Effective participation by the psychiatrist in this multidisciplinary setting requires a working familiarity with the concepts and procedures of pediatric neurology, speech and language pathology, psychological assessment, and special educational programming.

Communication Disorders

The development of spoken language has a profound influence on many other aspects of development, including general cognition, play, educational achievement, peer relations, and emotional and behavioral development (Cohen 2001). Even in relatively mild forms, communication disorders impede adaptation and are highly associated with a variety of serious problems, including increased risk of psychiatric disorders, poor peer relations, poor performance in school, and poor vocational functioning (Cantwell and Baker 1991; Cohen 2001).

■ Definition

The American Speech-Language-Hearing Association (1993) defines *communication disorder* as "an impairment in the ability to receive, send, process, and comprehend concepts or verbal, nonverbal, and graphic symbol systems" (p. 40). The association further divides communication disorders into speech disorders and language disorders. *Speech disorders* involve problems with articulation, fluency, or voice. Articulation disorder (phonological disorder in DSM-IV-TR) involves impairment in the intelligibility of speech resulting from difficulty with correct production of the sounds used in speech. With fluency disorder (stuttering in DSM-IV-TR), a child has difficulty maintaining the flow of speech, with difficulties noted in terms of rate and rhythm, as well as repetitions of speech parts. Voice disorder (coded in DSM-IV-TR under communication disorder not otherwise specified) involves age- or sex-inappropriate abnormalities in voice characteristics, such as quality, pitch, volume, resonance, tone, and duration.

Language disorder is defined as "the impaired comprehension and/or use of spoken, written, and/or other symbol systems"

(American Speech-Language-Hearing Association 1993, p. 40). It can involve the form, context, and/or function of language. The form of language includes phonology, morphology, and syntax; the context of language includes semantics; and the function of language includes pragmatics (American Speech-Language-Hearing Association 1993). The definitions of these components of language are included in Table 12–1. In DSM-IV-TR, language disorders are divided into expressive language disorder and mixed receptive–expressive language disorder. Throughout this chapter, the terms *communication disorder* and *language disorder* will be used more or less interchangeably.

According to DSM-IV-TR, children with *expressive language disorder* generally have adequate understanding of language but have difficulty using it to communicate. These are children whose expressive language (e.g., vocabulary, use of tense, word recall, sentence production) is significantly below expected for nonverbal intelligence and receptive language development, as measured by discrepancies between standardized tests of these functions (American Psychiatric Association 2000).

Children with *mixed receptive–expressive language disorder* manifest deficits in expression as well as in comprehension of language (e.g., understanding of words, sentences, or specific types of words, such as those used to describe spatial location). As a result, this form of communication disorder is more socially and academically disabling. DSM-IV-TR requires a significant discrepancy on standardized measures between both expressive and receptive language development and nonverbal intelligence in order to make this diagnosis. In all communication disorders, the deficit must interfere with school, work, or social functioning and must be distinct from other conditions in which language delay is an associated feature, such as the pervasive developmental disorders (American Psychiatric Association 2000).

In DSM-IV-TR, *phonological disorder* is described as the failure to use age-appropriate and expected speech sounds, often resulting in speech that sounds immature for age. The diagnosis is made by considering articulatory proficiency relative to age as well as the consistency of any deficit. The primary clinical finding in a child who has phonological disorder is decreased intelli-

Table 12–1. Components of language

Form of language

Phonology	A language's sound system and accompanying rules governing the combination of sounds; phonemes are the basic sound components of speech
Morphology	The system that governs the structure and formation of words in a language; morphemes are the smallest meaningful linguistic units
Syntax	The system that governs the order and combination of words to form sentences, clauses, and phrases, and the relationships among elements of a sentence

Context of language

Semantics	The system that governs the meaning of words and sentences

Function of language

Pragmatics	The system that combines the above language components into functional and socially appropriate communication

gibility of speech production in the context of normal sentence production and comprehension (e.g., errors of sound production, use, representation, or organization, such as substitutions and omissions; American Psychiatric Association 2000). In DSM-IV-TR, *stuttering* is essentially a disturbance in the age-appropriate fluency and patterning of speech, including characteristics such as repetitions of syllables or words, prolongations of sounds, pauses between or within words, interjections, tension associated with word production, and word substitutions (American Psychiatric Association 2000).

In DSM-IV-TR, communication disorders focus on spoken language and understanding of spoken language. Disorders of reading and written expression are classified separately under learning disorders, although they are significantly associated with disorders of language and communication. In fact, some professionals in the field prefer to use the term *language-based learning disabilities* when discussing disorders of reading and written expression, in acknowledgement of the relationship between spoken and written language and the frequent comorbidity of communication problems in children with these disorders (American Speech-Language-Hearing Association 2002).

◼ History

Our understanding of language disorders has evolved in the past century as the result of contributions from many disciplines, including speech and language pathology, neurology, psychiatry, educators of the deaf and of children with developmental disabilities, and neuropsychology. The term *developmental dysphasia* came into use to describe deficient, delayed, and/or partial acquisition of language, as distinguished from acquired

aphasias caused by focal lesions of the brain (Rapin and Allen 1988; Zangwill 1987). Investigators attempted to devise empirical classifications of language disorders by studying large numbers of children with language problems on a range of linguistic and other cognitive and neurological variables and applying statistical techniques to separate them into clinically significant subgroups (Aram and Nation 1975; Aram et al. 1984). More recently, techniques such as functional magnetic resonance imaging are being used to identify neurological markers for language disorders (Paul 2001).

◼ Clinical Presentation

The linguistic phenomena that lead to clinical referrals depend on the type of deficit and the age of the child. For toddlers and preschoolers, primary considerations include whether the child speaks at all, how many words are in the child's spoken vocabulary and their intelligibility, whether the child understands simple directions, and whether the child is able to name objects. For school-age children, more common causes of referral include problems with comprehension, formulation, and spoken expression of the syntactically and semantically more complex material required for successful school functioning. For adolescents, the issue is more likely to involve the ability to formulate or comprehend abstract ideas, complex instructions, or metaphoric expressions in spoken or written language (Cohen 2001; Hummel and Feinstein 1997). Because of the dramatic changes in language capacities over time and the greatly increased complexity of the phenomena being evaluated, it is not surprising that nonspecialist clinicians are more likely to suspect a language disorder in the very young child than in the older child, unless the deficits in the older child are profound.

In *expressive language disorder*, very young children may have no spoken language at all, while older children may use developmentally immature forms of language, speak in short, telegraphic sentences, or rely heavily on contextual cues and nonverbal communication. These children tend to make syntactic or semantic errors in sentence construction. Word retrieval difficulties may result in circumlocutions, reliance on jargon, or word substitutions (Richardson 1989). Speech may appear awkward, incoherent, or unintelligible. Adolescents with expressive language disorder may also have difficulty with the pragmatic, social use of language.

Expressive language delays are most common in children younger than 3 years, with prevalence in this age range estimated at 10%–15%. These numbers decrease with age, and by school age, only 3%–7% of children present with this disorder. Developmental expressive language disorder is more common than the acquired form and more often occurs in boys than in girls, although this finding may be reflective of a referral bias (American Psychiatric Association 2000; Beitchman and Young 1997). Associated findings may include phonological disorder, erratic rate and rhythm of speech, learning disorders (particularly of written expression), developmental coordination disorder, enuresis, and neurological abnormalities (American Academy of Child and Adolescent Psychiatry 1998; American Psychiatric Association 2000).

Mixed receptive–expressive language disorder is not as prevalent as expressive language disorder, with approximately 5% of preschoolers and 3% of school-age children affected (American Psychiatric Association 2000). As with expressive language disorder, more boys than girls are thought to have this disorder, but this may again be an artifact of referral bias. Associated find-

ings may include auditory processing problems that interfere with language comprehension, phonological disorder, speech perception deficits, memory problems, learning disorders, developmental coordination disorder, enuresis, and neurological abnormalities (American Psychiatric Association 2000).

There is wide variation in the severity and degree of intelligibility in children with *phonological disorder*. Moderate-to-severe phonological disorder is estimated to affect 2% of early-school-age children in whom other organic causes are not identified; a somewhat higher prevalence is seen in the milder form of the disorder, with estimates of up to 20% reported (American Academy of Child and Adolescent Psychiatry 1998; American Psychiatric Association 2000). The disorder is more common in boys than in girls (American Psychiatric Association 2000). Many children with phonological disorder have associated nonlinguistic findings, including neurological soft signs, enuresis, developmental coordination disorder, and learning disorders (Cantwell and Baker 1987). Anywhere from 50%–70% of children with phonological disorder are reported to have general academic problems throughout school (Castrogiovanni 2002).

Stuttering begins early in life, usually between ages 2 and 7 years, and is often exacerbated by stress or anxiety. The prevalence of stuttering is 1% in young children, with more males affected than females, by a ratio of about 3:1 (American Psychiatric Association 2000; National Institute on Deafness and Other Communication Disorders 1997). Phonological disorder and expressive language disorder are seen more frequently in children who stutter than in the general population, with as many as 44% of children who stutter having one or both of these other communication disorders as well (American Psychiatric Association 2000; Arndt and Healey 2001). Some investigators have distinguished between "remediable" and "chronic perseverative" stuttering, noting that whereas children with remediable stuttering are able to learn and use techniques to overcome this problem, chronic perseverative stuttering involves problems that extend beyond developmental disfluency and are less amenable to treatment. Approximately two-thirds of children who stutter have the remediable form, while one in five have the chronic perseverative form (Cooper 1987, 1993).

Although disorders of the pragmatics of language are not yet represented separately in DSM-IV-TR, they have attracted considerable clinical and research attention, particularly because they are correlated with a variety of psychiatric disorders in children and adults (Baltaxe and Simmons 1988). Children (and adults) with poor pragmatics have a deficit in understanding the context and function of language, fail to track the listener's response to their talking, and appear socially impaired. Although these language impairments are frequently described in pervasive developmental disorders, several investigators have suggested that this disorder also exists separately from pervasive developmental disorders (Cohen 2001; Toppelberg and Shapiro 2000).

■ Relation to Psychiatric Disorders

A wide range of emotional and behavioral disorders have been described in children and adolescents with communication disorders. These may represent emotional reactions to the linguistic deficit, symptoms of concomitant psychiatric disorders, or manifestations of a common underlying neurological substrate. Signs of impulsivity, inattentiveness, aggressiveness, lack of self-confidence, low

self-esteem, social withdrawal, low frustration tolerance, anxiety, and social immaturity have been noted in younger children with communication disorders (American Psychiatric Association 2000; Cantwell and Baker 1987; Cohen 2001). Emotional problems also are common in adolescents with communication disorders. Symptoms may include anxiety, compulsiveness, withdrawal, aggressiveness, and rigidity (Beitchman et al. 1996; Cohen 2001).

About half of all children with language disorders seen in speech and language clinics also have an Axis I psychiatric disorder. In particular, associations have been found with attention-deficit/hyperactivity disorder, other disruptive behavior disorders, and anxiety disorders (Beitchman et al. 1986; Paul 2001). In their investigation of a group of children diagnosed with a communication disorder, Cantwell and Baker (1991) found a comorbid disruptive behavior disorder in 26% of the children, with attention-deficit/hyperactivity disorder the most common (found in 19% of the children), followed by oppositional defiant disorder and conduct disorder (in 7%). Anxiety disorders were found in 10% of the children. Children with mixed receptive–expressive language disorder are the most likely to have comorbid psychiatric disorders. Language disorders are more likely than speech disorders (phonological disorder or stuttering) to be associated with comorbid psychiatric conditions (Cantwell and Baker 1991; Stevenson 1996). Longitudinal data suggest that language problems at age 5 years place a child at risk for a variety of psychiatric disorders by age 19 years, including attention-deficit/hyperactivity disorder, antisocial personality disorder, criminal behavior, and substance use disorders (Beitchman et al. 1996, 1999).

It is extremely important to be aware that up to two-thirds of children seen in outpatient child psychiatry settings have language disorders that are too subtle to be detected by all but the most experienced psychiatrists without specialized evaluations (Paul 2001; Stevenson 1996). Cohen et al. (1993) found, in a group of children from outpatient child psychiatry clinics who were identified as having language disorders, that approximately 30% were previously undiagnosed. These children had less difficulty with expressive sentence formation, milder language difficulties overall, and higher rates of externalizing problems, such as delinquency, compared with children whose language disorders had been previously diagnosed. Unfortunately, many clinicians in mental health settings overlook speech and language problems and are unaware of the risks these disorders pose to development and outcome.

■ Diagnosis

The child psychiatrist should routinely take a careful history of language development and assess current level of linguistic functioning. A useful preliminary evaluation can be done in the context of the clinical interview and mental status examination. Specific areas that the clinician should observe include inner language, comprehension, production, phonation, and pragmatics (Rutter 1987). *Inner language* refers to the use of symbolization in the child's thought and can be evaluated most easily in younger children by observing play behavior for evidence of symbolic play. Language comprehension should be evaluated in terms of the child's ability to follow commands without gestures, answer questions both relevant to the situation and out of context, follow conversation, understand abstract language, and draw inferences. Language *production* involves an assessment of the amount, fluency, and intelligibility of speech produced. Additionally, specific components

of speech content to be evaluated include morphology, syntax, and semantics. *Phonation* is assessed by attending to the quality of the child's voice and includes pitch, volume, intonation, and prosody (melody of speech). *Pragmatic* language is gauged by observing the child's ability to use language for effective communication. This involves the child's ability to sustain a reciprocal conversation on a shared topic, to use nonverbal behaviors such as eye contact and gestures, to attend to nonverbal cues, and to both use and understand idiomatic expressions and metaphoric language appropriate to age (Rutter 1987).

If, in the course of the psychiatric evaluation, a speech or language impairment is suspected, referral for further specialized assessment is warranted. For both expressive language disorder and mixed receptive–expressive language disorder, diagnosis, as defined in DSM-IV-TR, is predicated on demonstrating a significant discrepancy between nonverbal cognitive functioning and language development. The assessment of cognitive and linguistic abilities requires psychometric testing, which should not be limited to merely comparing verbal and nonverbal dimensions on an intelligence test. Although an overall measure of intelligence (and a specific measure of nonverbal intelligence) is essential, such a measure will provide neither the specificity nor the sensitivity to detect or delineate many linguistic deficits. Standardized measures of linguistic functioning, usually conducted by a speech–language pathologist, are required. Table 12–2 provides a list of commonly used speech–language tests. (A list of intelligence tests is presented later in this chapter, in the section on learning disorders.) Of particular importance is the consideration of a child's cultural context, including bilingualism, in determining the most appropriate measures of functioning. In addition to linguistic and

Table 12–2.   Speech–language tests

Test	Age range (age expressed as year–month)	Functions assessed
Test batteries		
Clinical Evaluation of Language Fundamentals—Preschool, 2nd Edition (CELF-P-II; Semel et al. 2004)	3–0 to 6–11	Total language score, receptive and expressive language comprehension
Clinical Evaluation of Language Fundamentals—4th Edition (CELF-4; Semel et al. 2003)	5–0 to 21–11	Core language score, receptive and expressive language, language structure, language content, language content and memory, working memory
Preschool Language Scale—4th Edition (PLS-4; Zimmerman et al. 2002)	0–1 to 6–11	Total language score, auditory comprehension, expressive communication
Test of Adolescent and Adult Language—3rd Edition (TAAL-3; Hammill et al. 1994)	12–0 to 24–0	Receptive and expressive language, oral and written responses
Test of Early Language Development—3rd Edition (TELD-3; Hresko et al. 1999)	2–0 to 7–11	Early development of oral language in the areas of receptive and expressive language, syntax, and semantics
Test of Language Development—3rd Edition (TOLD-3), Versions I:3 and P:3 (Newcomer and Hammill 1997)	P:3: 4–0 to 8–11 I:3: 8–0 to 12–11	Receptive and expressive language (syntax, semantics, phonology), auditory discrimination and memory
Tests of specific speech–language abilities		
Arizona Articulation Proficiency Scale—3rd Edition (Fudala 2001)	1–5 to 18–0	Speech articulation of initial and final consonants, blends, vowels, and dipthongs
Comprehensive Test of Phonological Processing (CTOPP; Wagner et al. 1999)	5–0 to 24–11	Phonological awareness, phonological memory, rapid naming
Expressive and Receptive One-Word Picture Vocabulary Tests (EOWPVT, ROWPVT; Brownell 2000)	2–0 to 11–11	Expressive vocabulary, receptive vocabulary
Goldman-Fristoe Test of Articulation—2 (GFTA-2; Goldman and Fristoe 2000)	2–0 to 21	Speech articulation of consonant sounds, single word and conversational speech production
MacArthur-Bates Communicative Development Inventories (CDIs; Fensen et al. 1993)	0–8 to 2–6	Expressive and receptive language, parent interview format, infant and toddler forms
Peabody Picture Vocabulary Test—3rd Edition (PPVT-III; Dunn et al. 1997)	2–6 to 90+	Receptive vocabulary

Table 12–2. Speech–language tests *(continued)*

Test	Age range (age expressed as year–month)	Functions assessed
Tests of specific speech–language abilities *(continued)*		
Test of Auditory Comprehension of Language—3rd Edition (TACL-3; Carrow-Woolfolk 1999)	3–0 to 9–11	Auditory comprehension of vocabulary, grammatical morphemes, elaborated phrases and sentences
Test of Auditory Processing Skills—3rd Edition (TAPS-3; Martin and Brownell 2005)	4–0 to 18–1	Basic auditory skills, auditory memory, auditory cohesion
Test of Pragmatic Language (TOPL; Phelps-Terasaki and Phelps-Gunn 1992)	5–0 to 13–11	In-depth screen of pragmatic language

psychological testing, a hearing evaluation is an important part of the assessment.

A differential diagnosis of other conditions should be conducted before diagnosis of a communication disorder is made. Specifically, other causes of language disorders, such as hearing impairment, mental retardation, pervasive developmental disorders, and selective mutism, should be ruled out. Research suggests that language disorders can and do occur in mentally retarded individuals (Rondal 1987), and these children should receive both diagnoses if language function is impaired beyond what can be accounted for by the mental retardation.

Despite the fact that DSM-IV-TR currently uses a cognitive–linguistic discrepancy model for identification of language disorders, there are major operational problems with this approach (Aram et al. 1994; Fletcher and Morris 1986; Fletcher et al. 1998; Paul 2001). Discrepancy-based approaches do not address the issue of whether important functional or etiological differences exist between children whose language functioning is low but commensurate with nonverbal intelligence and children who meet the discrepancy criteria. Furthermore, there is debate about which tests to use, how large the discrepancy must be, which aspects of language are essential to the diagnosis, and how many linguistic capacities must be deficient and to what degree (Aram and Morris 1992). Additionally, diagnosis of infants and toddlers with a discrepancy-based approach is difficult, because assessment measures for this younger population are limited (Wetherby and Prizant 1997). It has been suggested that a more appropriate means of identification would be to simply target all children whose language skills are below those expected for age (American Academy of Child and Adolescent Psychiatry 1998; Paul 2001).

■ Etiology and Pathogenesis

The etiology of communication disorders is primarily biological, but family environment and sociological factors also clearly play a role (Cantwell and Baker 1991; Wetherby and Prizant 1997). Biological factors that have been demonstrated to influence the development of language include prenatal risk factors (e.g., exposure to intrauterine teratogens such as alcohol, drugs, or environmental toxins like lead), perinatal risk factors (e.g., anoxia, asphyxia, low birth weight), early childhood risk factors (e.g., recurrent persistent otitis media, childhood illnesses), and genetic and metabolic disorders. Important environmental risk factors include poverty, abuse or neglect, and psychiatric disorders in caregivers. Although individual risk factors may not play numerically important roles as etiological factors in language disorders, an important predictor is the accumulation of multiple risk factors, both biological and environmental (Paul 2001; Wetherby and Prizant 1997).

There is considerable evidence that hereditary factors are a prominent cause of language disorder, particularly expressive language disorder (American Academy of Child and Adolescent Psychiatry 1998; Bishop et al. 1995; Tomblin and Buckwalter 1994). Early language delay (as measured by vocabulary at age 2 years) is under strong hereditary influence, as documented by Dale et al. (1998) in a study of 3,000 twin pairs. The heritability of group differences for children whose vocabulary scores were in the lowest 5% was estimated at 73%. Shared environment was only a quarter as important for the language-delayed sample as for the entire sample. Twin research also documents an association between motor immaturity and specific language impairment in children (Bishop 2002). Much of the evidence for the role of specific genetic factors in language dysfunction (particularly regarding genes on chromosomes 6, 7, and 15) is reviewed in the section of this chapter on learning disorders.

Phonological disorder also has a strong heritable component, as noted in several studies (Lewis 1992; Lewis and Thompson 1992). Similarly, in stuttering there also appears to be a familial pattern. Half of people who stutter have other family members who also stutter (Felsenfeld 1998). Stuttering is more than three times more common in first-degree relatives of persons who stutter than in the general population, and a family history of other communication disorders increases the risk of stuttering. In families in which fathers stutter, approximately 10% of daughters and 20% of sons also stutter (American Psychiatric Association 2000).

As with the phonological-processing-deficit models of reading disorder, there is considerable evidence that the very rapid neural processing of speech sounds required to decode and comprehend spoken language is impaired in children with receptive language problems (Fitch et al. 1997). It is likely, however, that there are other neurological dysfunctions involved in language disorder that are not due to phonological deficits. Working-verbal-memory deficits appear to be a factor in phonological and semantic information processing for some children with receptive language disorder (Johnson 1994)

■ Treatment

Children meeting criteria for communication disorders are often eligible for special education services through the school system to address these deficits. Such services can include individual or group speech therapy or more intensive services such as special education classroom placement. The goals of intervention vary from child to child and may include elimination of the deficit (if possible), teaching specific strategies to change the deficit and increase skills, teaching compensatory coping strategies, or changing the child's environment (Paul 2001). Intervention approaches may include clinician-directed approaches (drill, drill play, and modeling), which follow a formal, behavioral approach to treatment; child-centered approaches (indirect language stimulation or facilitative play, and whole language), which are appropriate for children who are unassertive or refuse to participate in a clinician-directed approach; and hybrid approaches (focused stimulation, vertical structuring, milieu teaching, and script therapy), which combine aspects of the previous two approaches (Paul 2001).

Two commonly used methods for treating language impairments—imitation-based therapy and modeling therapy—have been shown to improve more than the specific targeted aspects of language taught (Leonard 1998). Language therapy is increasingly designed to be conducted in relevant social environments, where the focus is on functional language in transactional contexts (Schiefelbusch and Lloyd 1988; Wetherby and Prizant 1997). In addition, assisting caregivers to develop appropriate styles of communication with their children that encourage successful communicative interactions is an important identified treatment approach (Wetherby and Prizant 1997).

Fast ForWord, a computer-assisted intervention program developed by the Scientific Learning Corporation for children with language impairments and reading deficits, claims to improve a child's temporal auditory processing abilities. Training aims to increase a child's speech, nonspeech discrimination, and language comprehension skills, thereby affecting reading skills as well as spoken language (Merzenich et al. 1996; Tallal et al. 1996). Studies of this technique have found modest gains in oral and written language and pragmatics, as well as improvements in phonemic awareness, speaking, and syntax (Gillam et al. 2001; Thibodeau et al. 2001; Hook et al. 2001). Other available treatment

programs have also been shown to be effective, such as the Laureate Learning Systems and the Orton Gillingham programs, which also address both reading and spoken language deficits (Gillam et al. 2001; Hook et al. 2001).

The Lidcombe Program, a treatment approach developed for stuttering, is based on the principles of operant conditioning. Parents are taught how to use these principles on a day-to-day basis in natural contexts with their children, providing verbal contingencies in the form of praise for nonstuttered speech and occasional corrections for stuttering. Research suggests that this is a promising treatment method, leading to alleviation of symptoms in preschool children and low rates of relapse (Onslow et al. 2001; Woods et al. 2002).

When treating any comorbid psychiatric conditions, the presence of a language disorder should be taken into consideration, particularly in regard to verbally based forms of treatment, including traditional psychotherapy, as well as group treatment programs and family therapy. Language disorders present a significant impediment to effective communication in psychotherapy. Children and adolescents with language disorders are likely to have difficulty expressing themselves and understanding the information presented to them in these settings. Care should be taken not to misinterpret the behavior of the language-impaired child or adolescent (e.g., as oppositionality when in fact the observed behavior may be the result of not understanding information or not knowing how to respond).

■ Prognosis and Natural History

Most children with expressive and mixed receptive–expressive language disorders speak by the time they reach school age and have normal language abilities by late adolescence. However, significant language and learning deficits may persist for up to half of these children, particularly those with more severe initial impairment (Shapiro and Rich 1999). A 10-year systematic prospective study of children with language disorders as preschoolers (Aram et al. 1984) found that only 30% of these children had a normal academic course. The remainder had either repeated a grade or were in special education classes. Follow-up language testing of these children revealed that 62% had language scores that were significantly below average. Children diagnosed with mixed receptive–expressive language disorder have a poorer prognosis than those diagnosed with an expressive language disorder, with fewer children improving over time and a higher rate of learning disorders and psychiatric diagnoses (Cantwell and Baker 1991). Continuing language impairment can lead to academic failure, which can affect adult achievement in areas such as occupational and social functioning. In addition, decreased self-esteem, depression, and learned helplessness are risks, as well as insufficient social learning, leading to later social difficulties (Settle and Milich 1999; Weinberg et al. 1999). Children with language and learning disabilities have a 50% greater than average rate of school dropout (U.S. Department of Education 1995).

Spontaneous recovery of mild to moderate phonological disorder not due to a medical condition occurs by age 6 years in approximately 75% of cases and may be hastened by appropriate therapy. The prevalence by age 17 years is 0.5% (American Psychiatric Association 2000). Poorer prognoses are mostly seen in children with co-occurring problems, such as stuttering or hypernasality (Johnson 1980). Stuttering often resolves spontaneously by mid-adolescence, in 20%–80% of cases (American Psychiatric Association 2000). Children with remediable stuttering will be more likely to experience an alleviation of symptoms, whereas those with chronic perseverative stuttering will be more likely to continue to have symptoms (Cooper 1987, 1993).

Motor Skills Disorder

■ Definition and History

Motor delays and coordination problems not meeting criteria for medical conditions such as cerebral palsy have been identified in the literature for many years. Terms used have included "clumsiness syndrome," "dyspraxia syndrome," "poor coordination of developmental onset," and "specific motor developmental disorder" (Denckla and Roeltgen 1992). Currently, the term *developmental coordination disorder* is used in DSM-IV-TR and is defined as a significant impairment in either gross- or fine-motor coordination, as evidenced by delays in developmental motor milestones or difficulty with other expected motor tasks during development, such as fine and gross motor clumsiness, difficulty with sports activities, and poor handwriting. Skills fall significantly below expected for the child's age and intelligence. This disorder is distinct in DSM-IV-TR from medical conditions that cause motor difficulties, as well as other conditions with a common motor skills delay component, such as the pervasive developmental disorders (American Psychiatric Association 2000).

■ Clinical Presentation

Developmental coordination disorder is estimated to occur in up to 6% of 5- to 11-year-olds (American Psychiatric Association 2000). Typically, it is first diagnosed when parents notice a delay in development of specific motor skills or difficulty with skills once attempted. In addition to delays and deficits in motor skills, children with developmental coordination disorder often have associated delays of other developmental milestones. Other disorders commonly observed include learning and communication disorders (American Psychiatric Association 2000; Sugden and Wright 1998). When developmental coordination disorder is accompanied by a learning disorder, there is a correlation with greater severity of perceptual-motor dysfunction (Jongmans et al. 2003). In addition, comorbid conditions such as attention-deficit/hyperactivity disorder are frequently seen (Denckla and Roeltgen 1992). The co-occurrence of attention-deficit/hyperactivity disorder with developmental coordination disorder, when there is not a significant learning deficit or medical explanation for the motor delay, has been described in several countries as a distinct neurodevelopmental phenotype, referred to by the acronym *DAMP* (deficits in attention, motor control, and perception). This condition is seen in approximately half of children diagnosed with attention-deficit/hyperactivity disorder and half of children diagnosed with developmental coordination disorder (Gillberg 2003).

The clumsiness associated with developmental coordination disorder can lead to peer teasing that has a harmful emotional impact on these children, leading to social withdrawal, low self-esteem, anxiety, and feelings of incompetence and low self-efficacy. These children often do not participate in physically based social activities (Chen and Cohn 2003).

■ Diagnosis and Treatment

In addition to a medical evaluation to rule out potential medical causes of the motor impairment, a thorough history is necessary, as well as standardized testing and child observation. History information collected should include developmental motor milestones, as well as other early motor behaviors seen in infancy and toddlerhood, such as sucking, swallowing, crying, tracking, grasping, toileting, feeding, dressing, drawing, and others (Denckla and Roeltgen 1992). An evaluation by an occupational therapist can provide quantitative information about a child's fine and gross motor skills. Table 12–3 lists of some of the tests commonly used for the assessment of motor functioning.

Other conditions resulting in motor difficulties that should be ruled out before a diagnosis of developmental coordination disorder is made include neurological conditions that affect motor coordination and the pervasive developmental disorders. It is possible for a child to have a developmental coordination disorder if mental retardation is also present. However, it must be demonstrated that the motor deficits present are above what would be expected, given the diagnosis of mental retardation.

Treatment approaches fall into the broad categories of task-oriented versus process-oriented strategies. Process-oriented treatment is based on the underlying assumption that there is a deficit that needs to be addressed before functional skills can be taught; task-oriented treatment approaches focus on teaching functional skills (Sugden and Wright 1998). The primary treatment modality for motor skills disorder is occupational therapy. In the school setting, a child might also receive adaptive physical education for gross motor incoordination, or assistive technology resources for fine motor deficits, such as handwriting problems. Assistive technology services typically include keyboard-based strategies, such as use of a computer or portable keyboard, or dictation-based strategies, in which a child dictates orally to a scribe (Freeman et al. 2004).

Table 12–3.   Tests of motor functioning

Test	Age range (age expressed as year–month)	Functions assessed
Test batteries		
Bruininks-Oseretsky Test of Motor Proficiency (BOTMP; Bruininks 1978)	4–6 to 14–5	Gross and fine motor development; running speed and agility; balance; bilateral coordination; strength; upper-limb coordination, speed, and dexterity; response speed; visuomotor control
Peabody Developmental Motor Scale, 2nd Edition (PDMS-2; Folio and Fewell 2000)	Birth to 6–11	Total motor score, gross and fine motor scores; reflexes, stationary, locomotion, object manipulation, grasping, visuomotor integration
Toddler and Infant Motor Evaluation: A Standardized Assessment (T.I.M.E.; Miller and Roid 1994)	Birth to 3–6	Mobility, stability, motor organization, functional performance, social-emotional abilities
Tests of specific motor abilities		
Test of Gross Motor Development, 2nd Edition (TGMD-2; Ulrich 2000)	3–0 to 10–11	Gross motor skills: locomotor and object control measures
Beery-Buktenica Developmental Test of Visual-Motor Integration, 5th Edition (VMI; Beery et al. 2004)	2–0 to 18–11	Visuomotor perception; separate measures of visual perception and motor coordination

Learning Disorders

■ Definition

The National Joint Committee on Learning Disabilities (1997) defines learning disorders as a diverse group of conditions in which a specific area of learning is compromised, including skills in listening, speaking, reading, writing, reasoning, and mathematics. DSM-IV-TR defines learning disorders in a narrower manner, focusing on impairments in three specific academic areas (reading, writing, and mathematics). To meet diagnostic criteria for these conditions, scores on individually administered standardized tests of achievement must fall substantially below those expected for age, schooling, and intelligence in the identified skill area. Children with sensory or cognitive deficits (i.e., visual, linguistic, attention, memory) or mental retardation can be diagnosed with learning disorders, but the learning difficulty must be in excess of the difficulty usually associated with those deficits.

Children with *reading disorder* (commonly referred to as dyslexia) have poor reading ability (including rate, accuracy, and comprehension) often combined with spelling problems, poor writing, speech delay, or dyspraxia. These difficulties result in performance below the expected level given the child's age, intelligence, and level of education and interfere with functioning in settings that require reading. Researchers have further defined reading disorder as a neurobiological, language-based deficit in word recognition, spelling, and decoding, based on an underlying deficit in phonological processing (i.e., turning print into sound; Shaywitz 2003). Behavioral indicators of reading disorder include deficits in phonemic awareness, auditory processing and working memory, visual processing speed, and rapid automatic naming/fluency. These areas should be assessed, in addition to examining reading achievement scores (Bell et al. 2003).

Mathematics disorder is characterized by difficulty in mathematical calculation or reasoning, manifesting in a variety of difficulties, including problems with the linguistic, perceptual, attention, and mathematical skills needed to understand mathematical concepts. In *disorder of written expression,* the essential impairment is in writing ability, as demonstrated by the use of grammar and punctuation, organization, spelling, and handwriting (American Psychiatric Association 2000).

The Individuals with Disabilities Education Act (IDEA; U.S. Congress 1997), which included national mandates for special education services in the United States, defined "specific learning disabilities" for the purpose of eligibility for special education services. In this definition, difficulties in "understanding or in using language, spoken or written" are identified as the central deficit, with subsequent problems noted in "the ability to listen, think, speak, read, write, spell, or do mathematical calculations." To be eligible for the educational classification of a specific learning disability, learning problems cannot be the result of sensory or cognitive deficits; mental retardation; emotional disturbance; or environmental, cultural, or economic disadvantage. This is often interpreted to mean that only children of normal intelligence can

meet eligibility for a specific learning disability through the public schools.

■ History

Case studies of children with learning disabilities appeared as early as 1896 (Morgan). An early theoretical explanation for learning disabilities was offered by Orton (1937), who proposed that the problem was a failure to establish cerebral dominance during development. Orton later divided developmental disorders into alexia, agraphia, word deafness, motor aphasia, apraxia, and stuttering (Doris 1993). In the 1950s, Cruickshank (1967) studied a group of children with perceptual disabilities, attention deficit, poor motor coordination, and impulsivity. Because of their behavioral similarity to brain-damaged children, he described these children as having "minimal brain damage," despite the absence of any clear evidence of frank neurological problems. In the early 1960s, the term *minimal brain dysfunction* was coined to describe a syndrome with a variety of features, including specific learning deficits, perceptual–motor problems, poor coordination, hyperkinesis, impulsivity, equivocal neurological signs, and abnormal electroencephalographic findings (Clements and Peters 1962). Concurrently, the term *specific learning disability* was applied to describe the same population of children (Farnham-Diggory 1978).

During the 1970s, the focus was on the attentional deficits in children thought to have minimal brain dysfunction. However, it became increasingly clear that use of stimulant medication significantly reduced hyperactivity and improved attention but had no effect on specific learning problems (Silver 1986). Neurologists became involved in examining this population, who were assumed to have an underlying brain dysfunction (Kinsbourne 1973). However, the inability to identify "hard" neurological signs in most children continues to impede progress in establishing a role for neurological examination in the diagnosis of learning disorders. In recent years, functional magnetic resonance imaging, in concert with neuropsychological and linguistic tests, has begun to illuminate the brain mechanisms underlying these conditions (Shaywitz et al. 2000).

■ Clinical Presentation

Clinically, children with learning disorders present with poor academic achievement relative to their intelligence. Symptoms vary with level of intellectual functioning; children with higher IQs tend to show fewer neurological signs and fewer symptoms of motor skills and language disorders (Shepherd et al. 1989). Many children with learning disorders have difficulty with active information processing, which may manifest as difficulty in developing strategies for organizing, prioritizing, rehearsing, or presenting information, especially when it is linguistically based (American Academy of Child and Adolescent Psychiatry 1998). In many cases, by the time of referral for evaluation, the child not only has poor academic performance but also lacks the basic learning skills needed to comprehend or master the more advanced material he or she may be confronting in school.

Reading disorder is thought to occur in 2%–20% of children, accounting for up to 80% of all children with a diagnosed learning disorder (Shaywitz 2003; Shaywitz et al. 2000). Approximately 80% of those affected are boys (American Psychiatric Association 2000), although epidemiological research has failed to find a true sex difference (Flynn and Rahbar 1994; Shaywitz et al. 1990). *Mathematics disorder* is reported to occur in 1%–6% of

school-aged children, with higher rates in girls than in boys (American Academy of Child and Adolescent Psychiatry 1998). *Disorder of written expression* has been suggested to occur in 2%–8% of children, is more common in boys than in girls, and is usually reported in combination with other learning disorders (American Academy of Child and Adolescent Psychiatry 1998; American Psychiatric Association 2000).

Relative or absolute failure in school places a child at risk for development of a psychiatric disorder (Offord and Waters 1983). Furthermore, a negative emotional cycle often develops in which poor self-esteem, anxiety, depression, deficits in social competence, alienation, or rebellion further interfere with the child's ability to participate effectively in school (Beitchman and Young 1997; Bryan 1991). As with communication disorders, the rate of concurrent Axis I psychopathology is as high as 50% in children and adolescents with learning disorders. The combination of having both a learning and a language disorder may further increase the likelihood of an Axis I diagnosis (American Academy of Child and Adolescent Psychiatry 1998; Beitchman et al. 1986). Attention-deficit disorders are reported to occur in 20% or more of the population with learning disorders (Hinshaw 1992; Shaywitz and Shaywitz 1989). Conversely, 10%–25% of children diagnosed with a disruptive behavior disorder or depressive disorder have comorbid learning disorders (American Psychiatric Association 2000). In adolescents, there is also evidence of a significant relationship between conduct problems and learning disorders, with estimates that up to 85% of juvenile delinquents may have a diagnosable learning disorder (Klein and Mannuzza 2000; Moffitt 1995). A significant related risk is for the development of a substance use disorder (Karacostas and Fisher 1993).

■ Diagnosis

Learning disorders are frequently identified by the schools. However, in view of
the high rate of comorbidity between
learning disorders and psychiatric disorders, the child and adolescent psychiatrist
must always be vigilant to the substantial
possibility that children and adolescents
referred for psychiatric evaluation of emotional or behavioral problems may also
have an undetected learning disorder.
The first step in making the diagnosis of a
learning disorder involves establishing a
discrepancy between the academic skill or
skills in question and the child's intelligence, and then eliminating all other explanations for the discrepancy. To establish this discrepancy, a psychoeducational
evaluation is typically performed by a qualified psychologist, comparing scores on
standardized academic achievement tests
with scores on intelligence tests. Intelligence tests usually include both verbal
and nonverbal components; however,
when a child is already known to have a
communication disorder, consideration
of the use of a nonverbal intelligence test
may be appropriate. Table 12–4 briefly
lists some of the most commonly used intelligence and achievement tests. A significant difference between scores is frequently defined as a discrepancy of 1 to 2
standard deviations, with achievement
level lower than IQ.

The second part of the diagnostic procedure for learning disorders involves differential diagnosis. Other conditions often
resulting in poor academic performance
and associated with learning disorders include mental retardation, neurological
damage or disease, memory problems, and
Axis I psychiatric conditions, such as at-
tention-deficit/hyperactivity disorder and
communication disorders. In addition, factors such as sensory impairment, inadequate schooling, cultural factors, nonna-
tive English-speaking, and environmental
deprivation must be differentiated from
learning disorders. Learning disorder
should not be diagnosed if the academic
difficulties are due primarily to these factors, unless the difficulties seen are greater
than would be expected given these conditions alone. All children suspected of having a learning disorder should receive vision and hearing screening.

As with communication disorders, the
use of a discrepancy model to identify
learning disorders is controversial. Research suggests that use of an IQ–achievement discrepancy to diagnose learning
disorders may result in underdiagnosis
for children of average or low average IQ,
as well as for children with socioeconomic
deprivation and/or minority status (Fletcher et al. 1994, 1998). However, a more
appropriate method of identification has
not been agreed upon by the scientific
community (American Academy of Child
and Adolescent Psychiatry 1998). One
suggested alternative involves evaluation
of achievement in specific academic domains, with comparison to abilities that
are matched with the specific skill areas
(Fletcher et al. 1998; Zigmond 1993). As
with communication disorders, it has also
been suggested that any poor reader (the
same would apply for math and writing)
should be entitled to services (Shaywitz
2003).

■ Etiology and Pathogenesis

The etiology of learning disorders is unknown but presumed to include a variety
of neurocognitive deficits resulting in
disruptions of cognitive processing. Most
advances in understanding the neural
basis for learning disorders have been
based on the study of reading disorder.
There is considerable overlap in findings
with those from research in the language
disorders.

Table 12–4.   Intelligence and achievement tests

Test	Age range (age expressed as year–month)	Functions assessed
Infant cognitive development		
Bayley Scales of Infant and Toddler Development, 3rd Edition (Bayley-III; Bayley 2005)	0–1 to 3–6	Cognitive, language, motor, social-emotional, and adaptive behavior domains
Mullen Scales of Early Learning (Mullen 1995)	0–1 to 5–8	Visual reception, gross and fine motor, expressive and receptive language domains
Intelligence tests		
Kaufman Assessment Battery for Children—2nd Edition (KABC-II; Kaufman and Kaufman 2003a)	3–0 to 18–1	Sequential and simultaneous mental processing, planning and learning ability, knowledge; culturally fair
Stanford-Binet Intelligence Scale—5th Edition (SB5; Roid 2003)	2–0 to 85+	Full-scale IQ, verbal IQ, and nonverbal IQ; domains assessed: fluid reasoning, knowledge, quantitative reasoning, working memory, visuospatial processing
Wechsler Preschool and Primary Scale of Intelligence—3rd Edition (WPPSI-III; Wechsler 2002)	2–6 to 7–3	Full-scale IQ, verbal IQ, and performance IQ (nonverbal); visual processing speed and general language composites
Wechsler Intelligence Scale for Children—4th Edition (WISC-IV; Wechsler 2003)	6–0 to 16–11	Full-scale IQ, verbal comprehension, perceptual reasoning, visual processing speed, auditory working memory
Nonverbal intelligence tests		
Leiter International Performance Scale—Revised (LIPS-R; Roid and Miller 1996)	2–0 to 20–11	Nonverbal IQ, language-free; measure of visual perception, discrimination, and reasoning
Comprehensive Test of Nonverbal Intelligence (CTONI; Hammill et al. 1997)	6–0 to 90	Nonverbal intelligence screen; measure of analogical reasoning, categorical classification, sequential reasoning
Educational achievement test batteries		
Kaufman Test of Educational Achievement—2nd Edition (KTEA-II; Kaufman and Kaufman 2003b)	4–6 to 25–11	Reading, mathematics, spelling, written expression, oral language
Wechsler Individual Achievement Test—2nd Edition (WIAT-II; Psychological Corporation 2001)	4–0 to 85	Word reading, pseudoword decoding, reading comprehension, spelling, written expression, numerical operations, math reasoning, listening comprehension, oral expression

Table 12–4. Intelligence and achievement tests *(continued)*

Test	Age range (age expressed as year–month)	Functions assessed
Educational achievement test batteries *(continued)*		
Wide Range Achievement Test—3rd Edition (WRAT-3; Wilkinson 1993)	5–0 to 75–0	Screening measure for reading, spelling, and arithmetic
Woodcock-Johnson Psychoeducational Battery—3rd Edition (WJ-III; Woodcock et al. 2001)	3–0 to adult	Reading, writing, spelling, oral language, fluency, math
Tests of specific academic abilities		
Gray Oral Reading Tests, 4th Edition (GORT; Wiederholt and Bryant 1992)	6–0 to 18–11	Overall reading ability score; rate, accuracy, fluency, comprehension
KeyMath–Revised/NU: A Diagnostic Inventory of Essential Mathematics, Normative Update (Connolly 1997)	5–0 to 22–11	Assesses arithmetic abilities in the areas of basic concepts, operations, and applications
Test of Written Language—3rd Edition (TOWL-3; Hammill and Larsen 1995)	7–6 to 17–11	Overall writing score; contrived writing, spontaneous writing
Woodcock Reading Mastery Tests—Revised/Normative Update (WRMI-R/NU; Woodcock 1998)	5–0 to 75+	Reading readiness, basic reading skills, reading comprehension

There are numerous causes for poor reading, including both hereditary and environmental factors. Environmental factors with known associations to reading delays in children include prematurity, major perinatal adversity, poverty, malnutrition, poor schooling, early abuse and neglect, and parental substance abuse. However, it is becoming evident, with the accumulation of genetic studies, that hereditary factors also play an important role. The familial risk for reading disorder in first-degree relatives of children with reading disorder is between 35% and 45% (Pennington 1995; Shepherd and Uhry 1993). There is also considerable evidence for a link between reading disorder and attention-deficit/hyperactivity disorder on a hereditary basis (Beitchman and Young 1997). For example, Light et al. (1995) found that 70% of the covariance

between reading disability and attention-deficit/hyperactivity disorder was heritable. Stevenson et al. (1993) found that 75% of the comorbidity of spelling disability and attention-deficit/hyperactivity disorder was heritable.

Genetic loci on chromosomes 6 and 15 have been linked to some familial cases of reading disability (Grigorenko 1997). An abnormality of the *FOX P2* gene on chromosome 7 has recently been identified as causal of deficits in both phonological processing and grammatical usage (Lai et al. 2001).

Although single-gene causes are associated with some forms of familial reading impairment, most inherited variations in reading ability are due to polygenic influences. This perspective is supported by the findings of Shaywitz et al. (1996), who used an epidemiological approach to establish that children's reading abilities were spread along a continuum rather than split at categorical break points between normal and abnormal reading. This finding supports a multiple-risk model for variations in reading ability rather than a causal model that emphasizes categorical differences between normal and deficient readers. It is likely that there are no categorical differences between children at the lower end of the normal spectrum of reading disability and those classified as having a reading disorder (Shaywitz et al. 1992).

Considerable recent progress has been made in elucidating the functional neuroanatomical correlates of poor reading. These findings utilize functional neuroimaging and neurophysiological techniques to support and extend previously established findings regarding the importance of the temporoparietal region of the left brain (Galaburda et al. 1985; Rumsey 1987). Deficits in phonological processing, primarily a left-hemisphere function, are the most common neurocognitive impairments responsible for these conditions (Merzenich et al. 1996; Shaywitz et al. 2000; Tallal et al. 1996). Functional neuroimaging and electrophysiological techniques have to some extent clarified the brain pathways by which the various left-brain regions involved in reading decode and translate both written and auditory language (orthographic and phonetic units of information) from one modality to the other and then interface with brain centers more concerned with meaning (semantics). This involves pathways from the occipital lobe to the posterior superior temporal, middle temporal, supramarginal and angular gyri, and the inferior frontal region (Broca's area; Fulbright et al. 1997; Simos et al. 2000, 2001). Evidence suggests that children with dyslexia have an underactivation of the posterior region (Wernicke's area, angular gyrus, striate cortex), and an overactiva-

tion of the anterior region (inferior frontal gyrus; Shaywitz 2003). Extrastriate and basal temporal areas are also involved in the processing of visually presented written words into their component graphemes (Pugh et al. 1996).

■ Treatment

In the public school setting, children who meet educational criteria for a specific learning disability are eligible to receive special education services, such as resource support (individualized instruction by a special education teacher), special education classroom placement, or tutorial help. Specific treatment approaches for learning disorders vary in focus. Some address underlying perceptual, visuomotor, or phonemic awareness deficits, while others focus on presenting information in multiple sensory formats (American Academy of Child and Adolescent Psychiatry 1998; Merzenich et al. 1996; Tallal et al. 1996). Examples of programs often used include Fast ForWord (described earlier in this chapter, in the section on communication disorders), Orton Gillingham, and Lindamood Bell. Enhancing the child's attention and motivation for academic tasks is another method used, with attentional enhancement primarily addressed pharmacologically and motivational enhancement addressed with behavioral techniques.

In addition to treating the learning disorder, treatment of any comorbid psychiatric conditions should take into account the limitations imposed by the learning disorder itself. For example, a child or adolescent with marked deficits in receptive and expressive language might not be an ideal candidate for verbally based psychotherapy. In addition, evidence suggests that some children with learning disorders have significant social skills deficits; therefore, treatment should include identification and targeting of these deficits (Kavale and Forness 1996; Sheehan 2001).

Prognosis and Natural History

Federal laws mandating individualized educational programming have had a considerable effect on the education of children with learning disorders; therefore, it is difficult to differentiate the natural longitudinal course of these conditions from the effects of educational intervention. Furthermore, because most longitudinal studies have focused on reading disorders, fewer data are available for other types of learning disorders. One early study (Watson et al. 1982) found that only 25% of children with mild reading disorders and 5% of those with severe disorders early in elementary school read at grade level by the end of high school. When a diagnosis is made early, a child has a better chance of remediation. However, Klein and Mannuzza (2000) reported that even children with uncomplicated reading disorder (i.e., no concurrent psychiatric disorder) go on to have a greater prevalence of mood and substance use disorders at 16-year follow-up.

Summary

Communication, motor skills, and learning disorders are a heterogeneous set of neurocognitive deficits seen in significant numbers of children and adolescents. They constitute a major vulnerability factor for psychiatric disorder and are comorbid conditions in many youngsters with psychiatric disorder. Because of these considerations, language, motor, and learning skills should be carefully assessed during all psychiatric evaluations of children and adolescents. Treatment planning must address these deficits in skills as well as any other Axis I disorder and associated family problems. Untreated problems in these important domains of a child's development are likely to undermine both therapeutic efforts and ongoing successful psychosocial adaptation.

References

American Academy of Child and Adolescent Psychiatry: Practice parameters for the assessment and treatment of children and adolescents with language and learning disorders. J Am Acad Child Adolesc Psychiatry 37:46S–62S, 1998

American Psychiatric Association: Diagnostic and Statistical Manual of Mental Disorders, 4th Edition, Text Revision, Washington, DC, American Psychiatric Association, 2000

American Speech-Language-Hearing Association (Ad Hoc Committee on Service Delivery in the Schools): Definitions of communication disorders and variations. ASHA 35 (suppl 10): 40–41, 1993

American Speech-Language-Hearing Association: Language-based learning disabilities. Rockville, MD, American Speech-Language-Hearing Association, 2002. Available at: http://www.asha.org/speech/disabilities/Language-Based-Learning-Disabilities.cfm. Accessed May 24, 2003

Aram DM, Morris R: Validity of discrepancy criteria for identifying children with developmental language disorder. J Learn Disabil 25:549–554, 1992

Aram DM, Nation JE: Patterns of language behavior in children with developmental language disorders. J Speech Hear Res 18:229–241, 1975

Aram DM, Ekelman BL, Nation JE: Preschoolers with language disorders: 10 years later. J Speech Hear Res 27:232–244, 1984

Aram D, Morris R, Hall N, et al: Clinical and research congruence in identifying children with specific language impairment. J Speech Hear Res 37:824–830, 1994

Arndt J, Healey EC: Concomitant disorders in school-age children who stutter. Language, Speech, and Hearing Services in School (special issue) 32:68–78, 2001

Baltaxe CAM, Simmons JQ: Pragmatic deficits in emotionally disturbed children and adolescents, in Language Perspectives: Acquisition, Retardation and Intervention. Edited by Schiefelbusch R, Lloyd L. Austin, TX, Pro-Ed, 1988, pp 223–253

Bayley N: Bayley Scales of Infant and Toddler Development, 3rd Edition. San Antonio TX, Psychological Corporation, 2005

Beery KE, Buktenica NA, Beery NA: Beery-Buktenica Developmental Test of Visual-Motor Integration, 5th Edition. Odessa, FL, Psychological Assessment Resources, 2004

Beitchman JH, Young A: Learning disorders with a special emphasis on reading disorders: a review of the past 10 years. J Am Acad Child Adolesc Psychiatry 36:1020–1032, 1997

Beitchman JH, Nair R, Clegg M, et al: Prevalence of psychiatric disorders in children with speech and language disorders. J Am Acad Child Adolesc Psychiatry 25:528–535, 1986

Beitchman JH, Wilson B, Brownlie EB, et al: Long-term consistency in speech/language profiles, I: developmental and academic outcomes. J Am Acad Child Adolesc Psychiatry 35:804–814, 1996

Beitchman JH, Douglas L, Wilson B, et al: Adolescent substance use disorders: findings from a 14-year follow-up of speech/language-impaired and control children. J Clin Child Psychol 28:312–321, 1999

Bell SM, McCallum RS, Cox EA: Toward a research-based assessment of dyslexia: using cognitive measures to identify reading disabilities. J Learn Disabil 36:505–516, 2003

Bishop DV: Motor immaturity and specific speech and language impairment: evidence for a common genetic basis. Am J Med Genet 114:56–63, 2002

Bishop DVM, North T, Donlan C: Genetic basis of specific language impairments: evidence from a twin study. Dev Med Child Neurol 37:56–71, 1995

Brownell R: Expressive and Receptive One-Word Picture Vocabulary Tests. San Antonio, TX, Psychological Corporation, 2000

Bruininks RH: Bruininks-Oseretsky Test of Motor Proficiency. Austin, TX, ProEd, 1978

Bryan T: Social problems and learning disabilities, in Learning About Learning Disabilities. Edited by Wong BY. San Diego, CA, Academic Press, 1991, pp 195–229

Cantwell D, Baker L: Developmental Speech and Language Disorders. New York, Guilford, 1987

Cantwell DP, Baker L: Psychiatric and Developmental Disorders in Children With Communication Disorder. Washington, DC, American Psychiatric Press, 1991

Carrow-Woolfolk E: Test for Auditory Comprehension of Language, 3rd Edition. Circle Pines, MN, American Guidance Service, 1999

Castrogiovanni A: Communication Facts: Incidence and Prevalence of Communication Disorders and Hearing Loss in Children—2002 Edition. Rockville, MD, American Speech-Language-Hearing Association. Available at: http://professional. asha.org/resources/factsheets/children.cfm. Accessed May 24, 2003

Chen HF, Cohn ES: Social participation for children with developmental coordination disorder: conceptual, evaluation and intervention considerations. Phys Occup Ther Pediatr 23:61–78, 2003

Clements S, Peters J: Minimal brain dysfunctions in the school-age child. Arch Gen Psychiatry 6:185–197, 1962

Cohen NJ: Language impairment and psychopathology in infants, children, and adolescents, in Developmental Clinical Psychology and Psychiatry, Vol 45. Thousand Oaks, CA, Sage Publications, 2001, pp 1–38

Cohen NJ, Davine M, Horodesky N, et al: Unsuspected language impairment in psychiatrically disturbed children: relevance and language and behavioral characteristics. J Am Acad Child Adolesc Psychiatry 32:595–603, 1993

Connolly AJ: KeyMath, Revised: A Diagnostic Inventory of Essential Mathematics, Normative Update. Circle Pines, MN, American Guidance Service, 1997

Cooper EB: The chronic perseverative stuttering syndrome: incurable stuttering. J Fluency Disord 12:381–388, 1987

Cooper EB: Chronic perseverative stuttering syndrome: a harmful or helpful construct? American Journal of Speech-Language Pathology 3:11–22, 1993

Cruickshank WM: The Brain-Injured Child in Home, School, and Community. Syracuse, NY, Syracuse University Press, 1967

Dale PS, Simonoff E, Bishop DV, et al: Genetic influence on language delay in two-year-old children. Nat Neurosci 1:324–328, 1998

Denckla MB, Roeltgen DP: Disorders of motor function and control, in Handbook of Neuropsychology, Vol 6. Edited by Rapin I, Segalowitz SJ. Amsterdam, Elsevier, 1992, pp 455–476

Doris JL: Defining learning disabilities: a history of the search for consensus, in Better Understanding Learning Disabilities: New Views from Research and Their Implications for Education and Public Policies. Edited by Lyon GR, Gray DB, Kavanagh JF, et al. Baltimore, MD, Paul H Brookes, 1993, pp 97–115

Dunn LM, Dunn LM, Williams TK: Peabody Picture Vocabulary Test—III. Circle Pines, MN, American Guidance Service, 1997

Farnham-Diggory S: Learning Disabilities. Cambridge, MA, Harvard University Press, 1978

Felsenfeld S: What can genetic research tell us about stuttering treatment issues?, in Treatment Efficacy for Stuttering: A Search for Empirical Bases. Edited by Cordes AK, Ingham RJ. San Diego, CA, Singular Publishing Group, 1998, pp 51–65

Fensen L, Dale PS, Reznick JS, et al: MacArthur-Bates Communicative Development Inventories. Baltimore, MD, Paul H Brookes, 1993

Fitch RH, Miller S, Tallal P: Neurobiology of speech perception. Ann Rev Neurosci 20:331–353, 1997

Fletcher J, Morris R: Classification of disabled learners: beyond exclusionary definitions, in Handbook of Cognitive, Social, and Neuropsychological Aspects of Learning Disabilities. Edited by Ceci S. Hillsdale, NJ, Lawrence Erlbaum, 1986, pp 55–80

Fletcher JM, Shaywitz S, Shankweiler D, et al: Cognitive profiles of reading disability: comparison of discrepancy and low achievement definitions. Journal of Educational Psychology 86:6–23, 1994

Fletcher JM, Francis DJ, Shaywitz SE, et al: Intelligence testing and the discrepancy model for children with learning disabilities. Learning Disabilities Research and Practice 13: 186–203, 1998

Flynn JM, Rahbar MH: Prevalence of reading failure in boys compared to girls. Psychology in the Schools 31:66–71, 1994

Folio MR, Fewell RR: Peabody Developmental Motor Scales, 2nd Edition. Austin, TX, ProEd, 2000

Freeman AR, MacKinnon JR, Miller LT: Assistive technology and handwriting problems: what do occupational therapists recommend? Can J Occup Ther 71:150–160, 2004

Fudala JB: Arizona Articulation Proficiency Scale, 3rd Edition. Los Angeles, CA, Western Psychological Services, 2001

Fulbright RK, Shaywitz SE, Shaywitz BA, et al: Neuroanatomy of reading and dyslexia. Child Adolesc Psychiatr Clin North Am 6:431–445, 1997

Galaburda AM, Sherman GR, Rosen GD, et al: Developmental dyslexia: four consecutive patients with cortical anomalies. Ann Neurol 18:222–233, 1985

Gillam RB, Crofford JA, Gale MA, et al: Language change following computer-assisted language instruction with Fast ForWord or Laureate Learning Systems software. Am J Speech-Lang Pathology (Special Forum on Fast ForWord) 10:231–247, 2001

Gillberg C: Deficits in attention, motor control, and perception: a brief review. Arch Dis Child 88:904–910, 2003

Goldman R, Fristoe M: Goldman-Fristoe Test of Articulation, 2nd Edition. Circle Pines, MN, American Guidance Service, 2000

Grigorenko EL, Wood FB, Meyer MS, et al: Susceptibility loci for distinct components of developmental dyslexia on chromosomes 6 and 15. Am J Hum Genet 60:27–39, 1997

Hammill DD, Larsen SC: Test of Written Language, 3rd Edition. Circle Pines, MN, American Guidance Service, 1995

Hammill DD, Brown VL, Larsen SC, et al: Test of Adolescent and Adult Language, 3rd Edition. Austin, TX, ProEd, 1994

Hammill DD, Pearson NA, Wiederholt JL: Comprehensive Test of Nonverbal Intelligence. San Antonio, TX, Psychological Corporation, 1997

Hinshaw SP: Externalizing behavior problems and academic underachievement in childhood and adolescence: causal relationships and underlying mechanisms. Psychol Bull 111:127–155, 1992

Hook PE, Macaruso P, Jones S: Efficacy of Fast ForWord training on facilitating acquisition of reading skills by children with reading difficulties—a longitudinal study. Annals of Dyslexia 51:75–96, 2001

Hresko WP, Reid DK, Hammill DD: Test of Early Language Development, 3rd Edition. Circle Pines, MN, American Guidance Service, 1999

Hummel L, Feinstein C: Developmental language disorders in school-age children, in Handbook of Child and Adolescent Psychiatry, Vol 2: The Grade-School Child: Development and Syndromes. Edited by Kernberg PF, Bemporad JR (Noshpitz JD, editor-in-chief). New York, Wiley, 1997, pp 420–435

Johnson J: Cognitive abilities of children with language impairment, in Specific Language Impairments in Children. Edited by Watkins R, Rice M. Baltimore, MD, Paul H Brookes, 1994, pp 107–121

Johnson JP: Nature and Treatment of Articulation Disorders. Springfield, IL, Charles C Thomas, 1980

Jongmans MJ, Smits-Engelsman BC, Schoemaker MM: Consequences of comorbidity of developmental coordination disorders and learning disabilities for severity and pattern of perceptual-motor dysfunction. J Learn Disab 36:528–537, 2003

Karacostas DD, Fisher GL: Chemical dependency in students with and without learning disabilities. J Learn Disabil 26:213–219, 1993

Kaufman AS, Kaufman NL: Kaufman Assessment Battery for Children, 2nd Edition. Circle Pines, MN, American Guidance Service, 2003a

Kaufman AS, Kaufman NL: Kaufman Test of Educational Achievement, 2nd Edition. Circle Pines, MN, American Guidance Service, 2003b

Kavale KA, Forness SR: Social skill deficits and learning disabilities: a meta-analysis. J Learn Disabil 29:226–237, 1996

Kinsbourne M: School problems. Pediatrics 52:697–710, 1973

Klein RG, Mannuzza S: Children with uncomplicated reading disorders grown up: a prospective follow-up into adulthood, in Learning Disabilities: Implications for Psychiatric Treatment. Edited by Greenhill LL (Review of Psychiatry Series; Oldham JO, Riba MB, series eds.). Washington, DC, American Psychiatric Press, 2000, pp 1–31

Lai CSL, Fisher SE, Hurst JA, et al: A forkhead-domain gene is mutated in a severe speech and language disorder. Nature 413:519–523, 2001

Leonard LB: Children With Specific Language Impairment. Cambridge, MA, MIT Press, 1998

Lewis BA: Pedigree analysis of children with phonology disorders. J Learn Disabil 25:586–597, 1992

Lewis BA, Thompson LA: A study of developmental speech and language disorders in twins. J Speech Hear Res 35:1086–1094, 1992

Light JG, Pennington BF, Gilger JW, et al: Reading disability and hyperactivity disorder; evidence for a common genetic etiology. Dev Neuropsychol 11:323–335, 1995

Martin N, Brownell R: Test of Auditory Processing Skills, 3rd Edition. Austin, TX, ProEd, 2005

Merzenich MM, Jenkins WM, Johnston P, et al: Temporal processing deficits of language-learning impaired children ameliorated by training. Science 271:77–81, 1996

Miller LJ, Roid GH: Toddler and Infant Motor Evaluation: A Standardized Assessment. San Antonio, TX, Psychological Corporation, 1994

Moffitt TE: The neuropsychology of conduct disorder. Dev Psychopathol 5:135–151, 1995

Morgan WP: A case of congenital word-blindness. BMJ 2:1378, 1896

Mullen EM: Mullen Scales of Early Learning. Circle Pines, MN, American Guidance Service, 1995

National Institute on Deafness and Other Communication Disorders: NIDCD fact sheet: Stuttering. NIH Publication No. 97-4232. Bethesda, MD, 1997

National Joint Committee on Learning Disabilities: Operationalizing the NJCLD definition of learning disabilities for ongoing assessment in schools. February 1, 1997. Available at: http://www.ldonline.org/njcld/operationalizing.html. Accessed May 24, 2003

Newcomer P, Hammill DD: Test of Language Development, 3rd Edition, Primary and Intermediate Versions. Austin, TX, Pro-Ed, 1997

Offord DR, Waters BG: Socialization and its failure, in Developmental-Behavioral Pediatrics. Edited by Levine MD, Carey WB, Crocker AC, et al. Philadelphia, PA, WB Saunders, 1983, pp 650–682

Onslow M, Menzies RG, Packman A: An operant intervention for early stuttering: the development of the Lidcombe program. Behav Modif 25:116–139, 2001

Orton ST: Reading, Writing and Speech Problems in Children. New York, WW Norton, 1937

Paul R: Language Disorders from Infancy Through Adolescence: Assessment and Intervention, 2nd Edition. St. Louis, MO, Mosby, 2001

Pennington BF: Genetics of learning disabilities. J Child Neurol 10 (suppl 1):S69–S77, 1995

Phelps-Terasaki D, Phelps-Gunn T: Test of Pragmatic Language. Austin, TX, ProEd Inc, 1992

Psychological Corporation: Wechsler Individual Achievement Test, 2nd Edition. San Antonio, TX, Harcourt Assessment, 2001

Pugh KR, Shaywitz BA, Shaywitz SE, et al: Cerebral organization of component processes in reading. Brain 119:1221–1238, 1996

Rapin I, Allen DA: Syndromes in developmental dysphasia and adult aphasia, in Language, Communication, and the Brain. Edited by Plum F. New York, Plenum, 1988, pp 57–75

Richardson SO: Developmental language disorder, in Comprehensive Textbook of Psychiatry, 5th Edition, Vol 2. Edited by Kaplan HI, Sadock BJ. Baltimore, MD, Williams & Wilkins, 1989, pp 1812–1817

Roid GH: Stanford-Binet Intelligence Scales, 5th Edition. Itasca, IL, Riverside Publishing, 2003

Roid GH, Miller L: The Leiter International Performance Scale—Revised. Wood Dale, IL, Stoelting, 1996

Rondal J: Language development and mental retardation, in Language Development and Disorders. Edited by Yule W, Rutter M. Philadelphia, PA, JB Lippincott, 1987

Rumsey JM, Berman KF, Denckla MB, et al: Regional cerebral blood flow in severe developmental dyslexia. Arch Neurol 44:1144–1150, 1987

Rutter M: Assessment objectives and principles, in Language Development and Disorders. Edited by Yule W, Rutter M. Philadelphia, PA, JB Lippincott, 1987, pp 295–311

Schiefelbusch RL, Lloyd LL: Language Perspectives: Acquisition, Retardation and Intervention. Austin, TX, Pro-Ed, 1988

Schoenbrodt L, Kumin L, Sloan J: Learning disabilities existing concomitantly with communication disorder. J Learn Disabil 30:264–281, 1997

Semel E, Wiig EH, Secord WA: Clinical Evaluation of Language Fundamentals, 4th Edition. San Antonio, TX, Psychological Corporation, 2003

Semel E, Wiig EH, Secord WA: Clinical Evaluation of Language Fundamentals, Preschool Version, 2nd Edition. San Antonio, TX, Psychological Corporation, 2004

Settle SA, Milich R: Social persistence following failure in boys and girls with LD. J Learn Disabil 32:201–212, 1999

Shapiro J, Rich R: Facing learning disabilities in the adult years. New York, Oxford Press, 1999

Shaywitz BA, Shaywitz SE: Learning disabilities and attention disorders, in Pediatric Neurology: Principles and Practice, Vol 2. Edited by Swaiman KF. St. Louis, MO, CV Mosby, 1989, pp 857–890

Shaywitz BA, Pugh KR, Fletcher JM, et al: What cognitive and neurobiological studies have taught us about dyslexia, in Learning Disabilities: Implications for Psychiatric Treatment. Edited by Greenhill L (Review of Psychiatry Series; Oldham JM and Riba MB, series eds.). Washington, DC, American Psychiatric Press, 2000, pp 59–96

Shaywitz SE: Overcoming Dyslexia. New York, NY, Alfred A. Knopf, 2003

Shaywitz SE, Shaywitz BA, Fletcher JM, et al: Prevalence of reading disability in boys and girls: results of the Connecticut Longitudinal Study. JAMA 264:998–1002, 1990

Shaywitz SE, Escobar MD, Shaywitz BA, et al: Evidence that dyslexia may represent the lower tail of a normal distribution of reading ability. N Engl J Med 326:145–150, 1992

Shaywitz SE, Fletcher JM, Shaywitz BA: A conceptual model and definition of dyslexia, findings emerging from the Connecticut Longitudinal Study, in Language, Learning, and Behavior Disorders: Developmental, Biological and Clinical Perspectives. Edited by Beitchman J, Cohen N, Konstantareas M, et al. New York, Cambridge University Press, 1996, pp 199–223

Sheehan JA: Social skills training with children and adolescents: an overview and guidelines. Unpublished doctoral dissertation, West Hartford, CT, University of Hartford, 2001 [Dissertation Abstracts International 62:2078, 2001]

Shepherd MJ, Uhry JK: Reading disorder. Child Adolesc Psychiatr Clin N Am 2:193–208, 1993

Shepherd MJ, Charnow DA, Silver LB: Developmental reading disorder, in Comprehensive Textbook of Psychiatry, 5th Edition, Vol 2. Edited by Kaplan HI, Sadock BJ. Baltimore, MD, Williams & Wilkins, 1989, pp 1790–1796

Silver AA, Hagin RA: Prevention of learning disorders, in Prevention of Mental Disorders, Alcohol and Other Drug Use in Children and Adolescents. Edited by Shaffer D, Silverman M, Anthony V. Washington, DC, Office of Substance Abuse Prevention (Monogr No 2), U.S. Department of Health and Human Services, 1989, pp 413–442

Silver LB: The "magic cure": a review of the current controversial approaches for treating learning disabilities. American Journal of the Disabled Child 140:1045–1052, 1986

Simos PG, Breier JI, Wheless JW, et al: Brain mechanisms for reading: the role of the superior temporal gyrus in word and pseudoword naming. Neuroreport 11:2443–2447, 2000

Simos PG, Breier JI, Fletcher JM, et al: Age-related changes in regional brain activation during phonological decoding and printed word recognition. Dev Neuropsychol 19:191–210, 2001

Stevenson J: Developmental changes in the mechanisms linking language disabilities and behavior disorders, in Language, Learning, and Behavior Disorders: Developmental, Biological, and Clinical Perspectives. Edited by Beitchman JH, Cohen NJ, Konstantareas MM, et al. New York, Cambridge University Press, 1996, pp 78–99

Stevenson J, Pennington BF, Gilger JW, et al: Hyperactivity and spelling disability: testing for shared genetic aetiology. J Child Psychol Psychiatry 34:1137–1152, 1993

Sugden DA, Wright HC: Motor coordination disorders in children, in Developmental Clinical Psychology and Psychiatry, Vol 39. Thousand Oaks, CA, Sage Publications, 1998

Tallal P, Miller SL, Bedi G, et al: Language comprehension in language-learning impaired children improved with acoustically modified speech. Science 271:81–84, 1996

Thibodeau LM, Friel-Patti S, Britt L: Psychoacoustic performance in children completing Fast ForWord training. Am J Speech-Lang Pathology 10:248–257, 2001

Tomblin JB, Buckwalter PR: Studies of the genetics of specific language impairment, in Specific Language Impairments in Children. Edited by Watkins R, Rice M. Baltimore, MD, Paul H Brookes, 1994, pp 7–34

Toppelberg CO, Shapiro T: Language disorders: a 10-year research update review. J Am Acad Child Adolesc Psychiatry 39:143–152, 2000

Ulrich DA: Test of Gross Motor Development, 2nd Edition. Austin, TX, ProEd, 2000

U.S. Congress: Amendments to the Individuals With Disabilities Education Act. Washington, DC, U.S. Government Printing Office, 1997

U.S. Department of Education: Seventeenth Annual Report to Congress on the Implementation of the Individuals With Disabilities Education Act. Washington, DC, U.S. Office of Special Education Programs, 1995

Wagner R, Torgesen J, Rashotte C: Comprehensive Test of Phonological Processing (CTOPP). Austin, TX, ProEd, 1999

Watson BU, Watson CS, Fredd R: Follow-up studies of specific reading disability. J Am Acad Child Psychiatry 21:376–382, 1982

Wechsler D: Wechsler Preschool and Primary Scale of Intelligence, 3rd Edition. San Antonio, TX, Psychological Corporation, 2002

Wechsler D: Wechsler Intelligence Scale for Children, 4th Edition. San Antonio, TX, The Psychological Corporation, 2003

Weinberg WA, Gallagher LS, Harper CR, et al: The impact of school on academic achievement. Child Adolesc Psychiatr Clin N Am 6:593–606, 1999

Wetherby AM, Prizant BM: Speech, language, and communication disorders in young children, in Handbook of Child and Adolescent Psychiatry, Vol 1: Infants and Preschoolers: Development and Syndromes. Edited by Greenspan S, Wieder S, Osofsky J (Noshpitz JD, editor-in-chief). New York, Wiley, 1997, pp 473–491

Wiederholt L, Bryant BR: Gray Oral Reading Tests, 4th Edition. Circle Pines, MN, American Guidance Service, 1992

Wilkinson GS: Wide Range Achievement Test, 3rd Edition. Wilmington, DE, Jastak Associates, 1993

Woodcock RW: Woodcock Reading Mastery Tests, Revised, Normative Update. Circle Pines, MN, American Guidance Service, 1998

Woodcock RW, McGrew KS, Mather N: Woodcock-Johnson, 3rd Edition, Tests of Achievement. Itasca, IL, Riverside, 2001

Woods S, Shearsby J, Onslow M, et al: Psychological impact of the Lidcombe Program of early stuttering intervention. Int J Lang Commun Disord 37:31–40, 2002

Zangwill OL: The concept of developmental dysphasia, in Developmental Dysphasia. Edited by Wyke MA. London, Academic Press, 1987

Zigmond N: Learning disabilities from an educational perspective, in Better Understanding Learning Disabilities: New Views from Research and Their Implications for Education and Public Policies. Edited by Lyon GR, Gray DB, Kavanagh JF, et al. Baltimore, MD, Paul H Brookes, 1993, pp 251–272

Zimmerman IL, Steiner VG, Pond RE: Preschool Language Scale, 4th Edition. San Antonio, TX, The Psychological Corporation, 2002

Self-Assessment Questions

Select the single best response for each question.

12.1 In language, *morphology* is defined as

    A. A language's sound system and accompanying rules governing the combination of sounds.

    B. The system that governs the structure and formation of words in a language.

    C. The system that governs the order and combination of words to form sentences.

    D. The system that governs the meaning of words and sentences.

    E. The system that combines the language components into functional and socially appropriate communication.

12.2 Which of the following communication disorders disproportionately affects males?

    A. Developmental (versus acquired) expressive language disorder.

    B. Mixed receptive–expressive language disorder.

    C. Phonological disorder.

    D. Stuttering.

    E. All of the above.

12.3 Which of the following statements concerning the etiology of communication disorders is *false?*

    A. The etiology is primarily due to family environment and sociological factors.

    B. Exposure to intrauterine teratogens may adversely affect language development.

    C. Anoxia and asphyxia have been implicated in the development of communication disorders.

    D. Important environmental risk factors for the development of communication disorders include poverty and abuse or neglect.

    E. Early childhood risk factors that have been implicated in communication disorders include persistent otitis media and other childhood illnesses.

12.4 All of the following statements concerning developmental coordination disorder are correct *except*

    A. The disorder occurs in up to 6% of 5- to 11-year-olds.

    B. The clumsiness associated with this disorder can lead to peer teasing.

    C. Children with developmental coordination disorder seldom have associated delays of other developmental milestones.

    D. Comorbid conditions such as attention-deficit/hyperactivity disorder (ADHD) are frequently seen in children with developmental coordination disorder.

    E. The coordination deficits may continue throughout life.

12.5 Which of the following statements concerning the clinical presentation of learning disorders is *false?*

A. Reading disorder occurs in 2%–20% of children.

B. Reading disorder accounts for up to 80% of all children diagnosed with a learning disorder.

C. An equal proportion of boys and girls are diagnosed with a reading disorder.

D. Disorder of written expression is more common in boys than in girls.

E. Mathematics disorder is reported to occur in 1%–6% of school-age children.

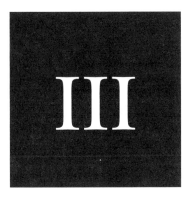

Psychiatric Disorders

Schizophrenia and Other Psychotic Disorders

Luke Y. Tsai, M.D.

Donna J. Champine, M.D.

Historical Background

The term *schizophrenic syndrome of childhood* (or its synonym *childhood schizophrenia*) has a different meaning from the term *schizophrenia in childhood*. The former term, proposed by the British Working Party (Creak et al. 1961) and later adopted in DSM-II (American Psychiatric Association 1968), was intended to apply to a wide spectrum of patients, including those with autism, schizophrenia, disintegrative psychosis, and other childhood psychoses. Thus, it is clear that data derived from studies (mostly conducted before 1980) that used the diagnostic criteria for childhood schizophrenia are not very meaningful, because they failed to make any distinction between autism and schizophrenia in childhood and because they had methodological flaws (e.g., standardized, well-defined diagnostic criteria were not used, and diagnostic criteria used for children were less restrictive than those applied to adult schizophrenic patients).

In DSM-III (American Psychiatric Association 1980) the term *schizophrenia in childhood and adolescence* was introduced to apply to children and adolescents in whom clear symptoms of schizophrenia, as found in adult patients with schizophrenia, are present.

For the purposes of this chapter, the definition and diagnostic criteria for schizophrenia in childhood are the same as those described in DSM-IV-TR (American Psychiatric Association 2000) for adult schizophrenia. There are at least three good reasons to use the adult criteria. First, there is now convincing evidence supporting the view that infantile autism and schizophrenia in childhood are two distinct disorders. Second, it is clear that schizophrenia, as described in the adult literature, can begin in childhood. Third, according to DSM-IV-TR, children and adolescents display the same symptoms as do adults diagnosed with schizophrenia.

Current Diagnostic Criteria for Schizophrenia

The diagnosis of schizophrenia in children and adolescents is currently made by using the criteria outlined in DSM-IV-TR. According to DSM-IV-TR, the active phase of the illness is characterized by the presence of at least two of the following symptoms, each present for a significant portion of time during a 1-month period: 1) delusions, 2) hallucinations, 3) disorganized speech, 4) grossly disorganized or catatonic behavior, and 5) negative symptoms (e.g., affective flattening, alogia, avolition). Only one symptom is needed, however, if the delusions are bizarre or if the hallucinations involve either a voice giving a running commentary on the person's behavior or thinking or two or more voices conversing. If treatment results in a resolution of the symptoms, then the duration of acute-phase symptoms can be less than 1 month.

In addition to the symptoms described above, there must also be a marked deterioration in social or occupational functioning present for a significant amount of time since the onset of the disturbance. This requirement is modified in child and adolescent schizophrenia, for which the criterion is "failure to achieve expected level of interpersonal, academic, or occupational achievement" (American Psychiatric Association 2000, p. 312).

Also included in DSM-IV-TR is the requirement that signs of the disturbance be present for at least 6 months, with at least 1 month of active-phase symptoms (fewer if successfully treated). The 6-month duration may include periods of prodromal or residual symptoms.

In making a diagnosis of schizophrenia, mood disorders and schizoaffective disorders must be ruled out. Because adolescents with bipolar disorder often present at onset with manic episodes with psychosis, this distinction becomes especially important in making a diagnosis in adolescents (American Academy of Child and Adolescent Psychiatry 2001). Psychosis due to a general medical condition, medication, or illicit drug use should also be ruled out.

Diagnostic Criteria for Other Psychotic Disorders

DSM-IV-TR diagnostic criteria for the other psychotic disorders, including schizophreniform disorder, schizoaffective disorder, delusional disorder, brief psychotic disorder, shared psychotic disorder, psychotic disorder due to a general medical condition, substance-induced psychotic disorder, and psychotic disorder not otherwise specified, are discussed below under "Differential Diagnosis."

Epidemiology

■ Prevalence

The true incidence of schizophrenia in childhood is unknown. Population studies have suggested that the prevalence may be less than 1 in 1,000 (reviewed by Werry 1979). In a study of prevalence in children between ages 2 and 12 in North Dakota (population 110,723 at time of the study), no patients with schizophrenia were found. However, within the next year, 2 of the children were reevaluated by the investigators and met DSM-III criteria for schizophrenia. Thus, point prevalence in North Dakota was 0.19 in 10,000 for this age group (Burd and Kerbeshian 1987). In the study in Dunedin, New Zealand (a prospective longitudinal study in which each subject was evaluated with a variety of measures, including the Diagnostic Interview Schedule for Children), no cases of schizophrenia were reported in a sample of 792 children (Anderson et al. 1987).

Sex Ratio

Spencer and Campbell (1994) reported a male-to-female ratio of 3.8:1 in a sample of 24 children.

It appears that age may determine the sex ratio in schizophrenia occurring in childhood. Although most studies have shown a higher male-to-female ratio, as age increases, the ratio tends to even out. Adult studies have suggested that the onset of schizophrenia is 5 years earlier in males than in females (American Academy of Child and Adolescent Psychiatry 2001). Therefore the reported male predominance in early-onset schizophrenia may be a cross-sectional effect (American Academy of Child and Adolescent Psychiatry 2001).

Socioeconomic Status

Schizophrenic children probably tend to come from families of lower social class, just as adults with schizophrenia do (Rutter 1972). However, most available studies have a selection bias toward inpatient samples (American Academy of Child and Adolescent Psychiatry 2001).

Premorbid Functioning

Many studies have reported that the majority of patients with childhood-onset schizophrenia have premorbid abnormalities. A variety of general, nonspecific behavioral symptoms, social problems, cognitive and academic difficulties, speech and language problems, developmental delays, and specific diagnoses of other mental disorders before the onset of schizophrenia have been described (Alaghband-Rad et al. 1995; Asarnow and Ben-Meir 1988; Spencer and Campbell 1994; Werry et al. 1991).

Although schizophrenia can be preceded by a variety of developmental delays and symptoms, these symptoms usually do not meet DSM-IV-TR criteria for autism.

Clinical and neurobiological characterization of children with childhood-onset schizophrenia is ongoing at the National Institute of Mental Health (NIMH) (Alaghband-Rad et al. 1995; Frazier et al. 1994; Gordon et al. 1994; McKenna et al. 1994a, 1994b). Alaghband-Rad et al. (1995) reviewed premorbid histories of 23 children with onset of schizophrenia before age 12 years (all of whom met DSM-III criteria) and compared the results with childhood data of subjects with adult-onset schizophrenia. Specific developmental disabilities and transient early symptoms of autism, especially motor stereotypies, were common. Compared with childhood characteristics of subjects with adult-onset schizophrenia, the subjects with childhood onset showed greater delay in language development, more premorbid speech and language disorders, disruptive behavior disorders, and learning disorders. Although they acknowledged the selection and ascertainment bias present in their sample, the authors concluded that childhood-onset schizophrenia might represent a more malignant form of the disorder.

Age at Onset

Schizophrenia seldom becomes apparent in children before age 9 years (Russell et al. 1989; Thomsen 1996). In a study of 312 youths in Denmark who were hospitalized for schizophrenia over a 13-year period, Thomsen (1996) found only 28 children younger than age 15 and only 4 children younger than age 13.

Adult literature on schizophrenia suggests that the average age at onset in males is 5 years earlier than in females. Loranger (1984) examined consecutive discharges from a hospital. It was found that 39% of the men had their first psychotic symptoms by age 19 years, whereas

23% of women had their first psychotic symptoms by age 19 years.

■ Type of Onset

The onset in childhood-onset schizophrenia is usually insidious, with acute onset observed in perhaps 25% of cases (Werry 1992). In a sample of 24 children younger than 12 years, 23 had insidious onset of schizophrenia, whereas only 1 had subacute onset (Spencer et al. 1994). Of 17 hospitalized schizophrenic subjects, ages 7–13 years, studied by Asarnow and Ben-Meir (1988), 8 had insidious onset, 8 had chronic onset, and 1 had acute onset. Gordon et al. (1994) reported similar figures. Thus, acute onset is relatively rare in childhood. In a study of 29 children and adolescents who met DSM-III criteria for schizophrenia with onset before age 12 years, Alaghband-Rad et al. (1997) found that males were more likely than females to have had an insidious onset.

■ Deterioration in Functioning

For adults, one of the DSM-IV-TR diagnostic criteria for schizophrenia is marked deterioration in functioning in the areas of work, social relationships, and self-care. However, the equivalent criterion for children and adolescents is failure to reach the expected level of interpersonal, academic, or social achievement. Russell et al. (1989) reported that all 35 subjects with schizophrenia in their sample (ages 4–13 years) exhibited a marked deterioration from a previous level of functioning, which was verified by parents: the child either required psychiatric hospitalization or showed severe deterioration in behavior in school.

Clinical Symptoms

A review of studies of the phenomenology of psychotic illnesses in children and ado-

lescents reveals that for both childhood-onset and adolescent-onset schizophrenia, the same symptoms that have been noted in adults are present. Schizophrenia has been described as having two broad sets of symptom clusters, positive and negative, both of which also are described in children and adolescents. Positive symptoms include hallucinations, delusions, and thought disorder. Negative symptoms are deficit symptoms, such as flattened affect, amotivation, and alogia (American Psychiatric Association 1997).

■ Hallucinations

Hallucinations are the most frequently reported positive symptoms. Russell and colleagues (1989) reported that auditory hallucinations were present in about 80% of patients. Other investigators reported hallucinations in up to 100% of children with schizophrenia who were age 13 years or younger (Spencer and Campbell 1994). Visual hallucinations were reported in between 30.3% (Kolvin et al. 1971) and 50% (Green and Padron-Gayol 1986) of patients and were usually accompanied by auditory hallucinations. A small percentage of children with schizophrenia reported tactile hallucinations (Green and Padron-Gayol 1986; Russell et al. 1989; Spencer and Campbell 1994).

■ Delusions

Werry et al. (1994) and Russell (1994) reported that children with schizophrenia had fewer delusions than did adults with schizophrenia. Other studies reported frequencies of delusions ranging from 43.8% (Green and Padron-Gayol 1986) to 100% (Spencer and Campbell 1994). Although the types of delusions were not always specified, Russell et al. (1989) found that persecutory and somatic delusions were most common (about 20% each), whereas thought control and religious delusions were rare (3%) in children ages 4–13 years. Russell et al. (1989) noted that the delusions of older children were more complex than those of younger children.

■ Affective Disturbances

Affective disturbance was common in children with schizophrenia. Affective disturbance was also reported by Russell et al. (1989) in 74% and by Spencer et al. (1994) in 87.5% of children with schizophrenia. Flattened affect, a negative symptom, has also been consistently reported in early-onset schizophrenia, although catatonic symptoms may be less frequent (Green et al. 1992; Werry 1992).

■ Thought Disorder

Thought disorder has been reported to be present in between 40% (Russell et al. 1989) and 100% (Watkins et al. 1988) of children with schizophrenia younger than 13 years. Various investigators (Arboleda and Holzman 1985; Caplan 1994) have discussed problems of assessing thought disorder in children. Caplan and associates (1990) developed the Kiddie Formal Thought Disorder Rating Scale, an instrument that operationalized the four DSM-III criteria for formal thought disorder (i.e., illogical thinking, loose associations, incoherence, and poverty of content of speech) for use with children. Two of the measures, illogical thinking and loose associations, were reliable in differentiating 14 schizophrenic and 3 schizotypal children from 15 psychiatrically healthy children matched by gender and mental age (Caplan et al. 1990). Caplan and colleagues (2001) compared thought disorder and associated cognitive variables in 115 children with attention-deficit/hyperactivity disorder (ADHD), 88 children with schizophrenia, and 190 psychiatrically healthy children. Compared with the healthy children, the subjects in both the ADHD and the schizophrenic groups exhibited thought disorder, although the subjects with ADHD had a narrower range of less severe thought disorder than did the schizophrenic children. The authors concluded that thought disorder in childhood was not specific to schizophrenia and reflected impaired development of communication skills.

■ Cognitive Impairment

Most schizophrenic children function in the low average to average range of intelligence. Mean IQ scores in four studies reviewed by Volkmar (1996) ranged from 82 (SD=12.5) to 94 (SD=10.5). In a brief review of studies and a discussion of cognitive delays in early-onset schizophrenia, it is noted that 10%–20% of children with early-onset schizophrenia have IQs in the borderline to mentally retarded range (American Academy of Child and Adolescent Psychiatry 2001). Determining whether delays are due to the impact of illness on cognitive functioning or whether they existed premorbidly is difficult because premorbid test results are often not available. Schizophrenia is associated with cognitive deficits that produce functional impairment (American Academy of Child and Adolescent Psychiatry 2001). Bedwell et al. (1999) investigated postpsychotic decline in Full-Scale IQ during adolescence for 31 patients with childhood-onset schizophrenia to determine whether the decline noted was due to a dementing process or failure to acquire new information and skills. Subjects had significant declines in scores on three postpsychotic subtest scales, including picture arrangement, information, and block design. However, there was no decline in the raw scores (which are not age corrected) for any subtest. The authors concluded that the decline during adolescence in full-scale IQ of patients with childhood-onset schizophrenia reflected an inability to acquire new information and abilities rather than dementia.

■ Language, Communication, and Information Processing

Language and communication deficits are described widely in the literature (Baltaxe and Simmons 1995; Caplan et al. 2000). Information-processing problems in children with schizophrenia have been observed (Asarnow et al. 1994).

■ Neurobiological Deficits

Briefly, neuroimaging studies have shown a progressive increase in ventricular size in subjects over 2 years (Rapoport et al. 1997); a decrease in cortical gray matter during adolescence, especially in the frontal and temporal regions (Rapoport et al. 1999); correlation of smaller total cerebral volumes with negative symptoms (Alaghband-Rad et al. 1997); and frontal lobe dysfunction consistent with that noted in adults (Thomas et al. 1998). These findings are described in more detail below under "Neuroanatomical Factors." It should be noted, however, that none of these findings are diagnostic for schizophrenia. Therefore, the primary role for laboratory tests and neuroimaging studies in the assessment and diagnosis of childhood-onset schizophrenia is to rule out other medical disorders (American Academy of Child and Adolescent Psychiatry 2001).

Course and Outcome

DSM-IV-TR diagnostic criteria require continuous signs of disorder for a 6-month period, during which there is at least 1 month of active-phase symptoms. Schizophrenia is considered to be a phasic disorder in which there can be much individual variation. It is important for clinicians to be cognizant of the various phases of schizophrenia when making diagnostic or treatment decisions. The phases are as follows (American Academy of Child and Adolescent Psychiatry 2001):

- *Prodrome.* Before the onset of psychotic symptoms, most patients experience some degree of functional deterioration. There may be unusual behaviors, bizarre preoccupations, social withdrawal and isolation, poor academic performance, dysphoria, or problems with sleep and appetite (American Academy of Child and Adolescent Psychiatry 2001). Substance abuse, sometimes comorbid with an emerging psychosis in adolescents, may confuse the diagnostic picture. The length of the prodromal phase may be days to weeks or months to years (Werry and Taylor 1994). Distinguishing premorbid personality characteristics or cognitive/developmental deficits from the onset of symptoms may be difficult.
- *Acute phase.* During this phase, positive symptoms (i.e., hallucinations, delusions, thought disorder, and disorganized behavior) are predominant. This phase usually lasts 1–6 months, sometimes longer, and the length is affected by treatment response. Symptoms may shift from positive to negative during the course of treatment.
- *Recovery phase.* After the remission of acute-phase symptoms, there is often a continuing period (lasting several months) of impairment that is frequently characterized by negative symptoms of flattened affect, apathy, anergia, and social withdrawal (Remschmidt et al. 1991). Postpsychotic depressive disorder of schizophrenia may be seen in some patients and is characterized by dysphoria and flat affect. Positive symptoms may still be present to some degree.

- *Residual phase.* As recovery continues, patients may experience periods of several months or more between acute phases during which there are few positive symptoms but some degree of persisting impairment due to negative symptoms
- *Chronically ill patients.* Some patients remain chronically symptomatic over several years despite appropriate treatment (Asarnow et al. 1994; Eggers and Bunk 1997; Maziade et al. 1996; McClellan et al. 1993). The availability of atypical antipsychotic medications offers some hope; clozapine has been effective in some cases of treatment-resistant schizophrenia (Sporn and Rapoport 2001).

Some youths with schizophrenia experience only one cycle of these phases, although most have more (Asarnow et al. 1994; McClellan et al. 1993; Werry et al. 1991). Werry and Taylor (1994) noted that recovery was incomplete in 80% of cases in which youths had had more than one episode.

Schulz et al. (1998) reviewed outcome studies in childhood-onset and adolescent-onset schizophrenia. They cited a study conducted in Germany with a large population of adolescent-onset patients who were assessed 5–11 years after onset of illness (Krausz and Muller-Thomsen 1993). Many were judged to have continuous illness and required ongoing care. Anxiety and suicidality were issues of comorbidity at follow-up. Females in this study had a better overall outcome than males.

Eggers (1989) studied a group of 57 patients with childhood schizophrenia for a mean follow-up period of 16 years. The age at onset of illness in the children ranged from 7 to 13 years. In terms of outcome, 20% had complete remission, 30% had good to satisfying social adaptation, and 50% remained significantly impaired. Diagnostically, 28% were identified as having schizoaffective disorder according to ICD-9 criteria (World Health Organization 1977). Eggers and Bunk (1997) reported on a 42-year follow-up of a subset of the cohort described above, consisting of 44 subjects. Overall, the outcome for patients with childhood onset was poor, with 50% judged to be poorly remitted. However, 25% had complete remission. Insidious onset and onset before 12 years of age were associated with a poorer outcome, and none of the patients with insidious onset had a full remission.

Maziade and colleagues (1996) conducted a study designed to examine the presence and stability across life of the positive and negative symptom distinction in childhood-onset schizophrenia and to identify factors predictive of long-term outcome for childhood-onset schizophrenia. Across a 14.8-year follow-up period, two separate factors corresponding to the positive and negative symptom dimensions were identified. The best childhood predictors of adult outcome were premorbid functioning and severity of positive and negative symptoms during acute episodes. However, the presence of premorbid developmental problems and premorbid nonpsychotic behavioral disturbances was not related to severity of outcome.

Symptom dimensions of childhood-onset schizophrenia were described by Bunk and colleagues (1999) in a study focusing on the clinical features of 44 patients at onset of illness during their first episode and at follow-up assessment 42 years after onset. All of the subjects were rediagnosed with DSM-IV criteria (American Psychiatric Association 1994) and symptomatology evaluated with the Positive and Negative Syndrome Scale for Schizophrenia (PANSS) (Kay et al. 1987) at onset and at follow-up. Factor analysis revealed five symptom dimensions (factors) at the onset of psychosis: cognitive symptoms, social withdrawal, antisocial behavior, excitement, and reality distortion. At follow-up, a five-factor solution was also found, but the dimensions differed from those identified at onset; the follow-up factors were positive, negative, excitement, cognitive, and anxiety/depression components. The first psychotic episode of childhood-onset schizophrenia was accompanied by symptoms that were less specific, such as social withdrawal and antisocial behavior, whereas in later stages the symptom dimensions changed to those recognized in adult-onset schizophrenia. In general, positive and global symptoms decreased over the course of the illness, but the frequency of negative symptoms did not change.

Diagnostic Issues

The diagnosis of schizophrenia in younger children or in children with developmental disabilities is challenging for a number of reasons. Difficulties in communication, developmental changes in thought processes, changing conceptions of reality, and the nature of expression of symptoms in younger children may complicate the diagnostic picture. Appropriate studies to rule out endocrinological, metabolic, neurological, infectious, or toxic causes of psychosis, as well as genetic studies, may be needed. Evaluation over several sessions, using information from multiple informants (including family and collaborative sources), in addition to direct mental status examination of the child, may be necessary in making the diagnosis.

It is important to note that hallucinations in children are not necessarily a sign of schizophrenia but can also be seen in a variety of other conditions in healthy children (Pilowsky and Chambers 1986). In preschool children, hallucinations must be distinguished from sleep-related phenomena and from other developmental phenomena such as imaginary friends or fantasy figures (Volkmar 1996). At times of stress and anxiety, transient hallucinations in preschool children might be observed. Often, these hallucinations are visual or tactile and have their onset at night, although they can also occur when the child is fully awake (Volkmar 1996). However, in school-age children, hallucinations may be more persistent and are often associated with more serious disorders (Russell et al. 1989). In this age group, the content of hallucinations and delusions frequently reflects developmental concerns (Volkmar 1996). Hallucinations may involve monsters, pets, or toys. Delusions often involve aspects of identity and are not as systematic or complex as those in adults (Russell et al. 1989).

Cultural and religious factors need to be considered when diagnosing schizophrenia because cultural and religious beliefs, taken out of context, may be misconstrued as psychotic symptoms. Clinician biases may also influence diagnostic decisions. Kilgus et al. (1995) found that African American youths were less likely to receive mood, anxiety, or substance abuse diagnoses and were more likely to be described as having either an organic or a psychotic illness.

Differential Diagnosis

■ Autistic Disorder

Most individuals with autism do manifest prodromal or residual symptoms similar to those seen in schizophrenia, such as social isolation, impairment in role functioning or grooming, and inappropriate affect. Many higher-functioning autistic individuals exhibit illogical thinking, incoherence, and poverty in content of speech. Their lack of nonverbal communication may be seen as blunt affect. Inappropriate laughing or weeping in autism, due to inability to comprehend the meaning of events, may be interpreted as labile or abnormal affect. Some higher-functioning verbal autistic persons have strange beliefs (e.g., believing that there is no air in other states), idiosyncratic interests (e.g., spending an enormous amount of time studying dinosaurs), or sensory experiences (e.g., seeing other people's faces in the air when alone in the room) bordering on delusions or hallucinations. These symptoms, however, are qualitatively different from those seen in schizophrenic patients. These "schizophrenic symptoms" seen in autism may be caused by underdevelopment of cognitive and language/speech functions in autistic individuals, whereas the schizophrenic symptoms in schizophrenic patients represent a deviance in previously relative normal cognitive and language/speech development. Autistic individuals tend to answer "yes" to questions they do not quite understand or tend to interpret meanings of words literally. Often an autistic person may talk or laugh to himself or herself while looking at something the observer cannot identify or while having funny thoughts that he or she does not know how to share with the observer. This tends to be interpreted as listening to voices or seeing visions. Some autistic adolescents or adults continue to have childlike fantasies of being an inanimate object, an animal, or a character of a fairy tale, which may be mistaken for delusions, whereas the tendency of others to make irrelevant remarks or to talk excessively on their favorite topics may lead to a mistaken diagnosis of thought disorder.

However, individuals with schizophrenia can be differentiated from higher-functioning autistic people on the basis of such factors as age at onset, developmental history, clinical features, and family history. Almost all persons with autism have an onset before age 5 years, whereas most often the onset of schizophrenia in childhood is during the preadolescent or adolescent period.

In a study of patterns involving intellectual functioning (as measured by factor scores on the Wechsler Intelligence Scale for Children—Revised), Asarnow and colleagues (1987) found that schizophrenic and autistic children did not significantly differ on the verbal and perceptual organization factors but that the schizophrenic children had significantly lower scores on the freedom from distraction factor (including attention, short-term memory, visuomotor coordination, speed of responding, and mental arithmetic) than the nonretarded (higher-functioning) autistic children. The only subtest on which the autistic children scored significantly lower than the schizophrenic children was the comprehension subtest.

■ Schizophreniform Disorder, Brief Psychotic Disorder, Psychotic Disorder Not Otherwise Specified

Children presenting with schizophreniform disorder, brief psychotic disorder, or psychotic disorder not otherwise specified may appear to have schizophrenia but do not meet DSM-IV-TR criteria for schizophrenia. Children with schizophreniform disorder have duration of illness less than 6 months, and with time they may receive a diagnosis of schizophrenia. Also, diagnosis of schizophreniform disorder does not require a decline in functioning (American Psychiatric Association 2000).

Children with a diagnosis of brief psychotic disorder experience psychotic symptoms for at least 1 day but usually less than 1 month; these symptoms often follow a severe precipitating stress. The children subsequently return to their premorbid level of functioning. It is emphasized, however, that the onset of psychosis in schizophrenic children may also be in response to stress.

Psychotic patients whose symptoms do not meet specified DSM-IV-TR diagnostic criteria are classified as having psychotic disorder not otherwise specified, a relatively common diagnosis in hospitalized adolescents (Armenteros et al. 1995; Kafantaris et al. 1992). This diagnosis may be used when there is insufficient information to decide between a diagnosis of schizophrenia and other psychotic disorders or when the presenting symptoms may possibly be substance induced or the result of a general medical condition that has not yet been determined. This type of uncertainty is more likely early in the course of a disorder.

■ Personality Disorders

Children and adolescents who later develop schizotypal, borderline, schizoid, and paranoid personality disorders may exhibit transient psychotic symptoms. Comprehensive evaluation of these children and adolescents should focus on clarifying whether schizophrenic symptomatology and deterioration of daily functioning are present.

■ Affective Disorders

It is important to distinguish between schizophrenia and mood disorders with psychotic features when diagnosing children and adolescents. Psychotic depressive disorders may present with mood-congruent or mood-incongruent psychotic features in the form of hallucinations or delusions (American Academy of Child and Adolescent Psychiatry 1998a). Chambers et al. (1982) found that about 48% of prepubertal children with major depressive disorder had hallucinations of any type and that 36% reported complex auditory hallucinations. Delusions, however, were described as rare in major depressive disorder with onset in childhood (Puig-Antich et al. 1985).

At times it may be difficult to distinguish bipolar affective disorder from schizophrenia in adolescence (Werry et al. 1994). A study by McKenna et al. (1994a) delineates subsequent diagnoses in a group of patients thought to have childhood-onset schizophrenia on referral to NIMH for an ongoing study. On subsequent evaluation, 27% were diagnosed with a primary mood disorder.

Making an accurate diagnosis of schizoaffective disorder can be difficult. Although retrospective evaluation of a temporal relationship between mood episodes and psychotic symptoms can be a problem, overlap of the two is what distinguishes schizoaffective disorder from bipolar disorder in DSM-IV-TR (Calderoni et al. 2001). The presence of psychotic symptoms in the presence of mood symptoms is a criterion for diagnosis of schizoaffective disorder. If mood symptoms are depressive and resemble the negative symptoms of schizophrenia, then the diagnosis of schizoaffective disorder could be missed. Likewise, it can be difficult to distinguish the activation of mania from the agitation and disorganization of schizophrenia (Carlson et al. 2000).

■ Organic Syndromes

Patients presenting with psychotic symptoms should also receive a thorough medical evaluation, including a neurological examination, to rule out an organic etiology. Although the list of potential etiological organic conditions and neuropsychiatric conditions that could cause or contribute to a psychotic presentation is very long, the following, among other conditions, have been associated with psychotic symptoms and should be routinely considered: 1) seizure disorders; 2) delirium; 3) central nervous system lesions, including brain tumors, vascular lesions, congenital malformations, and head trauma; 4) metabolic and endocrine disorders (e.g., hypothyroidism, Wilson's disease); 5) neurodegenerative disorders (Huntington's disease, lipid storage disorders); 6) developmental disorders; 7) toxic encephalopathies (including those caused by abuse of substances such as amphetamines, cocaine, hallucinogens, phencyclidine, alcohol, and cannabis; those caused by solvents, heavy metals, and environmental toxins; and those caused by medications such as stimulants, corticosteroids, and anticholinergic agents); 8) infectious diseases (such as human immunodeficiency virus infection, encephalitis, and meningitis); and 9) autoimmune disorders (e.g., systemic lupus erythematosus).

■ Substance Abuse

The issue of substance abuse warrants careful consideration in the differential diagnosis of early-onset schizophrenia. There is a significant rate of comorbid substance abuse in adolescents with schizophrenia, as great as 50% in some studies (McClellan and McCurry 1998). Diagnosis is sometimes complicated by the presence of active substance use or abuse at the first onset of psychiatric symptoms. Many different types of substance-related disorders may produce symptoms similar to those of schizophrenia. Sustained amphetamine or cocaine use may produce hallucinations or delusions (American Psychiatric Association 2000). Phencyclidine use may produce a mixture of both positive and negative symptoms. 3,4-Methylenedioxymethamphetamine (MDMA), also known as ecstasy, has been associated with neurotox-

icity. It is known that cannabis use can exacerbate the symptoms of schizophrenia (Hall and Degenhardt 2000).

Ideally, it is recommended that the clinician try to observe the individual during a sustained period (at least 4 weeks) of abstinence, although this is often difficult to accomplish (American Psychiatric Association 2000). Therefore, the clinician may need to rely on other evidence, such as whether psychotic symptoms appear to be exacerbated by the substance use and diminished when it has been discontinued; level of functioning before the onset of substance use; and severity of psychotic symptoms in relation to the amount and duration of substance use. A thorough knowledge of characteristic symptoms produced by particular substances is also needed if the clinician is to distinguish the effects of substance use from psychotic symptoms (American Psychiatric Association 2000).

■ Other Nonpsychotic Conditions

Youths with conduct disorder and other emotional disorders that are nonpsychotic may report psychotic-like symptoms and may therefore be misdiagnosed as having a primary psychotic disorder such as schizophrenia (Hornstein and Putnam 1992; McClellan and McCurry 1999). However, compared with psychotic youths, this group has lower rates of negative symptoms, thought disorder, and bizarre behavior (McClellan and McCurry 1999).

■ Anxiety Disorders

Famularo et al. (1992) reported significantly higher rates of psychotic symptoms in children with posttraumatic stress disorder than in control subjects. Children with posttraumatic stress disorder who report psychotic-like symptoms may be describing dissociative or anxiety phenomena such as intrusive thoughts or worries, depersonalization, or derealization (Altman et al. 1997). It is important to keep in mind that children with schizophrenia also may have been maltreated, so the diagnosis of schizophrenia should not be ruled out just on the basis of an abuse history (McClellan and McCurry 1999).

Children and adolescents with obsessive-compulsive disorder may experience intrusive thoughts and ritualistic behaviors that at times are difficult to distinguish from psychosis. For example, fears related to contamination by germs or toxic chemicals may be a paranoid delusion, an obsessive symptom, or even a realistic response to the threat of biochemical warfare, depending on the circumstances. Generally, individuals with obsessive-compulsive disorder recognize their symptoms as being products of their own obsessive thinking or as being unreasonable (American Academy of Child and Adolescent Psychiatry 1998b). However, in children, insight into the nature of symptoms is not always apparent, and lack of insight does not preclude a diagnosis of obsessive-compulsive disorder.

Etiology

The etiology of schizophrenia is unknown, and the relative roles of genetic, neurobiological, and environmental and psychosocial influences remain controversial.

■ Genetic Factors

Cytogenetic Abnormalities

Specific cytogenetic abnormalities have recently been examined in a cohort from the ongoing NIMH study of childhood-onset schizophrenia (Nicolson et al. 1999). Five of 47 patients with childhood-onset schizo-

phrenia were found to have cytogenetic abnormalities, including a girl with Turner's syndrome, a boy with a balanced translocation of chromosomes 1 and 7 (Yan et al. 2000), and two girls and a boy with velocardiofacial syndrome (22q11 deletion). Burgess et al. (1998) reported on an association between trinucleotide expansions and childhood-onset schizophrenia. Other studies have investigated a dopamine D_4 receptor polymorphism in association with catatonic schizophrenia (Kaiser et al. 2000) and a neurotrophin gene polymorphism in relation to hippocampal volume in psychoses (Kunugi et al. 1999).

Familial Patterns

Several studies reported an increased family history of schizophrenia and schizophrenia-spectrum disorders—including schizoaffective, schizotypal, and paranoid personality disorders—in patients diagnosed with childhood-onset schizophrenia (Asarnow et al. 2001; Green et al. 1992; Kendler et al. 1993; McClellan and McCurry 1998; McClellan et al. 1993; Werry et al. 1991). Earlier studies had shown increased prevalence of schizophrenia in family members, as demonstrated in offspring (Gottesman et al. 1987; Mirsky et al. 1985) and in siblings (Gottesman and Shields 1972), as well as in adoption studies (Heston 1966; Kety et al. 1994) and twin studies (Gottesman and Shields 1972; Gottesman et al. 1987). Whereas the risk of developing schizophrenia is not greater than 1% in the general population, it is 10%–15% if one parent has schizophrenia (Kendler and Diehl 1993).

Nicolson and colleagues (2000) reported the results of a recent screening of first-degree relatives of the NIMH cohort. Nineteen relatives younger than 18 years were given the Diagnostic Interview Schedule for Children and Adolescents, and 105 relatives older than 17 years were administered the Schedule for Affective Disorders and Schizophrenia and the Structured Clinical Interview for DSM-IV Personality Disorders. Two first-degree relatives were determined to have schizophrenia, and one was determined to have schizoaffective disorder. Approximately 25.7% of first-degree relatives assessed had either paranoid or schizotypal personality disorder; 42.6% of the probands had at least one relative with a schizophrenia-spectrum disorder. Asarnow and colleagues (2001) found an increased lifetime morbid risk for schizophrenia (4.95% ± 2.16%) and schizotypal personality disorder (4.2% ± 2.06%) in the parents of probands with childhood schizophrenia compared with the parents of subjects with ADHD and community control subjects. There is remarkable similarity in the disorders that do and do not aggregate in the parents of patients with adult-onset schizophrenia and in the parents of probands with childhood-onset schizophrenia, a finding that provides support for the hypothesis of etiological continuity between adult-onset and childhood-onset schizophrenia.

In a study of Danish identical and fraternal discordant twins, the risk of schizophrenia in the offspring of the nonschizophrenic co-twins of identical twins was the same as in the offspring of the schizophrenic twin. In contrast, the offspring of the nonschizophrenic co-twins of fraternal twins had a risk for schizophrenia much below the risk in the offspring of the schizophrenic twin (Gottesman and Bertelsen 1989). These results suggest that environmental events may trigger the development of schizophrenia. They may also explain the etiology for childhood-onset schizophrenia: in an individual who has the genetic predisposition, an environmental trigger—such as birth trauma, prematurity, low birth weight, or viral illness in utero or even in the first

few years of life—may spark the onset of schizophrenia in childhood. Further research in this area may clarify the genetic contributions to childhood-onset schizophrenia and better elucidate the biological/environmental (including psychosocial) risk factors and their interaction with genetics as they affect ongoing neurodevelopment.

■ Risk Factors

Several risk factors have been examined in childhood schizophrenia for evidence of greater predominance and severity. These risk factors include obstetrical complications, gender, pubertal development, medical conditions, and neurological signs.

Obstetrical Complications

A number of studies have noted an excess of prenatal and perinatal complications in patients with schizophrenia (Nicolson et al. 2000). Patients with adult-onset schizophrenia have been reported to have higher rates of obstetrical complications compared with their siblings or healthy control subjects (Gunther-Genta et al. 1994; O'Callaghan et al. 1993), although results are not consistent (Done et al. 1991). A reanalysis of original data from a number of studies has suggested that birth complications were greater in patients with an earlier onset of illness (Verdoux et al. 1997); however, other investigators have found no differences in obstetrical complications between patients with childhood-onset schizophrenia and sibling control subjects (Nicolson et al. 2000). Therefore, although obstetrical complications may play a role in some patients in the development of schizophrenia, they may not be more salient in childhood-onset cases (Nicolson et al. 2000).

Pubertal Development

In many neurodevelopmental theories of schizophrenia, a brain change at puberty that triggers the onset of schizophrenia is proposed (Keshavan et al. 1994; Weinberger 1987). A prediction of this model is that in childhood-onset schizophrenia there would be some physical or endocrine manifestation of early puberty or an acceleration of developmental brain changes (Jacobsen and Rapoport 1998). Most prospective studies of childhood-onset schizophrenia have not mentioned pubertal status of the samples (Green et al. 1992; Russell 1994; Spencer and Campbell 1994; Werry et al. 1994). There was no clear relationship between onset of psychosis and indices of sexual development for childhood-onset schizophrenia.

Medical Conditions

Kolvin et al. (1971) reported that 2 of 33 children with onset of psychosis between ages 5 and 12 also had temporal lobe epilepsy. One long-term follow-up study of 100 children with temporal lobe epilepsy found that 10% developed schizophrenia in adulthood (Lindsay et al. 1979). Caplan et al. (1993) noted that children with complex partial seizure disorders had significantly more illogical thinking and used fewer linguistic cohesive devices, findings similar to those noted in children with childhood-onset schizophrenia.

Neurological Signs

Several studies have documented a variety of neurological soft signs or motor dysfunctions in subjects at high risk for schizophrenia; impaired fine motor coordination is among the signs most frequently reported (Erlenmeyer-Kimling and Cornblatt 1987; Marcus et al. 1985; Rieder and Nichols 1979). Jacobsen and Rapoport (1998) noted a higher frequency of neuro-

logical dysfunction—including movement disorders, poor sensory integration, and impaired coordination—in the NIMH childhood-onset schizophrenia cohort. Karp et al. (2001) reported that neurological signs decreased with age in control subjects but did not decrease in children with schizophrenia. The researchers concluded that this finding suggested a delay in or failure of normal brain maturation in the children with schizophrenia.

■ Neuroanatomical Factors

Computed Tomographic Studies

Schulz et al. (1983) used computed tomography to study ventricular enlargement in adolescents with schizophrenia and in medical control subjects and patients with personality disorder. The adolescent schizophrenic patients (average age, 16 years), who had been ill for less than 2 years, had greater ventricular brain ratios compared with both of the other groups. In the schizophrenic teenagers, ventricular brain ratio was not related to length of illness. Jennings and colleagues (1985) found that ventricular brain ratio in psychotic adolescents was inversely correlated with the dopamine metabolite homovanillic acid and with the serotonin metabolite 5-hydroxyindoleacetic acid.

Magnetic Resonance Imaging Studies

Researchers are using magnetic resonance imaging (MRI) with increasing frequency to study the schizophrenic population. In a comprehensive review of neuroimaging findings in child and adolescent psychiatric disorders, including childhood-onset schizophrenia, Hendren and colleagues (2000) summarized MRI findings and suggested that brain changes in childhood-onset schizophrenia appeared to occur in two waves: 1) early in neurodevelopment, with asymmetries, basal ganglia reductions, and nonspecific reductions in overall brain size associated with negative symptoms; and 2) in adolescence, with reductions in frontal and temporal structures and ventricular enlargement associated with positive symptoms. Some of the MRI studies supporting these conclusions are briefly reviewed below.

Cerebellum. Jacobsen et al. (1997a) studied 24 adolescents with schizophrenia and 52 matched control subjects. Volumes of the cerebellar vermis, midsagittal area, and inferior posterior lobe were significantly smaller in subjects with schizophrenia, and no correlation with neuroleptic exposure was found. Keller et al. (2003) reported that childhood-onset schizophrenia is associated with significant progressive loss of cerebellar volume during adolescence.

Cerebral hemispheres and ventricles. Several studies have found smaller total cerebral volume in children with childhood-onset schizophrenia (Frazier et al. 1996; Jacobsen et al. 1997b; Rapoport et al. 1997, 1999). Rapoport and colleagues, in a 1997 study (replicated in 1999), scanned subjects (mean age at first scan, 14.8 years) at initial admission and again 2 years later, using identical equipment and measurement methods. Children with childhood-onset schizophrenia showed a significantly greater decrease in total cerebral volume and increase in ventricular volume than did control subjects. Jacobsen and colleagues (1998a) also found decreased total cerebral volume in 10 schizophrenic adolescents with childhood onset compared with control subjects at 2-year follow-up (Frazier et al. 1996; Rapoport et al. 1997). Cerebral asymmetry, with the right hemisphere larger than the left, across groups was also noted. In contrast to the studies cited above (the NIMH group), Hendren et al. (1995) and Yeo et al. (1997) found

no differences in the childhood-onset schizophrenia group in overall brain volume, total ventricular volume, or frontal area. They found a reversal of normal asymmetry in the childhood-onset schizophrenia-spectrum group. However, the group studied by Hendren et al. (1995) was younger and had less severe symptoms than the NIMH group.

Temporal lobe structures. Jacobsen et al. (1996a) found that children with childhood-onset schizophrenia had larger volumes of the superior temporal lobe gyrus and its posterior segment and that they displayed a trend toward larger temporal lobe volumes compared with control subjects. In 1998, Jacobsen and associates published data after rescanning part of the original group and control subjects. The researchers found that the schizophrenic subjects had significantly greater decreases in volume in the right temporal lobe, bilateral superior temporal gyrus, posterior superior temporal gyrus, right anterior superior temporal gyrus, and left hippocampus (Jacobsen et al. 1998a). Greater decreases in hippocampal volume over the follow-up interval were associated with greater negative symptoms at baseline and greater delusions at follow-up. In a longitudinal study of 15 original subjects from the same cohort, Rapoport and colleagues (1999) noted decreases in frontal and parietal lobe gray matter volumes, with greater decreases in children with schizophrenia. The subjects with schizophrenia also showed decreases in temporal gray matter. Hendren et al. (1995) and Yeo et al. (1997) found smaller amygdala and reduced temporal cortex volumes in children with schizophrenia-spectrum disorder. Findling et al. (1996) found no differences in hippocampal volume between adolescents with childhood-onset schizophrenia and control subjects.

Thalamic area.   Frazier et al. (1996) reported smaller midsagittal thalamic areas in children with schizophrenia than in control subjects. Rapoport et al. (1997) noted a significant decrease on the rescanned midsagittal thalamic area among the schizophrenic group but no change in control subjects.

Corpus callosum.   The only two studies of the corpus callosum in childhood-onset schizophrenia had conflicting results. Jacobsen et al. (1997b) reported larger corpus callosum areas in 25 adolescents with childhood-onset schizophrenia, whereas Yeo et al. (1997) reported reduced corpus callosum areas in younger children (mean age, 11 years) with schizophrenia-spectrum disorders.

Cavum septi pellucidi.   In a study by Nopoulos and colleagues (1998), there was a significantly higher frequency of enlarged cavum septi pellucidi in adolescents with childhood-onset schizophrenia than in matched control subjects.

Magnetic Resonance Spectroscopy Studies

Several magnetic resonance spectroscopy studies have reported abnormalities in the frontal lobes in childhood-onset schizophrenia groups, with lower N-acetylaspartate/creatine ratios (Bertolino et al. 1998; Brooks et al. 1998). The role of N-acetylaspartate has not yet been firmly established.

Positron Emission Tomographic Studies

In a positron emission tomographic study, Gordon and colleagues (1994) found decreased right parietal metabolism in children with schizophrenia compared with control subjects on an auditory continuous-performance task, possibly secondary to poor attentional performance. Jacobsen and colleagues (1997c) used positron emission tomography with an auditory continuous-performance task to study 16 adolescents with childhood-onset schizophrenia and 26 matched control subjects and found no hypofrontality in either group.

Summary of Neuroanatomical Factors

In general, results from neuroimaging studies indicate consistency in the structures found to be abnormal but some inconsistencies in the nature of the abnormalities (Hendren et al. 2000).

■ Infectious Disease and Immunological Factors

Infectious Diseases

Some investigators had reported findings of association between maternal infections (particularly influenza) during pregnancy and the development of childhood-onset schizophrenia (Mednick et al. 1988; O'Callaghan et al. 1991). However, other studies reported that maternal influenza was not associated with an increased risk for the development of schizophrenia (Erlenmeyer-Kimling et al. 1994; Morgan et al. 1997; Selten et al. 1999). Buka and colleagues (2001) found that the offspring of mothers with elevated levels of total IgG and IgM immunoglobulins and antibodies to herpes simplex virus type 2 are at increased risk for the development of schizophrenia and other psychotic illnesses in adulthood.

Autoimmune Diseases

In an investigation of the immune system in childhood-onset schizophrenia, Jacobsen and colleagues (1998b) compared 8 schizophrenic children and 51 ethnically matched control subjects for frequencies of human leukocyte antigens (HLAs) that had previously been reported to be associated with schizophrenia or autoimmune disorders. Results showed no significant differences between schizophrenic and healthy subjects in the frequency of any of the antigens tested.

■ Neurophysiological Factors

Event-Related Potential Studies

Studies of event-related potentials and neurophysiological tests in schizophrenic children suggest some dysfunction in the prefrontal cortex (Asarnow et al. 1986).

Eye-Tracking Studies

A study of eye tracking in adolescents with schizophrenia reported significantly greater catch-up saccade amplitude and a trend for lower gain in this population (Friedman et al. 1993). Jacobsen et al. (1996b) examined smooth-pursuit eye movements in children with schizophrenia compared with psychiatrically healthy subjects and subjects with ADHD. Schizophrenic children exhibited significantly greater impairments in smooth-pursuit eye movements compared with either subjects with ADHD or healthy control subjects, and the pattern of abnormalities in smooth-pursuit movements was similar to that seen in adult-onset schizophrenia. Kumra et al. (2001) reported that schizophrenic children exhibited a pattern of eye-tracking dysfunction similar to that reported for adult patients.

Autonomic Function Studies

Autonomic function was examined in 21 subjects (mean age, 14.1 years) with childhood-onset schizophrenia and in 54 age-matched control subjects. The study revealed that abnormalities in autonomic functioning in the patients with childhood-onset schizophrenia included high levels of resting activity, impaired response to novel stimuli, and failure to stop responding to familiar stimuli (Zahn et al. 1997). This pattern is also seen in adults with chronic schizophrenia, thus providing support for the hypothesis of continuity between child and adult forms of the disorder.

■ Neuropsychological Factors

In assessing neuropsychological functioning in childhood-onset schizophrenia, Asarnow et al. (1994) found that children with schizophrenia perform poorly on tasks involving fine motor speed or tasks requiring attention or short-term memory. They do not, however, exhibit impairment in rote language skills and simple perceptual processing tasks. In studies using the Span of Apprehension Task, children with schizophrenia had delayed initiation of serial search or carried out the serial search more slowly than did nonschizophrenic children. Data from a study examining adolescents with schizophrenia suggested deficits in attention, short-term memory, and recent long-term memory (Friedman et al. 1996). Karatekin and Asarnow (1998) investigated both verbal and spatial working memory in children with childhood-onset schizophrenia, children with ADHD, and age-matched healthy control subjects. Both children with schizophrenia and children with ADHD showed deficits in verbal and spatial working memory. The results suggest that in both disorders the capacity of sensory buffers may be diminished or the availability or allocation of resources to the central executive may be limited.

Jacobsen and Rapoport (1998) reported that children with schizophrenia showed a significant deterioration in intellectual functioning during the time between the premorbid period and after the onset of psychosis. Furthermore, the subjects' IQ scores continued to decline 24–48 months after the onset of psychosis. This pattern is different from that noted in adults with schizophrenia. This pattern of intellectual decline and insidious onset seems to suggest that there may be an ongoing pathological process that continually erodes brain function in childhood-onset schizophrenia, in contrast to a fixed lesion that may underlie the adult-onset disorder (Breslin and Weinberger 1991; Weinberger 1987).

■ Neurolinguistic Factors

Baltaxe and Simmons (1995) examined communication characteristics and specific language deficits in 47 children diagnosed with childhood-onset schizophrenia using DSM-III-R criteria. Standardized tests and formal measures were used to assess impairment in specific areas, including pragmatics, receptive and expressive vocabulary and syntax, abstract language, auditory processing, and speech production. Results indicated that pragmatics, prosody, auditory processing, and abstract language showed the greatest impairment. Communication deficits in the group with childhood-onset schizophrenia were found to be similar to the phenomenology reported in studies of the communication characteristics of adult-onset schizophrenia.

■ Psychological and Social Factors

No evidence exists that psychological or social factors cause schizophrenia. However, environmental risks are thought to interact with biological and genetic risk factors and thus affect the timing, severity, and course of the illness. Psychosocial stressors, including high expressed emotion within the family environment, are believed to contribute to onset or exacerbation of acute episodes and may influence relapse rates (American Psychiatric Association 1997). In general, interactions among psychological, social, and illness factors are believed to be complex and "bidirectional" (American Academy of Child and Adolescent Psychiatry 2001).

■ Summary of Etiology

Neurodevelopmental theory can be conceptualized in at least three ways. One theory is that in a normally developing brain, some insult, such as birth trauma or viral infection, occurs during the critical period of brain development. This insult may change the brain structure, with the subsequent development of schizophrenic behaviors. The second theory is that the actual development of the fetal brain is defective in a way that may not be apparent in the earlier years and that certain stresses during maturation may trigger the onset of the schizophrenic behavior. The third theory is that there is a genetic predisposition to schizophrenia that is expressed as a disruption of fetal brain areas undergoing rapid development in the second trimester of intrauterine life. These disruptions in neural development can result in an increased vulnerability to certain complications of pregnancy and delivery, and the combination of these factors may produce periventricular damage. Data from recent genetic research; neuroimaging studies; studies of familial associations and risk factors; and studies of vulnerability, protective factors, and stressful life events as well as their interactions continue to add to a growing body of evidence supporting a neurodevelopmental perspective and a genetic–environment interaction model for the development of childhood-onset schizophrenia.

Treatment

There is little research available regarding the effectiveness of various treatments for children and adolescents with schizophrenia. However, given the strong evidence for continuity between the childhood-onset and adult-onset forms of the disorder, it is assumed by many that the treatments used in adults will also apply to children, provided that modifications are made that take into account age, developmental stage, and other individual circumstances. In clinical practice, careful assessment of a child's strengths, weaknesses, and environmental resources is critical in treatment planning. Combined modalities for an individual patient will likely be required and may include psychoeducation of patient and family, individual therapy, group therapy, parent counseling, family therapy, special education services, community support services, case management, vocational training, and psychopharmacology as deemed appropriate. Within the school setting, services offered may include teacher consultant services, resource room services, self-contained classroom services, speech and language therapy, occupational therapy, physical therapy, and social work services. Vocational training during secondary years may also need to be considered. Individualized educational plans will need to be developed for each child in accordance with his or her specific needs as assessed by a multidisciplinary evaluation team.

Nonpharmacological Therapies

Psychoeducational interventions aimed at family functioning, problem-solving and communication skills, and relapse prevention have been shown to decrease relapse rates in adults with schizophrenia. Social skills training has been reported to be helpful in enhancing socialization and vocational skills (Heinssen et al. 2000). In terms of individual therapy, supportive psychotherapy may be of benefit to some children. Behavior modification procedures may also be useful in reducing levels of maladaptive behavior. More recently, cognitive-behavioral therapy techniques have been shown to be efficacious in the care of patients with chronic psychiatric illnesses (Buckley et al. 2000). This approach was noted to be helpful in the management of suicidality in young people with a first epi-

sode of schizophrenia (Buckley et al. 2000). In a literature review, McClellan and Werry (1994) noted that certain combined treatments that are effective in adult patients might also be effective in younger schizophrenic patients. These treatments are family treatment programs combined with administration of psychoactive agents (Falloon 1992; Goldstein 1989) and family therapy and pharmacotherapy combined with social skills training (Falloon 1992).

Psychopharmacotherapy

Conventional Antipsychotics

There have been very few controlled trials using antipsychotic medications in children and adolescents with schizophrenia. Poole and colleagues (1976) conducted a randomized, double-blind, placebo-controlled study of haloperidol and loxapine in 75 adolescents (ages 13–18 years) with schizophrenia. Results supported a modest but significant superiority of these medications over placebo, but high rates of sedation and extrapyramidal side effects were noted in the active medication groups. Only one double-blind, placebo-controlled study has involved prepubertal schizophrenic patients (Spencer and Campbell 1994). In this study, 16 hospitalized children (ages 5.5–11.75 years) had a good response to haloperidol: 12 showed marked improvement, and 4 showed mild or moderate improvement as measured by the Global Clinical Judgments consensus scale (Spencer and Campbell 1994). Persecutory ideation and delusions, hallucinations, ideas of reference, and other thinking disorders, as measured by the Child Psychiatric Rating Scale, were significantly reduced in patients who received haloperidol in dosages ranging from 0.5 to 3.5 mg/day (mean, 1.9 mg/day). The most common side effects were sedation, acute dystonia, and extrapyramidal symptoms. Older children, children with higher IQs, and those with later onset of schizophrenia showed greater response to haloperidol (Spencer and Campbell 1994). These findings were confirmed when the sample was enlarged to 24 children (Spencer et al. 1994).

Atypical Antipsychotics

Recently, an increasing number of new-generation atypical antipsychotics have been developed, the prototype of which is clozapine. Since their development, these agents have been widely used in the treatment of children and adolescents with schizophrenia. A comprehensive review of all identified published and unpublished studies of the use of antipsychotic medications in children and adolescents from 1996 onward addresses efficacy and tolerability (Bryden et al. 2001). Most of the studies reported reasonable treatment response, but problems with excessive weight gain, sedation, and some degree of extrapyramidal side effects are noted with many of these medications. Studies involving the use of clozapine, risperidone, olanzapine, and quetiapine in children and adolescents are briefly discussed below.

Clozapine. Although some of the newer atypical neuroleptics may have more benign side-effect profiles, clozapine is often the drug of choice in nonresponders or partial responders (Sporn and Rapoport 2001). Kumra et al. (1996) reported on a 6-week double-blind, parallel randomized study of haloperidol and clozapine in 21 patients with treatment-refractory childhood-onset schizophrenia. Clozapine was superior to haloperidol for treatment of both positive and negative symptoms. However, clozapine was associated with severe side effects, including blood dyscrasias, seizures, excessive weight gain, and a significant increase in liver enzymes, necessitating discontinuation in several patients. Turetz et al. (1997) conducted an open trial of clozapine (mean dosage, 227

mg/day) in 11 children ages 9–13 years with treatment-refractory schizophrenia and found significant improvements in both positive and negative symptoms as measured by the Brief Psychiatric Rating Scale (BPRS) (Overall and Gorham 1962) and the PANSS (Kay et al. 1987). Adverse effects, including sedation, sialorrhea, and weight gain, were noted in both of the studies mentioned above (Kumra et al. 1996; Turetz et al. 1997). Tolerability of clozapine may be enhanced by administering it at low initial dosages with subsequent slow dosage increases (Bryden et al. 2001).

There are several other reports of open studies or case reports of the use of clozapine (Birmaher et al. 1992; Blanz and Schmidt 1993; Frazier et al. 1994, 2003; Kumra et al. 1996; Remschmidt et al. 1994). The role of clozapine in the treatment of children and adolescents with schizophrenia and its long-term efficacy and safety in this age group remain to be determined in large samples of patients under adequately controlled, double-blind conditions.

Risperidone. Risperidone has a profile similar to that of clozapine and is reported to exert therapeutic effects on both positive and negative symptoms in adults with schizophrenia (Marder and Meibach 1994). Several reports, mainly open trials and case studies, suggest that risperidone may also be efficacious in the treatment of children and adolescents. In 3 patients ages 11–17 years with schizophrenia, Simeon et al. (1995) found marked improvement associated with administration of risperidone at dosages ranging from 2 to 6 mg/day (taken in two divided doses). Paranoid ideation, impulsivity, and aggressive behavior were among the symptoms most responsive to risperidone. The patients did not experience untoward effects. In another study of a diagnostically heterogeneous group of 10 patients, all improved clinically with risperidone (2–6 mg/day), but untoward effects were noted in 8 patients and extrapyramidal symptoms were observed in 6 (Mandoki 1995). Two of the 10 patients, ages 10 and 17 years, had a diagnosis of schizophrenia. In a letter to the editor, Cozza and Edison (1994) reported significant improvement in two adolescents within 1 week of treatment with risperidone. Extrapyramidal side effects associated with risperidone appear to be dose related (Cozza and Edison 1994; Fras and Major 1995).

Armenteros et al. (1997), in an open pilot study, treated 10 youths (ages 12–18 years) with acute schizophrenia for a 6-week period with risperidone dosages of 4–10 mg/day. Significant reductions in both positive and negative symptoms as assessed by the PANSS, BPRS, and Clinical Global Impression (CGI) Scale were noted. Side effects included weight gain (8 subjects with a mean weight increase of 4.5 kg), mild somnolence (in 8 subjects), dystonic reaction (in 2 subjects), parkinsonism (in 3 subjects), blurred vision (in 1 subject), and poor concentration (in 1 subject). Extrapyramidal signs were noted to be minimal at smaller doses and increased at doses greater than 6 mg. Quintana and Keshavan (1995) reported on four children (ages 12–17 years) who received risperidone treatment. Of the four subjects, three responded well to risperidone at dosages of 4–5 mg/day with improvement in positive and negative symptoms. Relatively few side effects were reported. In a retrospective review of 16 children with schizophrenia or schizoaffective disorder, many of whom had previously undergone failed trials of typical agents, Grcevich and colleagues (1996) reported that 15 had a significant reduction in BPRS scores.

Olanzapine.   Sholevar et al. (2000) described the use of olanzapine in 15 hospi-

talized schizophrenic children ages 6–13 years. The majority of patients improved with olanzapine treatment. It was noted that age was inversely correlated with positive response to olanzapine, and patients with no history of antipsychotic use did better than those who had previously undergone a failed medication trial. Kumra et al. (1998) studied eight children diagnosed with schizophrenia and compared sequential trials of clozapine and olanzapine. Olanzapine led to a 17% reduction in BPRS scores and a 27% improvement in negative symptoms. However, 8 weeks after initiating olanzapine treatment, the effect size was smaller than the effect size at 6 weeks with clozapine treatment. There are several other open-label studies of olanzapine (Grothe et al. 2000; Mozes et al. 2003; Ross et al. 2003).

Quetiapine.   Quetiapine was introduced in 1997. It has not yet been studied much in children and adolescents with schizophrenia. McConville et al. (2000) studied quetiapine at doses of 100 mg given twice daily and 400 mg given twice daily in 10 children with psychoses, ages 12.3–15.9 years. Improvement in both positive and negative symptoms was observed. Adverse events included postural tachycardia and insomnia, but there were no extrapyramidal symptoms and no increase in prolactin levels.

Ziprasidone.   In 2001, ziprasidone was approved by the U.S. Food and Drug Administration (FDA). It had been studied in pediatric patients before its release. Sallee and colleagues (2000), reporting on a pilot study of 28 children with Tourette's disorder, noted side effects of mild somnolence but no weight gain or extrapyramidal symptoms (other than akathisia in one patient).

Side effects of atypical neuroleptic treatment.   In general, sedation and anticholinergic effects are frequently noted with use of the atypical antipsychotic medications. Extrapyramidal symptoms and neuroleptic malignant syndrome are rare, but they do occur. Buck (2001) noted that each agent in the atypical class can potentially cause serious adverse side effects. Clozapine has been associated with agranulocytosis and seizures, and frequent regular blood sampling is needed if this medication is used. Risperidone and ziprasidone have been associated with prolongation of the QT interval, which can increase the risk of cardiac arrhythmia and sudden death. Quetiapine has been associated with elevations in liver enzyme levels. The atypical antipsychotics in general have been associated with increased prolactin levels, weight gain, hyperglycemia, and new-onset or worsening diabetes. Increasing clinical evidence suggests that diabetes occurs at higher-than-expected rates in patients with schizophrenia who are treated with atypical antipsychotics. The most evidence exists for clozapine, followed by olanzapine. There have been numerous case reports of patients treated with clozapine or olanzapine developing diabetic ketoacidosis—which significantly increases the risk of death—shortly after initiation of treatment (Henderson 2002). Patients treated with atypical antipsychotics should be routinely screened for diabetes and other metabolic disorders. Close monitoring of blood glucose levels, lipid profiles, blood pressure, and changes in body weight is highly recommended in patients treated with atypical antipsychotics.

Research Issues

The current understanding of the etiology and treatment of childhood-onset and adolescence-onset schizophrenia is still quite limited because it is a relatively rare disorder. It is critical to have a multidisciplinary collaborative study at many major research institutions. Such a multicenter study should also include centers from other countries of various racial or ethnic groups. Such a study should examine the similarities and differences between childhood-onset and late adolescence–onset schizophrenia in terms of phenomenology, risk factors, and neurobiological and psychosocial factors. Such studies will provide answers to the question of whether childhood-onset schizophrenia is the same or different from adult-onset schizophrenia. Prospective longitudinal studies of subjects with childhood-onset schizophrenia will provide further data to answer this question. Family and genetic studies based on molecular genetic technologies should also be actively pursued so that effective treatment or prevention of childhood-onset schizophrenia can become possible soon.

In the meantime, carefully designed studies are critically needed to examine the treatment efficacy of the newly developed atypical neuroleptics because there are opponents of medication treatment of schizophrenia who constantly challenge the practice of using medications in individuals with schizophrenia. The medication studies should include short-term and long-term assessment of both treatment efficacy and adverse effects of these new neuroleptics.

References

Alaghband-Rad J, McKenna K, Gordon CT: Childhood-onset schizophrenia: the severity of premorbid course. J Am Acad Child Adolesc Psychiatry 34:1273–1283, 1995

Alaghband-Rad J, Hamburger SD, Giedd JN, et al: Childhood-onset schizophrenia: biological markers in relation to clinical characteristics. Am J Psychiatry 154:64–68, 1997

Altman H, Collins M, Mundy P: Subclinical hallucinations and delusions in nonpsychotic adolescents. J Child Psychol Psychiatry 38:413–420, 1997

American Academy of Child and Adolescent Psychiatry: Practice parameters for the assessment and treatment of children and adolescents with depressive disorders. J Am Acad Child Adolesc Psychiatry 37 (suppl): 63S–83S, 1998a

American Academy of Child and Adolescent Psychiatry: Practice parameters for the assessment and treatment of children and adolescents with obsessive-compulsive disorder. J Am Acad Child Adolesc Psychiatry 37 (suppl):27S–45S, 1998b

American Academy of Child and Adolescent Psychiatry: Practice parameters for the assessment and treatment of children and adolescents with schizophrenia. J Am Acad Child Adolesc Psychiatry 40 (suppl):4S–23S, 2001

American Psychiatric Association: Diagnostic and Statistical Manual of Mental Disorders, 2nd Edition. Washington, DC, American Psychiatric Association, 1968

American Psychiatric Association: Diagnostic and Statistical Manual of Mental Disorders, 3rd Edition. Washington, DC, American Psychiatric Association, 1980

American Psychiatric Association: Diagnostic and Statistical Manual of Mental Disorders, 4th Edition. Washington, DC, American Psychiatric Association, 1994

American Psychiatric Association: Practice guidelines for the treatment of patients with schizophrenia. Am J Psychiatry 154 (suppl):1–63, 1997

American Psychiatric Association: Diagnostic and Statistical Manual of Mental Disorders, 4th Edition, Text Revision. Washington, DC, American Psychiatric Association, 2000

Anderson JC, Williams S, McGee R, et al: DSM-III disorders in preadolescent children. Arch Gen Psychiatry 44:69–76, 1987

Arboleda C, Holzman PS: Thought disorder in children at risk for psychosis. Arch Gen Psychiatry 42:1004–1013, 1985

Armenteros JL, Fennelly BW, Hallin A, et al: Schizophrenia in hospitalized adolescents: clinical diagnosis, DSM-III-R, DSM-IV and ICD-10 criteria. Psychopharmacol Bull 31:383–387, 1995

Armenteros JL, Whitaker AH, Welikson M, et al: Risperidone in adolescents with schizophrenia: an open pilot study. J Am Acad Child Adolesc Psychiatry 36:694–700, 1997

Asarnow JR, Ben-Meir S: Children with schizophrenia spectrum and depressive disorders: a comparative study of premorbid adjustment, onset pattern and severity of impairment. J Child Psychol Psychiatry 29:477–488, 1988

Asarnow R, Sherman T, Strandburg R: The search for the psychobiological substrate of childhood-onset schizophrenia. J Am Acad Child Psychiatry 26:601–614, 1986

Asarnow RF, Tanguay PE, Bott L, et al: Patterns of intellectual functioning in nonretarded autistic and schizophrenic children. J Child Psychol Psychiatry 28:273–280, 1987

Asarnow RF, Asamen J, Granholm E, et al: Cognitive/neuropsychological studies of children with a schizophrenic disorder. Schizophr Bull 20:647–669, 1994

Asarnow RF, Nuechterlein KH, Fogelson D, et al: Schizophrenia and schizophrenia-spectrum personality disorders in the first-degree relatives of children with schizophrenia: the UCLA family study. Arch Gen Psychiatry 58:581–588, 2001

Baltaxe CA, Simmons JQ 3rd: Speech and language disorders in children and adolescents with schizophrenia. Schizophr Bull 21:677–692, 1995

Bedwell JS, Keller B, Smith AK, et al: Why does postpsychotic IQ decline in childhood-onset schizophrenia? Am J Psychiatry 156:1996–1997, 1999

Bertolino A, Kumra S, Callicott JH, et al: Common pattern of cortical pathology in childhood-onset and adult-onset schizophrenia as identified by proton magnetic resonance spectroscopic imaging. Am J Psychiatry 155:1376–1383, 1998

Birmaher B, Baker R, Kapur S, et al: Clozapine for the treatment of adolescents with schizophrenia. J Am Acad Child Adolesc Psychiatry 31:160–164, 1992

Blanz B, Schmidt MH: Clozapine for schizophrenia (letter). J Am Acad Child Adolesc Psychiatry 32:223–224, 1993

Breslin NA, Weinberger DR: Neurodevelopmental implications of findings from brain imaging studies of schizophrenia, in Fetal Neural Development and Adult Schizophrenia. Edited by Mednick SA, Cannon TD, Barr CE, et al. New York, Cambridge University Press, 1991, pp 199–215

Brooks WM, Hodde-Vargas J, Vargas LA, et al: Frontal lobe of children with schizophrenia spectrum disorders: a proton magnetic resonance spectroscopic study. Biol Psychiatry 43:263–269, 1998

Bryden K, Carrey N, Kutcher S: Update and recommendations for the use of antipsychotics in early onset psychoses. J Child Adolesc Psychopharmacol 11:113–130, 2001

Buck ML: Using the atypical antipsychotic agents in children and adolescents. Pediatric Pharmacotherapy 7(8):1–5, 2001

Buckley PF, Buchanan RW, Tamminga CA, et al: Schizophrenia research: a progress report, summarizing proceedings of the 1999 International Congress on Schizophrenia Research. Schizophr Bull 26:411–419, 2000

Buka SL, Tsuang MT, Torrey EF, et al: Maternal infections and subsequent psychosis among offspring. Arch Gen Psychiatry 58:1032–1037, 2001

Bunk D, Eggers C, Klapal M: Symptom dimensions in the course of childhood-onset schizophrenia. Eur Child Adolesc Psychiatry 8 (suppl 1):129–135, 1999

Burd L, Kerbeshian J: A North Dakota prevalence study of schizophrenia presenting in childhood. J Am Acad Child Adolesc Psychiatry 26:347–350, 1987

Burgess CE, Lindblad K, Sidransky E, et al: Large CAG/CTG repeats are associated with childhood-onset schizophrenia. Mol Psychiatry 3:321–327, 1998

Calderoni D, Wudarsky M, Bhangoo R, et al: Differentiating childhood-onset schizophrenia from psychotic mood disorders. J Am Acad Child Adolesc Psychiatry 40:1190–1196, 2001

Caplan R: Thought disorder in childhood. J Am Acad Child Adolesc Psychiatry 33:605–615, 1994

Caplan R, Perdue S, Tanguay PE, et al: Formal thought disorder in childhood-onset schizophrenia and schizotypal personality disorder. J Child Psychol Psychiatry 31:169–177, 1990

Caplan R, Guthrie D, Shields WD, et al: Communication deficits in children undergoing temporal lobectomy. J Am Acad Child Adolesc Psychiatry 32:604–611, 1993

Caplan R, Guthrie D, Tang B, et al: Thought disorder in childhood schizophrenia: replication and update of concept. J Am Acad Child Adolesc Psychiatry 39:771–778, 2000

Caplan R, Guthrie D, Tang B, et al: Thought disorder in attention-deficit hyperactivity disorder. J Am Acad Child Adolesc Psychiatry 40:965–972, 2001

Carlson GA, Bromert EJ, Sievers S: Phenomenology and outcome of subjects with early and adult-onset psychotic mania. Am J Psychiatry 157:213–219, 2000

Chambers WJ, Puig-Antich J, Tabrizi MA, et al: Psychotic symptoms in pre-pubertal major depressive disorder. Arch Gen Psychiatry 39:921–927, 1982

Cozza SJ, Edison DL: Risperidone in adolescents (letter). J Am Acad Child Adolesc Psychiatry 33:1211, 1994

Creak M, Cameron K, Cowie V, et al: Schizophrenic syndrome in childhood. BMJ 2:889–890, 1961

Done DJ, Johnstone EC, Frith CD, et al: Complications of pregnancy and delivery in relation to psychosis in adult life: data from the British perinatal mortality survey sample. BMJ 302:1576–1580, 1991

Eggers C: Schizoaffective psychosis in childhood: a follow-up study. J Autism Dev Disord 19:327–334, 1989

Eggers C, Bunk D: The long-term course of childhood-onset schizophrenia: a 42-year follow-up. Schizophr Bull 23: 105–117, 1997

Erlenmeyer-Kimling L, Cornblatt B: High-risk research in schizophrenia: a summary of what has been learned. J Psychiatr Res 21:401–411, 1987

Erlenmeyer-Kimling L, Folgenovic Z, Hrabak-Zerjavic V, et al: Schizophrenia and prenatal exposure to the 1957 A2 influenza epidemic in Croatia. Am J Psychiatry 151:1496–1498, 1994

Falloon IRH: Psychotherapy for schizophrenic disorders: a review. Br J Hosp Med 48:164–170, 1992

Famularo R, Kinscherff R, Fenton T: Psychiatric diagnoses of maltreated children: preliminary finding. J Am Acad Child Adolesc Psychiatry 31:863–867, 1992

Findling RL, Friedman L, Henny JT, et al: Hippocampal volume in adolescent schizophrenia. Schizophr Res 18:185–188, 1996

Fras I, Major LF: Clinical experience with risperidone (letter). J Am Acad Child Adolesc Psychiatry 34:833, 1995

Frazier JA, Gordon CT, McKenna K, et al: An open trial of clozapine in 11 adolescents with childhood-onset schizophrenia. J Am Acad Child Adolesc Psychiatry 33:658–663, 1994

Frazier JA, Giedd JA, Hamburger SD, et al: Brain anatomic magnetic resonance imaging in childhood-onset schizophrenia. Arch Gen Psychiatry 53:617–624, 1996

Frazier JA, Cohen LG, Jacobsen L, et al: Clozapine pharmacokinetics in children and adolescents with childhood-onset schizophrenia. J Clin Psychopharmacol 23:87–91, 2003

Friedman L, Schulz SC, Jesberger JA: Smooth pursuit eye movement performance in adolescent-onset psychosis. Schizophr Res 9:157, 1993

Friedman L, Findling RL, Buch J, et al: Structural MRI and neuropsychological assessments in adolescent patients with either schizophrenia or affective disorders. Schizophr Res 18:189–190, 1996

Goldstein MJ: Psychosocial treatment of schizophrenia, in Schizophrenia: Scientific Progress. Edited by Schulz SC, Tamminga CA. New York, Oxford University Press, 1989, pp 318–324

Gordon CT, Frazier JA, McKenna K, et al: Childhood-onset schizophrenia: an NIMH study in progress. Schizophr Bull 20:697–712, 1994

Gottesman II, Bertelsen A: Confirming unexpressed genotypes for schizophrenia: risks in the offspring of Fischer's Danish identical and fraternal discordant twins. Arch Gen Psychiatry 46:867–872, 1989

Gottesman II, Shields J: Schizophrenia and Genetics: A Twin Study Vantage Point. New York, Academic Press, 1972

Gottesman II, McGuffin P, Farmer AE: Clinical genetics as clues to the "real" genetics of schizophrenia: a decade of modest gains while playing for time. Schizophr Bull 13:23–47, 1987

Grcevich SJ, Findling RL, Rowane WA, et al: Risperidone in the treatment of children and adolescents with schizophrenia: a retrospective study. J Child Adolesc Psychopharmacol 6:251–257, 1996

Green WH, Padron-Gayol M: Schizophrenic disorder in childhood: its relationship to DSM-III criteria, in Biological Psychiatry 1985. Edited by Shagass C, Josiassen RC, Bridger WH, et al. New York, Elsevier, 1986, pp 1484–1486

Green WH, Padron-Gayol M, Hardesty AS, et al: Schizophrenia with childhood-onset: a phenomenological study of 38 cases. J Am Acad Child Adolesc Psychiatry 31:968–976, 1992

Grothe DR, Calis KA, Jacobsen L, et al: Olanzapine pharmacokinetics in pediatric and adolescent inpatients with childhood-onset schizophrenia. J Clin Psychopharmacol 20:220–225, 2000

Gunther-Genta F, Bovet P, Hohlfeld P: Obstetric complications and schizophrenia: a case-control study. Br J Psychiatry 164:165–170, 1994

Hall W, Degenhardt L: Cannabis use and psychosis: a review of clinical and epidemiological evidence. Aust N Z J Psychiatry 34:26–34, 2000

Heinssen RK, Liberman RP, Kopelowicz A: Psychosocial skills training for schizophrenia: lessons from the laboratory. Schizophr Bull 26:21–46, 2000

Henderson DC: Atypical antipsychotic-induced diabetes mellitus. CNS Drugs 16(2):77–89, 2002

Hendren RL, Hodde-Varges J, Yeo RA, et al: Neuropsychophysiological study of children at risk for schizophrenia: a preliminary report. J Am Acad Child Adolesc Psychiatry 34:1284–1291, 1995

Hendren RL, De Backer I, Pandina GJ: Review of neuroimaging studies of child and adolescent psychiatric disorders from the past 10 years. J Am Acad Child Adolesc Psychiatry 39:815–827, 2000

Heston LL: Psychiatric disorders in foster home reared children of schizophrenic mothers. Br J Psychiatry 112:819–825, 1966

Hornstein JL, Putnam FW: Clinical phenomenology of child and adolescent dissociative disorders. J Am Acad Child Adolesc Psychiatry 31:1077–1085, 1992

Jacobsen LK, Rapoport J: Research update: childhood-onset schizophrenia: implications of clinical and neurobiological research. J Child Psychol Psychiatry 39:101–113, 1998

Jacobsen LK, Giedd JN, Vaituzis AC, et al: Temporal lobe morphology in childhood-onset schizophrenia. Am J Psychiatry 153:355–361, 1996a

Jacobsen LK, Hong WL, Hommer DW, et al: Smooth pursuit eye movements in childhood-onset schizophrenia: comparison with attention-deficit hyperactivity disorder and normal controls. Biol Psychiatry 40:1144–1154, 1996b

Jacobsen LK, Giedd JN, Berquin PC, et al: Quantitative morphology of the cerebellum and fourth ventricle in childhood-onset schizophrenia. Am J Psychiatry 154:1663–1669, 1997a

Jacobsen LK, Giedd JN, Vaituzis AC, et al: Quantitative magnetic resonance imaging of the corpus callosum in childhood-onset schizophrenia. Psychiatry Res 68:77–86, 1997b

Jacobsen LK, Hamburger SD, Van Horn JD, et al: Cerebral glucose metabolism in childhood-onset schizophrenia. Psychiatry Res 75:131–144, 1997c

Jacobsen LK, Giedd JN, Castellanos FX, et al: Progressive reduction of temporal lobe structures in childhood-onset schizophrenia. Am J Psychiatry 155:678–685, 1998a

Jacobsen LK, Mittleman BB, Kumra S, et al: HLA antigens in childhood-onset schizophrenia. Psychiatry Res 78:123–132, 1998b

Jennings WS, Schulz SC, Narasimhachari N, et al: Brain ventricular size and CSF monoamine metabolites in an adolescent inpatient population. Psychiatry Res 16:87–94, 1985

Kafantaris V, Ernst M, Samuel R, et al: Psychotic disorders in hospitalized adolescents: diagnostic issues (abstract), in Scientific Proceedings, 39th Annual Meeting of the American Academy of Child and Adolescent Psychiatry, Washington, DC, October 20–25, 1992. Washington, DC, American Academy of Child and Adolescent Psychiatry, 1992, p 63

Kaiser R, Konneker M, Henneken M, et al: Dopamine D_4 receptor 48-bp repeat polymorphism: no association with response to antipsychotic treatment, but association with catatonic schizophrenia. Mol Psychiatry 5:418–424, 2000

Karatekin C, Asarnow RF: Working memory in childhood-onset schizophrenia and attention-deficit/hyperactivity disorder. Psychiatry Res 17:165–176, 1998

Karp BI, Garvey M, Jacobsen LK, et al: Abnormal neurologic maturation in adolescents with early onset schizophrenia. Am J Psychiatry 158:118–122, 2001

Kay SR, Fishbein A, Opier LA: The positive and negative syndrome scale (PANSS) for schizophrenia. Schizophr Bull 13:261–276, 1987

Keller A, Castellanos FX, Vaituzis AC, et al: Progressive loss of cerebellar volume in childhood-onset schizophrenia. Am J Psychiatry 160:128–133, 2003

Kendler KS, Diehl SR: The genetics of schizophrenia: a current, genetic-epidemiologic perspective, in Special Report: Schizophrenia 1993 (NIMH Publ No 93-3499). Edited by Shore D. Rockville, MD, U.S. Department of Health and Human Services, 1993, pp 87–111

Kendler KS, McGuire M, Gruenberg AM, et al: The Roscommon Family Study, I: methods, diagnosis of probands, and risk of schizophrenia in relatives. Arch Gen Psychiatry 50:527–540, 1993

Keshavan MS, Anderson S, Pettegrew JW: Is schizophrenia due to excessive synaptic pruning in the prefrontal cortex? The Feinberg hypothesis revisited. J Psychiatr Res 28:239–265, 1994

Kety SS, Wender PH, Jacobsen B, et al: Mental illness in the biological and adoptive relatives of schizophrenic adoptees: replication of the Copenhagen study in the rest of Denmark. Arch Gen Psychiatry 51:442–455, 1994

Kilgus MD, Pumariega AJ, Cuffe SP: Influence of race on diagnosis in adolescent psychiatric inpatients. J Am Acad Child Adolesc Psychiatry 34:67–72, 1995

Kolvin I, Ounsted C, Humphrey M, et al: Studies in the childhood psychoses, II: the phenomenology of childhood psychoses. Br J Psychiatry 118:385–395, 1971

Krausz M, Muller-Thomsen T: Schizophrenia with onset in adolescence: an 11-year follow-up. Schizophr Bull 19:831–841, 1993

Kumra S, Frazier JA, Jacobsen LK, et al: Childhood-onset schizophrenia: a double-blind clozapine-haloperidol comparison. Arch Gen Psychiatry 53:1090–1097, 1996

Kumra S, Jacobsen LK, Lenane M, et al: Childhood-onset schizophrenia: an open label study of olanzapine in adolescents. J Am Acad Child Adolesc Psychiatry 37:377–385, 1998

Kumra S, Sporn A, Hommer DW, et al: Smooth pursuit eye-tracking impairment in childhood-onset psychotic disorders. Am J Psychiatry 158:1291–1298, 2001

Kunugi H, Hattori M, Nanko S, et al: Dinucleotide repeat polymorphism in the neurotrophin-3 gene and hippocampal volume in psychoses. Schizophr Res 37:271–273, 1999

Lindsay J, Ounsted C, Richards P: Long-term outcome in children with temporal lobe seizures, II: marriage, parenthood, and sexual indifference. Dev Med Child Neurol 21:433–440, 1979

Loranger AW: Sex difference in age at onset of schizophrenia. Arch Gen Psychiatry 41:157–161, 1984

Mandoki MW: Risperidone treatment of children and adolescents: increased risk of extrapyramidal side effects? J Child Adolesc Psychopharmacol 5:49–67, 1995

Marcus J, Hans SL, Lewow E, et al: Neurological findings in high-risk children: childhood assessment and 5-year follow-up. Schizophr Bull 11:85–100, 1985

Marder SR, Meibach RC: Risperidone in the treatment of schizophrenia. Am J Psychiatry 151:825–835, 1994

Maziade M, Bouchard S, Gingras N, et al: Long-term stability of diagnosis and symptom dimensions in a systematic sample of patients with onset of schizophrenia in childhood and early adolescence, II: postnegative distinction and childhood predictors of adult outcome. Br J Psychiatry 169:371–378, 1996

McClellan J, McCurry C: Neurocognitive pathways in development of schizophrenia. Semin Clin Neuropsychiatry 3:320–332, 1998

McClellan J, McCurry C: Early onset psychotic disorders: diagnostic stability and clinical characteristics. Eur Child Adolesc Psychiatry 8 (suppl 2):1S–7S, 1999

McClellan J, Werry J: Practice parameters for the assessment and treatment of children and adolescents with schizophrenia. J Am Acad Child Adolesc Psychiatry 33:616–635, 1994

McClellan JM, Werry S, Ham M: A follow-up study of early onset psychosis: comparison between outcome diagnoses of schizophrenia, mood disorder and personality disorders. J Autism Dev Disord 23:243–262, 1993

McConville B, Arvanitis L, Thyrum PT, et al: Pharmacokinetics, tolerability and clinical effectiveness of quetiapine fumarate in adolescents with selected psychotic disorders. J Clin Psychiatry 61:252–260, 2000

McKenna K, Gordon CT, Lenane M, et al: Looking for childhood-onset schizophrenia: the first 71 cases screened. J Am Acad Child Adolesc Psychiatry 33:636–644, 1994a

McKenna K, Gordon CT, Rapoport JL: Childhood-onset schizophrenia: timely neurobiological research. J Am Acad Child Adolesc Psychiatry 33:771–781, 1994b

Mednick SA, Machon RA, Huttunen MO, et al: Adult schizophrenia following prenatal exposure to an influenza epidemic. Arch Gen Psychiatry 45:189–192, 1988

Mirsky AF, Silberman EK, Latz A, et al: Adult outcomes of high-risk children: differential effects of town and kibbutz rearing. Schizophr Bull 11:150–154, 1985

Morgan V, Castle D, Page A, et al: Influenza epidemics and incidence of schizophrenia, affective disorder and mental retardation in Western Australia: no evidence of a major effect. Schizophr Res 26:25–39, 1997

Mozes T, Greenberg Y, Spivak B, et al: Olanzapine treatment in chronic drug-resistant childhood-onset schizophrenia: an open-label study. J Child Adolesc Psychopharmacol 13:311–317, 2003

Nicolson R, Giedd J, Lenane M, et al: Clinical and neurobiological correlates of cytogenetic abnormalities in childhood-onset schizophrenia. Am J Psychiatry 156:1575–1579, 1999

Nicolson R, Lenane M, Singaracharlu S, et al: Premorbid speech and language impairments in childhood-onset schizophrenia: association with risk factors. Am J Psychiatry 157:794–800, 2000

Nopoulos PC, Giedd JN, Andreasen NC, et al: Frequency and severity of enlarged cavum septi pellucidi in childhood-onset schizophrenia. Am J Psychiatry 155:1074–1079, 1998

O'Callaghan E, Sham P, Takei N, et al: Schizophrenia after prenatal exposure to 1958 A_2 influenza epidemic. Lancet 337:1248–1250, 1991

O'Callaghan, Gibson T, Colohan HA, et al: Risk of schizophrenia in adults born after obstetric complications and their association with early onset of illness: a controlled study. BMJ 305:1256–1259, 1993

Overall JE, Gorham DR: The Brief Psychiatric Rating Scale. Psychol Rep 10:799–812, 1962

Pilowsky D, Chambers WJ (eds): Hallucinations in Childhood. Washington, DC, American Psychiatric Press, 1986

Poole D, Bloom W, Mielke DH, et al: A controlled evaluation of Loxitane in seventy-five adolescent schizophrenic patients. Curr Ther Res Clin Exp 19:99–104, 1976

Puig-Antich J, Ryan N, Rabinovich H: Affective disorders in childhood and adolescence, in Diagnosis and Psycho-pharmacology of Childhood and Adolescent Disorders. Edited by Wiener J. New York, Wiley, 1985, pp 113–150

Quintana H, Keshavan M: Case study: risperidone in children and adolescents with schizophrenia. J Am Acad Child Adolesc Psychiatry 34:1292–1296, 1995

Rapoport JL, Giedd J, Kumra S, et al: Childhood-onset schizophrenia. Progressive ventricular change during adolescence. Arch Gen Psychiatry 54:897–903, 1997

Rapoport JL, Giedd JN, Blumenthal J: Progressive cortical change during adolescence in childhood-onset schizophrenia: a longitudinal magnetic resonance imaging study. Arch Gen Psychiatry 56:649–654, 1999

Remschmidt H, Martin M, Schulz E, et al: The concept of positive and negative schizophrenia in child and adolescent psychiatry, in Negative Versus Positive Schizophrenia. Edited by Marneros A, Andreasen NC, Tsuang MT. New York, Springer-Verlag, 1991, pp 219–242

Remschmidt HE, Schulz E, Martin M: An open trial of clozapine in thirty-six adolescents with schizophrenia. J Child Adolesc Psychopharmacol 4:31–41, 1994

Rieder RO, Nichols PL: Offspring of schizophrenics, III. Arch Gen Psychiatry 36:665–674, 1979

Ross RG, Novins D, Farley GK, et al: A 1-year open-label trial of olanzapine in school-age children with schizophrenia. J Child Adolesc Psychopharmacol 13:301–309, 2003

Russell AT: The clinical presentation of childhood-onset schizophrenia. Schizophr Bull 20:631–646, 1994

Russell AT, Bott L, Sammons C: The phenomenology of schizophrenia occurring in childhood. J Am Acad Child Adolesc Psychiatry 28:399–407, 1989

Rutter M: Childhood schizophrenia reconsidered. J Autism Child Schizophr 2:315–337, 1972

Sallee FR, Kurlan R, Goetz CG, et al: Ziprasidone treatment of children and adolescents with Tourette's syndrome: a pilot study. J Am Acad Child Adolesc Psychiatry 39:292–299, 2000

Schulz SC, Koller MM, Kishore PR, et al: Ventricular enlargement in teenage patients with schizophrenia spectrum disorder. Am J Psychiatry 140:1592–1595, 1983

Schulz SC, Findling RL, Wise A, et al: Child and adolescent schizophrenia. Psychiatr Clin North Am 21:43–56, 1998

Selten JP, Brown AS, Moons KG, et al: Prenatal exposure to the 1957 influenza pandemic and non-affective psychosis in the Netherlands. Schizophr Res 38:85–91, 1999

Sholevar EH, Baron DA, Hardie TL: Treatment of childhood-onset schizophrenia with olanzapine. J Child Adolesc Psychopharmacol 10:69–78, 2000

Simeon JG, Carrey NJ, Wiggins DM, et al: Risperidone effects in treatment-resistant adolescents: preliminary case reports. J Child Adolesc Psychopharmacol 5:69–79, 1995

Spencer EK, Campbell M: Children with schizophrenia: diagnosis, phenomenology, and pharmacotherapy. Schizophr Bull 20:713–725, 1994

Spencer EK, Alpert M, Pouget ER, et al: Baseline characteristics and side-effect profile as predictors of haloperidol treatment outcome in schizophrenic children. Paper presented at National Institute of Mental Health New Clinical Drug Evaluation Unit 34th annual meeting, Marco Island, FL, May–June 1994

Sporn A, Rapoport J: Childhood-onset schizophrenia. Child and Adolescent Psychopharmacology News 2:1–6, 2001

Thomas MA, Ke Y, Levitt J: Preliminary study of frontal lobe ^{1}H MR spectroscopy in childhood-onset schizophrenia. J Magn Reson Imaging 8:841–846, 1998

Thomsen PS: Schizophrenia with childhood and adolescent onset: a nationwide register-based study. Acta Psychiatr Scand 94:187–193, 1996

Turetz M, Mozes T, Toren P, et al: An open trial of clozapine in neuroleptic-resistant childhood-onset schizophrenia. Br J Psychiatry 170:507–510, 1997

Verdoux H, Geddes JR, Takei N, et al: Obstetric complications and age at onset in schizophrenia: an international collaborative meta-analysis of individual patient data. Am J Psychiatry 154:1220–1227, 1997

Volkmar FR: Childhood schizophrenia, in Child and Adolescent Psychiatry, A Comprehensive Textbook. Edited by Lewis M. Baltimore, MD, Williams & Wilkins, 1996, pp 629–635

Watkins JM, Asarnow RF, Tanguay PE: Symptom development in childhood-onset schizophrenia. J Child Psychol Psychiatry 29:865–878, 1988

Weinberger DR: Implications of normal brain development for the pathogenesis of schizophrenia. Arch Gen Psychiatry 44:660–669, 1987

Werry JS: The childhood psychoses, in Psychopathological Disorders of Childhood, 2nd Edition. Edited by Quay HC, Werry JS. New York, Wiley, 1979, pp 41–89

Werry JS: Child and adolescent (early onset) schizophrenia: a review in light of DSM-III-R. J Autism Dev Disord 22: 601–624, 1992

Werry JS, Taylor E: Schizophrenia and allied disorders, in Child and Adolescent Psychiatry: Modern Approaches, 3rd Edition. Edited by Rutter M, Taylor EA, Hersov LA. Boston, MA, Blackwell Scientific, 1994, pp 594–615

Werry JS, McClellan JM, Chard L: Childhood and adolescent schizophrenic, bipolar, and schizoaffective disorders: a clinical and outcome study. J Am Acad Child Adolesc Psychiatry 30:457–465, 1991

Werry JS, McClellan JM, Andrews LK, et al: Clinical features and outcome of child and adolescent schizophrenia. Schizophr Bull 20:619–630, 1994

World Health Organization: International Classification of Diseases, 9th Revision. Geneva, World Health Organization, 1977

Yan WL, Guan XY, Green ED, et al: Childhood-onset schizophrenia/autistic disorder and t(1;7) reciprocal translocation: identification of a BAC contig spanning the translocation breakpoint at 7q21. Am J Med Genet 96:749–753, 2000

Yeo RA, Hodde-Vargas J, Hendren RL, et al: Brain abnormalities in schizophrenia-spectrum children: implications for a neurodevelopmental perspective. Psychiatr Res 76:1–13, 1997

Zahn TP, Jacobsen LK, Gordon CT, et al: Autonomic nervous system markers of psychopathology in childhood-onset schizophrenia. Arch Gen Psychiatry 54:904–912, 1997

Self-Assessment Questions

Select the single best response for each question.

13.1 The diagnosis of schizophrenia with childhood onset

  A. Is a common presentation for this disorder.
  B. Is five times more likely in females than in males.
  C. Requires no mood disorder exclusion.
  D. Can be made when signs of disturbance have been present for at least 3 months.
  E. May have a prevalence of less than 1 in 1,000.

13.2 In regard to National Institute of Mental Health studies comparing patients with childhood-onset schizophrenia and patients with adult-onset schizophrenia, all of the following findings are correct *except*

  A. Childhood-onset patients showed greater delay in language development than did adult-onset patients.
  B. Childhood-onset patients evidenced more disruptive behavior disorders than did adult-onset patients.
  C. Childhood-onset patients evidenced more learning disorders than did adult-onset patients.
  D. Childhood-onset patients evidenced few motor stereotypes.
  E. Childhood-onset schizophrenia appears to represent a more malignant form of the disorder.

13.3 Which phase of illness in schizophrenic patients is best described by the following definition: "A 1- to 6-month (or longer) period when symptoms of hallucinations, delusions, thought disorder, or disorganized behavior are predominant?"

  A. Prodrome.
  B. Acute phase.
  C. Recovery phase.
  D. Residual phase.
  E. Chronicity.

13.4 Which of the following statements concerning the differential diagnosis of childhood psychotic disorders is *true?*

  A. The diagnostic criteria for schizophreniform disorder require an illness duration of less than 6 months.
  B. Once a diagnosis of schizophreniform disorder is made, a diagnosis of schizophrenia can never be given.
  C. A diagnosis of schizophreniform disorder requires the presence of a decline in function.
  D. Brief psychotic disorder requires a symptom duration of at least 1 month but no more than 6 months.
  E. The diagnosis of psychotic disorder not otherwise specified is very rare in the hospitalized adolescent population.

13.5 Magnetic resonance imaging (MRI) studies in children with schizophrenia have reported all of the following findings *except*

A. Decreases in total cerebral volume.

B. Cerebral asymmetry.

C. Decreases in ventricular volume.

D. Increases in temporal lobe volume.

E. Decreases in midsagittal thalamic area.

14

Mood Disorders

Elizabeth B. Weller, M.D.

Angelica L. Kloos, D.O.

Ronald A. Weller, M.D.

Early-onset mood disorders exert a major impact on social, emotional, and occupational functioning. They are associated with significant morbidity and mortality, lengthy course, and risk for recurrence, usually persisting into adulthood (Birmaher et al. 1996a; Emslie et al. 1997b; Lewinsohn et al. 1994b; Strober et al. 1993). They also contribute to significant psychosocial morbidity with potentially debilitating effects on growth and development. This can include impairment in family and peer relationships and poor school performance (Fleming and Offord 1990; Kashani et al. 1987b; Puig-Antich et al. 1993). In addition, these youngsters are also at increased risk for substance abuse, legal difficulties, and hospitalizations (Akiskal et al. 1985; Lewinsohn et al. 1995; Strober et al. 1995). Depressed children and adolescents are at increased risk for both suicide attempts and suicide completions (Brent 1987; Pfeffer et al. 1991a). More than 90% of adolescents who commit suicide have an associated psychiatric illness, most often a mood disorder. This fact alone highlights the importance of preventive measures aimed at the detection of mood disorders as early as possible (Bhatara 1992).

In the past, childhood mood disorders were often misdiagnosed or underdiagnosed (E.B. Weller et al. 1995). In fact, childhood depression was not officially recognized in the United States until the 1975 National Institute of Mental Health (NIMH) Conference on Depression in Childhood (Schulterbrandt and Raskin 1977), which concluded that adult criteria could be used to diagnose depression in children if appropriate modifications were made to accommodate for age and stage of development. As a result, mood disorders in children and adolescents are now receiving much more attention but continue to present diagnostic problems. Many young children lack the language capacity to verbally express their emotions. Often these children present with somatic symptoms such as headaches and stomachaches or complaints of "not feeling well." Thus, they are seen in primary care clinics rather than in mental health centers.

The clinical presentation of bipolar disorder in children very often shows similarities with externalizing disorders, such as attention-deficit/hyperactivity disorder (ADHD), oppositional defiant disorder and conduct disorder. It is now accepted that bipolar disorder in prepubertal children is frequently comorbid with externalizing disorders and can present in a rapid-cycling or "mixed" picture (Kovacs and Pollock 1995; Tillman et al. 2003). Previously, children and adolescents with mood disorders were often diagnosed with adjustment disorder, conduct disorder, ADHD, or schizophrenia (Akiskal and Weller 1989).

Diagnostic Criteria and Clinical Presentations

■ Major Depressive Disorder

Approximately 2.5% of children and 8.3% of adolescents in the United States have depression (Birmaher et al. 1996a). In DSM-IV-TR (American Psychiatric Association 2000), a major depressive episode is characterized by five or more of the following symptoms that have been present during the same 2-week period and represent a change from previous functioning: 1) depressed mood most of the day (can be irritable mood in children and adolescents), 2) markedly diminished interest or pleasure in all (or almost all) activities, 3) changes in appetite or weight change (which can include a failure to meet expected growth rates [E.B. Weller et al. 2000]), 4) insomnia or hypersomnia, 5) psychomotor agitation or retardation, 6) fatigue or loss of energy, 7) feelings of worthlessness or excessive or inappropriate guilt, 8) diminished ability to think or concentrate, 9) recurrent thoughts of death.

These symptoms should represent a change from the individual's previous level of functioning and should cause distress or impairment. The symptoms must not be due to the effects of medications, alcohol or drug abuse, or a general medical condition. Uncomplicated bereavement is also specifically excluded from the diagnosis of major depressive disorder. A major depressive episode is considered to have ended when the symptoms have diminished below the threshold for diagnosis or have been resolved completely for at least 2 consecutive months. DSM-IV-TR allows the current or most recent episode to be specified as mild, moderate, severe without psychotic features, severe with psychotic features, in partial remission, in full remission, chronic, with catatonic features, with melancholic features, with atypical features, and with postpartum onset. The longitudinal course may be specified as a single episode, recurrent with full interepisode recovery, recurrent without full interepisode recovery, and with seasonal pattern (American Psychiatric Association 2000, p. 356).

It is important to note that although the criteria used to diagnose depressive episodes in children may be similar to those for adults, the methods for eliciting the information necessary to make the diagnosis vary with age. Children are less able to describe the chronological details of inner mood states, and are often unable to explain either current or recent moods (Angold et al. 1996). In children, particularly under the age of 14 years, it is crucial to obtain information on symptoms and behaviors from various informants, including the child, parents, teachers, school counselors, and pediatricians (E.B. Weller et al. 2000).

Although the essential features of major depression are similar in children, adolescents, and adults, there are noticeable differences in phenomenology. Younger children, unable to express emotions as adequately as adolescents and adults, tend to present with more somatic complaints, psychomotor agitation, and, at times, mood-congruent hallucinations. With age, these symptoms begin to decrease, but self-esteem seems to worsen. Among adolescents, antisocial behavior, substance use, restlessness, "grouchiness," aggression, social withdrawal, problems with family and school, and feelings of wanting to leave home, or feelings of not being understood and approved of are more frequent. In adolescence the phenomenology of major depression is similar to that of adult major depression (Kessler et al. 2001). Birmaher et al. (1996a) suggest that symptoms of "endogenicity"—melancholia, psychosis, suicide attempts, lethality of suicide attempts, and impairment of functioning—increase with age. The details of presentation of major depressive disorder according to age are described below.

Infants

Literature on the clinical presentation of mood disorders in infants is very limited. Spitz (1946) and Bowlby (1951) described the moods of children who had been separated from their primary caretakers at an early age. These children look depressed, cry a lot, react slowly to stimuli, and exhibit retarded movements. They may have sleep and appetite disturbances. In institutionalized infants and toddlers, this clinical picture has been called hospitalism.

Preschool-Age Children

In preschool children, pathologically prolonged states of emotional arousal in response to minimal stimuli and episodic frenzied activity with minor symptoms of depression have been described by Carlson (1983). Kashani and Carlson (1987) noted preschoolers with depression look very sad, have limited verbal communica-

tion, and appear slowed down. They appear to "lack a twinkle in their eyes" (E.B. Weller et al. 2004a).

School-Age Children

School-age children are able to describe symptoms such as depressed mood ("low, down in the dumps" or "wanting to be nothing when I grow up"), trouble concentrating, poor performance in school, irritability, crying, and suicidal thoughts that are often unknown to their parents. Because of the myth that children younger than age 10 years do not attempt suicide, suicide attempts by young children are often mistakenly characterized as accidents. Somatic symptoms may coexist with depressive symptoms in school-age children. The most common complaints are headaches and abdominal pain/discomfort. Such depressed children are often seen by pediatricians or family physicians, who after extensive medical evaluation and laboratory work may conclude that nothing is wrong or "it's all in the head" (E.B. Weller et al. 2004a).

Adolescents

By adolescence, somatic complaints and depressed appearance decrease in frequency and are commonly replaced by symptoms of anhedonia, diurnal variation, hopelessness, psychomotor retardation, and delusions (Carlson and Kashani 1988b). Ryan et al. (1987) reported that anhedonia, hopelessness, hypersomnia, weight change, and drug abuse were more common in adolescents than in children. There was no significant difference in the severity of suicidal ideation between depressed adolescents and children, but adolescents chose significantly more lethal methods in their attempts.

Often the presenting problem in a depressed adolescent is an overt behavioral problem, and the accompanying depression may not be detected. An early study of the phenomenology associated with depressed mood in adolescents found that most looked sad only when discussing their depression (Inamdar et al. 1979). Teenagers usually desire to be with their friends and be involved in extra-curricular activities. When adolescents become depressed, their symptoms often evolve into boredom, apathy, and lack of attention to their friends and interests. They may become socially withdrawn and often report feeling lonely and unloved (Inamdar et al. 1979). They tend to have few friends, poor peer relationships (Goodyer et al. 1989; Puig-Antich et al. 1985a, 1985b), and negative self-esteem (Asarnow 1988). There is some evidence that the social skills deficits and psychological morbidity associated with major depressive disorder in adolescents may persist after recovery from the depressive episode (Rao et al. 1995).

Poor school performance, a change in grades, or academic failure may be important markers of adolescent depression related to impaired concentration, fatigue, and withdrawal. Conduct disorders, promiscuous sexual behavior, and substance abuse are also common among depressed adolescents and often complicate the clinical picture. Drug abuse is the presenting symptom in approximately 20% of adolescents with a mood disorder (E.B. Weller and Weller 1990).

Adolescents with major depression have a twofold to fourfold greater risk for depression as young adults (Pine et al. 1998). Adolescent major depressive disorder can co-occur with conduct, anxiety, and substance use disorders both at onset and at follow-up, and the rates of these comorbid disorders may be high in patients with severe major depressive disorder, potentially confounding disorder severity with comorbidity. Children with major depressive disorder have persistent social functioning deficits in comparison with psychiatrically healthy children (Puig-Antich et al. 1985b).

Gender and Major Depressive Disorder

Epidemiological studies have documented gender differences in the prevalence of depressed mood, depressive syndromes, and depressive disorders. However, gender is not believed to affect recovery from major depression (Kovacs et al. 1984a, 1997; McCauley et al. 1993) or its recurrence (Kovacs et al. 1984b; Rao et al. 1995). Gender was also reported to have an impact on symptom presentation. Specifically, in epidemiological, community, and some clinical samples, girls reported higher levels of depressive symptoms than boys (Allgood-Merten et al. 1990; Avison and Mcalpine 1992) and were more likely than boys to complain of depressed mood (Compas et al. 1997). Girls with depressive disorders have more inwardly directed symptoms related to feeling sad and anxious, whereas depressed boys may have higher rates of irritability and acting-out behaviors such as running away, theft, or substance abuse (Ostrov et al. 1989). In community samples, girls had lower self-worth or poorer self-esteem than boys (Avison and Mcalpine 1992). Lewinsohn et al. (1999) reported that females were more likely to develop major depressive disorder and adjustment disorder in young adulthood, whereas males were more likely to develop nonaffective Axis I disorders and Axis II psychopathology. Additional research is needed to determine whether gender effects are detectable on other clinical parameters of major depressive disorder during adolescence or later in development.

■ Dysthymic Disorder

Diagnostic criteria for dysthymic disorder in children and adolescents require the presence of a persistent depressed or irritable mood that occurs for most of the day, for more days than not, and for at least 1 year. This varies from the criteria for adults, for which the duration of the mood disturbance must be at least 2 years. As with major depressive disorder, the symptoms must result in clinically significant distress or impairment in functioning or require markedly increased effort to maintain a previous level of functioning. During the initial 1-year interval, a major depressive episode must not be present (American Psychiatric Association 2000). After the initial year, major depressive episodes may be superimposed on the dysthymic disorder. This is referred to as "double depression."

Early-onset dysthymic disorder has a protracted course (mean episode length is 4 years) and is associated with increased risk for subsequent major depressive disorder (76%), bipolar disorder (13%), and substance abuse (15%) (Kovacs et al. 1984a, 1984b, 1994; Lewinsohn et al. 1991). Children with dysthymic disorder usually have their first episode of major depressive disorder 2–3 years after the onset of dysthymia. Kovacs et al. (1994) theorized that dysthymic disorder is one of the "gateways" to the development of recurrent mood disorders. Results from their longitudinal prospective study revealed several characteristics of dysthymic disorder. Dysthymic disorder presented at an earlier age than major depressive disorder. Dysthymia also had frequent symptoms of mood dysregulation, low rates of anhedonia and neurovegetative symptoms, and greater overall risk for subsequent mood disorder. After the first episode of major depressive disorder, the clinical course of the initially dysthymic youths was similar to the course of the comparison subjects with regard to rates of recurrent major depression, bipolar disorder, and certain nonaffective disorders. The authors concluded that childhood-onset dysthymic disorder is an early marker of recurrent mood disorder.

Teenagers with dysthymic disorder may have significant academic, social, and psychological deficits, including hopelessness and low self-esteem (Kashani et al. 1989). The interval between the onset of dysthymia and the first major depression provides a window of opportunity for intervention and possible prevention of later episodes (Kovacs et al. 1994).

■ Bipolar Disorder

Bipolar disorder is a chronic and recurrent condition. It often begins in adolescence and is associated with marked impairment in family, social, and occupational functioning. Compared with adults, children and adolescents with bipolar disorder may have a more prolonged early course and be less responsive to treatment (McGlashan 1988; Strober et al. 1995). Bipolar disorder lifetime prevalence rates as high as 1% (Lewinsohn et al. 1995) have been reported.

Bipolar I disorder requires the existence of a manic or mixed episode. A manic episode is defined in DSM-IV-TR as a distinct period of "abnormally and persistently elevated, expansive, or irritable mood" (American Psychiatric Association 2000, p. 357). A mixed episode is characterized by "rapidly alternating moods with symptoms of a manic episode and a major depressive episode" (American Psychiatric Association 2000, p. 362). The duration of the mood disturbance should be at least 1 week. The episode should be severe enough to require hospitalization, cause marked impairment in functioning, or have psychotic features. During the period of mood disturbance, at least three (or four if the mood is irritable rather than elevated or expansive) of the following symptoms must be present: 1) inflated self-esteem or grandiosity, 2) decreased need for sleep, 3) more talkativeness than usual or pressure to keep talking, 4) flight of ideas or racing thoughts, 5) distractibility, 6) increased goal-directed activity or psychomotor agitation, and 7) excessive involvement in pleasurable activities that have a high potential for painful consequences (American Psychiatric Association 2000, p. 362).

Bipolar II disorder is characterized by one or more major depressive episodes accompanied by at least one hypomanic episode, which is defined as "a distinct period during which there is an abnormally and persistently elevated, expansive, or irritable mood that lasts at least 4 days" (American Psychiatric Association 2000, p. 365). It should be accompanied by a minimum of three (if the mood is elevated or expansive) or four (if the mood is irritable) of the above-mentioned seven manic symptoms. A hypomanic episode, in contrast to a manic episode, is not severe enough to require hospitalization and does not cause a marked impairment in social or other important areas of functioning.

Cyclothymic disorder, a bipolar disorder of milder clinical symptomatology is described as a chronic and fluctuating mood disorder. The onset is usually in adolescence or early adult life and is characterized by "numerous periods of hypomanic and depressive symptoms" (American Psychiatric Association 2000, p. 398). Both the hypomanic and depressive symptoms must be insufficient in number, severity, duration, and pervasiveness to meet full criteria for a manic or major depressive episode. In children and adolescents, symptoms must be present for an initial period of at least 1 year and there should not be a symptom-free interval longer than 2 months. As with dysthymic disorder, cyclothymic disorder is characterized as a chronic but less se-

vere mood disorder. Unlike dysthymic disorder, however, cyclothymic disorder is not frequently diagnosed in clinical settings.

Although the adult DSM-IV-TR criteria for diagnosing child and adolescent depressive disorders have proven to be fairly reliable, the same can not be said for the adult DSM-IV-TR criteria for classifying manic episodes in children and adolescents. A retrospective review by R.A. Weller et al. (1986) found that nearly half of children who met criteria for mania had been misdiagnosed with such disorders as schizophrenia. Diagnosing bipolar disorder in children and adolescents can be a difficult task because of several factors. First, when manic symptoms initially appear in adolescence, they may build up gradually or be less severe and thus not receive clinical attention. The first episode of a mood disorder in adolescents with bipolar disorder is often not a manic episode. Of the 18 adolescents with bipolar disorder in a community sample of 1,709 adolescents, the disorder began with a manic or hypomanic episode in only 1 (5.5%); it started with a major or minor depressive episode in 11 (61.1%); and in 6 (33.3%) the first episode could not be determined (Lewinsohn et al. 1995). McGlashan (1988) noted that a delay of up to 5 years often occurs between the onset of symptoms during adolescence and an episode of sufficient severity to require hospitalization or treatment. As a result of the variation in presentation and diagnostic overlap with other disorders (such as externalizing disorders), there are no large-scale, long-term studies to determine the exact prevalence of early-onset bipolar disorder. Recent literature has called for diagnostic criteria that are more developmentally appropriate and provide more validity and reliability (Coyle et al. 2003).

Second, an "atypical" clinical presentation of mania in children and adolescents may be common. In general, psychotic symptoms, suicidal attempts, inappropriate sexual behavior, and a "stormy" first year of illness were reported by E.B. Weller et al. (1995) as common symptoms of child and adolescent mania. Kovacs and Pollock (1995) reported some youngsters with mania show serious acting-out behaviors, including burglary, stealing, vandalism, and a history of school suspensions. Behavioral symptoms that masked bipolar disorder were reported by Isaac (1992). In his study of 12 adolescents (ages 13–19 years) with behavioral disorders, 8 were found to have the characteristics of bipolar disorder on follow-up.

Infants and Preschool-Age Children

Symptoms of mania vary among age groups. Episodes of manic behavior have been reported in children as young as 1 year of age. In preschool-age children, explosive and unmanageable temper tantrums, sexual joking, and nightmares with violent imagery were described by Popper (1984).

School-Age Children

Mania in school-age children is characterized by pressured speech, which is difficult or impossible to interrupt. Children frequently describe racing thoughts in very concrete terms. For example, children state that they are not able to get anything done because their thoughts keep running in their head "like a wound-up motor." Increased motor activity and goal-directed behavior, involvement in pleasurable activities with a high level of danger, hypersexuality, disordered sleep patterns with decreased need for sleep, high activity levels in the bedroom before sleep, and other symptoms are typical for manic school-age children (Varanka et al. 1988). In addition, children with manic episodes do not present with the same dis-

crete periods as seen in adults. The time course for manic episodes in early-onset bipolar disorder has been described as highly variable, often with a chronic, non-episodic, and rapid-cycling presentation (Geller and Luby 1997; Wozniak et al. 1995).

Adolescents

Carlson et al. (1994) and Carlson and Kashani (1988a) reported manic symptoms to be common in adolescence, but full-blown bipolar disorder may be rare. Developmental issues and symptom overlap with more frequent childhood psychiatric disorders pose additional challenges in diagnosis (Bowring and Kovacs 1992). Irritability and an unpredictable and labile mood are more common than euphoria. Mixed or dysphoric episodes (McElroy et al. 1992) and psychotic features (Ballenger et al. 1982) are also common among the more severely ill teenagers with bipolar disorder.

Phenomenology

Patients who have early-onset bipolar disorder have higher rates of psychotic features than those with an older age at onset (Joyce 1984; McElroy et al. 1997; McGlashan 1988). Early onset of symptoms often indicates a more severe course of illness. Carlson et al. (2000) used data from an epidemiologically derived sample to assess similarities and differences in psychopathology in subjects with early-onset bipolar disorder (i.e., hospitalized with a first episode of psychotic mania between ages 15 and 20 years) and those with adult onset (i.e., age over 30 when hospitalized with a first episode). Several noteworthy findings come from this study. First, male subjects predominated in the early-onset group: 69.6% of subjects in the early-onset group were male, while only 26.6% of subjects in the adult-onset group were male. Additionally, subjects with early-onset psychotic mania were significantly more likely to have had a clinically significant behavior disorder in childhood and more frequently demonstrated poor school performance. The early-onset subjects were significantly more likely to have a substance use disorder at the onset of their mood disorder and were significantly more likely to report paranoid (100% vs. 80%) and grandiose (73.9% vs. 40%) delusions. However, the likelihood of mood-incongruent psychotic symptoms, formal thought disorders, or hallucinations did not differ between the groups. Early-onset subjects also experienced fewer remissions and spent more time in the hospital during the 24-month follow-up period than adult-onset subjects. Manic episodes recurred more frequently in early-onset subjects (64.7% vs. 12.5%), and depressive episodes recurred more frequently in adult-onset subjects (62.5% vs. 17.6%). At the 6-month research consensus diagnosis conference, 100% of the adult-onset subjects but only 81.8% of the early-onset group were identified as having bipolar disorder. Mixed episodes were much more likely to be experienced by early-onset subjects (26.1% vs. 3.3%) and were the most difficult to diagnose. They were often initially diagnosed as psychosis not otherwise specified, drug-induced psychosis, or schizoaffective disorder.

Children and adolescents with bipolar disorder may have a more prolonged early course and be less responsive to treatment than adults (McGlashan 1988; Strober et al. 1995). This may be due to the fact that adolescents with bipolar disorder frequently present with mixed features, psychotic symptoms, and comorbid behavior/substance abuse. These all predict a more refractory response to lithium. In a 5-year prospective, naturalistic, follow-up study of 54 adolescents with bipolar disorder, 2 subjects never achieved complete remission (Strober et al. 1995). Of the remaining

52 subjects who recovered from their index episode, 23 had a relapsing course (either major depression or mania), and 11 of these subjects had two or more additional episodes. Recovery from the index episode took longer for patients with depression (median time to recovery, 26 weeks) than for patients with either mania (median recovery time, 9 weeks) or mixed episodes (median recovery time, 11 weeks). Long-term studies of hospitalized bipolar patients suggest the short-term course is not necessarily predictive of ultimate functioning, especially in young people (Carlson et al. 1977; McGlashan 1988). Thus, follow-up is needed.

Comorbidity and Differential Diagnosis

Comorbidity in children and adolescents with mood disorders is the rule rather than the exception. In general, comorbid diagnoses appear to influence the risk for recurrent episodes, duration of the symptoms, suicide attempts or suicidal behavior, functional outcome, response to treatment, and utilization of mental health services (Brent et al. 1993; Kovacs et al. 1993; Lewinsohn et al. 1995).

■ Major Depressive Disorder

Clinical (Kovacs et al. 1984b; Ryan et al. 1987) and epidemiological studies (Angold and Costello 1993; Bird et al. 1988; Kashani et al. 1987a; Rohde et al. 1991) have found that 40%–70% of depressed children and adolescents have comorbid psychiatric disorders. At least 20%–50% have two or more comorbid diagnoses. The most frequent comorbid diagnoses are dysthymic disorder (30%–80%), anxiety disorders (30%–80%), disruptive disorders (10%–80%), and substance abuse (20%–30%). Major depressive disorder is more likely to occur after the onset of other psychiatric disorders (except for substance abuse) (Biederman et al. 1995; Kovacs et al. 1989; Reinherz et al. 1993a). However, conduct problems may develop as a complication of the depression and may persist after the depression remits (Kovacs et al. 1988). In general, comorbidities are associated with a more severe and persistent course of depression (Birmaher et al. 1996b) and are therefore important to recognize and address in treatment.

Kovacs et al. (1984a) first reported the association between major depressive disorder and dysthymia in children. Among a group of referred 8- to 13-year-old children, 38% of those with major depressive disorder had underlying dysthymia, and 57% of those with dysthymia had concurrent major depressive disorder. In a community sample of adolescents (ages 14–18 years), 33% of those with major depressive disorder also had a diagnosis of dysthymic disorder, but only 7% of those with dysthymic disorder also had major depressive disorder (Lewinsohn et al. 1991). These figures are higher than those reported in adults (Keller and Shapiro 1982). In particular, youth with double depression (major depressive disorder and dysthymic disorder) have been found to have more severe and longer depressive episodes, a higher rate of comorbid disorders, more suicidality, and worse social impairment than youths with either major depressive disorder or dysthymic disorder alone (Ferro et al. 1994; Kovacs et al. 1994; Lewinsohn et al. 1991).

The comorbidity of depression and anxiety may also have clinical implications, as evidenced by studies showing increased severity and duration of depressive symptoms, increased risk for substance abuse, increased suicidality, poor response to psychotherapy, and more psychosocial problems with the presence of comorbid anxiety (Brent et al. 1988, 1993; Kovacs et al. 1989).

Depressive and externalizing disorders often are comorbid and may represent more serious psychopathology than either condition alone. In clinical samples, 36%–80% of depressed juveniles meet criteria for conduct disorder (Ferro et al. 1994; Kovacs et al. 1988). In an epidemiological study, more than 50% of children and adolescents with mood disorder also had conduct disorder or oppositional defiant disorder (Bird et al. 1988). Youth with both depressive and conduct disorders have been reported to be at increased risk for suicide (Brent et al. 1988) and to have less favorable short-term clinical outcomes (Harrington et al. 1991). According to Asarnow (1988), child psychiatric inpatients with these comorbid diagnoses had worse peer relationships than the ones with depression but no conduct disorder. Young adults who had depression and conduct problems in childhood reported greater social dysfunction in adulthood than those who had depression only (Harrington et al. 1991). Depressed patients with comorbid disruptive disorders were reported as having worse short-term outcome, fewer melancholic symptoms, fewer recurrences of depression, a lower familial aggregation of mood disorders, a higher incidence of adult criminality, more suicide attempts, higher levels of family criticism, and a higher response to placebo than patients with major depressive disorder who did not have disruptive disorders (Harrington et al. 1991; Hughes et al. 1990; Kutcher et al. 1989; Puig-Antich et al. 1989b).

Substance use disorder is often comorbid with depressive disorders in adolescents. Rao et al. (1995) examined demographic, clinical, and biological factors associated with the development of substance use disorders. Twenty-eight adolescents (mean age: 15.4 ± 1.3 years) with unipolar major depression and no history of substance use disorders were compared with 35 group-matched psychologically healthy control subjects. After 7 years of follow-up, risk for substance use disorders was high in both groups (34.6% in the depressed group vs. 24.2% in the control group). Depressed adolescents had an earlier onset of substance use disorders and greater psychosocial impairment than did control subjects.

More than 60% of depressed adolescents appear to have comorbid personality disorders, with borderline personality disorder accounting for 30% of all diagnosed comorbid personality disorders (Kutcher et al. 1989). After the depression has remitted, however, personality disorder symptoms are often no longer evident. This indicates the value of giving only provisional or no personality disorder diagnoses in children and adolescents in general and during acute depressive episodes in particular.

Several disorders are included in the differential diagnosis. In the school-age child, adjustment disorder with depressed mood in response to a circumscribed noxious event in a child's life (e.g., parents' divorce or sibling's birth) must be considered in the differential diagnosis of depression. Children with adjustment disorder with depressed mood do not satisfy criteria for a major depressive episode but may have a few depressive symptoms. Normal bereavement should also be in the differential diagnosis because 39% of children who experience the death of a parent satisfy criteria for major depression in the 3 months after the death of a parent (E.B. Weller and Weller 1990).

Another important consideration is substance-induced mood disorder with depressive features. This is diagnosed when the depressed mood is due to the physiological effects of a medication (such as steroids), a drug of abuse, expo-

sure to a toxin, or other somatic treatment. A substance-induced mood disorder with depressive features is distinguished from a major depressive disorder or other depressive disorders by considering the onset, course, and clinical presentation (E.B. Weller et al. 2004b). Substance-induced mood disorder with depressive features arises only in association with the states of withdrawal or intoxication, whereas primary depressive disorders may precede the onset of substance use or may occur during times of sustained abstinence. Because the use of alcohol and illegal drugs is widespread among adolescents, this factor must always be considered in the differential diagnosis. Medically or psychiatrically ill youngsters are likely to be taking prescribed medications. It is crucial to examine the patient's list of medications (including over-the-counter medications) and dosages to rule out drug–drug interactions, toxicity, and pharmacologically induced depressive symptoms (E.B. Weller et al. 2004b).

Many medical conditions can produce symptoms of depression. Such conditions include malignancy, brain injury, infection, endocrine disorders, metabolic abnormalities, acquired immunodeficiency syndrome (AIDS), multiple sclerosis, and chronic fatigue syndrome. Migraine headaches (which frequently begin during adolescence) may be associated with shifts in mood, depression, and irritability. Seizure disorders should be considered in the differential diagnosis of depressive disorders because focal seizures in individuals with brain damage may present as sudden fluctuations in mood. Children and adolescents with intracranial tumors may develop not only seizures but also increased intracranial pressure, which may present initially as a change in mood. Apathy, bradykinesia, and anhedonia are most commonly seen in individuals with right-hemisphere problems, frontal lobe damage, or disorders of dopaminergic transmission. Patients who are 25% above or below ideal body weight or have other clinical indicators should be tested for thyroid and adrenal dysfunction. Testing for mononucleosis is also recommended for depressed children and adolescents. Those in high-risk groups should be tested for human immunodeficiency virus (HIV) (E.B. Weller et al. 2004b).

Infants or toddlers who look sad, seem depressed or apathetic, and are not gaining weight should be evaluated for organic failure to thrive. The differential diagnosis would include central nervous system, hormonal, metabolic, and gastrointestinal disorders. In the absence of organic reasons for failure to thrive, etiologies such as neglect, abuse, and Munchausen syndrome by proxy should be considered. Hospitalization may be helpful in clarifying the diagnosis, because children whose failure to thrive is nonorganic quickly improve their affect and gain weight under the care of nurturing professionals. The clinician also must carefully assess these children's primary caretakers (usually mothers), who often have undiagnosed depression, so that they can be treated and thus be better able to care effectively and safely for their children. Similarly, in the depressed preschool child, a malignancy or neglect and abuse (both physical and sexual) must be ruled out when considering the diagnosis of depression (E.B. Weller and Weller 1990).

The excessive weight loss and emaciated appearance of an anorexic adolescent combined with a history of intense fear of gaining weight and disturbance in body image help to differentiate anorexia nervosa from a depressive disorder. Hyperphagia may be present in both bulimia nervosa and major depressive disorder. However, the inappropriate compensatory behaviors (vomiting, excessive exercise, or use of purgatives) and characteristic preoccupation with body shape and weight are not typically seen in patients with depressive disorders (E.B. Weller et al. 2004b).

When there is a history of psychotic symptoms (such as delusions, hallucinations, or disorganized speech or behavior), their severity, scope, duration, and prominence in relation to mood symptoms must be determined. This is necessary to differentiate a mood disorder with psychotic features from a psychotic disorder such as schizophrenia.

■ Bipolar Disorder

The occurrence of comorbid psychiatric disorders in bipolar disorder is high. A recent review suggested the occurrence of comorbid disorders with bipolar disorder is nearly 100% (Kessler et al. 2001). The most frequent comorbid diagnosis was ADHD. It was seen in 27%–90% of children and 30% of adolescents with bipolar disorder. Conduct disorder, anxiety disorders, substance abuse, and personality disorders are also frequently reported as comorbid with bipolar disorder. These common comorbidities often affect the outcome and treatment course of bipolar disorder (Kim and Miklowitz 2002).

Due to the diagnostic complexity of bipolar disorder in children and adolescents, many conditions must be considered in the differential diagnosis. Many medical conditions can mimic symptoms of bipolar illness. Manic symptoms can result from a variety of neurological disorders such as: head trauma, multiple sclerosis, and temporal lobe seizures. Manic episodes and bipolar disorders have been reported to occur after traumatic brain injury. However, their occurrence is less frequent than that of depressive episodes following brain injury.

Damage to the basal region of the right temporal lobe and right orbitofrontal cortex in patients with a family history of bipolar disorder appears to predispose to the development of mania (E.B. Weller et al. 2004b).

Use of various medications (e.g. steroids, antidepressants, stimulants) and illicit substances (e.g., amphetamines, cocaine) has been associated with manic symptoms and should be considered in the differential diagnosis of mania. The classic example is that of euphoric mood, decreased need for sleep, decreased appetite, grandiosity, and increased goal-directed activity, which are associated with cocaine intoxication. In the intoxicated state, the symptoms are indistinguishable from those of acute mania. However, without repeated administration of cocaine, the euphoric effects are short-lived and are followed by symptoms of dysphoria referred to as the "crash." Antidepressant-induced mania has been well described in adult psychiatric literature and has also been reported in adolescents (Achamallah and Decker 1991; Rosenberg et al. 1992).

Sexual abuse is especially important as a differential diagnosis during the childhood years because manic hypersexuality is often manifested in children by self-stimulatory behaviors, including frequent masturbation in public. Therefore, it is essential to obtain a careful history of sexual abuse and exposure to inappropriate adult sexual behaviors (E.B. Weller et al. 2004a).

Children and adolescents with bipolar disorder are frequently misdiagnosed as having schizophrenia. Mood-incongruent hallucinations, paranoia, and thought disorders have been reported to be associated with bipolar disorder (E.B. Weller et al. 2004b). However, in contrast to bipolar disorder, children with schizophrenia usually have an insidious onset

of illness, lack the engaging quality associated with mania, and are less likely to have a family history of mania. In the past, psychotic mood disorders in youth were frequently misdiagnosed as schizophrenia (Ferro et al. 1994; R.A. Weller et al. 1986). Some clinicians have argued that, if in doubt, a mood disorder should be diagnosed rather than schizophrenia, as schizophrenia is generally believed to have a less favorable prognosis and a poorer response to treatment (E.B. Weller and Weller 1991).

Lewinsohn and colleagues (1995) also found a high degree of comorbidity between bipolar disorder and disruptive behavioral disorders. The difficulty in differentiating childhood mania from conduct disorder is not surprising, because juvenile mania is frequently mixed (dysphoric). It also can be associated with affective storms, or prolonged and aggressive temper outbursts (Carlson 1983, 1984; Davis 1979), which can include threatening or attacking behavior toward family members, children, adults, and teachers. Children with conduct disorder and children with mania often become involved in dangerous acts with painful consequences. However, children with mania are typically mischievous rather than vindictive and calculating. Their conflicts with authority usually result from poor judgment and grandiosity (E.B. Weller et al. 1995).

Children and adolescents with bipolar disorder have high rates of comorbid ADHD. Systematic studies of children and adolescents found rates of ADHD ranging from 57% to 98% in bipolar patients (Geller et al. 1995; West et al. 1995; Wozniak et al. 1995). A leading source of diagnostic confusion in prepubertal mania is the symptom overlap with ADHD. Because distractibility, impulsivity, hyperactivity, and emotional lability can be present in both ADHD and bipolar disorder, the differential diagnosis can be difficult (Carlson 1984). Although ADHD and mania should be considered in the differential diagnosis of both disorders, they can and frequently do coexist, which adds to the diagnostic difficulty (Biederman et al. 1996).

ADHD differs from mania in several respects. The onset of ADHD is typically in the preschool age when the child starts to walk or early elementary school years (i.e., before age 7 years), whereas the onset of mania is more common after puberty. The sleep disturbance and overactivation associated with ADHD are chronic and are part of the child's baseline behavior. The sleep disturbance in mania is associated with the onset of the mood disturbance and is often described as a diminished need for sleep instead of inability to sleep. ADHD is not associated with psychosis, flight of ideas, euphoria, or grandiosity, which are common symptoms in mania. In contrast, children with ADHD usually display low self-esteem. The overactivity of a manic child is goal directed, whereas that of a child with ADHD is often disorganized and haphazard (E.B. Weller et al. 2004a). Wozniak et al. (1995) reported that juvenile mania is often comorbid with ADHD and recommended examining overlapping symptoms to determine the robust quality of the diagnosis.

The often observed high rate of comorbidity of substance abuse/dependence and bipolar disorder is important to consider, because "secondary" substance use may be more amenable to treatment and have a better prognosis (Geller and Luby 1997; Winokur et al. 1995). In addition, comorbidity of mood and substance use disorders has been correlated with increased suicide risk in older adolescents and young adults (Rich et al. 1986, 1990).

Epidemiology

Depressive disorders affect 0.3% of preschoolers, 1%–2% of elementary school-age children, and 5% of adolescents (Anderson et al. 1987; Bird et al. 1988). However, no large-scale epidemiological studies have been done on the prevalence of major depressive disorder in prepubertal children. Two percent of a sample of 9-year-old children from the general population were reported to be depressed (Kashani et al 1983). In specialized populations, depression was reported in 7% of children admitted to pediatric hospitals for medical reasons (Kashani et al. 1981) and in 40% of children in pediatric neurology clinics presenting with headaches (Ling et al. 1970).

In the United States, 1.3 million adolescents between the ages of 15 and 19 years experience depression each year (Angold et al. 1998). Population studies have found prevalence rates of depression between 0.4% and 8.3% in adolescents (Lewinsohn et al. 1993a, 1994c). The lifetime prevalence rate of major depressive disorder in adolescents has been estimated to range from 15% to 20%, which is comparable to the lifetime rate of major depressive disorder in adults (Kessler et al. 1994; Lewinsohn et al. 1986, 1993a, 1993b).

Several studies have reported on the prevalence of major depressive disorder in adolescents. Kashani et al. (1987a) used a structured interview to assess a community sample of 150 adolescents. The prevalence was 4.7% for major depressive disorder and 3.3% for dysthymic disorder. Further epidemiological studies on dysthymic disorder have reported point prevalence rates from 1.6% to 8.0% in adolescents (Kashani et al. 1987a, 1987b; Lewinsohn et al. 1993a, 1994c). Lewinsohn et al. (1993a) studied point prevalence, lifetime prevalence, 1-year incidence and comorbidity of depression with other disorders in a randomly selected sample of 1,710 high school students. Of this population, 9.6% met criteria for a current depressive disorder, more than 33% had experienced a depressive disorder over their lifetimes, and 31.7% of the latter had experienced a second disorder.

Before puberty, major depressive disorder occurs at approximately the same rate in girls as in boys, whereas in adolescents, the female-to-male ratio is estimated to be approximately 2:1, similar to the ratio reported in adults (Fleming and Offord 1990; Kessler et al. 1994; Lewinsohn et al. 1994b). Lewinsohn et al. (1993a) reported an overall 1-year first incidence of major depression in 112 high school students ages 14–18 years to be 5.26% (7.14% for females and 4.35% for males). For dysthymia, the rates were 0.13% for females and 0% for males. Kashani et al. (1987b) reported that among depressed adolescents ages 14–16 years, girls outnumbered boys by a ratio of 5:1. Whitaker et al. (1990) studied a sample of 356 high school students and also found depressive disorders to be more common in girls than in boys. The combined lifetime prevalence rates for both sexes in this study were 4.0% for major depression and 4.9% for dysthymia. These researchers also found that the pattern of sex distribution of depression observed in adults does not appear until puberty, when the rate of depression quadruples in girls and doubles in boys. They postulated that the youngsters with an earlier age at onset of depression appear to have a first major depressive episode of longer duration and of greater severity than those with later age at onset (Clarke et al. 1995; Garland and Weiss 1995; Lewinsohn et al. 1994b). The incidence of major depressive disorder in adolescents observed in several

studies was significantly higher than that reported in many adult studies. In adolescents, annual incidence rates of 1.1% for males and 2.0% for females were reported in the Epidemiologic Catchment Area study (Eaton et al. 1989; Marangell et al. 1997). Similarly, Weissman and colleagues (1993), in a cross-cultural study, demonstrated rates of major depression and dysthymia that were higher in females than in males.

The following general conclusions can be drawn. There is a tendency for major depressive disorders to have a higher incidence among adolescents than among preschool or prepubertal children (Kashani et al. 1987a). Discrepancies between the prevalence and incidence rates of major depression in adolescents and adults may be explained by the use of different methodologies. It is possible that adolescents may have a lower threshold for reporting depressive symptoms.

There are reports indicating that the incidence of depression is greater among those from lower socioeconomic classes. Some researchers have also found an association between the incidence of depression and major life events such as health problems, family disorder, conflict with parents, or death of a parent (Lewinsohn et al. 1994d; Reinherz et al. 1993b). For example, remarriage of a parent for males and death of a parent for females significantly increased the risk of developing major depressive disorder (Reinherz et al. 1993b). However, Lewinsohn et al. (1994c) found that the death of a parent or living with fewer than two biological parents did not increase risk for depression in adolescents. Therefore, it is currently unclear if undesirable life events or family structure are always associated with increased incidence of major depressive disorder. E.B. Weller et al. (2004a) reported that 33% of adolescents experience depression within the first year of a parent's death, most often within the first 3 months of the death.

Available data on bipolar disorder in childhood and adolescence are mostly derived from patient samples. In comparison to major depressive disorder, bipolar disorder is much less common in the general population. Lifetime prevalence is estimated as 0.4%–1.6% among adults. Carlson and Kashani (1988a) studied 150 adolescents in a community sample and found that 20 (13.3%) had periods of at least 2 days during which they experienced four or more manic symptoms. None of these adolescents exhibited sufficient impairment to meet criteria for a manic episode, but 3 (1.5%) appeared to qualify for a diagnosis of bipolar II disorder or cyclothymia.

Lewinsohn et al. (1995) conducted an epidemiological study using a community sample of adolescents. Subjects were randomly selected Oregon high school students who were assessed with a structured diagnostic interview—the Schedule for Affective Disorders and Schizophrenia for School-Age Children (K-SADS)—at two different times: at baseline ($n=1{,}709$) and at follow-up approximately 1 year later ($n=1{,}507$). Bipolar disorder was diagnosed in 18 subjects after the two evaluations. Thus, the prevalence of bipolar disorder was approximately 1%. Of the 18 subjects with bipolar disorder, 2 met full DSM-III-R (American Psychiatric Association 1987) criteria for a lifetime manic episode (bipolar I disorder), 11 met criteria for bipolar II disorder, and 5 received a diagnosis of cyclothymia. An additional 5.7% of the sample reported having experienced a distinct period of abnormally and persistently elevated, expansive, or irritable mood. However they never met criteria for bipolar disorder on follow-up.

The lifetime prevalence of bipolar dis-order is thought to approach 1% by adolescence (Lewinsohn et al. 1995). Current data on the prevalence of bipolar disorder in childhood and adolescence are based on relatively small community surveys or retrospective data and have yielded varying results. In a retrospective study involving 200 adult patients with well-established diagnoses of bipolar disorder, 0.5% reported the age at onset of their illness to have been between 5 and 9 years; 7.5% reported their onset between 10 and 14 years (Loranger and Levine 1978). In a review of 898 cases from 1977 to 1985, Goodwin and Jamison (1990) reported that 3 (0.3%) patients had onset of illness before age 10 years. However, in other studies of adults with bipolar disorder, a childhood onset was reported in up to 59% of subjects (Lish et al. 1994). Furthermore, an increasingly earlier onset of bipolar disorder in more recently born cohorts has been suggested (Gershon et al. 1987). In a recent study, Geller et al. (1998b) reported that the mean age at onset of bipolar disorder in the children they studied was 8.1 ± 3.5 years. Burke et al. (1990) found that most of their bipolar patients had an onset between the ages of 15 and 19 years.

The male-to-female ratio of bipolar disorder in children has been addressed in a few studies. Although bipolar disorder in adulthood affects both sexes equally, reports of mania in childhood suggest prepubertal-onset mania may be more common in boys than in girls particularly in the hospitalized patients (Geller et al. 1998b; Varanka et al. 1988).

Etiology and Pathogenesis

■ Biological Factors

Growth Hormone

Depressed children and adolescents had hyposecretion of growth hormone after various challenges, including insulin-induced hypoglycemia and oral administration of clonidine, levodopa, desmethylimipramine, and growth hormone–releasing hormone (Jensen and Garfinkel 1990; Ryan et al. 1994). Furthermore, blunted growth hormone response to insulin-induced hypoglycemia was reported to persist after remission of a major depressive episode. This might be a "trait" or "scar" marker for major depressive disorder (Ryan et al. 1994). These authors suggested that dysregulation in growth hormone secretion in depression may reflect changes in the central noradrenergic receptors or may be secondary to changes in other neurotransmitters such as somatomedin and somatostatin, which may be altered in some depressed patients.

Cortisol and ACTH

Cortisol has been postulated to have some role in the etiology of depression. However, dysregulation of the hypothalamic-pituitary-adrenal axis in depressed children and adolescents has not been systematically studied, and findings have varied. Some depressed individuals may have abnormal cortisol regulatory mechanisms, with a tendency to hypersecrete corticotropin-releasing hormone (CRH) or cortisol in response to stressful stimuli. Birmaher et al. (1996c) found no significant differences between prepubertal children with major depressive disorder and non-depressed control subjects in baseline or post-CRH stimulation levels of either cortisol or adrenocorticotropic hormone (ACTH). However, the depressed inpatients and subjects in melancholic subgroups were found to secrete significantly less overall ACTH. Abnormalities in ACTH secretion in response to CRH have also been observed in abused children, with the nature of the ACTH disturbances being affected by both past history of

abuse and current stressors (De Bellis et al. 1994). Some studies (Casat and Powell 1988; Puig-Antich et al. 1989a) have found that severely depressed and suicidal children and adolescents may manifest cortisol hypersecretion (Pfeffer et al. 1991b).

Thyroid Hormones

Dorn et al. (1996) examined thyroid hormone concentrations and their influence on mood and behavior in adolescents with depression. They concluded that free T_4 concentrations were lower in depressed adolescents, which suggested a relationship between negative behaviors and dysfunction of the hypothalamic-pituitary-thyroid axis. The same study also found a trend for concentrations of immunoreactive morning thyroid-stimulating hormone (TSH) to be lower in the depressed group.

Melatonin

There are only a few studies on melatonin levels in major depression in youth, and results are inconsistent.

Neurotransmitters

Major depressive disorder.   Norepinephrine and serotonin are the major biogenic amines that are believed to play an important role in the regulation of mood and consequently in the pathophysiology of depression. The major classes of antidepressants—which include monoamine oxidase inhibitors (MAOIs), tricyclic antidepressants (TCAs), and selective serotonin reuptake inhibitors (SSRIs)—appear to function by restoring regulation of the dysregulated neurotransmitter system in the brain (Ryan 1990). A possible relationship between dopamine and serotonin and mood disorders has been demonstrated in adults. It has been postulated that high levels of sex hormones during puberty may decrease the effectiveness of TCAs (Kutcher et al. 1994).

Bipolar disorder. In bipolar disorder, the Na+-K+-ATPase hypothesis (el Mallakh and Li 1993) proposes that the manic symptoms of flight of ideas, irritability, distractibility, and high energy are related to a decrease in the activity of the Na+-K+-ATPase pump, which results in increased neuronal excitability. Bipolar depression is hypothesized to be secondary to a larger decrease in pump activity and a subsequent decrease in neurotransmitter release. Guanine nucleotide binding proteins (Tappia et al. 1997) have been postulated to play an important role in the molecular etiology of bipolar disorder (Schreiber and Avissar 1991). This hypothesis is based on the finding that lithium attenuates the functioning of G-protein and dampens the oscillatory system, thereby resulting in a more stable state (Manji 2003).

Sleep Abnormalities

Depressed children and adolescents frequently report disturbed sleep (Goetz et al. 1987). However, electroencephalographic studies have had varying results and have not found consistent sleep changes paralleling those observed in adults with depression.

■ Genetic Factors

Major Depressive Disorder

Twin studies support the presence of a genetic factor in the etiology of depression. Concordance rates for depression are much higher in monozygotic twins (54%) (McGuffin and Katz 1989) than in dizygotic twins (24%) (Carlson and Abbott 1995). Adult twin studies also indicate that mood disorders are strongly heritable, with a much stronger genetic component for bipolar disorder than for major depressive disorder.

Several reports (Kutcher and Marton 1991; Mitchell et al. 1989) indicate that early-onset depression is associated with increased familial aggregation. Lifetime prevalence rates in the first-degree relatives of depressed youths have ranged from 17% (Strober 1984) to 46% (Mitchell et al. 1989; Todd et al. 1993). Lifetime rates of affective disorders in the first-degree relatives of depressed inpatient adolescents were significantly higher than expected rates in the general population (Strober 1984). Weissman et al. (1984a) reported that first-degree relatives of depressed adolescents who were suicidal may have increased lifetime rates of suicidal behavior.

Overall, family studies have consistently reported a twofold to threefold increase in the lifetime rates of depressive disorders in the relatives of depressed subjects compared with healthy control subjects (Gershon et al. 1982; Weissman et al. 1982, 1984b, 1984c). Early-onset depression (age 20 years or younger) is associated with the greatest risk for depression in family members (Puig-Antich et al. 1989b; Weissman et al. 1984c).

The lifetime risk for major depressive disorder in children of depressed parents ranged from 15% (Orvaschel et al. 1988) to 45% (Hammen et al. 1990). Factors in the depressed parent such as early onset and recurrence of depression appear to contribute to the highest risk for major depressive disorder in their children (Orvaschel 1990; Warner et al. 1995; Weissman et al. 1988). The risk for depression also increased when both parents had a mood disorder. Children of depressed parents are not only at high risk to develop depression but are also at increased risk to have other psychopathology, including anxiety and disruptive disorders (Hammen et al. 1990; Keller et al. 1988; Orvaschel et al. 1988; Warner et al. 1995; Weissman et al. 1987, 1988).

The familial aggregation of depression suggests a family genetic component for depression. However, it is possible that a vulnerability to depression and anxiety may be what is actually inherited. Thus, certain environmental stressors may be required for one of these disorders to be manifested (Kendler 1995; Warner et al. 1995).

Bipolar Disorder

Bipolar disorder may have the strongest genetic component of any psychiatric disorder. The concordance rate is much higher in monozygotic twins (65%) than in dizygotic twins (14%) (Nurnberger and Gershon 1982). Family studies of adolescent-onset bipolar disorder have found increased rates of bipolar disorder among relatives. Furthermore, early onset was associated with a higher prevalence of illness in family members (Rice et al. 1987; Strober 1992; Strober et al. 1988). Todd et al. (1993) found elevated rates of mood disorders and increased severity of mood disorders in relatives of children with bipolar affective disorder and major depressive disorder. Earlier onset and increased numbers of suicide attempts were also observed. Kutcher and Marton's (1991) study of bipolar adolescents ages 13–19 years found a significantly higher prevalence of bipolar illness in the first-degree relatives. Relatives of bipolar probands had significantly higher rates of bipolar disorder than relatives of unipolar probands. Rates of unipolar illness and other psychiatric disorders were not increased. The rate of bipolar illness in the first-degree relatives of adolescent probands was approximately 15%.

Strober et al. (1988) noted that significantly increased aggregation of bipolar I disorder in first-degree relatives and decreased antimanic response to lithium carbonate were two variables that distinguished adolescent bipolar probands with childhood-onset psychiatric illness from those who had no childhood-onset psychiatric disorders. As a general principle, it is assumed that early age at onset predicts a higher familial loading in bipolar mood disorder (Strober 1992).

Genetic studies have also suggested that environmental factors—particularly nonshared intrafamilial and extra familial environmental experiences—have an important impact. These factors include differences in how individual parents treat each of their children (Kendler 1995; Plomin 1994). Individuals at high genetic risk appear to be more sensitive to the effects of adverse environment than individuals at low genetic risk (Kendler 1995). It has also been suggested environmental effects may be, at least in part, under genetic influence (Plomin 1994).

■ Structural Brain Abnormalities

New brain imaging techniques allow the identification of structural brain abnormalities in patients with mood disorders. However, the number of studies on brain imaging in bipolar children and adolescents is very limited.

Magnetic resonance imaging studies of older adults with major depressive disorder have documented decreases in frontal lobe volume relative to age- and sex-matched comparison subjects (Coffey et al. 1993). Because the frontal lobe continues to undergo substantial maturational changes during adolescence (Jernigan et al. 1991), several authors have questioned whether a decrease in frontal lobe volume occurs in early-onset depression. Steingard et al. (1996) measured frontal lobe and lateral ventricular volume in 125 children and adolescents (ages 6–17 years) who were hospitalized for a depressive disorder. Hospitalized psychiatric patients without depressive symptoms served as a comparison group. There was decreased frontal lobe volume and increased ventricular volume in depressed subjects compared with nondepressed subjects. These results are consistent with magnetic resonance imaging findings of reduced frontal lobe volume (Coffey et al. 1993) and reduced volume of structures adjacent to the lateral ventricles, such as the putamen (Husain et al. 1991) and caudate nucleus (Krishnan et al. 1992) in adults with major depression.

Botteron et al. (1995) suggested there are structural differences in the central nervous system between young manic individuals and healthy subjects. The authors assessed ten consecutively referred 8- to 16-year-old manic and five psychiatrically healthy subjects. Magnetic resonance scans of four manic subjects and one control subject showed ventricular or white matter abnormalities. There were significant positive correlations between increasing age and both right and left ventricular volumes. Two of the eight manic subjects and no control subjects had confluent subcortical hyperintensities. Subjective review of scans and the structured ratings suggested that there were neuromorphometric differences between these children and adolescents with bipolar disorder and healthy children and adolescents.

Chang et al. (2004) compared functional magnetic resonance imaging (fMRI) results of 12 boys ages 9–18 years with a diagnosis of bipolar disorder and at least one parent with bipolar disorder with fMRI results of 10 age- and IQ-matched healthy male controls. The two groups completed various cognitive and affective tasks while undergoing fMRI. The children and adolescents with bipolar disorder appeared to have underlying abnormalities in the regulation of prefrontal-subcortical circuits.

■ Psychological Theories

There are several psychological theories on mood disorders. None alone provides a full explanation of the etiology and pathogenesis of mood disorders in children and adolescents.

Psychoanalytic Model

Psychoanalytic theory suggests that depression results from aggression turned inward after the loss of an ambivalently loved object. Gabbard (1995) identified four key points in the psychodynamic understanding of depression: 1) disruption of the early infant-mother relationship during the oral phase increases an individual's vulnerability to depression in later life; 2) depression can be related to either real or imagined loss; 3) introjection, a defense mechanism in which the person internalizes the lost object, is used to cope with the distress connected to the loss of the departed object; 4) because of mixed feelings of love, hatred, and anger toward the lost object, feelings of anger are directed inward toward the self.

Few scientific data are available to support this model. A transition from grief to pathological depression occurs in no more than 10%–15% of children and 2%–5% of adults (Akiskal and McKinney 1975). In a study of children and adolescents who lost a parent, one-third experienced depression within the first 8 weeks. Bereaved children who became depressed had abnormal dexamethasone suppression test results similar to outpatient depressed children (E.B. Weller et al. 1990).

Cognitive-Behavioral Models

In Beck's (1967) model, distorted, negative thoughts characteristic of depressed individuals are seen as underlying the depression. The cognitive model redefines depression in terms of the cognitive triad: pessimistic, deprecatory thoughts about 1) oneself, 2) one's experiences, and 3) one's future. Research with children and adolescents supports the validity and clinical utility of this model in youth (Brent et al. 1997). This model led to the development of treatment strategies aimed at modifying maladaptive cognitive patterns, which have proved to be a major advance in the treatment of depression.

Studies of depressed children and adolescents have found maladaptive attributional styles (Asarnow and Bates 1988; Seligman et al. 1984; Summerville et al. 1992), cognitive distortions (Kendall et al. 1990), and negative self-concept (Hammen 1988; Lewinsohn et al. 1994d), as well as social skills deficits, impaired problem solving, and passive or avoidant coping strategies (Adams and Adams 1991). Although these factors may not be specific to depression, they are important because they typically serve as targets of treatment in cognitive-behavioral therapy (CBT).

Learned Helplessness Model

The learned helplessness model (Seligman and Peterson 1986) connects depression to the experience of uncontrollable life events. In relation to depression, the learned helplessness model describes deficits in all areas of human responsiveness—cognitive, emotional, and motivational.

Self-Control Model

Rehm's (1977) self-control model proposes that depressed persons have deficiencies in self-monitoring, self-evaluation, and self-reinforcement that result in cognitive distortions that lead to depression. The depressed individual's misperceptions create selective attention to negative events and misattribution of personal success and failure. These result in maladaptive behavioral styles such as focusing attention on short-term rather than long-term consequences, setting unrealistic goals, engaging in excessive self-punishment, and applying inadequate positive self-reinforcement.

■ Social and Environmental Factors

Major Depressive Disorder

Studies of depressed adults, offspring of depressed parents, and depressed youth have reported a modest but significant relationship between stressful life events and depression in both clinical and community samples. The family interactions in these patients were characterized by increased conflict, rejection, problems with communication, less expression of affect, less support, and more child abuse than the family interactions of nondepressed control subjects (Kaufman 1991; Williamson et al. 1995). Furthermore, depressive symptoms in high school–age students correlated positively with higher levels of stress and negatively with higher levels of social support (Gore et al. 1992).

There are several mechanisms by which abnormal family interactions might lead to depression. Abnormal early interactions between mother and child may cause children to develop patterns of handling stress that predispose them to depression. Family conflict is also thought to be a trigger of depression in susceptible individuals. Other factors such as lack of parental affect, irritability directed toward the child, and child abuse may also contribute to increased vulnerability to depression or other psychopathology in children (Adrian and Hammen 1993). Finally, depressed children may generate conflicts that contribute to the maintenance of their parents' depression and their own depression or create conflicts in an otherwise normally functioning family.

Several studies of children (Banez and Compas 1990; Mullins et al. 1985) and adolescents (Swearingen and Cohen 1985) examined the relationship between stressful life events and symptoms of depression. Overall, these studies found that life events were positively correlated with symptoms of depression, which suggested that life events might play a causal role in the development of depressive symptoms. Specific events—including loss, divorce, bereavement, and exposure to suicide—

individually or in combination with other risk factors (e.g., lack of support) have been associated with the onset of depression (Brent et al. 1993; E.B. Weller and Weller 1991).

Exposure to suicide has been described as a severe, stressful event associated with a threefold increase in acute and recurrent major depressive disorder in friends, siblings, and mothers of the suicide victims (Brent et al. 1988, 1993). The risk of developing depression was proportional to the individual's closeness to the victim and the intensity of the exposure. Factors such as history of additional interpersonal losses, additional stressors, family psychiatric history, and prior psychopathology (including depression) also increased the risk for depression.

Lewinsohn et al. (1994c) examined psychosocial risk factors thought to be associated with depression in a community sample of 1,508 adolescents. Depressed teenagers were more likely to have a history of current or past mental illness (especially anxiety and substance use disorders), to have made a suicide attempt, to show greater pessimism and personal attributions for failure, to have a more negative body image, to have lower self-esteem, to be overly emotionally dependent on others, to be more self-conscious, to use less effective coping skills, to report less social support from family and friends, and to smoke cigarettes than nondepressed peers. Factors that were not associated with being depressed but that were predictive of subsequent depression included conflict with parents, dissatisfaction with grades, and failure to do homework. Neither major life events nor "daily hassles" appeared to act as triggers for future depression. The authors concluded that stressful events were characteristically present in depressed adolescents before, during, and after an episode of depression.

A major limitation of the research on stressful life events in early-onset depression is the fact that much of the research has focused on cross-sectional correlational data obtained from self-report checklists. Therefore, it is difficult to establish a causal relationship between the stressful events and depression because such events could be either a cause or a result of the depression. Studies using an adaptation of the adult Life Event and Difficulty Schedule Interview (Brown and Harris 1989) for use in children and adolescents found significantly more severe and nonsevere stressful life events (especially in the areas of romantic relationships, education, relationships with friends or parents, work, and health) in depressed youths 12 months before the onset of depression compared with psychiatrically healthy control subjects (Goodyer et al. 1985, 1988).

Bipolar Disorder

Although biological factors figure more prominently in the etiology of bipolar disorder, psychological and environmental influences are also important and may be involved in precipitating manic episodes. Psychodynamic theories of bipolar illness have focused on mania as a defensive reaction to depression (Gabbard 1995). Other explanations of mania include the view that manic euphoria is a compensatory reaction to profound depression or an unconscious wish fulfillment of narcissistic aspirations. The grandiose and expansive style of manic individuals is viewed as a compensatory reaction to their true feelings of extremely low self-esteem.

In summary, even less is speculated about the etiology of early-onset bipolar disorder than about the etiology of juvenile-onset depression. Most research has focused on biological mechanisms, but psychological, social, and environmental factors are also thought to play a role in precipitating episodes of mania and depression. Advances in molecular biology and neuroimaging have opened the door to further study in these areas and will certainly contribute to the future understanding of mood disorders. It must be emphasized that all of these theories contribute to the understanding of the etiology of depression and serve as some of the components of the biopsychosocial model of mood disorders (E.B. Weller et al. 2004b).

Treatment

Depressive symptomatology, even at a subsyndromal level, may predict the eventual development of a full-blown depressive episode (Clarke et al. 1995; Prien and Kupfer 1986). Therefore, treating subsyndromal depressive symptomatology may prevent relapse and the need for more extensive treatment (Clarke et al. 1995; Kroll et al. 1996). Treatment may be divided into acute treatment, continuation treatment, and maintenance treatment. The setting selected for care is generally the least restrictive environment. Currently, treatment is oriented more to outpatient models. However, the safety and psychosocial circumstances of the child or adolescent are important considerations. Hospitalization should be considered when the child or adolescent is actively suicidal or homicidal, frankly psychotic, volatile, aggressive, or at risk for ongoing abuse or neglect if returned to the home environment. In addition, hospitalization may be appropriate when children and adolescents require medication but adequate observation or supervision is not possible because of either the psychosocial situation or complicated general medical conditions. Aggression, deterioration in symptomatic and functional status, and family discord are the main predictors or correlates of inpatient hospitalization for children and adolescents (Costello et al. 1991; Gutterman et al. 1993).

The first steps in treating a child or adolescent patient are to establish rapport and to develop a therapeutic alliance. The youth and his or her family should always be informed and educated about the diagnosis and possible choices for treatment modalities that are evidence based. As evidence-based medicine progresses, it will be determined whether pharmacotherapy, psychotherapy, or a combination of the two will provide the best treatment.

■ Major Depressive Disorder

Biological and Pharmacological Treatments

Despite insufficient evidence of safety and efficacy from randomized double-blind, placebo-controlled trials, antidepressant medications continue to be widely prescribed for children and adolescents. In 2004, it was estimated that 1 million American children were taking SSRIs, a 50% increase since 1999. In addition, it was estimated that the number of SSRI prescriptions for preschool children has increased the greatest (Ward 2004). Between 1996 and 1997 alone, the number of children ages 5 years and younger taking SSRIs jumped 500%, from 8,000 to 40,000 (Hughes et al. 1999). Arguments supporting the practice of prescribing antidepressants to children and adolescents with depression include 1) the well-studied efficacy of antidepressants in treating depression in adults, 2) the evidence for continuity between adolescent and adult depression (Harrington et al. 1990), and 3) the significant morbidity and mortality rates of adolescent depression (Kye and Ryan 1995).

However, in response to recent concern over the potential risk for increased suicidal behavior, controlled studies of antidepressants in children and adolescents are in high demand. The suggested pharmacological approaches for children and adolescents with depressive disorders are based primarily on data available from adult studies, as well as anecdotal, clinical, and research experience. There have been attempts to explain the weak response to antidepressants among youth with major depressive disorder. There is some evidence that juvenile mood disorders may be more refractory to pharmacological intervention than adult mood disorders (Ambrosini et al. 1993). Another problem in evaluating the efficacy of treatment is the fact that the average length of a depressive episode in community samples is 6 months, and in clinical samples is 8 months (Kovacs 1996; Lewinsohn et al. 1994b). However, the majority of clinical trials on either pharmacological or psychosocial treatments of depression in children and adolescents have been of 4–16 weeks in duration. This may be too brief a time to completely treat a depressive episode. As a result, there are relatively low response rates (50%–60%) with the briefer psychosocial or pharmacological treatments, as well as a relatively high rate of relapse on follow-up (Brent et al. 1998; Emslie et al. 1998; Vostanis et al. 1996; Wood et al. 1996). In regard to methodology, some have suggested that doses may have been inadequate and that too few patients were studied. In addition, the changing hormonal status of children and adolescents compared with adults was postulated to account for the poor response to TCAs, but there has been no convincing evidence that sex hormones can consistently augment antidepressant response (E.B. Weller et al. 2004b).

Selective serotonin reuptake inhibitors.
Even though SSRIs have been available for more than a decade, there are only five published placebo-controlled trials of the

efficacy and safety of SSRIs in children and adolescents: two double-blind, randomized, placebo-controlled trials of fluoxetine (Emslie et al. 1997a, 2002); a randomized, controlled study of the efficacy of paroxetine, imipramine, and placebo (Keller et al. 2001); a multicenter randomized, double-blind, placebo-controlled trial of sertraline (Wagner et al. 2003); and a randomized, placebo-controlled trial of citalopram (Wagner et al. 2004).

Emslie et al. (1997a) evaluated the comparative efficacy, safety, and tolerability of fluoxetine compared with placebo in 96 child and adolescent outpatients with nonpsychotic major depressive disorder. This study found fluoxetine to be superior to placebo in the acute-phase treatment of major depressive disorder in child and adolescent outpatients. At 8 weeks, 56% of those treated with fluoxetine were rated as "much" or "very much" improved on the Clinical Global Impressions (CGI) scale, compared with only 33% of those receiving placebo. In addition, after 5 weeks of treatment, weekly measurements of depression severity (Children's Depression Rating Scale—Revised [CDRS-R] scores) began to vary significantly between the two groups. The results of this study were confirmed in a second study of 219 outpatients, ages 8–17 years, given an 8-week trial of fluoxetine versus placebo (Emslie 2002). In this second study, response rates, defined as CGI ratings of "much" or "very much" improved, were 52% for fluoxetine versus 37% for placebo. In addition, the fluoxetine-treated group again showed significantly greater improvement of CDRS-R scores at endpoint than did those treated with placebo.

Keller et al. (2001) conducted a multicenter double blind, randomized, parallel-design comparison of paroxetine with placebo and imipramine in 275 adolescents who met the DSM-IV (American Psychiatric Association 1994) criteria for a current episode of major depression of at least 8 weeks' duration. Paroxetine was significantly more effective than placebo as determined by 1) a Hamilton Rating Scale for Depression (Ham-D) total score of 8 or less, 2) a CGI score of 1 (very much improved) or 2 (much improved), and 3) improvements in the depressed mood items of the Ham-D and the K-SADS-L (juvenile version of the Schedule for Affective Disorders and Schizophrenia for Adolescents—Lifetime Version). The response to imipramine was not significantly different from placebo for any measure. Based on these results, the authors suggested that paroxetine, at a mean dose of 28 mg, was well tolerated and effective for major depression in adolescents. However, Birmaher et al. (2000) examined the sample as to the presence of comorbid psychiatric diagnoses, and reported depressed adolescents with comorbid ADHD did better on imipramine than paroxetine.

Wagner et al. (2003) conducted a multicenter, randomized, double-blind, placebo-controlled trial to determine the efficacy and safety of sertraline. A flexible dose of 50–200 mg/day was used in 376 children and adolescents ages 6–17 years. All had a DSM-IV diagnosis of major depressive disorder. At the conclusion of a 10-week trial, the authors found sertraline to be significantly superior to placebo. Response rate was 69% for sertraline-treated subjects versus 59% for those treated with placebo. Sertraline was well tolerated. Common adverse reactions (gastrointestinal upset and agitation) occurred in 5% of subjects.

A multicenter randomized, placebo-controlled, double-blind study was conducted to determine the efficacy and safety of citalopram (Wagner et al. 2004). One hundred and seventy-four depressed children and adolescents, ages 7–17 years, were treated for 8 weeks with either citalopram (20–40 mg/day) or placebo. The response rate for citalopram (36%) was significantly greater than placebo (24%). Citalopram was generally well tolerated: the only adverse effects to occur at frequencies of greater than 10% were rhinitis (13.5%), nausea (13.5%), and abdominal pain (11.2%).

In summary, despite insufficient double-blind controlled trials of the safety and efficacy of SSRIs for depressed youth, available data suggest that serotonergic agents may be beneficial for depressive states in youth, but treatment should be maintained for at least 8–10 weeks. However, due to recent issues concerning SSRIs specifically, and antidepressants in general, in regard to potential suicidality, prescribing physicians must exercise caution. Fluoxetine is currently the only SSRI approved by the U.S. Food and Drug Administration (FDA) to treat depression in children older than 8 years. The FDA has also recently published a "black box" warning on all antidepressants, indicating an increased risk of suicidality in children and adolescents given antidepressant medications. In addition, the FDA has requested that all antidepressant medications be packaged in specific quantities. With each prescription, patients should also receive a medication guide, alerting them to the increased risk of suicidal thinking and behavior; patients should also receive close follow-up when initiating medication or altering dosages (FDA News 2004).

SSRI pharmacokinetics. Fluoxetine is a phenylpropylamine, paroxetine is a phenylpiperidine, and sertraline is a naphthaleneamine. Fluvozamine is a valerophenone oxime. In vitro, sertraline and paroxetine are more potent inhibitors of serotonin uptake than is fluoxetine. None of the SSRIs appreciably inhibit noradrenaline uptake in vitro. Sertraline appears to inhibit dopamine up-take to a greater extent than do the other SSRIs. Whether these relative differences have any clinical significance is unknown. Paroxetine, fluvoxamine, and sertraline have inactive metabolites, but the primary metabolite of fluoxetine, norfluoxetine, is reported to be four times more potent than fluoxetine in inhibiting serotonin reuptake (E.B. Weller et al. 2004b).

Fluoxetine, paroxetine, and sertraline are more than 90% plasma protein bound. Fluvoxamine is about 77% plasma protein bound at drug concentrations up to 4,000 ng/mL. The half-life of fluoxetine is 2 days after a single dose and 8 days after repeated dosing. Norfluoxetine, fluoxetine's active metabolite, has a half-life of 7–19 days. The half-lives of other SSRIs range from 12 to 36 hours. Although there is substantial individual variability in steady-state levels, the SSRIs appear to have a wide therapeutic range; thus, steady-state levels are thought to have little clinical significance in adults. Whether children and adolescents are different in this regard is not known (Preskorn 1997).

The SSRIs are metabolized in the liver by the cytochrome P450 (CYP) isoenzyme system and differentially inhibit the CYP isoenzymes, which can lead to drug-drug interactions with drugs that are metabolized by the same isoenzyme (DeVane 1994).

In children and adolescents, there is little information available on the impact of age on absorption, metabolism, therapeutic levels, or possible drug interactions. However, to achieve the same serum levels in children compared with adults, it has been suggested that the relative dosage (milligrams per kilogram) needs to be higher (Birmaher et al. 2003).

Other nontricyclic antidepressants. Bupropion, venlafaxine, trazodone, and nefaz-odone all have different mechanisms of action. Bupropion (an aminoketone) undergoes extensive biotransformation to three metabolites that are pharmacologically active. Increased incidence of side effects may be associated with increased levels of the metabolite hydroxy-bupropion. Side effects may worsen if bupropion is combined with fluoxetine. Bupropion is primarily noradrenergic and anticholinergic. Antihistaminic and orthostatic hypotensive effects are negligible. Concerns about seizures in bulimic adults have limited the use of bupropion. However, seizures were rare in adults when divided doses were used and dosages were below 450 mg/day. Bupropion has a half-life in adults of 10–21 hours, and it is quickly absorbed. Pharmacological data are not available for children and adolescents, but it might be expected that multiple daily doses would be even more important to use in children than in adults because the half-life is presumably shorter. Dosages used in studies of ADHD range from 3.0 to 6.0 mg/kg/day (Conners et al. 1996).

Venlafaxine (a phenylethylamine) inhibits reuptake of both serotonin and norepinephrine. Similar to the SSRIs, venlafaxine has no significant affinity for muscarinic, cholinergic, histaminic, or α_1-adrenergic receptors. It has a relatively short half-life in adults (3–7 hours) and is given in divided doses. Venlafaxine is a much less potent inhibitor of CYP 2D6 isoenzymes than SSRIs in vitro (Conde Lopez et al. 1997). Venlafaxine is one of the few newer antidepressants to have pharmacokinetic data for children and adolescents (Derivan et al. 1995). However, a double-blind, placebo-controlled study of 33 depressed subjects between the ages of 8 and 17 years was unable to attribute improvement of depressive symptoms to venlafaxine drug therapy (Mandoki et al. 1997).

Nefazodone (a phenylpiperazine) is in the same chemical class as trazodone. The antidepressant activity of nefazodone is presumed to be linked to the potentiation of serotonergic activity. Nefazodone works at both sites of the serotonin (5-hydroxytryptamine [5-HT]) receptors. It blocks the 5-HT$_2$ receptor (postsynaptic) and inhibits serotonin reuptake (presynaptic). Nefazodone has no significant affinity for α_2-adrenergic, α-adrenergic, histaminergic, dopaminergic, or cholinergic receptors and has weak α_1-adrenergic blocking activity (E.B. Weller et al. 2004b).

Studies conducted using nefazodone have been encouraging. Findling et al. (2000) conducted an 8-week open-label trial of nefazodone in 28 depressed children and adolescents to determine its pharmacokinetics and safety. It was relatively well tolerated by subjects. Wilens et al. (1997) reported improvement in seven children and adolescents with treatment-refractory and highly comorbid juvenile mood disorders who were treated with nefazodone for a mean of 13 weeks at a mean daily dosage of 357 ± 151 mg (3.4 mg/kg). The risk of life-threatening liver failure has limited the use of nefazodone.

Tricyclic antidepressants. Studies of TCAs in adults with major depressive disorder have established their efficacy in acute (Morris and Beck 1974) and maintenance treatment (Frank et al. 1990). However, literature reviews (Ambrosini et al. 1993; Kye and Ryan 1995) and a meta-analysis of 12 randomized controlled trials of TCAs in patients ages 6–18 years (Hazell et al. 1995) found that TCAs were no more effective than placebo in the treatment of depression in children and adolescents. However, it should be remembered that fewer than 300 children and adolescents have been studied in well-designed double blind,

placebo-controlled studies of TCAs in depressed children and adolescents, whereas thousands of adults have been treated in such controlled trials (E.B. Weller et al. 2004b). In the past, TCAs were considered the first line of treatment for depressive disorders. After the introduction of SSRIs and following reports of possible cardiovascular risk and sudden death associated with the use of TCAs, their use in psychiatric practice has greatly decreased.

Open trials in depressed children have found that 60%–80% respond to TCAs (Geller et al. 1986; Preskorn et al. 1982; Puig-Antich et al. 1979). A small study (*n*=22) by Preskorn et al. (1987) reported a statistically significant but clinically small antidepressant effect of imipramine in depressed prepubertal children with comorbid anxiety disorder. Also, depressed children who had abnormal dexamethasone suppression test results did better with imipramine than with placebo (Hughes et al. 1990).

To identify relevant studies that evaluated cardiovascular effects of TCAs, Wilens et al. (1996) performed a systematic search of the literature from 1967 to 1996. TCA treatment was associated with minor increases in systolic and diastolic blood pressure; in heart rate; and in the electrocardiographic conduction parameters PR, QRS, and QTc. Holter electrocardiographic monitoring and exercise testing also revealed minor treatment effects. Some electrocardiographic changes related to specific TCAs emerged. Few age-related electrocardiographic differences in TCA-treated children, adolescents, or adults were detected. Electrocardiographic abnormalities were associated with relatively higher serum TCA levels. The authors interpreted those data as suggesting a fatality rate of 1% associated with TCA overdose, primarily due to cardiovascular and central nervous system events. There was a statistically significant higher relative risk of fatality reported with desipramine compared with the other TCAs in adults (Kapur et al. 1992). By 2001, eight cases of sudden death were reported in children treated with TCAs, five of whom were on desipramine and two on imipramine (Varley 2001).

Monoamine oxidase inhibitors. In adults, MAOIs may be more effective than TCAs for depression with atypical features (Thase et al. 1995). MAOIs have several limitations, including drug–diet and drug–drug interactions and lack of published data demonstrating efficacy in children and adolescents (E.B. Weller et al. 2004b).

There are only a few studies on the use of MAOIs in adolescents. Ryan et al. (1988) reported the efficacy of irreversible mixed MAOIs from a chart review of 23 depressed adolescents, 21 of whom had not responded to treatment with heterocyclic antidepressants. Treatment with MAOIs alone or in combination with heterocyclic antidepressants resulted in 70% having "good" or "fair" response. Dietary noncompliance was a significant problem in 80% of the subjects during the study. Because of the relatively high risk of noncompliance with the tyramine-free diet in a population with high impulsivity and potential for substance use, Ryan et al. (1988) suggested the risks of MAOI treatment outweighed the potential therapeutic benefits in unreliable patients or families. In adolescents, the most important foods to avoid are pepperoni and sausage. Small amounts of chocolate may sometimes be eaten without causing a problem (E.B. Weller et al. 2000).

The selective reversible MAOIs have advantages over the classic MAOIs in terms of dangerousness, side effects, drug interactions, and cognitive effects. Furthermore, the absence of detrimental effects on cog-

nitive function of moclobemide in young adults (Hindmarch and Kerr 1992) is a significant advantage for children, for whom learning is an important task. In general, these agents are reserved for use only in the most responsible adolescents with the most treatment-resistant depression.

Summary. Currently, there is some confusion as to which pharmacotherapies are best for a depressed child or adolescent. The Texas Children's Medication Algorithm Project (Hughes et al. 1999) created a systematic pharmacological approach to depressed youngsters. They suggest that an SSRI be used, with caution, as a first-line treatment. If there is no response after a significant trial of treatment, another SSRI may be tried. If there is still not an adequate response, SSRI therapy may be augmented with medications such as buspirone, lithium, or another antidepressant. Alternatively, SSRI treatment could be discontinued and monotherapy with a different agent, such as bupropion, mirtazapine, or nefazodone could be tried. If there is still no response, combining or augmenting these antidepressants may be tried. If they fail, an MAOI may then be tried. If the above medications do not produce a significant response, a trial of electroconvulsive therapy (ECT) should be considered. To use ECT in children and adolescents, two additional child and adolescents psychiatrists need to agree that it is indicated. Currently, ECT is provided mostly by adult psychiatrists because of high malpractice coverage and they are often quite reluctant to consider ECT in children or adolescents. ECT should be seriously considered in depressed children and adolescents who have been adequately treated with multiple antidepressants and cognitive-behavioral therapy without remission, especially when they have a family history of depression that has responded only to

ECT. However, it should be remembered that the only SSRI approved by the FDA for depression in children and adolescents is fluoxetine, and there are limited scientific data to support these recommendations.

In regard to duration of pharmacotherapy, discontinuation could be considered 6–9 months after symptom resolution (unless the patient develops intolerable adverse reactions to medication). Medications should not be abruptly stopped but gradually tapered.

Psychological and Social/Environmental Treatments

Psychotherapy (including family therapy) may be effective in preschoolers. If psychotherapy is used for a depressed child, the clinician should take an active role rather than waiting for a depressed child to talk. Engaging games such as the Talking, Feeling, and Doing Games, as well as mutual storytelling are helpful. Supportive therapy with the child and the family can be productive, especially when accompanied by education about the illness. The clinician must not blame the child or the family for having caused the depression. Many families are eager to cooperate when the depression is described in terms of an illness model. As the acute phase of the illness abates, patients and families are often more open to work on family interactions that might be perceived as stressful by the depressed child and the family (E.B. Weller et al. 2004a).

Psychosocial treatments for adolescent depression may be divided into five general types: cognitive, behavioral, psychodynamic, group, and family (McCracken and Cantwell 1992).

Cognitive and behavioral therapies. Cognitive therapies for depression were initially derived from the work of Beck et al. (1979) and Ellis and Bernard (1983). Cognitive therapy is an active, problem-oriented treatment that seeks to identify and change maladaptive beliefs, attitudes, and behaviors that contribute to emotional distress. Cognitive models propose that a number of processes—including negativistic expectancies, dysfunctional attitudes or beliefs, biased attentional processes, cognitive distortions, problem-solving deficits, social skills deficits, and negativistic attributional style—may play a role in the development and maintenance of depressive disorders among adults.

Behavioral therapies for adolescent depression focus on the principles of operant conditioning and learning theories. According to behavioral theory, a depressed adolescent may be subject to the following types of influences, either singly or in combination: 1) an environment with a paucity of positive reinforcers, 2) an environment with an excess number of aversive contingencies, 3) a lack of skills to elicit positive reinforcement from others, and 4) involvement in behaviors that offend others (Lewinsohn et al. 1994a). The goal of behavior therapy is to teach skills and modify contingencies that will change the quality of the teenager's interaction with the environment.

Only a few well-designed investigations of nonpharmacological interventions such as cognitive-behavioral therapy (CBT) in children and adolescents with major depressive disorder have been published. CBT was effective in the treatment of depressed adolescents with dysphoric features. A meta-analysis by Reinecke et al. (1998) reported that CBT might be useful for reducing dysphoria among adolescents and treatment gains are maintained over time. Adolescent studies have employed various types of therapy, including CBT and relaxation therapy (Reynolds and Coats 1986) or self-control therapy and behavior therapy (Stark et al. 1987) versus a control therapy. In both studies active treatment groups provided a significant decrease in depressive or dysphoric symptoms compared to control groups at both initial and follow-up evaluations.

Kahn et al. (1990) investigated the efficacy of short-term CBT, relaxation, and self-modeling interventions for depressive symptoms in middle-school students ages 10–14 years. Subjects were randomly assigned to one of these three active treatments or to a waiting-list control group. All three active treatments significantly reduced dysphoria compared to control subjects.

CBT may have some advantages over other psychotherapeutic techniques. A study comparing 12–16 weeks of individual CBT, nondirective supportive psychotherapy, and systemic behavior family therapy in a group of 107 clinically referred, depressed adolescents showed CBT to be most efficacious for adolescent major depressive disorder in a clinical setting. CBT had the most rapid reduction in interviewer-rated and self-reported depression and the greatest increases in parent-rated treatment credibility (Brent et al. 1997). Lewinsohn et al. (1990) investigated the efficacy of two versions of a cognitive-behavioral intervention for depression. Fifty-nine high school students who met DSM-III (American Psychiatric Association 1980) criteria and Research Diagnostic Criteria for depression were randomly assigned to one of three conditions: adolescent and parent therapy, adolescent-only therapy, and waiting-list control. Adolescents in both treatment groups improved significantly more than the control subjects on self-report measures of dysphoria. Improvement was maintained at 2 years posttreatment.

Finally, Wood et al. (1996) studied the effectiveness of brief individual CBT and relaxation training for clinically depressed adolescent outpatients. A combination of cognitive, social problem solving, and symptom-focused interventions was associated with significant reductions in dysphoria and improved general adjustment. Patients who received CBT were more likely to remit from their depressive disorder than control patients.

Findings from community studies of children and adolescents designated as "at risk" as a result of having depressive symptoms have been promising. Short-term CBT was associated with a reduced risk of subsequent depression (Clarke et al. 1995). However, studies on long-term results are needed given the high risk of relapse (Harrington et al. 1990; Kovacs et al. 1984b; Rao et al. 1995). The relapse rate after the conclusion of CBT is high. Wood et al. (1996) found that more than 40% of adolescents who responded to CBT had relapsed within 6 months of remission. Brent et al. (1997) reported that approximately one-third of subjects admitted to a comparative trial of three psychosocial treatments (one of which was CBT) had a recurrence during the follow-up period. Moreover, data from other studies suggest that social impairment persists after remission of acute symptoms (Puig-Antich et al. 1985b), often into adulthood (Rao et al. 1995).

Continuity of CBT was assessed in a pilot study (Kroll et al. 1996) of continuation cognitive-behavioral therapy (CBT-C) for adolescents who remitted from major depressive disorder. There were fewer relapses in the group of adolescents who had continuation CBT for 6 months after remission than in a historical control group. In another study, 107 adolescents who met DSM-III-R criteria for major depression were randomly assigned to CBT, systemic behavioral family therapy, or nondirective supportive therapy for 12–16 weeks of acute treatment. At the end of acute treatment, CBT was found to be superior (Brent et al. 1999). Subjects were followed up periodically for 24 months after the end of acute treatment. Fifty-seven (53.3%) of the 107 randomized adolescents received additional treatment beyond that provided in the clinical trial. Median time to additional treatment from intake was 7.2 months. The rates of additional treatment and the times to additional treatment were similar in the three treatment groups despite the superior efficacy of CBT in the acute phase. The severity of the index depressive episode and comorbid dysthymia were predictors of additional treatment in the acute phase. In the follow-up period, the severity of depressive symptoms, the presence of disruptive disorders, and family problems predicted additional treatment. The authors emphasized the need to consider the treatment of an adolescent depressive episode in two phases: acute and continuation.

Prevention of depression in children and adolescents at high risk of developing depression—such as the offspring of depressed parents (Beardslee et al. 1993) and children with depressive symptoms but not a full-blown clinical depression (e.g., Dohrenwend et al. 1980; Weissman et al. 1992)—is an important goal. Studies of high school students (Clarke et al. 1995) and younger students (Jaycox et al. 1994) with subclinical symptoms of depression found that cognitive interventions reduced depressive symptoms and lowered the risk of developing depression up to 2 years after the intervention.

The Treatment for Adolescents with Depression Study (TADS) was a 12-week, multisite, double-blind, placebo-controlled study of 493 adolescents (ages 12–17 years) with a diagnosis of major depressive disorder. There were four treatment groups: 1) medication (fluoxetine) only, 2) CBT alone, 3) CBT with fluoxetine, and 4) placebo. The combination treatment group had a 71% response

rate, compared with a 61% response rate for fluoxetine alone, a 43% response rate for CBT alone, and 34.8% response for placebo. The combination of cognitive-behavioral therapy and fluoxetine had a response rate twice that of placebo (March et al. 2004).

Psychodynamic psychotherapy.   Psychodynamic psychotherapy for adolescent depression emphasizes the importance of object loss and self-critical internal representations and includes a reduction in the use of maladaptive defense mechanisms, resolution of past psychological trauma, and greater acceptance of the realistic limitations of one's family and one's own abilities. The aim of psychodynamic psychotherapy is not only to relieve the symptoms of depression but also to ensure maintenance of improvement and prevention of relapse through modification of the individual's adaptive style and personality organization. Evidence on the effects of psychodynamic psychotherapy in the treatment of adolescent depression is limited to case studies (Bemporad 1988; Kestenbaum and Kron 1987).

Interpersonal psychotherapy (IPT) is derived from psychodynamic therapy for depression in adults. It is a brief treatment directed toward the relief of symptoms through the resolution of interpersonal problems and social maladaptation associated with the onset of depression. There are four interpersonal problem areas: interpersonal deficits, interpersonal role conflicts, abnormal grief, and difficult role transitions (Klerman et al. 1984). The technique has been subsequently modified for use in depressed adolescents (Mufson et al. 1994). The most significant modifications were the addition of a fifth problem area (single-parent families) and involvement of the parents in all phases of therapy. Feedback from the school was also incorporated to ensure school attendance and to monitor performance. The duration of treatment was decreased from 16 to 12 weeks. Brief telephone sessions were allowed when the adolescent was unable to keep an appointment. Mufson et al. (1994) found that depressive symptoms, as measured by Beck Depression Inventory scores and the Milton Rating Scale for Depression, decreased significantly over the course of treatment. The most dramatic decline in symptoms occurred between weeks 8 and 12. Although these results were encouraging, no control group was used and sample size was small.

In another study (Mufson and Fairbanks 1996), depressed adolescents who received 12 weeks of modified interpersonal psychotherapy in an open clinical trial were followed up. Of the 10 adolescents who participated in the follow-up evaluation, only 1 met criteria for a mood disorder. The majority reported few depressive symptoms and had maintained improvement in social functioning, despite experiencing a significant number of negative life events. There were no reported hospitalizations, pregnancies, or suicide attempts. All of the adolescents were attending school regularly. Improvements that occurred during the 12-week open clinical trial were maintained for the next year. The positive results of these studies indicate that further study of interpersonal psychotherapy in children and adolescents is warranted.

Group therapy. Some consider group therapy the treatment of choice for adolescent depression because the developmental tasks of adolescence include emotional separation and individuation from parents and identification with a peer group (Scheidlinger 1985). Fine et al. (1991) compared two forms of short-term group therapy for depressed adolescents: a therapeutic support group (TSG) and a social skills group (SSG). Subjects in the TSG shared common problems, developed new ways to cope with stressful situations, and provided mutual support. SSG subjects focused on learning a variety of specific skills such as assertiveness, conversational skills, recognizing feelings, giving and receiving positive and negative feedback, social problem solving, and negotiating to resolve conflict. One session was devoted to each target skill. The authors hypothesized SSG would be more effective in reducing depressive symptoms. However, the subjects in the TSG improved significantly more than those in the SSG, as measured by a number of instruments. Adolescents treated with TSG therapy had significantly greater reductions in their depressive symptoms and increases in self-concept. However, these group differences were no longer evident at 9-month follow-up. Adolescents in the TSG maintained improvement. Those in the SSG caught up. However, this study was limited by the lack of a control group and the use of concurrent therapy by some subjects.

Another group intervention for depressed adolescents is the Adolescent Coping With Depression course (Clarke et al. 1990; Lewinsohn et al. 1994a). This course consists of 16 didactic sessions, each 2 hours in duration, conducted over an 8-week period. Group leaders teach adolescents methods of controlling their depressed mood through a variety of skills. In addition, a separate treatment format has been developed for the parents of depressed teenagers (Lewinsohn et al. 1991). The authors reported an 80% response rate, with no relapse over 2 years, when maintenance therapy was used.

Family therapy. Family therapy may be an important part of the treatment of depressed adolescents, although research in this area has been limited. The structural family therapy approach focuses on the relationship between family dysfunction and adolescent psychopathology. This approach emphasizes the understanding of the meaning or function of an adolescent's symptom within the context of the family unit (Minuchin 1974). Minuchin described enmeshed parent–child relationships that may perpetuate a chronic dysphoric mood in the child. Treatment in the family systems approach concentrates on the various aspects of the system that support or reinforce the depression. Family psychoeducational approaches are also being developed.

■ Bipolar Disorder

Bipolar disorder is a chronic and recurrent condition with high rates of morbidity and impairment in family, school, and social environment. Therefore, early and appropriate treatment is needed.

Biological and Pharmacological Treatments

Treatment of childhood bipolar disorder remains remarkably understudied despite an increasing body of literature documenting its occurrence (Botteron and Geller 1995; Kafantaris 1995). Because there are limited published double-blind, placebo-controlled medication studies on mania in children or adolescents (Geller and Luby 1997), clinicians are tempted to extrapolate from studies of adults. However, extrapolation from treatment of major depressive disorder in adults to children has not always been useful. Unfortunately, most clinicians have to make pharmacological treatment decisions based on the studies of adults and their own clinical experience. This situation will persist until systematic controlled studies are conducted in children and adolescents. Currently, a variety of mood stabilizers have been used to treat bipolar disorders in children and adolescents.

Lithium. Lithium carbonate has been recommended in the treatment of bipolar disorder in children (Youngerman and Canino 1978). Although lithium has been effective in adults (Schou 1968) and in some adolescents with mania (Strober et al. 1990), only a few studies have examined the efficacy of lithium in prepubertal children (DeLong and Aldershof 1987; Varanka et al. 1988). Lithium is approved by the FDA for treatment of bipolar disorder in adolescents who are 12 years and older. However, it has been used in younger children with bipolar disorder. Lithium is reported to have a shorter half-life in children than in adults (Vitiello et al. 1988). The literature on lithium suggests it can be given to children with the same safety precautions used in adults. These include monitoring renal, thyroid, calcium, and phosphorus indices at 6-month intervals (Fetner and Geller 1992; Khandelwal et al. 1984). However, a double-blind, placebo-controlled study of lithium in aggressive children found that some children develop cognitive impairment at low plasma levels (Silva et al. 1992). This was also noted in a double-blind, placebo-controlled study of lithium in depressed children at risk for developing bipolar disorder (Geller et al. 1994).

Because of the chronic course, rapid cycling, and mixed features often observed in childhood bipolar disorder, which are similar to the features that predict poor response in older individuals (Himmelhoch and Garfinkel 1986; Hsu 1986; Keller et al. 1993), the optimal duration of antimanic treatments has not been established. However, there is evidence to support long-term maintenance with lithium because subjects who discontinued lithium relapsed three times more often compared to those who continued lithium (Strober et al. 1990, 1995). Some researchers assert that it can be difficult to restabilize patients on lithium after interruptions in treatment (Ahrens et al. 1995; Schou 1995).

Numerous case reports and case series of lithium treatment for bipolar disorder in children and adolescents have suggested lithium is effective (E.B. Weller et al. 1986). In prepubertal children, open trials of lithium for bipolar disorder have reported response rates similar to those seen in adults (DeLong and Aldershof 1987; Varanka et al. 1988). In a small double-blind, randomized, placebo-controlled prospective study of lithium in 25 adolescents (13 on lithium and 12 on placebo), Geller et al. (1998a) reported that lithium may be helpful in the treatment of bipolar disorder in adolescents with comorbid substance abuse. This study suggests that substance abuse decreased in those adolescents who were on lithium but does not report in detail what was the outcome of the bipolar disorder. A study by Strober et al. (1988) found a stronger response to lithium in patients without pre-pubertal onset of psychopathology.

The distribution and elimination of lithium have been systematically studied in children and adolescents. Findings parallel observations in adults. However, evidence suggests a shorter elimination half-life and higher total clearance in children. Side-effect data are available from case reports, small case series, and systematic reporting of side effects in small, controlled efficacy studies. Common lithium side effects in children include nausea, diarrhea, tremor, enuresis, fatigue, ataxia (Silva et al. 1992), leukocytosis, and malaise. Renal, ocular, thyroid, neurological, dermatological, and cardiovascular side effects are less common. Changes in weight and growth, diabetes, and hair loss can also occur (Rosenberg et al. 1994). Children younger than age 6 years may experience neurological side effects relatively more frequently (Hagino et al. 1995).

Khandelwal et al. (1984) found no impairment in renal function in four adolescents who received lithium for 3–5 years. There is a concern regarding lithium therapy in sexually active adolescents, as it has been associated with a variety of congenital abnormalities, especially Ebstein's anomaly. However, a prospective study by Jacobson et al. (1992) reported that the risk for Ebstein's anomaly and other birth defects might be lower than was previously thought. As with adults, a medical evaluation and baseline laboratory studies should be performed before initiating lithium therapy in adolescents. Lithium levels, serum electrolytes, thyroid function and renal function should be monitored periodically. The patient and family should be educated about the use of other medications (e.g., diuretics) may affect lithium levels. Females should be advised to avoid pregnancy and breast-feeding while taking lithium (E.B. Weller et al. 2004b).

The therapeutic range for lithium blood levels is considered to be 0.6–1.2 mEq/L, based on adult data. This is usually achieved within five half-lives, but ultimately depends on the individual's lithium excretion rate. The narrow therapeutic range of lithium and the potential for significant toxicity must always be remembered.

Two approaches to calculate the dosage for lithium in children and adolescents with bipolar disorder have been published: a weight-based method (E.B. Weller et al. 1986) and a kinetics-based method (Geller and Fetner 1989). According to E.B. Weller et al. (1986), in 6- to 12-year-old children, a dosage of 30 mg/kg/day in three divided doses will produce a lithium level of 0.6–1.2 mEq/L within 5 days. Because children are often phobic of blood draws, lithium levels can be monitored using saliva levels (E.B. Weller et al. 1987). Geller and Fetner (1989) found that a single-dose,

kinetics-based method using a 600-mg lithium test dose predicted serum lithium levels in children.

Anticonvulsants.   Anticonvulsants are
also used in the acute and prophylactic
treatment of bipolar disorder in children
and adolescents. They were reported to
be most useful in the management of
mixed states and rapid-cycling bipolar
disorder (Keck and McElroy 1996; Post et
al. 1990). Although both carbamazepine
and valproate are used extensively in children and adolescents with bipolar disorder, controlled studies of these medications in this age group are still lacking.

Carbamazepine.   Carbamazepine is
FDA approved for the treatment of simple
and complex absence seizures and trigemi-
nal neuralgia in adults, but has not yet been
approved for the treatment of any psychiatric disorders in children. Several double-
blind, placebo-controlled studies showed
efficacy for carbamazepine in acute mania
in adults (Post et al. 1996). To our knowledge, no controlled studies have been published on carbamazepine in children and
adolescents with mood disorders. Nevertheless, it is frequently used in younger
patients with bipolar disorder, especially
when there are contraindications to lithium or intolerance to lithium.

The majority of reports of carbamazepine use in children and adolescents are
in those with comorbid ADHD or conduct disorder (some of whom also had
neurological disorders). Carbamazepine
was reported to be effective in seven
manic adolescents who were nonrespon-
sive to lithium (Hsu 1986), and it appeared safe and effective in treatment for
acute mania and long-term maintenance
treatment in three patients with juvenile-
onset bipolar I disorder (Woolston 1999).

Carbamazepine is usually started with a
low dose (100 mg twice a day for children
younger than 8 years), which is adjusted

upward on the basis of side effects to
achieve a blood level of 6–12 mcg/mL
(Ballenger 1988; Post et al. 1987). In children, the maintenance dose is usually 10–
20 mg/kg daily (200–600 mg/day) administered in divided doses. In adolescents,
maintenance dosage may go as high as
1,200 mg/day or more (Pedley et al. 1995;
Viesselman et al. 1993). Because of its effect on hepatic CYP, carbamazepine can
induce its own metabolism as well as that of
other hepatically metabolized medications,
which can result in lower than expected
blood levels. Plasma levels should be
checked 2–4 days after achieving a steady-
state plasma concentration. A baseline
complete blood cell count should be obtained, and differential platelet and reticulocyte counts should be periodically monitored for possible bone-marrow suppression (E.B. Weller et al. 2004b).

Common side effects are drowsiness,
loss of coordination, and vertigo. Other
potential side effects include hematological, dermatological, hepatic, and pancreatic effects. Twenty-seven cases of aplastic
anemia and 10 cases of agranulocytosis
(Ryan et al. 1999) have been reported with
carbamazepine use. Weakness, headache,
nausea, edema, and lethargy in children
taking carbamazepine may be associated
with the syndrome of inappropriate antidiuretic hormone secretion. Water retention and hyponatremia may result. Caution
should be observed with adolescent females, as there is an increased incidence of
congenital anomalies, including neural
tube defects, in the offspring of women
who took carbamazepine during pregnancy (Jones et al. 1989; Rosa 1991).

In children with seizure disorders,
cognitive and behavioral effects such as
impaired performance in learning and
memory tasks, irritability, agitation, insomnia, and emotional lability have been
reported (Carpenter and Vining 1993).
However, Stores et al. (1992) found no

significant cognitive or behavior effects after 1 year of therapy with either carbamazepine or valproate.

Valproic acid.   Valproate has been successfully used in treating mania in adults (Bowden et al. 1996). Several single case reports and small open series suggest valproic acid may be an effective mood stabilizer in children and adolescents. In three open studies, the addition of valproate to previously ineffective psychotropic treatments in hospitalized adolescents resulted in improvement (Papatheodorou and Kutcher 1993; West et al. 1994; Whittier et al. 1995).

There are a few open, uncontrolled studies of valproate on bipolar disorder. In one study, 42 children and adolescents (mean age: 11.4 years) with bipolar I and bipolar II disorder, with mixed or classic manic episodes, were randomized to treatment with valproate, lithium, or carbamazepine (Kowatch et al. 2000). Response rates were 46% for valproate, 34% for lithium, and 34% for carbamazepine. All three mood stabilizers were for the most part well tolerated. A multicenter double-blind, placebo-controlled study in its open label phase of 40 children and adolescents, ages 7–19 years, showed a greater than 50% improvement in the mania rating scale with divalproex in 61% of subjects. Unfortunately, there were not enough subjects during the placebo-controlled phase to see whether divalproate was superior to placebo (Wagner et al. 2002).

Common side effects of valproate are sedation, nausea, vomiting, appetite and weight gain, tremor, hepatic toxicity, hyperammonemia, blood dyscrasias, alopecia, decreased serum carnitine, neural tube defects, pancreatitis, hyperglycemia, and menstrual changes (Rosenberg et al. 1994). Hepatic toxicity (which may lead to death) appears to occur almost exclusively in young children, especially those younger than 2 years of age, who have been treated with a combination of anticonvulsants (Bryant and Dreifuss 1996; Silberstein and Wilmore 1996). The potential association with major congenital malformations also appears to be high with valproate. Emerging studies are demonstrating a significant risk for spina bifida, pulmonary atresia, and multiple anomalies when exposed to valproate monotherapy during pregnancy (Holmes 2004).

There is concern valproate may induce a metabolic syndrome characterized by obesity, hyperinsulinemia, lipid abnormalities, polycystic ovaries, and hyperandrogenism, particularly in younger women exposed peripubertally. In a cohort of mentally retarded Finnish women taking valproate for seizures, 80% of the women who began valproate before age 20 years had polycystic ovaries or an elevated serum testosterone concentration, as compared to the 27% of women taking other antiepileptics. In regard to women older than 20 years, 56% of those taking valproate had polycystic ovaries or elevated serum testosterone compared to 20% of those on other antiepileptics (Isojarvi et al. 1993). Isojarvi et al. (1998) found the severity of metabolic syndrome was reduced when valproate was replaced with lamotrigine in 16 women (suggesting a partial reversibility). The generalizability of these findings to psychiatric populations is unknown because reports of this syndrome, so far, are confined to women with epilepsy.

Other anticonvulsants.   Lamotrigine, gabapentin, and topiramate have been approved for treatment of epilepsy in adults. Lamotrigine has been reported to have moderate to marked mood-stabilizing effects in adults with bipolar disorder (Fatemi et al. 1997). Kusumakar and Yatham (1997) studied 22 adolescents with bipolar disorder who were refractory to treatment with a combination of divalproex and another mood stabilizer and an antidepressant. When lamotrigine was combined with divalproex in a 6-week open trial, 72% had a positive response by week 4. A 13-year-old boy with bipolar disorder responded to a combination of gabapentin and carbamazepine (Soutullo et al. 1998). Topiramate studies were discontinued in adult bipolar patients due to lack of efficacy. As a result studies in adolescents were also halted. However a retrospective chart review by Delbello et al. (2002a) reported topiramate might be an effective adjunctive therapy for children and adolescents with bipolar disorder.

Antipsychotics. Traditional antipsychotic medications have proven to be useful in the treatment of adults. However, research is limited in children and adolescents due to the fear of adverse events such as tardive dyskinesia and extrapyramidal symptoms (Worrel et al. 2000). Atypical medications, including clozapine, olanzapine, risperidone, and quetiapine, and aripiprazole have shown some promise as effective treatments in children and adolescents with bipolar disorder.

Clozapine was effective in an adolescent with bipolar disorder (Fuchs 1994) and in five children and adolescents with mixed mania who did not respond to treatment with other neuroleptics (Kowatch et al. 1995). Preliminary work found clozapine had significant antimanic and antidepressant effects in schizoaffective and bipolar patients who failed traditional medication (Worrel et al. 2000). A case series by Masi et al. (2002) reported a response to clozapine as either monotherapy or as adjunctive therapy in 10 adolescent inpatients with acute mania who had failed to improve on mood stabilizers or typical antipsychotics. The most common side effects of clozapine were sedation and weight gain (Fuchs 1994; Kowatch et al. 1995). The average weight gain in the case series by Masi

et al. (2002) was 6.96 kg at 6-month follow-up. The initial weekly blood draws required to monitor for clozapine-induced agranulocytosis hinder this agent's widespread use in children and adolescents.

Soutullo et al. (1999) reported moderate to marked improvement in 5 of 7 manic adolescents (mean age: 12–17 years) who were treated with olanzapine. An open-label study by Frazier et al. (2001) found an overall response rate of 61% in 23 children and adolescents, ages 5–14 years, with bipolar disorder. Mean weight gain in this study was 5 kg over the course of 8 weeks. Common side effects of olanzapine include somnolence, agitation and insomnia.

In a double-blind, placebo-controlled study of 156 adults, risperidone was found to be an effective adjunctive treatment to mood stabilizers for rapidly reducing manic symptoms (Sachs et al. 2002). A 3-week multicenter, double-blind, placebo-controlled trial of 259 adults demonstrated risperidone to be an effective and well-tolerated monotherapy for the acute treatment of mania (Hirschfeld et al. 2004). While no controlled studies such as these have been completed in children and adolescents, a retrospective chart review by Frazier et al. (1999) suggests that risperidone may be effective in treating the dysphoric aggression displayed in manic children. The weight gain with risperidone was an average of 1.2 kg per month over 6 months, without a tendency to plateau, in a chart review by Martin et al. (2000).

Preliminary data suggest quetiapine may be an effective and well-tolerated adjunctive treatment to divalproex for adolescent mania (Delbello et al. 2002b). As with all atypical antipsychotics, patients on quetiapine should be monitored for neuroleptic malignant syndrome, tardive dyskinesia, and weight gain. Common side effects for quetiapine include somnolence, dizziness, dry mouth, elevated liver transaminases, and constipation.

Patients on atypical antipsychotics should be alerted to the potential for weight gain and development of metabolic syndrome. Ratzoni et al. (2002) examined 50 Israeli adolescents on risperidone ($n = 21$), olanzapine ($n = 21$), and haloperidol ($n = 8$). After 12 weeks, olanzapine caused the greatest relative average weight gain, at 11.1%. The relative average weight gains on risperidone and haloperidol treatments were 6.6% and 1.5%, respectively (Ratzoni et al. 2002). Vreeland et al. (2003) suggested counseling patients and their parents about the risks and benefits of therapy before initiating treatment with an antipsychotic. Patients should also be encouraged to exercise and eat healthy food. Their weight, fasting plasma glucose, body mass index, waist circumference, and lipid profile should be monitored (Vreeland et al. 2003).

Other pharmacological treatments and electroconvulsive therapy. Other medications used in the treatment of adult bipolar disorder (e.g., calcium channel blockers, clonidine, L-thyroxine) have not been systematically studied in children or adolescents. ECT has been found to be an effective treatment for acute mania in adults (Lish et al. 1994; Prien and Potter 1990). Current literature suggests a 75%–100% response rate to ECT in mood disorders (American Academy of Child and Adolescent Psychiatry 2004). However, ECT has been underutilized, largely because of stigma and campaigns by groups with a bias against the treatment. Campbell (1952) reported favorable results in adolescents treated with ECT. More recently, Schneekloth et al. (1993) also reported remission of bipolar symptoms in adolescents after ECT. Potential side effects of ECT include mild cognitive impairment, transient effects on short-term memory, anxiety reactions, disinhibitions, and altered seizure threshold (Bertagnoli and Borchardt 1990). The cur-

rent American Academy of Child and Adolescent Psychiatry (2004) practice parameters suggest that ECT be considered after a failure to respond to two or more trials of pharmacotherapy or when symptoms preclude waiting for a response to medication. In the United States, use of ECT in a child or adolescent requires that two board-certified child and adolescent psychiatrists (other than the treating child and adolescent psychiatrist) recommend the treatment.

Psychological and Social/Environmental Treatments

The practice guidelines for treatment of adult patients with bipolar disorder (Lish et al. 1994) list eight specific interventions essential for psychiatric management of bipolar disorder: 1) developing and maintaining rapport, 2) monitoring the patient's mood and behavior, 3) providing information and education about bipolar disorder, 4) enhancing compliance with medication and other treatments, 5) promoting regular patterns of sleep and daily activities, 6) promoting integration and adaptation to the psychosocial effects of bipolar disorder, 7) recognizing new episodes early, and 8) minimizing the morbidity and academic, social, and interpersonal consequences of bipolar disorder.

The same principles may be applied to treatment of bipolar disorder in children and adolescents, but developmental considerations should be taken into account. Involvement of the family in treatment is essential. Although medication treatment is considered essential for managing acute episodes and maintenance, psychosocial treatments are a mainstay of therapy between acute episodes and are aimed at reducing morbidity and preventing relapse. An additional factor to be considered in treatment is the fact that bipolar disorder is often comorbid with other conditions such as disruptive behavior disorders, substance abuse, and learning disabilities. Each of these additional problems requires specifically targeted interventions (Lofthouse and Fristad 2004; E.B. Weller et al. 2004b).

Prognosis

Major depressive disorder in children and adolescents causes significant morbidity and mortality (Fleming and Offord 1990; McCracken and Cantwell 1992). Depression is a major factor in adolescent suicide (Brent 1987; Kovacs et al. 1993; Pfeffer et al. 1991a) and is a common cause of school failure and school dropout (Weinberg et al. 1973). Adolescents with bipolar disorder are at increased risk for suicide relative to children with other psychiatric illnesses (Brent et al. 1988, 1993). Depression in children and adolescents is also associated with an increased risk of suicidal behaviors, homicidal ideation, tobacco use, and abuse of alcohol and other substances during later adolescence (Deykin et al. 1992; Kandel et al. 1986) and adulthood (Rao et al. 1995). During a 5-year follow-up, 11 of 54 bipolar adolescents made suicide attempts that required medical attention (Strober et al. 1995).

Early-onset bipolar disorders have a greater chronicity than do adult-onset bipolar disorders and are less responsive to treatment (McGlashan 1988; Strober et al. 1995). Likewise, longitudinal studies have shown that adolescent depression is associated with a high risk of recurrent illness. In addition, adolescents with depression are at increased risk of developing bipolar disorder. Approximately half of affected persons experience significant impairment relative to their premorbid state (McGlashan 1988; Werry et al. 1991).

Prospective studies have demonstrated that even after recovery from major depressive disorder, children and adolescents may continue to show subclinical symptoms of depression, negative attributions, impairment in interpersonal relationships, increased smoking, impairment in global functioning, early pregnancy, and increased physical problems (Kandel and Davies 1986; Puig-Antich et al. 1985a, 1985b, 1993; Rao et al. 1995; Rohde et al. 1994; Strober et al. 1993). Adolescents with two or more depressive episodes appear to have poorer functioning, whereas adolescents with nonrecurrent major depressive disorder may have good psychosocial outcomes similar to nondepressed control subjects (Rao et al. 1995; Warner et al. 1995).

Disturbed psychosocial functioning is a severe consequence of major depressive disorder. Geller et al. (2001a) compared the adult psychosocial functioning of subjects with prepubertal major depressive disorder (mean age: 10.3 ± 1.5 years at baseline) to that of a psychiatrically healthy comparison group (mean age: 20.7 ± 2.0 years) after follow-up into adulthood. The time between baseline and follow-up was 9.9 ± 1.5 years. In the prepubertal major depressive disorder group, subjects with major depressive disorder, bipolar disorder, or substance use disorders during the previous 5 years had significantly worse psychosocial functioning than the healthy comparison group subjects at follow-up. Impairment in psychosocial functioning included significantly worse relationships with parents, siblings, and friends; significantly worse functioning in home, school, and work settings; and poorer overall quality of life and global social adjustment.

Relapse of depression in children and adolescents is common (Kovacs et al. 1984a, 1984b). One study (Kovacs et al. 1984b) reported that 26% of adolescents relapsed within 1 year, and 40% within 2 years of their initial depressive episode.

Two-thirds of subjects with major depression and dysthymic disorder had a subsequent episode by 5 years. A significant number of the adolescents also had school-related problems, including academic failure and peer relationship problems, suggesting that the recurrence rate has significantly hampered successful development in several areas (Kovacs et al. 1984b). A similar study in children showed approximately 80% of hospitalized depressed children were rehospitalized within 2 years of discharge (Asarnow et al. 1988). Several other follow-up studies reported a generally poor prognosis for depressed adolescents. There was a high risk for future episodes of mood disorders and chronic psychosocial problems (Garber et al. 1988; Kandel and Davies 1986). Follow-up studies in hospitalized depressed children and adolescents also reported chronicity and recurrence of depression (Welner et al. 1979).

Geller et al. (1994) have suggested that children with prepubertal major depressive disorder may in fact have bipolar disorder but have not yet had their first manic episode. Data from these authors' 2- to 5-year follow-up study of subjects with prepubertal major depressive disorder from their nortriptyline study indicated 31.6% had their diagnoses changed to bipolar disorder.

Geller et al. (2001b) followed up 100 subjects from an earlier study who were treated for childhood depression (Geller et al. 1992). At follow-up, significantly more of the subjects who had a prepubertal diagnosis of major depressive disorder had bipolar I disorder (33.3%) than did comparison subjects (0%). Subjects who had prepubertal diagnoses of major depressive disorder also had significantly higher rates of any bipolar disorder (48.6% vs. 7.1%), major depressive disorder (36.1% vs. 14.3%), substance use disorder (30.6% vs. 10.7%), and suicidality (22.2% vs. 3.6%) in comparison with nondepressed comparison subjects (Geller et al. 2001b).

Puig-Antich et al. (1985a, 1985b) reported impaired psychosocial functioning in subjects who had prepubertal major depressive disorder. More recently, Geller et al. (2000) reported impaired psychosocial functioning in subjects with prepubertal and early adolescent bipolar disorder phenotype.

The only naturalistic prospective follow-up study of mania involved 54 adolescents with bipolar disorder. All but 2 recovered from their initial episode over a 5-year period (Strober et al. 1995). Of the 54 adolescents, 24 (44%) had a relapsing course and 11 (20%) experienced two or more episodes during the 5-year follow-up. Furthermore, rate of recovery was influenced by the polarity of the index episode. Subjects with an index depressive episode took longer to recover (median, 26 weeks) than did subjects with cycling (median, 15 weeks), mixed (median, 11 weeks), or pure manic (median, 9 weeks) episodes.

Geller et al. (2001c) reported that the 1-year recovery rate of 89 bipolar subjects (mean age: 10.9 years) was 37.1%. The 1-year relapse rate for the same group was 38.3%. The low recovery rate and high relapse rate in this study supported a hypothesis of risk factors for poor outcome that was based on similarities between the characteristics of the prepubertal and early adolescent bipolar disorder phenotype (long episode duration and high prevalence of mixed mania, psychosis, and rapid cycling) and those of severe bipolar disorder in adults.

Research Issues

Some progress has been made during the past 15 years in the study of mood disorders in children and adolescents. The reconsideration of diagnostic criteria, better description of the clinical picture (particularly with regard to the so-called atypical features), the development of diagnostic instruments, improved knowledge on short- and long-term prognosis, and the beginning of controlled treatment studies on child and adolescent mood disorders are all important developments. However, much work remains to be done. There needs to be more emphasis on research in the etiopathogenesis of both depressive disorder and bipolar disorder. The interconnections between major depressive disorder and bipolar disorder also need further study (E.B. Weller et al. 2004b).

Mood disorders have been understudied in preschool-age and school age children. In particular, there is little research on treatment. Despite this, clinicians are using antidepressants, mood stabilizers, anticonvulsants and atypical antipsychotics in an effort to help these children. More double-blind, placebo-controlled studies are needed in this age group to document the safety and efficacy of these medications (E.B. Weller et al. 2004a).

Psychosocial and pharmacological treatments are vital to improve the acute and long-term course of mood disorders in children and adolescents. However, further research is needed to refine treatment strategies with an emphasis on prevention of recurrence. The high incidence of parental mental health problems indicates the need for further research on concurrent treatment of parents and youth with mood disorders. Also, more research is needed on the treatment of dysthymia, double depression, psychotic depression, and refractory depression (Birmaher et al. 1996b).

References

Achamallah NS, Decker DH: Mania induced by fluoxetine in an adolescent patient. Am J Psychiatry 148:1404–1405, 1991

Adams M, Adams J: Life events, depression, and perceived problem solving alternatives in adolescents. J Child Psychol Psychiatry 32:811–820, 1991

Adrian C, Hammen C: Stress exposure and stress generation in children of depressed mothers. J Consult Clin Psychol 61:354–359, 1993

Ahrens B, Grof P, Moller HJ, et al: Extended survival of patients on long-term lithium treatment. Can J Psychiatry 40:241–246, 1995

Akiskal HS, McKinney W: Overview of recent research in depression: integration of 10 conceptual models into a comprehensive clinical frame. Arch Gen Psychiatry 32:285, 1975

Akiskal HS, Weller EB: Mood disorders and suicide in children and adolescents, in Comprehensive Textbook of Psychiatry. Edited by Kaplan HI, Sadock BJ. Baltimore, MD, Williams & Wilkins, 1989, pp 1981–1994

Akiskal HS, Downs J, Jordan P, et al: Affective disorders in referred children and younger siblings of manic-depressives: mode of onset and prospective course. Arch Gen Psychiatry 42:996–1003, 1985

Allgood-Merten B, Lewinsohn PM, Hops H: Sex differences and adolescent depression. J Abnorm Psychol 99:55–63, 1990

Ambrosini PJ, Bianchi MD, Rabinovich H, et al: Antidepressant treatments in children and adolescents, I: affective disorders. J Am Acad Child Adolesc Psychiatry 32:1–6, 1993

American Academy of Child and Adolescent Psychiatry: Practice parameter for use of electroconvulsive therapy with adolescents. J Am Acad Child Adolesc Psychiatry 43:1521–1539, 2004

American Psychiatric Association: Diagnostic and Statistical Manual of Mental Disorders, 3rd Edition. Washington, DC, American Psychiatric Association, 1980

American Psychiatric Association: Diagnostic and Statistical Manual of Mental Disorders, 3rd Edition, Revised. Washington, DC, American Psychiatric Association, 1987

American Psychiatric Association: Diagnostic and Statistical Manual of Mental Disorders, 4th Edition. Washington, DC, American Psychiatric Association, 1994

American Psychiatric Association: Diagnostic and Statistical Manual of Mental Disorders, 4th Edition, Text Revision. Washington, DC, American Psychiatric Association, 2000

Anderson JC, Williams S, McGee R, et al: DSM-III disorders in preadolescent children: prevalence in a large sample from the general population. Arch Gen Psychiatry 44:69–76, 1987

Angold A, Costello EJ: Depressive comorbidity in children and adolescents: empirical, theoretical, and methodological issues. Am J Psychiatry 150:1779–1791, 1993

Angold A, Erkanli A, Costello EJ, et al: Precision, reliability and accuracy in the dating of symptom onsets in child and adolescent psychopathology. J Child Psychol Psychiatry 37:657–664, 1996

Angold A, Costello EJ, Worthman CM: Puberty and depression: the roles of age, pubertal status and pubertal timing. Psychol Med 28:51–61, 1998

Asarnow JR: Peer status and social competence in child psychiatric inpatients: a comparison of children with depressive, externalizing, and concurrent depressive and externalizing disorders. J Abnorm Child Psychol 16:151–162, 1988

Asarnow JR, Bates S: Depression in child psychiatric inpatients: cognitive and attributional patterns. J Abnorm Child Psychol 16:601–615, 1988

Asarnow JR, Goldstein MJ, Carlson GA, et al: Childhood-onset depressive disorders: a follow-up study of rates of rehospitalization and out-of-home placement among child psychiatric inpatients. J Affect Disord 15:245–253, 1988

Avison WR, Mcalpine DD: Gender differences in symptoms of depression among adolescents. J Health Soc Behav 33:77–96, 1992

Ballenger JC: The use of anticonvulsants in manic-depressive illness. J Clin Psychiatry 49:21–25, 1988

Ballenger JC, Reus VI, Post RM: The "atypical" clinical picture of adolescent mania. Am J Psychiatry 139:602–606, 1982

Banez GA, Compas BE: Children's and parents' daily stressful events and psychological symptoms. J Abnorm Child Psychol 18:591–605, 1990

Beardslee WR, Salt P, Porterfield K, et al: Comparison of preventive interventions for families with parental affective disorder. J Am Acad Child Adolesc Psychiatry 32:254–263, 1993

Beck AT: Depression: Clinical, Experimental and Theoretical Aspects. New York, Harper, 1967

Beck AT, Rush AJ, Shaw B, et al: Cognitive States of Depression. New York, Guilford, 1979

Bemporad JR: Psychodynamic treatment of depressed adolescents. J Clin Psychiatry 49 (suppl):26–31, 1988

Bertagnoli MW, Borchardt CM: A review of ECT for children and adolescents. J Am Acad Child Adolesc Psychiatry 29:302–307, 1990

Bhatara VS: Early detection of adolescent mood disorders. S D J Med 45:75–78, 1992

Biederman J, Faraone S, Mick E, et al: Psychiatric comorbidity among referred juveniles with major depression: fact or artifact? J Am Acad Child Adolesc Psychiatry 34:579–590, 1995

Biederman J, Faraone S, Mick E, et al: Attention-deficit hyperactivity disorder and juvenile mania: an overlooked comorbidity? J Am Acad Child Adolesc Psychiatry 35:997–1008, 1996

Bird HR, Canino G, Rubio-Stipec M, et al: Estimates of the prevalence of childhood maladjustment in a community survey in Puerto Rico: the use of combined measures. Arch Gen Psychiatry 45:1120–1126, 1988

Birmaher B, Ryan ND, Williamson DE, et al: Childhood and adolescent depression: a review of the past 10 years, I. J Am Acad Child Adolesc Psychiatry 35:1427–1439, 1996a

Birmaher B, Ryan ND, Williamson DE, et al: Childhood and adolescent depression: a review of the past 10 years, II. J Am Acad Child Adolesc Psychiatry 35:1575–1583, 1996b

Birmaher B, Dahl RE, Perel J, et al: Corticotropin-releasing hormone challenge in prepubertal major depression. Biol Psychiatry 39:267–277, 1996c

Birmaher B, McCafferty JM, Bellew KM, et al: Comorbid ADHD and other disruptive behavior disorders as predictors of response in adolescents treated for major depression. Abstract presented at American Psychiatric Association Annual Meeting, Chicago, IL, May 2000

Birmaher B, Axelson D, Monk K, et al: Fluox-etine for the Treatment of Childhood Anxi-ety Disorders. J Am Acad Child Adolesc Psy-chiatry 42: 415-423, 2003

Botteron KN, Geller B: Pharmacological treat-ment of childhood and adolescent mania. Child Adolesc Psychiatr Clin N Am 4:283–304, 1995

Botteron KN, Vannier MW, Geller B, et al: Pre-liminary study of magnetic resonance imag-ing characteristics in 8- to 16-year-olds with mania. J Am Acad Child Adolesc Psychiatry 34:742–749, 1995

Bowden CL, Janicak PG, Orsulak P, et al: Re-lation of serum valproate concentration to response in mania. Am J Psychiatry 153:765–770, 1996

Bowlby J: Maternal Care and Mental Health, 2nd Edition. Geneva, World Health Organi-zation, 1951

Bowring MA, Kovacs M: Difficulties in diag-nosing manic disorders among children and adolescents. J Am Acad Child Adolesc Psychiatry 31:611–614, 1992

Brent DA: Correlates of the medical lethality of suicide attempts in children and adoles-cents. J Am Acad Child Adolesc Psychiatry 26:87–91, 1987

Brent DA, Perper JA, Goldstein CE, et al: Risk fac-tors for adolescent suicide: a comparison of adolescent suicide victims with suicidal inpa-tients. Arch Gen Psychiatry 45:581–588, 1988

Brent DA, Perper JA, Moritz G, et al: Psychiat-ric risk factors for adolescent suicide: a case-control study. J Am Acad Child Adolesc Psy-chiatry 32:521–529, 1993

Brent DA, Holder D, Kolko D, et al: A clinical psy-chotherapy trial for adolescent depression comparing cognitive, family, and supportive therapy. Arch Gen Psychiatry 54:877–885, 1997

Brent DA, Kolko DJ, Birmaher B, et al: Predic-tors of treatment efficacy in a clinical trial of three psychosocial treatments for adolescent depression. J Am Acad Child Adolesc Psychi-atry 37:906–914, 1998

Brent DA, Kolko DJ, Birmaher B, et al: A clini-cal trial for adolescent depression: predic-tors of additional treatment in the acute and follow-up phases of the trial. J Am Acad Child Adolesc Psychiatry 38:263–270, 1999

Brown GW, Harris TO: Life Events and Illness. New York, Guilford, 1989

Bryant AE 3rd, Dreifuss FE: Valproic acid he-patic fatalities, III: U.S. experience since 1986. Neurology 46:465–469, 1996

Burke KC, Burke JD, Regier DA, et al: Age at onset of selected mental disorders in five community populations. Arch Gen Psychi-atry 47:511–518, 1990

Campbell J: Manic-depressive psychoses in chil-dren. J Nerv Ment Dis 116:424–439, 1952

Carlson GA: Bipolar affective disorders in child-hood and adolescence, in Affective Disor-ders in Childhood and Adolescence. Edited by Cantwell DP, Carlson GA. New York, Spec-trum, 1983, pp 61–83

Carlson GA: Classification issues of bipolar dis-orders in childhood. Psychiatr Dev 2:273–285, 1984

Carlson GA, Abbott SF: Mood disorders and sui-cide, in Comprehensive Textbook of Psychi-atry, 4th Edition. Edited by Kaplan HI, Sa-dock BJ. Baltimore, MD, Williams & Wilkins, 1995, pp 2367–2391

Carlson GA, Kashani JH: Manic symptoms in a non-referred adolescent population. J Affect Disord 15:219–226, 1988a

Carlson GA, Kashani JH: Phenomenology of major depression from childhood through adulthood: analysis of three studies. Am J Psychiatry 145:1222–1225, 1988b

Carlson GA, Davenport YB, Jamison K: A com-parison of outcome in adolescent- and later-onset bipolar manic-depressive illness. Am J Psychiatry 134:919–922, 1977

Carlson GA, Fennig S, Bromet EJ: The confu-sion between bipolar disorder and schizo-phrenia in youth: where does it stand in the 1990s? J Am Acad Child Adolesc Psychiatry 33:453–460, 1994

Carlson GA, Bromet EJ, Sievers S: Phenomenol-ogy and outcome of subjects with early and adult-onset psychotic mania. Am J Psychiatry 157:213–219, 2000

Carpenter RO, Vining EPG: Antiepileptics (anticonvulsants), in Practitioner's Guide to Psychoactive Drugs for Children and Adolescents. Edited by Werry JS, Aman MG. New York, Plenum, 1993, pp 321–346

Casat CD, Powell K: The dexamethasone suppression test in children and adolescents with major depressive disorder: a review. J Clin Psychiatry 49:390–393, 1988

Chang K, Adleman N, Dienes K, et al: Anomalous prefrontal-subcortical activation in familial pediatric bipolar disorder: a functional magnetic resonance imaging investigation. Arch Gen Psychiatry 61:781–792, 2004

Clarke GN, Lewinsohn PM, Hops H: Instructive Manual for the Adolescent Coping With Depression Course. Eugene, OR, Castalia, 1990

Clarke GN, Hawkins W, Murphy M, et al: Targeted prevention of unipolar depressive disorder in an at-risk sample of high school adolescents: a randomized trial of a group cognitive intervention. J Am Acad Child Adolesc Psychiatry 34:312–321, 1995

Coffey CE, Wilkinson WE, Weiner RD, et al: Quantitative cerebral anatomy in depression: a controlled magnetic resonance imaging study. Arch Gen Psychiatry 50:7–16, 1993

Compas BE, Oppedisano G, Connor JK, et al: Gender differences in depressive symptoms in adolescence: comparison of national samples of clinically referred and nonreferred youths. J Consult Clin Psychol 65:617–626, 1997

Conde Lopez VJ, Ballesteros Alcalde MC, Franco Martin MA, et al: [Critical evaluation of the use of antidepressants in childhood] (Spanish). Actas Luso Esp Neurol Psiquiatr Cienc Afines 25:105–117, 1997

Conners CK, Casat CD, Gualtieri CT, et al: Bupropion hydrochloride in attention deficit disorder with hyperactivity. J Am Acad Child Adolesc Psychiatry 35:1314–1321, 1996

Costello AJ, Dulcan MK, Kalas R: A checklist of hospitalization criteria for use with children. Hosp Community Psychiatry 42:823–828, 1991

Coyle JT, Pine DS, Charney DS, et al: Depression and bipolar disorder support alliance consensus statement on the unmet needs on diagnostic and treatment of mood disorders in children and adolescents. J Am Acad Child Adolesc Psychiatry 42:1494–1503, 2003

Davis RE: Manic-depressive variant syndrome in childhood: a preliminary report. Am J Psychiatry 136:702–706, 1979

De Bellis MD, Chrousos GP, Dorn LD, et al: Hypothalamic-pituitary-adrenal axis dysregulation in sexually abused girls. J Clin Endocrinol Metab 78:249–255, 1994

Delbello MP, Kowatch RA, Warner J, et al: Adjunctive topiramate treatment for pediatric bipolar disorder: a retrospective chart review. J Child Adolesc Psychopharmacol 12:323–330, 2002a

Delbello MP, Schwiers H, Rosenberg, HL, et al: A double-blind, randomized, placebo-controlled study of quetiapine as adjunctive treatment for adolescent mania. J Am Acad Child Adolesc Psychiatry 41:1216–1224, 2002b

DeLong GR, Aldershof AL: Long-term experience with lithium treatment in childhood: correlation with clinical diagnosis. J Am Acad Child Adolesc Psychiatry 26:389–394, 1987

Derivan A, Entsuah AR, Kikta D: Venlafaxine: measuring the onset of antidepressant action. Psychopharmacol Bull 31:439–447, 1995

DeVane CL: Pharmacokinetics of the newer antidepressants: clinical relevance. Am J Med 97:13S–23S, 1994

Deykin EY, Buka SL, Zeena TH: Depressive illness among chemically dependent adolescents. Am J Psychiatry 149:1341–1347, 1992

Dohrenwend BP, Shrout PE, Egri G, et al: Nonspecific psychological distress and other dimensions of psychopathology. Measures for use in the general population. Arch Gen Psychiatry 37:1229–1236, 1980

Dorn LD, Burgess ES, Dichek HL, et al: Thyroid hormone concentrations in depressed and nondepressed adolescents: group differences and behavioral relations. J Am Acad Child Adolesc Psychiatry 35:299–306, 1996

Eaton WW, Dryman A, Sorenson A, et al: DSM-III major depressive disorder in the community: a latent class analysis of data from the NIMH epidemiologic catchment area programme. Br J Psychiatry 155:48–54, 1989

Ellis A, Bernard M: Rational-Emotive Approaches to the Problems of Childhood. New York, Plenum, 1983 el Mallakh RS, Li R: Is the Na(+)-K(+)-ATPase the link between phosphoinositide metabolism and bipolar disorder? J Neuropsychiatry Clin Neurosci 5:361–368, 1993

Emslie GJ, Rush AJ, Weinberg WA, et al: A double-blind, randomized, placebo-controlled trial of fluoxetine in children and adolescents with depression. Arch Gen Psychiatry 54:1031–1037, 1997a

Emslie GJ, Rush AJ, Weinberg WA, et al: Recurrence of Major Depressive Disorder in Hospitalized Children and Adolescents. J Am Acad Child Adolesc Psychiatry 36:785–792, 1997b

Emslie GJ, Walkup JT, Pliszka SR, et al: Nontricyclic antidepressants: current trends in children and adolescents. J Am Acad Child Adolesc Psychiatry 38:517–528, 1999

Emslie GJ, Heiligenstein JH, Wagner KD, et al: Fluoxetine for acute treatment of depression in children and adolescents: a placebo-controlled, randomized, clinical trial. J Am Acad Child Adolesc Psychiatry 41:1205–1215, 2002

Fatemi SH, Rapport DJ, Calabrese JR, et al: Lamotrigine in rapid-cycling bipolar disorder. J Clin Psychiatry 58:522–527, 1997

FDA News: FDA Launches a Multi-Pronged Strategy to Strengthen Safeguards for Children Treated With Antidepressant Medications (October 15, 2004). Retrieved on January 11, 2005 from http://www.fda.gov/bbs/topics/news/2004/NEW01124.html

Ferro T, Carlson GA, Grayson P, et al: Depressive disorders: distinctions in children. J Am Acad Child Adolesc Psychiatry 33:664–670, 1994

Fetner HH, Geller B: Lithium and tricyclic antidepressants. Psychiatr Clin North Am 15:223–224, 1992

Findling RL, Preskorn SH, Marcus RN, et al: Nefazodone pharmacokinetics in depressed children and adolescents. J Am Acad Child Adolesc Psychiatry 39:1008–1016, 2000

Fine S, Forth A, Gilbert M, et al: Group therapy for adolescent depressive disorder: a comparison of social skills and therapeutic support. J Am Acad Child Adolesc Psychiatry 30:79–85, 1991

Fleming JE, Offord DR: Epidemiology of childhood depressive disorders: a critical review. J Am Acad Child Adolesc Psychiatry 29:571–580, 1990

Frank E, Kupfer DJ, Perel JM, et al: Three-year outcomes for maintenance therapies in recurrent depression. Arch Gen Psychiatry 47:1093–1099, 1990

Frazier JA, Meyer MC, Biederman J, et al: Risperidone treatment for juvenile bipolar disorder: a retrospective chart review. J Am Acad Child Adolesc Psychiatry 38:960–965, 1999

Frazier JA, Biederman J, Tohen M, et al: A prospective open-label treatment trial of olanzapine monotherapy in children and adolescents with bipolar disorder. J Child Adolesc Psychopharmacol 11:239–250, 2001

Fuchs DC: Clozapine treatment of bipolar disorder in a young adolescent. J Am Acad Child Adolesc Psychiatry 33:1299–1302, 1994

Gabbard GO: Mood disorders: psychodynamic etiology, in Comprehensive Textbook of Psychiatry, 6th Edition. Edited by Kaplan HI, Sadock BJ. Baltimore, MD, Williams & Wilkins, 1995, pp 1116–1123

Garber J, Kriss MR, Koch M, et al: Recurrent depression in adolescents: a follow-up study. J Am Acad Child Adolesc Psychiatry 27:49–54, 1988

Garland EJ, Weiss M: Subgroups of adolescent depression. J Am Acad Child Adolesc Psychiatry 34:831–833, 1995

Geller B, Fetner HH: Children's 24-hour serum lithium level after a single dose predicts initial dose and steady-state plasma level (letter). J Clin Psychopharmacol 9:155, 1989

Geller B, Luby J: Child and adolescent bipolar disorder: a review of the past 10 years [published erratum appears in J Am Acad Child Adolesc Psychiatry 36:1642, 1997]. J Am Acad Child Adolesc Psychiatry 36:1168–1176, 1997

Geller B, Cooper TB, Chestnut EC, et al: Preliminary data on the relationship between nortriptyline plasma level and response in depressed children. Am J Psychiatry 143:1283–1286, 1986

Geller B, Cooper TB, Graham DL, et al: Pharmacokinetically designed double-blind placebo-controlled study of nortriptyline in 6- to 12-year-olds with major depressive disorder. J Am Acad Child Adolesc Psychiatry 31:34–44, 1992

Geller B, Fox LW, Clark KA: Rate and predictors of prepubertal bipolarity during follow-up of 6- to 12-year-old depressed children. J Am Acad Child Adolesc Psychiatry 33:461–468, 1994

Geller B, Sun K, Zimerman B, et al: Complex and rapid-cycling in bipolar children and adolescents: a preliminary study. J Affect Disord 34:259–268, 1995

Geller B, Cooper T, Sun K, et al: Double-blind and placebo-controlled study of lithium for adolescent bipolar disorders with secondary substance dependency. J Am Acad Child Adolesc Psychiatry 37:171–178, 1998a

Geller B, Williams M, Zimerman B, et al: Prepubertal and early adolescent bipolarity differentiate from ADHD by manic symptoms, grandiose delusions, ultra-rapid or ultradian cycling. J Affect Disord 51:81–91, 1998b

Geller B, Bolhofner K, Craney JL, et al: Psychosocial functioning in a prepubertal and early adolescent bipolar disorder phenotype. J Am Acad Child Adolesc Psychiatry 39:1543–1548, 2000

Geller B, Zimerman B, Williams M, et al: Adult psychosocial outcome of prepubertal major depressive disorder. J Am Acad Child Adolesc Psychiatry 40:673–677, 2001a

Geller B, Zimerman B, Williams M, et al: Bipolar disorder at prospective follow-up of adults who had prepubertal major depressive disorder. Am J Psychiatry 158:125–127, 2001b

Geller B, Craney JL, Bolhofner K, et al: One-year recovery and relapse rates of children with a prepubertal and early adolescent bipolar disorder phenotype. Am J Psychiatry 158:303–305, 2001c

Gershon ES, Hamovit J, Guroff JJ, et al: A family study of schizoaffective, bipolar I, bipolar II, unipolar, and normal control probands. Arch Gen Psychiatry 39:1157–1167, 1982

Gershon ES, Hamovit JH, Guroff JJ, et al: Birth-cohort changes in manic and depressive disorders in relatives of bipolar and schizoaffective patients. Arch Gen Psychiatry 44:314–319, 1987

Goetz RR, Puig-Antich J, Ryan N, et al: Electroencephalographic sleep of adolescents with major depression and normal controls. Arch Gen Psychiatry 44:61–68, 1987

Goodwin F, Jamison K: Manic-Depressive Illness. New York, Oxford University Press, 1990

Goodyer I, Kolvin I, Gatzanis S: Recent undesirable life events and psychiatric disorder in childhood and adolescence. Br J Psychiatry 147:517–523, 1985

Goodyer IM, Wright C, Altham PM: Maternal adversity and recent stressful life events in anxious and depressed children. J Child Psychol Psychiatry 29:651–667, 1988

Goodyer IM, Wright C, Altham PM: Recent friendships in anxious and depressed school age children. Psychol Med 19:165–174, 1989

Gore S, Aseltine RH Jr, Colton ME: Social structure, life stress and depressive symptoms in a high school-aged population. J Health Soc Behav 33:97–113, 1992

Gutterman EM, Markowitz JS, LoConte JS, et al: Determinants for hospitalization from an emergency mental health service. J Am Acad Child Adolesc Psychiatry 32:114–122, 1993

Hagino OR, Weller EB, Weller RA, et al: Untoward effects of lithium treatment in children aged four through six years. J Am Acad Child Adolesc Psychiatry 34:1584–1590, 1995

Hammen C: Self-cognitions, stressful events, and the prediction of depression in children of depressed mothers. J Abnorm Child Psychol 16:347–360, 1988

Hammen C, Burge D, Burney E, et al: Longitudinal study of diagnoses in children of women with unipolar and bipolar affective disorder. Arch Gen Psychiatry 47:1112–1117, 1990

Harrington R, Fudge H, Rutter M, et al: Adult outcomes of childhood and adolescent depression, I: psychiatric status. Arch Gen Psychiatry 47:465–473, 1990

Harrington R, Fudge H, Rutter M, et al: Adult outcomes of childhood and adolescent depression, II: links with antisocial disorders. J Am Acad Child Adolesc Psychiatry 30:434–439, 1991

Hazell P, O'Connell D, Heathcote D, et al: Efficacy of tricyclic drugs in treating child and adolescent depression: a meta-analysis. BMJ 310:897–901, 1995

Himmelhoch JM, Garfinkel ME: Sources of lithium resistance in mixed mania. Psychopharmacol Bull 22:613–620, 1986

Hindmarch I, Kerr J: Behavioural toxicity of antidepressants with particular reference to moclobemide. Psychopharmacology (Berl) 106 (suppl):S49–S55, 1992

Hirschfeld RM, Keck PE, Kramer M, et al: Rapid antimanic effect of risperidone monotherapy: a 3-week multicenter, double-blind, placebo-controlled trial. Am J Psychiatry 161: 1057–1065, 2004

Holmes LB: The North American Antiepileptic Drug Pregnancy Registry: a seven year experience (Abstract B-05). Oral presentation at: American Epilepsy Society 2004 Annual Meeting, New Orleans, LA, December 3–7, 2004

Hsu LK: Lithium-resistant adolescent mania. J Am Acad Child Psychiatry 25:280–283, 1986

Hughes CW, Preskorn SH, Weller E, et al: The effect of concomitant disorders in childhood depression on predicting treatment response. Psychopharmacol Bull 26:235–238, 1990

Hughes CW, Emslie GJ, Crismon ML, et al: The Texas children's medication algorithm project: report of the Texas consensus conference panel on medication treatment if childhood major depressive disorder. J Am Acad Child Adolesc Psychiatry 38:1442–1454, 1999

Husain MM, McDonald WM, Doraiswamy PM, et al: A magnetic resonance imaging study of putamen nuclei in major depression. Psychiatry Res 40:95–99, 1991

Inamdar SC, Siomopoulos G, Osborn M, et al: Phenomenology associated with depressed moods in adolescents. Am J Psychiatry 136: 156–159, 1979

Isaac G: Misdiagnosed bipolar disorder in adolescents in a special educational school and treatment program. J Clin Psychiatry 53:133–136, 1992

Isojarvi JI, Laatikainen TJ, Pakarinen AJ, et al: Polycystic ovaries and hyperandrogenism in women taking valproate for epilepsy. N Engl J Med 329:1383–1388, 1993

Isojarvi JI, Rattya J, Myllyla VV, et al: Valproate, lamotrigine, and insulin-mediated risks in women with epilepsy. Ann Neurol 43:446–451, 1998

Jacobson SJ, Jones K, Johnson K, et al: Prospective multicentre study of pregnancy outcome after lithium exposure during first trimester. Lancet 339:530–533, 1992

Jaycox LH, Reivich KJ, Gillham J, et al: Prevention of depressive symptoms in school children. Behav Res Ther 32:801–816, 1994

Jensen JB, Garfinkel BD: Growth hormone dysregulation in children with major depressive disorder. J Am Acad Child Adolesc Psychiatry 29:295–301, 1990

Jernigan TL, Trauner DA, Hesselink JR, et al: Maturation of human cerebrum observed in vivo during adolescence. Brain 114(pt 5): 2037–2049, 1991

Jones KL, Lacro RV, Johnson KA, et al: Pattern of malformations in the children of women treated with carbamazepine during pregnancy. N Engl J Med 320:1661–1666, 1989

Joyce PR: Age of onset in bipolar affective disorder and misdiagnosis as schizophrenia. Psychol Med 14:145–149, 1984

Kafantaris V: Treatment of bipolar disorder in children and adolescents. J Am Acad Child Adolesc Psychiatry 34:732–741, 1995

Kahn J, Kehle T, Enson W, et al: Comparison of cognitive-behavioral, relaxation, and self-modeling interventions for depression in middle-school students. School Psychology Review 9:196–211, 1990

Kandel DB, Davies M: Adult sequelae of adolescent depressive symptoms. Arch Gen Psychiatry 43:255–262, 1986

Kandel DB, Davies M, Karus D, et al: The consequences in young adulthood of adolescent drug involvement: an overview. Arch Gen Psychiatry 43:746–754, 1986

Kapur S, Mieczkowski T, Mann JJ: Antidepressant medications and the relative risk of suicide attempt and suicide. JAMA 268:3441–3445, 1992

Kashani JH, Barbero GJ, Bolander FD: Depression in hospitalized pediatric patients. J Am Acad Child Psychiatry 20:123–134, 1981

Kashani JH, McGee RO, Clarkson SE, et al: Depression in a sample of 9-year-old children: prevalence and associated characteristics. Arch Gen Psychiatry 40:1217–1223, 1983

Kashani JH, Beck NC, Hoeper EW, et al: Psychiatric disorders in a community sample of adolescents. Am J Psychiatry 144:584–589, 1987a

Kashani JH, Carlson GA, Beck NC, et al: Depression, depressive symptoms, and depressed mood among a community sample of adolescents. Am J Psychiatry 144:931–934, 1987b

Kashani JH, Reid JC, Rosenberg TK: Levels of hopelessness in children and adolescents: a developmental perspective. J Consult Clin Psychol 57:496–499, 1989

Kaufman J: Depressive disorders in maltreated children. J Am Acad Child Adolesc Psychiatry 30:257–265, 1991

Keck PE Jr, McElroy SL: Outcome in the pharmacological treatment of bipolar disorder. J Psychopharmacol 16:15S–23S, 1996

Keller MB, Shapiro RW: "Double depression": superimposition of acute depressive episodes on chronic depressive disorders. Am J Psychiatry 139:438–442, 1982

Keller MB, Beardslee W, Lavori PW, et al: Course of major depression in non-referred adolescents: a retrospective study. J Affect Disord 15:235–243, 1988

Keller MB, Lavori PW, Coryell W, et al: Bipolar I: a five-year prospective follow-up. J Nerv Ment Dis 181:238–245, 1993

Keller MB, Ryan ND, Strober M, et al: Efficacy of paroxetine in the treatment of adolescent major depression: a randomized, controlled trial. J Am Acad Child Adolesc Psychiatry 40:762–772, 2001

Kendall PC, Stark KD, Adam T: Cognitive deficit or cognitive distortion in childhood depression. J Abnorm Child Psychol 18:255–270, 1990

Kendler KS: Is seeking treatment for depression predicted by a history of depression in relatives? Implications for family studies of affective disorder. Psychol Med 25:807–814, 1995

Kessler RC, McGonagle KA, Zhao S, et al: Lifetime and 12-month prevalence of DSM-III-R psychiatric disorders in the United States. Results from the National Comorbidity Survey. Arch Gen Psychiatry 51:8–19, 1994

Kessler RC, Avenevoli S, Merikangas K: Mood disorders in children and adolescents: an epidemiologic perspective. Biol Psychiatry 49:1002–1014, 2001

Kestenbaum CJ, Kron L: Psychoanalytic intervention with children and adolescents with affective disorders: a combined treatment approach. J Am Acad Psychoanal 15:153–174, 1987

Khandelwal SK, Varma VK, Srinivasa Murthy R: Renal function in children receiving long-term lithium prophylaxis. Am J Psychiatry 141:278–279, 1984

Kim EY, Miklowitz DJ: Childhood mania, attention deficit hyperactivity disorder and conduct disorder: a critical review of diagnostic dilemmas. Bipolar Disord 4:215–225, 2002

Klerman GL, Weissman MM, Rounsaville BJ, et al: Interpersonal Therapies of Depression. New York, Basic Books, 1984

Kovacs M: Presentation and course of major depressive disorder during childhood and later years of the life span. J Am Acad Child Adolesc Psychiatry 35:705–715, 1996

Kovacs M, Pollock M: Bipolar disorder and comorbid conduct disorder in childhood and adolescence. J Am Acad Child Adolesc Psychiatry 34:715–723, 1995

Kovacs M, Feinberg TL, Crouse-Novak MA, et al: Depressive disorders in childhood, I: a longitudinal prospective study of characteristics and recovery. Arch Gen Psychiatry 41:229–237, 1984a

Kovacs M, Feinberg TL, Crouse-Novak M, et al: Depressive disorders in childhood, II: a longitudinal study of the risk for a subsequent major depression. Arch Gen Psychiatry 41:643–649, 1984b

Kovacs M, Paulauskas S, Gatsonis C, et al: Depressive disorders in childhood, III: a longitudinal study of comorbidity with and risk for conduct disorders. J Affect Disord 15:205–217, 1988

Kovacs M, Gatsonis C, Paulauskas SL, et al: Depressive disorders in childhood, IV: a longitudinal study of comorbidity with and risk for anxiety disorders. Arch Gen Psychiatry 46:776–782, 1989

Kovacs M, Goldston D, Gatsonis C: Suicidal behaviors and childhood-onset depressive disorders: a longitudinal investigation. J Am Acad Child Adolesc Psychiatry 32:8–20, 1993

Kovacs M, Akiskal HS, Gatsonis C, et al: Childhood-onset dysthymic disorder. Clinical features and prospective naturalistic outcome. Arch Gen Psychiatry 51:365–374, 1994

Kovacs M, Obrosky DS, Gatsonis C, et al: First-episode major depressive and dysthymic disorder in childhood: clinical and sociodemographic factors in recovery. J Am Acad Child Adolesc Psychiatry 36:777–784, 1997

Kowatch RA, Suppes T, Gilfillan SK, et al: Clozapine treatment of children and adolescents with bipolar disorder and schizophrenia: a clinical case series. J Child Adolesc Psychopharmacol 5:241–253, 1995

Kowatch RA, Suppes T, Carmody TJ, et al: Effect size of lithium, divalproex sodium, and carbamazepine in children and adolescents with bipolar disorder. J Am Acad Child Adolesc Psychiatry 39:713–720, 2000

Krishnan KR, McDonald WM, Escalona PR, et al: Magnetic resonance imaging of the caudate nuclei in depression: preliminary observations. Arch Gen Psychiatry 49:553–557, 1992

Kroll L, Harrington R, Jayson D, et al: Pilot study of continuation cognitive-behavioral therapy for major depression in adolescent psychiatric patients. J Am Acad Child Adolesc Psychiatry 35:1156–1161, 1996

Kusumakar V, Yatham LN: Lamotrigine treatment of rapid cycling bipolar disorder (letter; comment). Am J Psychiatry 154:1171–1172, 1997

Kutcher SP, Marton P: Affective disorders in first-degree relatives of adolescent onset bipolars, unipolars, and normal controls. J Am Acad Child Adolesc Psychiatry 30:75–78, 1991

Kutcher SP, Marton P, Korenblum M: Relationship between psychiatric illness and conduct disorder in adolescents. Can J Psychiatry 34:526–529, 1989

Kutcher S, Boulos C, Ward B, et al: Response to desipramine treatment in adolescent depression: a fixed-dose, placebo-controlled trial. J Am Acad Child Adolesc Psychiatry 33:686–694, 1994

Kye CH, Ryan ND: Pharmacological treatment of child and adolescent depression. Child Adolesc Psychiatr Clin N Am 4:261–281, 1995

Lewinsohn PM, Duncan EM, Stanton AK, et al: Age at first onset for nonbipolar depression. J Abnorm Psychol 95:378–383, 1986

Lewinsohn PM, Clarke GN, Hops H, et al: Cognitive-behavioral treatment for depressed adolescents. Behavioral Therapy 21:385–401, 1990

Lewinsohn PM, Rohde P, Seeley JR, et al: Comorbidity of unipolar depression, I: major depression with dysthymia. J Abnorm Psychol 100:205–213, 1991

Lewinsohn PM, Hops H, Roberts RE, et al: Adolescent psychopathology, I: prevalence and incidence of depression and other DSM-III-R disorders in high school students. J Abnorm Psychol 102:133–144, 1993a

Lewinsohn PM, Rohde P, Seeley JR, et al: Age-cohort changes in the lifetime occurrence of depression and other mental disorders. J Abnorm Psychol 102:110–120, 1993b

Lewinsohn PM, Clarke GN, Rohde P: Psychological approaches to the treatment of depression in adolescents, in Handbook of Depression in Children and Adolescents. Edited by Reynolds WM, Johnston HF. New York, Plenum, 1994a, pp 309–344

Lewinsohn PM, Clarke GN, Seeley JR, et al: Major depression in community adolescents: age at onset, episode duration, and time to recurrence. J Am Acad Child Adolesc Psychiatry 33:809–818, 1994b

Lewinsohn PM, Roberts RE, Seeley JR, et al: Adolescent psychopathology, II: psychosocial risk factors for depression. J Abnorm Psychol 103:302–315, 1994c

Lewinsohn PM, Rohde P, Seeley JR: Psychosocial risk factors for future adolescent suicide attempts. J Consult Clin Psychol 62:297–305, 1994d

Lewinsohn PM, Klein DN, Seeley JR: Bipolar disorders in a community sample of older adolescents: prevalence, phenomenology, comorbidity, and course. J Am Acad Child Adolesc Psychiatry 34:454–463, 1995

Lewinsohn PM, Rohde P, Klein DN, et al: Natural course of adolescent major depressive disorder, I: continuity into young adulthood. J Am Acad Child Adolesc Psychiatry 38:56–63, 1999

Ling W, Oftedal G, Weinberg W: Depressive illness in childhood presenting as severe headache. Am J Dis Child 120:122–124, 1970

Lish JD, Dime-Meenan S, Whybrow PC, et al: The National Depressive and Manic-Depressive Association (DMDA) survey of bipolar members. J Affect Disord 31:281–294, 1994

Lofthouse N, Fristad MA: Psychosocial interventions for children with early-onset bipolar spectrum disorder. Clin Child & Family Psychology Review 7:71–88, 2004

Loranger AW, Levine PM: Age at onset of bipolar affective illness. Arch Gen Psychiatry 35:1345–1348, 1978

Mandoki MW, Tapia MR, Tapia MA, et al: Venlafaxine in the treatment of children and adolescents with major depression. Psychopharmacol Bull 33:149–154, 1997

Manji H: Depression, III: treatments. Am J Psychiatry 160:24, 2003

Marangell LB, George MS, Callahan AM, et al: Effects of intrathecal thyrotropin-releasing hormone (protirelin) in refractory depressed patients. Arch Gen Psychiatry 54:214–222, 1997

March J, Silva S, Petrycki S, et al: Fluoxetine, cognitive-behavioral therapy, and their combination for adolescents with depression: Treatment for Adolescents with Depression Study (TADS) randomized controlled trial. JAMA 292:807–820, 2004

Martin A, Landau J, Leebens P, et al: Risperidone-associated weight gain in children and adolescents: a retrospective chart review. J Child Adolesc Psychopharmacol 10:259–268, 2000

Masi G, Mucci M, Millepiedi S, et al: Clozapine in adolescent inpatients with acute mania. J Child Adolesc Psychopharmacol 12:93–99, 2002

McCauley E, Myers K, Mitchell J, et al: Depression in young people: initial presentation and clinical course. J Am Acad Child Adolesc Psychiatry 32:714–722, 1993

McCracken J, Cantwell DP: Management of child and adolescent mood disorder. Child Adolesc Psychiatr Clin N Am 1:229–255, 1992

McElroy SL, Keck PE Jr, Pope HG Jr, et al: Clinical and research implications of the diagnosis of dysphoric or mixed mania or hypomania. Am J Psychiatry 149:1633–1644, 1992

McElroy SL, Strakowski SM, West SA, et al: Phenomenology of adolescent and adult mania in hospitalized patients with bipolar disorder. Am J Psychiatry 154:44–49, 1997

McGlashan TH: Adolescent versus adult onset of mania. Am J Psychiatry 145:221–223, 1988

McGuffin P, Katz R: The genetics of depression and manic-depressive disorder. Br J Psychiatry 155:294–304, 1989

Minuchin S: Families and Family Therapy. Cambridge, MA, Harvard University Press, 1974

Mitchell J, McCauley E, Burke P, et al: Psychopathology in parents of depressed children and adolescents. J Am Acad Child Adolesc Psychiatry 28:352–357, 1989

Morris JB, Beck AT: The efficacy of antidepressant drugs: a review of research (1958–1972). Arch Gen Psych 30:667–674, 1974

Mufson L, Fairbanks J: Interpersonal psychotherapy for depressed adolescents: a one-year naturalistic follow-up study. J Am Acad Child Adolesc Psychiatry 35:1145–1155, 1996

Mufson L, Moreau D, Weissman MM, et al: Modification of interpersonal psychotherapy with depressed adolescents (IPT-A): phase I and II studies. J Am Acad Child Adolesc Psychiatry 33:695–705, 1994

Mullins LL, Siegel LJ, Hodges K: Cognitive problem-solving and life event correlates of depressive symptoms in children. J Abnorm Child Psychol 13:305–314, 1985

Nurnberger JI, Gershon E: Genetics, in Handbook of Effective Disorders. Edited by Pakel ES. Edinburgh, Scotland, Churchill Livingstone, 1982, pp 126–145

Orvaschel H: Early onset psychiatric disorder in high risk children and increased familial morbidity. J Am Acad Child Adolesc Psychiatry 29:184–188, 1990

Orvaschel H, Walsh-Allis G, Ye WJ: Psychopathology in children of parents with recurrent depression. J Abnorm Child Psychol 16:17–28, 1988

Ostrov E, Offer D, Howard KI: Gender differences in adolescent symptomatology: a normative study. J Am Acad Child Adolesc Psychiatry 28:394–398, 1989

Papatheodorou G, Kutcher SP: Divalproex sodium treatment in late adolescent and young adult acute mania. Psychopharmacol Bull 29:213–219, 1993

Pedley TA, Scheuer ML, Walczak TS: Epilepsy, in Merritt's Textbook of Neurology. Edited by Rowland LP. Baltimore, MD, Williams & Wilkins, 1995, pp 845–869

Pfeffer CR, Klerman GL, Hurt SW, et al: Suicidal children grow up: demographic and clinical risk factors for adolescent suicide attempts. J Am Acad Child Adolesc Psychiatry 30:609–616, 1991a

Pfeffer CR, Stokes P, Shindledecker R: Suicidal behavior and hypothalamic-pituitary-adrenocortical axis indices in child psychiatric inpatients. Biol Psychiatry 29:909–917, 1991b

Pine DS, Cohen P, Gurley D, et al: The risk for early adulthood anxiety and depressive disorders in adolescents with anxiety and depressive disorders. Arch Gen Psychiatry 55:56–64, 1998

Plomin R: The Emanuel Miller Memorial Lecture 1993. Genetic research and identification of environmental influences. J Child Psychol Psychiatry 35:817–834, 1994

Popper C: Biological cyclicity in two preschool children. Conference proceedings, American Academy of Child and Adolescent Psychiatry, Los Angeles, CA, 1984

Post RM, Uhde TW, Roy-Byrne PP, et al: Correlates of antimanic response to carbamazepine. Psychiatry Res 21:71–83, 1987

Post RM, Kramlinger KG, Altshuler LL, et al: Treatment of rapid cycling bipolar illness. Psychopharmacol Bull 26:37–47, 1990

Post RM, Ketter TA, Denicoff K, et al: The place of anticonvulsant therapy in bipolar illness. Psychopharmacology 128:115–129, 1996

Preskorn SH: Clinically relevant pharmacology of selective serotonin reuptake inhibitors. An overview with emphasis on pharmacokinetics and effects on oxidative drug metabolism. Clinical Pharmacokinetics 32 (suppl 1): 1–21, 1997

Preskorn SH, Weller EB, Weller RA: Depression in children: relationship between plasma imipramine levels and response. J Clin Psychiatry 43:450–453, 1982

Preskorn SH, Weller EB, Hughes CW, et al: Depression in prepubertal children: dexamethasone nonsuppression predicts differential response to imipramine vs. placebo. Psychopharmacol Bull 23:128–133, 1987

Prien RF, Kupfer DJ: Continuation drug therapy for major depressive episodes: how long should it be maintained? Am J Psychiatry 143:18–23, 1986

Prien RF, Potter WZ: NIMH workshop report on treatment of bipolar disorder. Psychopharmacol Bull 26:409–427, 1990

Puig-Antich J, Perel JM, Lupatkin W, et al: Plasma levels of imipramine (IMI) and desmethylimipramine (DMI) and clinical response in prepubertal major depressive disorder: a preliminary report. J Am Acad Child Psychiatry 18:616–627, 1979

Puig-Antich J, Lukens E, Davies M, et al: Psychosocial functioning in prepubertal major depressive disorders, I: interpersonal relationships during the depressive episode. Arch Gen Psychiatry 42:500–507, 1985a

Puig-Antich J, Lukens E, Davies M, et al: Psychosocial functioning in prepubertal major depressive disorders, II: interpersonal relationships after sustained recovery from affective episode. Arch Gen Psychiatry 42:511–517, 1985b

Puig-Antich J, Dahl R, Ryan N, et al: Cortisol secretion in prepubertal children with major depressive disorder: episode and recovery. Arch Gen Psychiatry 46:801–809, 1989a

Puig-Antich J, Goetz D, Davies M, et al: A controlled family history study of prepubertal major depressive disorder. Arch Gen Psychiatry 46:406–418, 1989b

Puig-Antich J, Kaufman J, Ryan ND, et al: The psychosocial functioning and family environment of depressed adolescents. J Am Acad Child Adolesc Psychiatry 32:244–253, 1993

Rao U, Ryan ND, Birmaher B, et al: Unipolar depression in adolescents: clinical outcome in adulthood. J Am Acad Child Adolesc Psychiatry 34:566–578, 1995

Ratzoni G, Gothelf D, Brand-Gothelf A, et al: Weight gain associated with olanzapine and risperidone in adolescent patients: a comparative prospective study. J Am Acad Child Adolesc Psychiatry 41:337–343, 2002

Rehm LP: A self-control model of depression. Behavior Therapy 8:787–804, 1977

Reinecke MA, Ryan NE, DuBois DL: Cognitive-behavioral therapy of depression and depressive symptoms during adolescence: a review and meta-analysis. J Am Acad Child Adolesc Psychiatry 37:26–34, 1998

Reinherz HZ, Giaconia RM, Lefkowitz ES, et al: Prevalence of psychiatric disorders in a community population of older adolescents. J Am Acad Child Adolesc Psychiatry 32:369–377, 1993a

Reinherz HZ, Giaconia RM, Pakiz B, et al: Psychosocial risks for major depression in late adolescence: a longitudinal community study. J Am Acad Child Adolesc Psychiatry 32:1155–1163, 1993b

Reynolds WM, Coats KI: A comparison of cognitive-behavioral therapy and relaxation training for the treatment of depression in adolescents. J Consult Clin Psychol 54:653–660, 1986

Rice J, Reich T, Andreasen NC, et al: The familial transmission of bipolar illness. Arch Gen Psychiatry 44:441–447, 1987

Rich CL, Young D, Fowler RC: San Diego suicide study, I: young vs old subjects. Arch Gen Psychiatry 43:577–582, 1986

Rich CL, Sherman M, Fowler RC: San Diego Suicide Study: the adolescents. Adolescence 25:855–865, 1990

Rohde P, Lewinsohn PM, Seeley JR: Comorbidity of unipolar depression, II: comorbidity with other mental disorders in adolescents and adults. J Abnorm Psychol 100:214–222, 1991

Rohde P, Lewinsohn PM, Seeley JR: Are adolescents changed by an episode of major depression? J Am Acad Child Adolesc Psychiatry 33:1289–1298, 1994

Rosa FW: Spina bifida in infants of women treated with carbamazepine during pregnancy. N Engl J Med 324:674–677, 1991

Rosenberg DR, Johnson K, Sahl R: Evolving mania in an adolescent treated with low-dose fluoxetine. J Child Adolesc Psychopharmacol 2:299–306, 1992

Rosenberg DR, Holttum J, Gershon S: Textbook of Pharmacotherapy for Child and Adolescent Psychiatric Disorders. New York, Brunner/Mazel, 1994

Ryan ND: Pharmacotherapy of adolescent major depression: beyond TCAs. Psychopharmacol Bull 26:75–79, 1990

Ryan ND, Puig-Antich J, Ambrosini P, et al: The clinical picture of major depression in children and adolescents. Arch Gen Psychiatry 44:854–861, 1987

Ryan ND, Puig-Antich J, Rabinovich H, et al: MAOIs in adolescent major depression unresponsive to tricyclic antidepressants. J Am Acad Child Adolesc Psychiatry 27:755–758, 1988

Ryan ND, Dahl RE, Birmaher B, et al: Stimulatory tests of growth hormone secretion in prepubertal major depression: depressed versus normal children. J Am Acad Child Adolesc Psychiatry 33:824–833, 1994

Ryan ND, Bhatara VS, Perel JM: Mood stabilizers in children and adolescents. J Am Acad Child Adolesc Psychiatry 38:529–536, 1999

Scheidlinger S: Group treatment of adolescents: an overview. Am J Orthopsychiatry 55:102–111, 1985

Sachs GS, Grossman F, Ghaemi SN, et al: Combination of a mood stabilizer with risperidone or haloperidol for treatment of acute mania: a double-blind, placebo-controlled comparison of efficacy and safety. Am J Psychiatry 159:1146–1154, 2002

Schou M: Lithium in psychiatric therapy and prophylaxis. J Psychiatr Res 6:67–95, 1968

Schou M: Prophylactic lithium treatment of unipolar and bipolar manic-depressive illness. Psychopathology 28:81–85, 1995

Schneekloth TD, Rummans TA, Logan KM: Electroconvulsive therapy in adolescents. Convuls Ther 9:158–166, 1993

Schreiber G, Avissar S: Lithium sensitive G protein hyperfunction: a dynamic model for the pathogenesis of bipolar affective disorder. Med Hypotheses 35:237–243, 1991

Schulterbrandt JG, Raskin A: Depression in Childhood: Diagnosis, Treatment, and Conceptual Models. New York, Raven, 1977

Seligman ME, Peterson C: A learned helplessness perspective on child depression: theory and research, in Depression in Young People. Edited by Rutter M, Izard CE, Read PB. New York, Guilford, 1986, pp 223–249

Seligman ME, Peterson C, Kaslow NJ, et al: Attributional style and depressive symptoms among children. J Abnorm Psychol 93:235–238, 1984

Silberstein SD, Wilmore LJ: Divalproex sodium: migraine treatment and monitoring. Headache 36:239–242, 1996

Silva RR, Campbell M, Golden RR, et al: Side effects associated with lithium and placebo administration in aggressive children. Psychopharmacol Bull 28:319–326, 1992

Soutullo CA, Casuto LS, Keck PE Jr: Gabapentin in the treatment of adolescent mania: a case report. J Child Adolesc Psychopharmacol 8:81–85, 1998

Soutullo CA, Sorter MT, Foster KD, et al: Olanzapine in the treatment of adolescent acute mania: a report of seven cases. J Affect Disord 53:279–283, 1999

Spitz R: Anaclitic depression. Psychoanal Study Child 2:113–117, 1946

Stark KD, Reynolds WM, Kaslow NJ: A comparison of the relative efficacy of self-control therapy and a behavioral problem-solving therapy for depression in children. J Abnorm Child Psychol 15:91–113, 1987

Steingard RJ, Renshaw PF, Yurgelun-Todd D, et al: Structural abnormalities in brain magnetic resonance images of depressed children. J Am Acad Child Adolesc Psychiatry 35:307–311, 1996

Stores G, Williams PL, Styles E, et al: Psychological effects of sodium valproate and carbamazepine in epilepsy. Arch Dis Child 67:1330–1337, 1992

Strober M: Familial aspects of depressive disorders in early adolescence, in An Update of Childhood Depression. Edited by Weller EB, Weller RA. Washington, DC, American Psychiatric Association, 1984, pp 38–48

Strober M: Relevance of early age-of-onset in genetic studies of bipolar affective disorder. J Am Acad Child Adolesc Psychiatry 31:606–610, 1992

Strober M, Morrell W, Burroughs J, et al: A family study of bipolar I disorder in adolescence. Early onset of symptoms linked to increased familial loading and lithium resistance. J Affect Disord 15:255–268, 1988

Strober M, Morrell W, Lampert C, et al: Relapse following discontinuation of lithium maintenance therapy in adolescents with bipolar I illness: a naturalistic study. Am J Psychiatry 147:457–461, 1990

Strober M, Lampert C, Schmidt S, et al: The course of major depressive disorder in adolescents, I: recovery and risk of manic switching in a follow-up of psychotic and nonpsychotic subtypes. J Am Acad Child Adolesc Psychiatry 32:34–42, 1993

Strober M, Schmidt-Lackner S, Freeman R, et al: Recovery and relapse in adolescents with bipolar affective illness: a five-year naturalistic, prospective follow-up. J Am Acad Child Adolesc Psychiatry 34:724–731, 1995

Summerville MB, Abbate MF, Siegel AM, et al: Psychopathology in urban female minority adolescents with suicide attempts. J Am Acad Child Adolesc Psychiatry 31:663–668, 1992

Swearingen EM, Cohen LH: Measurement of adolescents' life events: the junior high life experiences survey. Am J Community Psychol 13:69–85, 1985

Tappia PS, Ladha S, Clark DC, et al: The influence of membrane fluidity, TNF receptor binding, cAMP production and GTPase activity on macrophage cytokine production in rats fed a variety of fat diets. Mol Cell Biochem 166:135–143, 1997

Thase ME, Trivedi MH, Rush AJ: MAOIs in the contemporary treatment of depression. Neuropsychopharmacology 12:185–219, 1995

Tillman R, Geller B, Bolhofner K, et al: Ages of onset of syndromal and subsyndromal comorbid DSM-IV diagnoses in a prepubertal and early adolescent bipolar disorder phenotype. J Am Acad Child Adolesc Psychiatry 42:1486–1493, 2003

Todd RD, Neuman R, Geller B, et al: Genetic studies of affective disorders: should we be starting with childhood onset probands? J Am Acad Child Adolesc Psychiatry 32:1164–1171, 1993

Varanka TM, Weller RA, Weller EB, et al: Lithium treatment of manic episodes with psychotic features in prepubertal children. Am J Psychiatry 145:1557–1559, 1988

Varley CK: Sudden death related to selected tricyclic antidepressants in children: epidemiology, mechanisms, and clinical implications. Paediatric Drugs 3:613–627, 2001

Viesselman JO, Yaylayan S, Weller EB, et al: Antidysthymic drugs (antidepressants and antimanics), in Practitioner's Guide to Psychoactive Drugs for Children and Adolescents. Edited by Werry JS, Aman MG. New York, Plenum, 1993, pp 239–268

Vitiello B, Behar D, Malone R, et al: Pharmacokinetics of lithium carbonate in children. J Clin Psychopharmacol 8:355–359, 1988

Vostanis P, Feehan C, Grattan E, et al: A randomized controlled out-patient trial of cognitive-behavioural treatment for children and adolescents with depression: 9-month follow-up. J Affect Disord 40:105–116, 1996

Vreeland B, Minsky S, Menza M, et al: A program for managing weight gain associated with atypical antipsychotics. Psychiatr Serv 54:1155–1157, 2003

Wagner KD, Weller EB, Carlson GA, et al: An open-label trial of divalproex in children and adolescents with bipolar disorder. J Am Acad Child Adolesc Psychiatry 41:1224–1230, 2002

Wagner KD, Ambrosinin P, Rynn M, et al: Efficacy of sertraline in the treatment of children and adolescents with major depressive disorder: two randomized control trials. JAMA 290:1033–1041, 2003

Wagner KD, Robb AS, Findling RL, et al: A randomized, placebo-controlled trial of citalopram for the treatment of major depression in children and adolescents. Am J Psychiatry 161:1079–1083, 2004

Ward R: To prescribe or not to prescribe. Psychology Today 37:17, 2004

Warner V, Mufson L, Weissman MM: Offspring at high and low risk for depression and anxiety: mechanisms of psychiatric disorder. J Am Acad Child Adolesc Psychiatry 34:786–797, 1995

Weinberg WA, Rutman J, Sullivan L, et al: Depression in children referred to an educational diagnostic center: diagnosis and treatment—preliminary report. J Pediatr 83:1065–1072, 1973

Weissman MM, Kidd KK, Prusoff BA: Variability in rates of affective disorders in relatives of depressed and normal probands. Arch Gen Psychiatry 39:1397–1403, 1982

Weissman MM, Gershon ES, Kidd KK, et al: Psychiatric disorders in the relatives of probands with affective disorders: the Yale University–National Institute of Mental Health Collaborative Study. Arch Gen Psychiatry 41:13–21, 1984a

Weissman MM, Leckman JF, Merikangas KR, et al: Depression and anxiety disorders in parents and children: results from the Yale family study. Arch Gen Psychiatry 41:845–852, 1984b

Weissman MM, Wickramaratne P, Merikangas KR, et al: Onset of major depression in early adulthood: increased familial loading and specificity. Arch Gen Psychiatry 41:1136–1143, 1984c

Weissman MM, Gammon GD, John K, et al: Children of depressed parents: increased psychopathology and early onset of major depression. Arch Gen Psychiatry 44:847–853, 1987

Weissman MM, Leaf PJ, Tischler GL, et al: Affective disorders in five United States communities [published erratum appears in Psychol Med 18:following 792, 1988]. Psychol Med 18:141–153, 1988

Weissman MM, Fendrich M, Warner V, et al: Incidence of psychiatric disorder in offspring at high and low risk for depression. J Am Acad Child Adolesc Psychiatry 31:640–648, 1992

Weissman MM, Bland R, Joyce PR et al: Sex differences in rates of depression: cross-national perspectives. J Affect Disord 29:77–84, 1993

Weller EB, Weller RA: Depressive disorders in children and adolescents, in Psychiatric Disorders in Children and Adolescents. Edited by Garfinkel BD. Philadelphia, PA, WB Saunders, 1990, pp 3–20

Weller EB, Weller RA: Mood disorders in prepubertal children, in Textbook of Child and Adolescent Psychiatry. Edited by Wiener JM. Washington, DC, American Academy of Child and Adolescent Psychiatry, 1991, pp 333–342

Weller EB, Weller RA, Fristad MA: Lithium dosage guide for prepubertal children: a preliminary report. J Am Acad Child Psychiatry 25:92–95, 1986

Weller EB, Weller RA, Fristad MA et al: Saliva lithium monitoring in prepubertal children. J Am Acad Child Adolesc Psychiatry 26:173-175, 1987

Weller EB, Weller RA, Fristad MA, et al: Dexamethasone suppression test and depressive symptoms in bereaved children: a preliminary report. J Neuropsychiatry Clin Neurosci 2:418–421, 1990

Weller EB, Weller RA, Fristad MA: Bipolar disorder in children: misdiagnosis, underdiagnosis, and future directions. J Am Acad Child Adolesc Psychiatry 34:709–714, 1995

Weller EB, Weller RA, Rowan AB, et al: Depressive disorders in children and adolescents, in Child and Adolescent Psychiatry: A Comprehensive Textbook. Edited by Melvin Lewis. Philadelphia, PA, Lippincott Williams & Wilkins, 2000, pp 767–781

Weller EB, Weller RA, Danielyan A: Mood disorders in prepubertal children, in Textbook of Child and Adolescent Psychiatry. Edited by Wiener JM, Dulcan M. Washington, DC, American Psychiatric Publishing, 2004a, pp 411–436

Weller EB, Weller RA, Danielyan A: Mood disorders in adolescents, in Textbook of Child and Adolescent Psychiatry. Edited by Wiener JM, Dulcan M. Washington DC, American Psychiatric Publishing, 2004b, pp 437–481

Weller RA, Weller EB, Tucker SG, et al: Mania in prepubertal children: has it been underdiagnosed? J Affect Disord 11:151–154, 1986

Welner A, Welner Z, Fishman R: Psychiatric adolescent inpatients: eight- to ten-year follow-up. Arch Gen Psychiatry 36:698–700, 1979

Werry JS, McClellan JM, Chard L: Childhood and adolescent schizophrenic, bipolar, and schizoaffective disorders: a clinical and outcome study. J Am Acad Child Adolesc Psychiatry 30:457–465, 1991

West SA, Keck PE, McElroy SL, et al: Open trial of valproate in the treatment of adolescent mania. J Child Adolesc Psychopharmacol 4:263–267, 1994

West SA, McElroy SL, Strakowski SM, et al: Attention deficit hyperactivity disorder in adolescent mania. Am J Psychiatry 152:271–273, 1995

Whitaker A, Johnson J, Shaffer D, et al: Uncommon troubles in young people: prevalence estimates of selected psychiatric disorders in a nonreferred adolescent population. Arch Gen Psychiatry 47:487–496, 1990

Whittier MC, West SA, Galli VB, et al: Valproic acid for dysphoric mania in a mentally retarded adolescent (letter). J Clin Psychiatry 56:590–591, 1995

Wilens TE, Biederman J, Baldessarini RJ, et al: Cardiovascular effects of therapeutic doses of tricyclic antidepressants in children and adolescents. J Am Acad Child Adolesc Psychiatry 35:1491–1501, 1996

Wilens TE, Spencer TJ, Biederman J, et al: Case study: nefazodone for juvenile mood disorders. J Am Acad Child Adolesc Psychiatry 36:481–485, 1997

Williamson DE, Birmaher B, Anderson BP, et al: Stressful life events in depressed adolescents: the role of dependent events during the depressive episode. J Am Acad Child Adolesc Psychiatry 34:591–598, 1995

Winokur G, Coryell W, Akiskal HS, et al: Alcoholism in manic-depressive (bipolar) illness: familial illness, course of illness, and the primary-secondary distinction. Am J Psychiatry 152:365–372, 1995

Wood A, Harrington R, Moore A: Controlled trial of a brief cognitive-behavioral intervention in adolescent patients with depressive disorders. J Child Psychol Psychiatry 37:737–746, 1996

Woolston JL: Case study: carbamazepine treatment of juvenile-onset bipolar disorder. J Am Acad Child Adolesc Psychiatry 38:335–338, 1999

Worrel JA, Marken PA, Beckman SE, et al: Atypical antipsychotic agents: a critical review. Am J Health Syst Pharm 57:238–255, 2000

Wozniak J, Biederman J, Kiely K, et al: Mania-like symptoms suggestive of childhood-onset bipolar disorder in clinically referred children. J Am Acad Child Adolesc Psychiatry 34:867–876, 1995

Youngerman J, Canino IA: Lithium carbonate use in children and adolescents: a survey of the literature. Arch Gen Psychiatry 35:216–224, 1978

Self-Assessment Questions

Select the single best response for each question.

14.1 Childhood mood disorders are often underdiagnosed or misdiagnosed for which of the following reasons?

  A. The belief, on the part of some clinicians, that a child's immature superego and personality structure do not permit the development of a mood disorder.
  B. Many children lack the capacity to express their emotions verbally.
  C. Many children present with somatic complaints that are diagnosed as physical illness.
  D. Parents who are bipolar are often underdiagnosed.
  E. All of the above.

14.2 Commonly presenting symptoms of depression in adolescents include

  A. Poor school performance.
  B. Social withdrawal.
  C. Substance abuse.
  D. Conduct disorder.
  E. All of the above.

14.3 Diagnosing bipolar disorder in adolescence may be challenging for all of the following reasons *except*

  A. Presenting symptoms are often minor or major depression.
  B. Severity of symptoms frequently results in hospitalization.
  C. Because symptoms may build up gradually, they frequently are overlooked.
  D. Inappropriate sexual behavior and other "atypical" presentations are common.
  E. Serious conduct behaviors, such as vandalism, may mask underlying manic symptoms.

14.4 In a study by Carlson et al. (2000) comparing patients with early-onset (between the ages of 15 and 20 years) and adult-onset bipolar disorder, which of the following findings was reported?

  A. Women predominated in the early-onset group.
  B. More remissions occurred during follow-up in the early-onset group than in the adult-onset group.
  C. Individuals in the early-onset group were more likely than those in the adult-onset group to have a substance use disorder.
  D. Patients with early-onset bipolar disorder had an increased risk of mood-incongruent psychotic symptoms.
  E. Depressive episodes occurred more frequently in the early-onset group.

14.5 Approximately 40%–70% of children and adolescents with major depressive disorder have a comorbid psychiatric disorder. All of the following are common
comorbid conditions *except*

A. Eating disorders.
B. Anxiety disorders.
C. Dysthymic disorder.
D. Disruptive behavior disorder.
E. Substance use.

14.6 Common side effects of lithium treatment in children and adolescents include all
of the following *except*

A. Diarrhea.
B. Tremor.
C. Leukopenia.
D. Fatigue.
E. Ataxia.

Attention-Deficit/ Hyperactivity Disorder

Bruce Waslick, M.D.

Laurence L. Greenhill, M.D.

The core symptoms of attention-deficit/ hyperactivity disorder (ADHD) have long been recognized and reported on by mental health specialists dealing with children and adolescents. Nevertheless, the diagnosis of ADHD continues to be controversial. In 1998 the National Institutes of Health convened a special consensus development conference to address the degree of controversy related to the disorder. The following sentences were included in the conference summary statement:

> The diverse and conflicting opinions about ADHD have resulted in confusion for families, care providers, educators, and policymakers. The controversy raises questions concerning the literal existence of the disorder, whether it can be reliably diagnosed, and, if treated, what interventions are the most effective. (National Institutes of Health 2000, p. 5)

ADHD remains one of the most intensively researched areas in child psychiatry, and the literature on this disorder is expanding in terms of recognizing and understanding adolescent and adult presentations of the disorder. Although the shift toward more interest in the biological basis of mental disorders is evident in studies examining molecular, genetic, neurochemical, and neuroimaging correlates of the disorder, more information also continues to be gathered on the psychological manifestations of the disorder and the effect of psychological interventions. In this chapter we summarize the clinical and research understandings of ADHD and present biological, psychological, and social perspectives that contribute to the evolving definition of this complex psychiatric disorder.

Diagnostic Considerations

In the DSM-IV-TR (American Psychiatric Association 2000) definition of ADHD, three core symptom clusters are identified (Table 15–1). Each of these symptom clusters is described below under "Clinical Description."

Important diagnostic features of the disorder include the following:

- *Discriminant validity of ADHD*—Although oppositional defiant disorder and conduct disorder are highly associated with ADHD, the distinction between these three behavior disorders is supported by empirical evidence (Fergusson et al. 1994; Halperin et al. 1993).
- *Early onset*—some symptoms must be present before age 7 years.
- *Duration of symptoms*—the symptoms must be present for at least 6 months.
- *Pervasiveness of symptoms*—the symptoms must be evident in at least two different environments, typically (in children) at school and at home.
- *Abnormality of the symptoms*—the symptoms are clearly inappropriate for the child's developmental age and are maladaptive in terms of functioning.

Also, a criterion requiring that the individual manifest "clinically significant impairment" in social, academic, or occupational functioning was added, eliminating persons who have appropriate symptoms, but no impairment, from receiving this diagnosis.

Establishing a diagnosis in child psychiatry requires that information from multiple sources be synthesized. Often, the information reported by adults (e.g., parents, teachers) of a child's behavioral problems and the individual child's self-report are significantly different (Bird et al. 1992). Children with behavior disorders report symptoms of their disruptive behavior with less frequency than do the adults around them, and self-reports of symptoms from young children (i.e., between ages 6 and 11 years) are not reliable (Schwab-Stone et al. 1994).

In general, teachers and parents tend to agree on the identification of a child with a behavior disorder, even though the correlation between their reports of individual symptoms is quite low (Biederman et al. 1993), possibly because of the differing contexts of the observations available to each informant (Pelham et al. 1992). The diagnosis of disruptive behavior disorder tends to be more valid if it is based on adult reports rather than on the child's self-report (Pelham et al. 1992). Further complicating the diagnostic assessment is the suggestion that individual parental psychopathology may influence the parent's reporting of the child's behavior—for example, the tendency of depressed mothers to report increased numbers of symptoms (Fergusson et al. 1993). Adults' reports of symptoms of ADHD may also be affected by the presence of comorbid conduct disturbance in the child (Abikoff et al. 1993) as well as by cultural factors (Mann et al. 1992).

Dimensional scales (e.g., the Child Behavior Checklist and Conners' Teacher Rating Scale) have been applied to the study of attentional and hyperactive disorders of childhood in an attempt to identify cases of disorder on the basis of cutoff points representing significant deviation from normality on the respective symptom scales (Achenbach and Edelbrock 1983; Collett et al. 2003; Goyette et al. 1978). Highly structured interviews (e.g., the Diagnostic Interview Schedule for Children [Shaffer et al. 2000]), corresponding to specific diagnostic classification systems such as DSM, also are used for research purposes. There is significant correlation between structured diagnostic interviews and well-established dimensional scales for

---

Table 15–1.   DSM-IV-TR diagnostic criteria for attention-deficit/hyperactivity disorder

---

A. Either (1) or (2):

  (1) six (or more) of the following symptoms of **inattention** have persisted for at least 6 months to a degree that is maladaptive and inconsistent with developmental level:

Inattention

  (a) often fails to give close attention to details or makes careless mistakes in schoolwork, work, or other activities

  (b) often has difficulty sustaining attention in tasks or play activities

  (c) often does not seem to listen when spoken to directly

  (d) often does not follow through on instructions and fails to finish schoolwork, chores, or duties in the workplace (not due to oppositional behavior or failure to understand instructions)

  (e) often has difficulty organizing tasks and activities

  (f) often avoids, dislikes, or is reluctant to engage in tasks that require sustained mental effort (such as schoolwork or homework)

  (g) often loses things necessary for tasks or activities (e.g., toys, school assignments, pencils, books, or tools)

  (h) is often easily distracted by extraneous stimuli

  (i) is often forgetful in daily activities

  (2) six (or more) of the following symptoms of **hyperactivity–impulsivity** have persisted for at least 6 months to a degree that is maladaptive and inconsistent with developmental level:

Hyperactivity

  (a) often fidgets with hands or feet or squirms in seat

  (b) often leaves seat in classroom or in other situations in which remaining seated is expected

  (c) often runs about or climbs excessively in situations in which it is inappropriate (in adolescents or adults, may be limited to subjective feelings of restlessness)

  (d) often has difficulty playing or engaging in leisure activities quietly

  (e) is often "on the go" or often acts as if "driven by a motor"

  (f) often talks excessively

Impulsivity

  (g) often blurts out answers before questions have been completed

  (h) often has difficulty awaiting turn

  (i) often interrupts or intrudes on others (e.g., butts into conversations or games)

B. Some hyperactive–impulsive or inattentive symptoms that caused impairment were present before age 7 years.

C. Some impairment from the symptoms is present in two or more settings (e.g., at school [or work] and at home).

D. There must be clear evidence of clinically significant impairment in social, academic, or occupational functioning.

E. The symptoms do not occur exclusively during the course of a pervasive developmental disorder, schizophrenia, or other psychotic disorder and are not better accounted for by another mental disorder (e.g., mood disorder, anxiety disorder, dissociative disorder, or a personality disorder).

Table 15–1.   DSM-IV-TR diagnostic criteria for attention-deficit/hyperactivity disorder *(continued)*

Code based on type:

314.01   Attention-deficit/hyperactivity disorder, combined type: if both criteria A1 and A2 are met for the past 6 months

314.00   Attention-deficit/hyperactivity disorder, predominantly inattentive type: if criterion A1 is met but criterion A2 is not met for the past 6 months

314.01   Attention-deficit/hyperactivity disorder, predominantly hyperactive–impulsive type: if criterion A2 is met but criterion A1 is not met for the past 6 months

Coding note: For individuals (especially adolescents and adults) who currently have symptoms that no longer meet full criteria, "In Partial Remission" should be specified.

Source.   Reprinted from the *Diagnostic and Statistical Manual of Mental Disorders*, 4th Edition, Text Revision. Washington, DC, American Psychiatric Association, 2000. Copyright 2000, American Psychiatric Association. Used with permission.

the identification of behavior disorders in children (Jensen et al. 1993a). There is active research focusing on attempts to move from diagnoses based on subjective reports toward the use of more objective neuropsychological tests and laboratory assessments (such as the Continuous Performance Test, described under "Inattention" below). However, these types of assessments currently represent at best research tools and sources of supplementary clinical information (Barkley et al. 1991).

No separate definition of the adult type of ADHD exists in DSM-IV-TR. A residual type of ADHD has been demonstrated to exist in adolescents and adults and may be an increasingly recognized and important clinical entity. Recent research reports of children with ADHD observed prospectively in longitudinal studies demonstrate the relative decrease in symptoms of behavioral overactivity and the relative persistence of attentional problems (Biederman et al. 2000; Denckla 1991; Shaffer 1994). There is also increasing evidence demonstrating that in some cases ADHD can present with an onset of symptoms after the age of 7 years, especially in patients with the inattentive subtype (Applegate et al. 1997; Barkley and Biederman 1997; Willoughby et al. 2000).

In summary, ADHD can be viewed as a developmental disorder with somewhat varying symptom presentations appearing at different life phases. There is increasing recognition that the different developmental phases of the disorder are not captured well in the present diagnostic classification systems and that this should be clarified in the future.

Clinical Description

Establishing the diagnosis of ADHD depends more on taking a good behavioral history and less on a direct mental status examination of the child in the office. Under direct questioning, the child will often deny being symptomatic and will not complain about any problem. The clinician must rely on reports from parents and teachers and should use direct observations of the patient's behavior only if it is conducted in a social situation, such as a classroom. Even after gathering a classic history of ADHD, little chaos and mayhem may be seen in the first one-to-one exchange with the child. How can the clinician make a diagnosis if the disorder cannot be validated by direct observation in the interview?

The diagnostic decision and choice of

treatment depend on the clinician's experience in working with other children with ADHD and common-sense clinical judgment. In addition, psychological reports can help by revealing attentional lapses during tedious repetitive tasks, such as the coding task of the Wechsler Intelligence Scale for Children–Revised (Wechsler 1974). One clinical rule of thumb, now made explicit in DSM-IV-TR, is that the signs of the disorder must be present to a moderate degree in at least two of three settings (e.g., home, school, and clinician's office).

Despite changes in the DSM classification system over the past 20 years, the diagnosis of ADHD has retained three key elements: 1) a developmentally inappropriate level of motor hyperactivity, 2) inattention at school, and 3) impulsivity with regard to rule-governed behavior (Barkley 1982; Carlson et al. 1986). The clinician's history-taking approach works best when the inquiry focuses on the positive signs of the disorder, exclusion criteria, severity measures, associated conditions, and family history. Such information is best collected from both parents together, if possible.

The behavioral traits in a child with ADHD often seem to be exaggerations of normal childhood activities. Signs of inattention and overactivity interact with the environmental setting and are age dependent. The younger the child, the more pervasive is the motor drivenness, and its appearance is less dependent on the setting. The preschool-age child with ADHD rapidly moves about the room and is stimulus driven to touch everything and manipulate each object in a haphazard manner. He or she climbs, jumps, and runs as if "driven by a motor" out of control. Birthday parties and peer-group get-togethers are quickly derailed by the child with ADHD, who becomes wild, overactive, noisy, and unmanageable if the occasion is unstructured.

The school-age child may show a narrower range of impulsive and overactive behaviors, with large group settings required to bring out the most severe disturbances. In class, the inattentiveness predominates; the child with ADHD appears to be daydreaming or preoccupied. The child squirms and moves restlessly about when seated. The inattentiveness seriously interferes with academic performance, as revealed in the child's sloppy handwriting, careless errors, and messy papers. At home, parents find that the child with ADHD does not listen, does not follow through on even the most simple requests, and is unable to complete homework.

Children with ADHD may have a history of long-standing difficulties with impulse control, high levels of motor activity, and disruptiveness in groups. Activity levels in children with ADHD are generally higher, even during sleep (Porrino et al. 1983). In physical education class, activity levels may be lower because children with ADHD have trouble modulating their behavior downward (in academic class) or upward (during a soccer game) as the social setting demands. On the playground during recess, these children may seem to be just as active as their playmates, yet other children often find that impulsivity and inattentiveness make them poor teammates (Porrino et al. 1983; Whalen et al. 1979, 1987). Situations involving self-paced work exert the greatest stress (Whalen et al. 1979).

In the following sections, we discuss the three cardinal features of the disorder in detail.

■ Hyperactivity

Although developmentally inappropriate levels of hyperactivity have been both emphasized and deemphasized (Carlson et al. 1986), the importance of the high activity level in children with ADHD has been supported by research in the past decades. Children with ADHD, compared with control children, display higher activity levels, particularly when carrying out structured, in-seat activities (Abikoff and Gittelman 1985a; Conners and Werry 1979). Naturalistic studies employing small, solid-state memory-activity monitors mounted on the belt or vest have also shown that children with ADHD manifest significantly higher levels of activity in the classroom, at home, and while sleeping at night than do children without ADHD (Porrino et al. 1983). Monitored activity levels fall to normal when stimulants are given to children with ADHD. The high levels of sleep activity in children with ADHD and the normalization of activity with stimulant treatment strengthen the concurrent validity of the syndrome.

The higher-than-usual level of motility makes the child with ADHD appear to be driven, restless, and never tiring. Although some degree of hyperactivity is found ordinarily in school-age boys (Lapouse and Monk 1953), the diagnosis of ADHD should be limited to a developmentally inappropriate degree of gross motor activity in the school and/or home setting. Sedentary activities—such as sitting in school or church, riding in the car, or even going to a movie—lead to high levels of noncompliance and restlessness. In the classroom—where children are asked to sit still, remain quiet, and work independently—children with ADHD squirm in their chairs, hum, make noises, and tap on their desks. This activity disturbs other children. Hyperactive children also enjoy climbing; for example, they will climb along kitchen counters when their peers choose to walk on the floor.

■ Inattention

To date, no standardized office procedure is established to validly measure specific attentional abnormalities in children. The inattention component is best determined by history. The clinician inquires about attentional problems by asking the parents or teacher if the child has a short attention span, difficulty concentrating, an inability to modulate attention in response to externally imposed demands, a problem in initiating tasks, or trouble selectively attending to relevant stimuli while filtering out unnecessary noise (Carlson et al. 1986). Distractibility may reflect not a breakdown in filtering out unwanted input but rather an active seeking out of more stimuli when the activity requiring attention produces boredom (Zentall and Meyer 1987).

Inattentive children have difficulty processing classwork. They cannot complete goal-directed work without frequent refocusing from another person. They spend more time off the task and out of their seat than do children with more normal attentional abilities. These children are typically oversolicitous with the teacher (calling out more often or trying to answer questions that are not understood). Whereas other children complete their assignment sheets, tests, and workbook drills, children with ADHD produce very little "product," even if they are the brightest in the class. Teachers become frustrated when a bright student produces scanty, poor-quality work.

At home, school-age children with ADHD often have trouble listening to adults. These children look away and do not make eye contact when speaking with an adult. In doing chores, they forget what they were asked to do and have difficulty carrying out multicommission commands. Following written instructions for constructing a model airplane requires effortful redirecting and maintenance of attention, from the instruction sheet to the model and back again. Faced with a multistep instruction sheet, children with ADHD may decide to slap together the model, based on only the picture on the box. As a result, important pieces are ignored or left out. In just such a manner, ADHD children always seem to be rushed, too busy, or "on the way in a hurry" to some other activity. In other instances, they may start several activities at once and finish none of them.

Laboratory-based research studies have used a number of procedures to monitor the task performance of children with ADHD and have claimed that these laboratory measures detect attentional difficulties that otherwise would be seen only in a classroom. The best known of such tests is the Continuous Performance Test (CPT), which measures sustained attention (Cornblatt et al. 1988; Sykes et al. 1972; Weingartner et al. 1980). This test requires the child to watch a computer screen continuously for 10–15 minutes. The child is instructed to pick out the correct target among a group of nontarget letters that flash on the screen and to press a key as soon as the correct letter or combination of letters is seen. A wide range of modifications have been employed to avoid floor and ceiling effects (Cornblatt et al. 1988), including visually degrading the stimuli on the screen, playing movie soundtracks over earphones during the visual task, and even varying the time between stimuli, depending on the performance of the child. The CPT has been shown to be sensitive to drug effects (Garfinkel et al. 1986) and to dose of drug (Cornblatt et al. 1987; Rapport et al. 1985).

However, laboratory-based measures of attention do not always correlate with classroom performance (DuPaul et al. 1992). Any laboratory tool used in a 1-to-1 (1 researcher with 1 child) situation cannot easily recreate the demand set of the 1-to-30 environment found in a classroom (1 teacher to 30 students). Douglas (1983) wisely pointed out that sustained attention, which is tracked by the CPT, does not tap other important attentional functions required in complex tasks, such as self-regulation, the extent to which attention is self-directed and organized, the amount of effort that is invested, or whether the approach to a task involves a search strategy or is just simple exploration. In addition, research has downplayed the role of a sustained attention deficit as the sole cognitive deficit in ADHD (Corkum and Siegel 1993; Solanto and Wender 1989; Swanson and Cantwell 1989).

Other laboratory measures have been used in research, and some find their way into a marketplace for practitioners. None of these tasks has been widely accepted for clinical work. One simple device tests motor steadiness; one group has been able to correlate diminishing error rates and the plasma levels of methylphenidate (Birmaher et al. 1989). A rugged, portable CPT has been marketed with normative data to support its utility as a screening device (Gordon and Mettelman 1988). The Paired-Associates Learning Task measures short-term memory and is also medication sensitive, showing significant correlations with stimulant blood levels (Kupietz et al. 1982). The quality of performance on this test at various dosages of methylphenidate, for example, has been used as an argument for choosing lower doses to optimize cognitive performance in the classroom (Sprague and Sleator 1977).

These laboratory measures are not diagnostically specific. Werry et al. (1987) reported no differences among children with ADHD, conduct disorder, or anxiety disorder in CPT results, suggesting that attentional dysfunction (as measured by CPT) is a nonspecific correlate of child psychopathology in general (Barkley 1991; Werry et al. 1987).

■ Impulsivity

Impulsivity means that the child acts without forethought of the consequences, appearing to be unaware of danger or the relationship between cause and effect. The child with ADHD is willing to "take dares" that other children would not.

Complex academic tasks—which require individual initiation, self-monitoring, organization, and self-pacing—may best reveal the impulsivity in children with ADHD. In particular, behavior during homework may be the most distressing of the child's "invisible handicaps." Even bright children with ADHD report the rapid onset of boredom during homework and a strong feeling that "I work in school, so why should I have to continue this stuff at home?" In addition, teachers may insist that the child with ADHD finish uncompleted classwork at home, which further burdens the child with the very tasks that he or she finds most difficult. Secondary behavior patterns often develop during the homework struggle, particularly avoidance routines, such as "forgetting" assignments, leaving important books at school, and even rushing through the homework without concern for errors. When such a child is unsupervised, he or she will start three other activities and not finish either the schoolwork or the other projects. Parents quickly become discouraged after spending much of their leisure time hovering over their child while he or she struggles with homework.

During the early years, the impulsivity of the child with ADHD may take the form of "stimulus drivenness," a robot-like behavior in which the child must pick up, touch, or manipulate every object in the room. This pressure drives toddlers from one toy to the next, disrupting all objects in their path. During school-age years, these children constantly interrupt others and refuse to wait their turn in games. The thoughtless, unpremeditated quality of the hyperkinetic child's rule breaking often leads such children into situations where they get caught "holding the bag," while the real instiga-

tors are long gone. As a result, the child with ADHD can land in trouble and be included with children who have long histories of conduct problems.

Research studies have had the challenge of operationalizing an "impulsivity" dimension, a concept that is inferential at best. Measures have been developed using a number of approaches, including direct observations of a child's self-control during interactions with adults and peers, inhibition of behavior (e.g., a "draw-a-line-slowly" task), and cognitive problem-solving measures (e.g., the Matching Familiar Figures Test) (Carlson et al. 1986). Direct observation studies have been most successful in tapping this impulsive dimension. These studies show that the child with ADHD interrupts others often, does not wait for his or her turn in games, and is disliked by potential peers.

Comorbidity

Comorbid disorders occurring with ADHD have become an area of intense clinical and research concern. Developmental, medical, educational, and psychiatric conditions have all been recognized to contribute to the presentation, longitudinal course, and prognosis of ADHD. In some cases, the comorbidity may be suspected to result from a genetic relationship; in other cases, the comorbidity may be associated with environmental correlates; and in still others, the comorbidity is not clearly accounted for by a known or suspected causative factor.

A number of psychiatric disorders have been commonly associated with ADHD in children and adults. Other disruptive behavior disorders, such as oppositional defiant disorder and conduct disorder, occur with a high frequency in children with ADHD, with as many as 30%–50% of children affected (Biederman et al. 1991). Anxiety and mood disorders co-occur with ADHD in some children and may affect the child's overall degree of impairment, the course of the disorder, and the necessary treatment plan (Jensen et al. 1993b). A high proportion of children with tic disorders also manifest symptoms of ADHD as well as other disorders, leading some to conclude that a genetic relationship may exist (Comings and Comings 1990). ADHD is being increasingly recognized in other populations of children with special needs, such as those with mental retardation (Aman et al. 1991). In adolescents, residual symptoms of ADHD may be associated with conduct problems, substance abuse, and mood and anxiety disorders (Klein and Mannuzza 1991). Patterns of comorbidity in adults with ADHD may approximate those seen in the childhood disorder, a circumstance that lends support to the validity of the diagnosis in adulthood (Biederman et al. 1993). A significant number of adults who abuse cocaine and seek treatment have histories of childhood ADHD, as well as other co-occurring present and past diagnoses (Hoegerman et al. 1993; Rounsaville et al. 1991).

Specific learning disorders have been associated with the diagnosis of ADHD in a subgroup of children (Cantwell and Baker 1991). In general and as a group, children with ADHD perform more poorly in educational settings than nonaffected children, even if they do not have a specific learning disorder (Faraone et al. 1993). However, an unrecognized learning disorder that is inappropriately attributed to the behavioral disturbance and left untreated, leading to unnecessary school failure, can have a detrimental effect on the child's overall functioning and self-esteem.

Evidence of minor neurological dysfunction is present in a subgroup of children with ADHD, which reinforces the concept that the disturbance represents subtle organic insults to the child's brain that impair psychological development and behavioral control (Mayes et al. 1994).

Evaluation and Differential Diagnosis

Children with ADHD should receive a complete medical evaluation and examination. On occasion, a standard physical examination may reveal neurological problems that completely explain the child's inattentiveness, restlessness, and impulsivity; for example, in the sensory area, children with partial deafness or very poor vision may appear inattentive and restless to a teacher. Nonspecific signs found during a careful neurological evaluation, on the other hand, probably contribute little to the evaluation of children with ADHD. These nonspecific signs, including minor physical anomalies, have been referred to as *soft neurological signs* (Shaffer and Greenhill 1979). Soft signs present as asymmetries in reflex findings, minor choreoathetoid movements, an inability to carry out rapid alternating movements, and generally poor coordination. They are subject to intertest and interrater reliability problems. Their presence does not aid in making the diagnosis of ADHD (Shaffer and Greenhill 1979). In fact, an epidemiological study showed that these soft signs predict persistence of a higher-than-normal prevalence of anxiety disorders, not ADHD (Shaffer et al. 1985).

Some medical problems may lead to overactive and inattentive behavior. Language disorders will produce aberrant behavior and at times are associated with motor hyperactivity and severe inattentiveness. Dermatological conditions, such as eczema and even pinworms, may produce restlessness and disruptiveness in grade-school children and to the teacher may appear to be a pure behavior disorder. Even more rare, Sydenham's chorea generates intense restlessness in children and requires careful workup and treatment. Finally, as many as 50%–60% of patients ages 6–18 years with Tourette's disorder also may have ADHD (Cohen and Leckman 1989). Stimulants, which cause a release of catecholamines in the central nervous system, can exacerbate motor tics in these patients (Lowe et al. 1982), possibly by further intensifying the putative hyperdopaminergic state found in Tourette's disorder.

The child's height and weight should be measured before any treatment—particularly if the child will be given stimulant medication, which may cause a temporary delay in weight gain. Other tests, such as computed tomography or magnetic resonance imaging, have no current role in routine clinical evaluation.

Age-appropriate hyperactivity may occur in children who show no impulsive or attentional problems. The high level of activity found in ADHD differs from that of other clinical states by its intense, non–goal-directed quality. Children who have a comorbid Axis I diagnosis of conduct disorder will have all the features of ADHD, but their high propensity for aggressivity differs from the more typical behavior in a child with ADHD only. The impulsivity of a child with conduct disorder has more of a calculating, premeditated quality not found in the reactive and impulsive misbehaviors of the hyperactive child.

Children with other psychiatric disorders (such as severe and profound mental retardation, schizophrenia, and mania)—who may display impulsivity, hyperactivity, and inattentiveness—may display the chaotic, stimulus-bound motor drivenness of children with ADHD, but because the symptoms are secondary to the primary diagnosis, these children are not diagnosed with ADHD.

Epidemiology

The most frequently cited epidemiological studies use different methodologies and examine somewhat different populations (see Scahill and Schwab-Stone 2000 for a comprehensive review). Disorder is variably defined by cutoffs on certain rating scales or by a categorical diagnosis based on structured or semistructured interviews of parents or teachers. These studies may or may not include information from children in the sample, depending on the age range. Because epidemiological literature has not yet been published on DSM-IV-TR–defined ADHD, the closest approximation of this information is in studies that have attempted to diagnose the disorder based on earlier DSM definitions using multiple sources.

The prevalence rate ranges from 1.9% to 14.4% (Scahill and Schwab-Stone 2000). DSM-IV-TR reports the frequently cited prevalence estimate of 3%–7% of school-age children. It is commonly accepted that the disorder is more common in boys than in girls, at a ratio ranging from 2.5:1 to 5.6:1. ADHD is most common in school-age children, and prevalence rates are lower in studies of older populations (McGee et al. 1990). Rates of the disorder may vary in different cultures and countries (Verhulst et al. 1993) and depending on whether the sample studied is urban, suburban, or rural (Shen et al. 1985; Zahner et al. 1993).

Etiology

No clear etiology appears to lead to all, or even most, cases of ADHD. The precise cause of the disorder is unknown. A number of biological and environmental correlates of the disorder have been implicated in individual cases and groups of children with ADHD.

■ Genetics

ADHD is a familial disorder and is likely to have a genetic component. Gene knockout strategies (i.e., eliminating the gene coding for the dopamine transport protein) have produced mice strains with high levels of behavioral hyperactivity (Gainetdinov and Caron 2001), suggesting a role for behavioral genetics in understanding important features of the disorder. Symptoms of the disorder are more highly correlated in identical than in fraternal twin pairs (Goodman and Stevenson 1989). Adoption studies have confirmed that ADHD tends to occur more frequently in first-degree biological relatives of adopted probands than in families in which adopted probands cohabitate (Hechtman 1994). Several studies have reported that relatives of proband children with ADHD are more likely to have the disorder than are relatives of comparison children without ADHD (Biederman et al. 1990), and this appears to be true for girls as well as boys (Faraone et al. 1991). Offspring of adults who have a history of childhood-onset ADHD are at high risk for the development of the disorder (Biederman et al. 1995). Increasing interest in genes expressing gene products related to the functioning of dopamine in the central nervous system has been stimulated by reports supporting the association of the 7-repeat allele of the D_4 dopamine receptor with the ADHD diagnosis in some but not all studies (Faraone et al. 2001) and by molecular genetic studies of the dopamine transporter protein (Madras et al. 2002). Some authors (Sprich-Buckminster et al. 1993) have suggested that familial and nonfamilial subtypes of ADHD exist, with the familial subtype being accounted for by mostly genetic mechanisms and the nonfamilial subtype caused by environmentally induced circumstances, such as perinatal complications. In summary, abnormalities in genes coding for proteins involved in central nervous system dopamine function have been implicated in a preliminary fashion in the etiology of ADHD, but definitive replications are currently lacking. Identifying genetic polymorphisms that convey an elevated risk for ADHD in children remains an area of intense research interest. Shastry (2004) has comprehensively reviewed the molecular genetics of ADHD.

■ Perinatal Complications

The concept that perinatal complications may have an etiological role in ADHD comes from two main areas of investigation. In animal-model studies of infant rats (Speiser et al. 1983) and monkeys (Sechzer et al. 1973) asphyxiated at or near birth, overactivity and attentional problems in exposed organisms were reported, but the correlation with human behavior is speculative. Retrospective human studies that compared individuals with a diagnosis of ADHD with children without such a diagnosis found that perinatal complications (e.g., antepartum hemorrhage, prolonged maternal labor, low Apgar scores at 1 minute) had occurred more frequently in affected than in nonaffected subjects (Chandola et al. 1992). Maternal smoking during pregnancy appears to be a risk factor for the development of ADHD in offspring (Milberger et al. 1997). Infants with low birth weight and manifesting evidence of white matter injury may be at increased risk for the development of ADHD over time as well (Whitaker et al. 1997).

■ Neurological Illness

Investigators have continued to study the role of neurological problems in the etiology of ADHD, including soft signs of neurological illness (Vitiello et al. 1990), poor motor coordination, and subtle signs of abnormal brain function (Ornoy et al. 1993). The term formerly used to describe this disorder, *minimal brain dysfunction*, was derived from these neurological observations. Reports of the onset of ADHD syndromes after closed head trauma support the role of organic factors in the etiology of the disorder. An uncontrolled, prospective follow-up study of children who had been afflicted with septic meningitis found that a high percentage of children had developed ADHD (Alon et al. 1979), lending support to the idea that early insult to the central nervous system may increase the risk for ADHD. Recent anatomical neuroimaging studies have supported the concept that the brains of children with ADHD are different, if perhaps in subtle ways, from those of children without ADHD and that the structural abnormalities may be correlated to neuropsychological deficits (Casey et al. 1997; Castellanos et al. 2001; Semrud-Clikeman et al. 2000). Loss of the normal asymmetry of the caudate nucleus and regional abnormalities in the architecture of the corpus callosum have been identified (Castellanos et al. 1994, 2002, 2003; Giedd et al. 1994; Hynd et al. 1993) and may serve as markers of the disorder in at least a subgroup of children. Functional neuroimaging studies, using functional magnetic resonance imaging and positron emission tomography, have been performed in adults (Matochik et al. 1993), adolescents (Ernst et al. 1997; Rubia et al. 1999; Zametkin et al. 1993) and children (Ernst et al. 1999) with ADHD. Although the results have been equivocal, findings have suggested that subjects with ADHD may show abnormalities in prefrontal cortex function

(Rubia et al. 1999) and disturbed central nervous system dopaminergic activity (Ernst et al. 1999). Animal models of neuronal hypoplasia, induced generally by exposure to chemical agents or locally by focal X-irradiation (Diaz-Granados et al. 1994; Mercugliano et al. 1990; Shaywitz et al. 1976), have produced individual organisms that manifest many behavioral similarities to human hyperactivity and inattentiveness (Altman 1987).

■ Diet

The role of diet in the onset or exacerbation of hyperactivity and behavioral problems remains somewhat controversial, because evidence exists both to support and to refute the effects of different dietary agents (Barling and Bullen 1985; Egger et al. 1992; Rowe and Rowe 1994). The studies that support the notion that diet influences behavioral problems have focused on the roles of preservatives and artificial dyes and on food allergies. Despite the fact that dietary factors most likely do not play a role in the vast majority of children with ADHD, teachers frequently believe that diet influences children with behavior disorders and will counsel parents to restrict suspected offending agents as a means of helping their child (DiBattista and Shepherd 1993).

■ Allergy

The idea that children with allergies or allergic-type illnesses (e.g., asthma, eczema) are at greater risk for developing ADHD does not appear to be supported by current evidence (Biederman et al. 1994; McGee et al. 1993; Roth et al. 1991).

■ Environmental Toxins

The role of exposure to toxins (e.g., heavy metals, illicit drugs, alcohol) prenatally or postnatally is currently speculative, although children and animals exposed to lead (Minder et al. 1994; Sobotka and Cook 1974) or prenatal alcohol use by mothers (Streissguth et al. 1994) can manifest many symptoms of hyperactivity and attentional problems during development.

■ Other Pediatric Illnesses

Although a study reporting on the increased incidence of ADHD in individuals with a genetically transmitted, generalized resistance to thyroid hormone may be describing a highly biologically determined subtype of the disorder (Hauser et al. 1993), the rate of thyroid abnormalities in clinically referred children with ADHD is very low (Elia et al. 1994). Routine screening with thyroid function tests of children with ADHD is not recommended in the absence of other indicators of thyroid disease. The symptoms of ADHD may be increased in children with histories of other medical illnesses, such as recurrent early childhood ear infections (Adesman et al. 1990; Arcia and Roberts 1993; Hagerman and Falkenstein 1987) and acquired sensorineural hearing loss (Kelly et al. 1993).

Natural History

■ Age at Onset

The age at onset in any individual case is often difficult to determine (see Barkley and Biederman 1997). Most studies of clinical populations (Sullivan et al. 1990), as well as prevalence-focused epidemiological studies (McGee et al. 1992), can provide only estimates of age at onset based on retrospective reports of the child or parent, and studies may or may not attempt to validate this estimate by collecting information from different sources, such as physician records or school reports. Prospective studies are needed that begin at a very early age and involve diag-

nostic assessments repeated at regularly spaced intervals. Parents' reports of the onset of their child's behavioral problems appear to be stable over time and may have good reliability (Green et al. 1991). Children have little capacity to provide valid estimates of the onset of the disorder, although retrospective assessments of the patient's behavior may be the clinical standard for diagnosing ADHD in adults (Ward et al. 1993). It is generally understood that the roots of the disorder (according to the DSM-IV-TR definition) begin in early childhood, with at least some symptoms being present before the age of 7 years, but this may be more true of children with prominent hyperactivity as opposed to those with the inattentive subtype (Applegate et al. 1997). With the increased use of preschool and day care services for children, the behavior disorders of this age group may be attracting more clinical and research attention (DuPaul et al. 2001; Lahey et al. 1998; McGee et al. 1991; Palfrey et al. 1985; Strayhorn and Weidman 1989).

■ Clinical Presentation

The child typically comes to the attention of mental health providers as a result of disruptive behavior at home or in a structured setting, such as school, or because of academic failure. Not all persons in the general population who meet criteria for ADHD come to clinical attention, and those who do seek clinical attention may be different from those who do not (Bird et al. 1993). Parents of children with ADHD may seek intervention from their pediatrician, from their family doctor, from personnel at the child's school, or from clergy members prior to eventual referral to a mental health specialist. Stimulant therapy in the United States is routinely prescribed by primary care physicians and pediatricians as well as by child psychiatrists (Hoagwood et al. 2000). It is likely that patients presenting to mental health clinicians have more severe ADHD with more comorbidity.

■ Duration of Disorder

In general, several studies suggest that some symptoms of ADHD—particularly hyperactivity—tend toward remission over time but that inattention problems are remarkably persistent (for example, see Biederman et al. 2000). The disorder is not episodic but rather chronic and enduring (Keller et al. 1992) and has been likened to other developmental disorders with their onset in childhood. Prospective studies of clinical samples report that at least some impairment from the disorder is present in most adolescents who had been referred for clinical treatment as school-age children (Barkley et al. 1991; Gittelman et al. 1985). Follow-up studies of referred cohorts (and control subjects) into adulthood report that impairment persists in a sizable percentage of patients and that complications of the disorder include lower academic and professional achievement and an increased risk for developing antisocial behavior and possibly substance abuse (Klein and Mannuzza 1991). Some studies suggest that there may be different outcomes for the different symptom cores: that inattention symptoms tend to predict problems with educational achievement, but prominent hyperactivity and impulsivity symptoms may place a child at greater risk for the development of antisocial outcomes (for example, see Babinski et al. 1999).

Treatment

The body of research devoted to the treatment of ADHD in children exceeds that of any other diagnosis in child psychiatry. With the publication of the main intent-to-treat results of the National Institute of Mental Health–funded multi-site Multimodal Treatment of ADHD (MTA) study (MTA Cooperative Group 1999), clearer guidelines about the central role of medication treatment are now available. Less clear is the role of psychotherapy and other psychosocial interventions as components of treatment plans for individual children with the disorder.

■ Medication

Psychostimulants

The psychostimulants are the first-line agents of choice for symptom suppression. Methylphenidate, amphetamine preparations, and magnesium pemoline have all demonstrated efficacy in double-blind, placebo-controlled studies of children with ADHD, and the literature reporting the efficacy of the use of these agents in children and adults is expanding (Greenhill et al. 1999; Spencer et al. 1996). Methylphenidate tends to be the most popular drug of first choice, although whether it has greater efficacy or safety compared with other stimulants has not been proved.

Methylphenidate, in its unmodified form, is a short-acting agent and a racemate that generally requires multiple daily doses. Dexmethylphenidate hydrochloride (Focalin) is the d-threo-enantiomer of short-acting racemic methylphenidate and is currently approved for use in the treatment of ADHD (Wigal et al. 2004). Recently there have been developed, by a variety of manufacturers, different preparations of long-duration methylphenidate medications (Concerta, Metadate CD, Ritalin-LA) using different medication-delivery technologies to increase the effective duration of the medication load delivered in single morning doses (Greenhill et al. 2002; Quinn et al. 2004; Stein et al. 2003; Swanson et al. 2003, 2004; Wilens et al. 2003; Wolraich et al. 2001). These long-acting methylphenidate preparations have become increasingly popular with patients, families, clinicians, and schools, because often children will get good benefit from single-morning dosing regimens, making the previously common midday at school dosing unnecessary. The duration of symptom suppression in responsive children ranges from 1 to 4 hours, with an average of 2 or 3 hours with immediate-release preparations (Srinivas et al. 1992) and up to 12 hours of effect with the newer long-acting preparations. Delivery of the medication on a daily basis is generally timed to match the child's schedule when peak demands are placed on behavioral control and ability to pay attention, which, for a child, is during school hours. "Rebound" periods of exacerbation of symptoms before the next dose were not uncommon with the short-acting preparations but seem less clinically significant with the longer-acting preparations. At times, this exacerbation of symptoms is problematic and requires more-frequent dosing or the use of long-acting methylphenidate preparations (Birmaher et al. 1989). In children of normal weight, it is usually recommended to begin the medication at a dosage of 5 mg two or three times a day and to increase the dosage every 3 days until therapeutic effects are sufficient, and then to give a trial to crossing over to longer-acting preparations of relatively equal potency as the required daily dose of short-acting stimulant. Some clinicians favor initiation of treatment with long-acting preparations from the outset of treatment. The limiting factor related to maximal dosage is generally untoward side effects, although the *Physicians' Desk Reference* (2001) recommends that dosages equivalent to 60 mg/day of immediate-release methylphenidate generally not be exceeded in children.

Dextroamphetamine is the amphetamine agent that until recently was most often used in the treatment of ADHD. Currently short-acting and longer-acting preparations of Adderall, which consists of a mixture of amphetamine salts, are also available for use with patients with ADHD. Short-acting amphetamine preparations probably have a somewhat longer half-life and duration of action than short-acting methylphenidate in children with ADHD, but multiple daily dosing remains essential for all short-acting stimulant preparations (Biederman et al. 2002b; Greenhill et al. 2003; McCracken et al. 2003). The efficacy rates and side-effect profile reported by most research studies are generally equivalent to those seen in studies of methylphenidate (Greenhill et al. 1999). The starting dosage is generally 2.5–5 mg twice a day, and the dosage is gradually increased until the desired clinical effects are obtained. The medication is FDA approved for children as young as 3 years. Dosages exceeding 40 mg/day are rarely needed. As is the case with methylphenidate, longer-acting preparations of dextroamphetamine (dextroamphetamine spansules) and Adderall (Adderall XR) are available for clinical use and may eliminate the need to administer an in-school dose for many children.

Magnesium pemoline has been less well studied than the other two more frequently used stimulants, but it appears to be effective in children with symptoms of ADHD (Conners and Taylor 1980) and can be used in patients whose conditions do not respond to other stimulants. It has been known to cause liver toxicity rarely (Pratt and Dubois 1990), and routine assessment of liver function tests before and during treatment is necessary. It has been clinically recognized that the onset of therapeutic effect may be delayed for a few weeks after initiation of pemoline therapy, which is unlike treatment with the other stimulants; however, this finding has been challenged in a pharmacokinetic/pharmacodynamic study (Sallee et al. 1992). Pemoline is a longer-acting agent and may need to reach a steady-state serum level for maximum effects. It can be given once a day, with a usual starting dose of 37.5 mg, advancing in increments of 18.75 mg every 3–5 days until the desired clinical benefit is observed. Because of the availability of other stimulant and nonstimulant medications that may have more robust positive effects and the association of this therapeutically inferior agent with potentially severe side effects, most clinicians are hesitant to use pemoline as a first-line agent, if at all, in the treatment of ADHD.

Side effects of stimulant medications include appetite suppression, weight loss, sleep problems, irritability, headache, stomachache, skin picking, rash, and occasional association with the development (or exacerbation) of tics. Although psychostimulants may lead to time-limited delay of growth in some children (MTA Cooperative Group 2004b), no long-term adverse effects on growth or achievement of final adult height are apparent (Biederman et al. 2003; Klein and Mannuzza 1988). Children treated with psychostimulants generally achieve their predicted adult size if they are followed up into adulthood. However, it is common in children treated with stimulants to allow drug holidays during vacations or weekends if the behavioral problems tend to be more severe and compromising in a school setting and the parents feel that a temporary drug-free state will not adversely affect the child or the family. Weekend drug holidays can free the child from the appetite-suppressant effects of the stimulants and can lead to increased calorie consumption on weekends, which prevents unwanted weight loss or delayed weight gain. Holidays from drugs in the summer or during vacations can also help the clinician to assess the degree of persistence of the symptoms by observing a drug-free state and can provide useful information about the need for continuing treatment with medication.

In general, based on the results of numerous controlled trials, approximately 70%–75% of children with ADHD are expected to benefit from initiation of treatment with stimulant medication (Greenhill et al. 1999). When treatment with one stimulant results in insufficient benefit, treatment with the other stimulants should be attempted before changing to a different class of medication. It has been reported that as many as 90% of children will respond to treatment with either methylphenidate or dextroamphetamine (Elia et al. 1991). Nevertheless, because of the high prevalence of ADHD in the population, many children with ADHD will require other treatments.

Atomoxetine

Atomoxetine (Strattera) is the first non-stimulant medication approved by the FDA for use in the treatment of ADHD. Controlled clinical trials suggest that it is more effective than placebo in the acute phase suppression of ADHD symptoms (Biederman et al. 2002a; Kelsey et al. 2004; Michelson et al. 2001, 2002, 2004). The fact that atomoxetine has low potential for illicit use or abuse and that it was approved for use as a noncontrolled substance make this agent appealing to both clinicians and parents. Some clinicians use atomoxetine as a first-line or as a preferred therapeutic agent for children and adolescents with ADHD. Others reserve it for patients who cannot tolerate stimulant therapy, for patients with treatment-resistant cases, or for patients with a high potential for misuse or abuse of stimulant medications. Definitive, well-designed head-to-head comparison trials of atomoxetine versus stimulant therapy are not currently available to inform clinicians regarding the relative risks and benefits of these different agents. The weight of the evidence would likely support that stimulants remain the agent of first choice for most patients with ADHD. Recent isolated reports of idiosyncratic reversible liver damage have raised awareness but have not changed clinical practice recommendations.

Tricyclic Antidepressants

Tricyclic antidepressants (TCAs) are considered a second-line agent in the treatment of ADHD. Of the TCAs, research supports the effectiveness of two agents in particular—imipramine and desipramine (Biederman et al. 1989a; Cox 1982; Gross 1973; Pliszka 1987)—and suggests the usefulness of a third—nortriptyline (Wilens et al. 1993a)—in treatment of the disorder. TCAs have been tested in patients who previously have not been offered medication treatment as well as in individuals who have responded poorly to psychostimulant trials (Biederman et al. 1989a). In general, tricyclic antidepressants appear to be well tolerated by most children and adolescents who take them for ADHD and other indications (enuresis, depression), although benign effects on heart rate and blood pressure have been seen in some groups of children (Biederman et al. 1989b; Wilens et al. 1993b). There has been concern about the safety of the use of desipramine in children, based on the occurrence of sudden death associated with treatment in a small number of children (Riddle et al. 1993). The exact nature of the association is currently unclear. Explanations that have been proposed range from chance occurrence to a heightened cardiotoxicity of the medication to the hearts of young patients (Walsh et al. 1994). In any event, caution is warranted in patients who develop signifi-

cant cardiovascular symptoms or changes in electrocardiographic parameters during the course of treatment. Younger patients appear to metabolize these agents more efficiently than do adults and may require twice- or three-times-a-day dosing to achieve maximal clinical benefit, as opposed to the once-a-day dosing that is often effective in adults.

Other Medications

Alpha-adrenergic agonists.   The use of clonidine (and the related agent guanfacine) for symptoms of ADHD has some scientific support, but because of the lack of replicated double-blind, placebo-controlled trials, alpha-adrenergic agonists are currently considered third-line agents. Alpha-adrenergic agents have been used in patients with ADHD alone or as an adjunct to stimulants for associated aggression or stimulant-induced sleep disturbance (Connor et al. 1999; Prince et al. 1996). They also appear to have efficacy in treating the symptoms of ADHD and tics in children with the comorbid diagnosis of Tourette's disorder (Scahill et al. 2001; Steingard et al. 1993). The most notable side effects include drowsiness and drug-induced hypotension. Clonidine should be slowly tapered during discontinuation because rebound hypertension may occur if it is suddenly discontinued in patients who have been taking significant doses for a prolonged time.

Other antidepressants.   Bupropion has shown some promise in the treatment of ADHD in children and adults (Barrickman et al. 1995; Conners et al. 1996; Wender and Reimherr 1990; Wilens et al. 2001), although it may worsen tics in children with tic disorder (Spencer et al. 1993). The role of monoamine oxidase inhibitors has scientific support (Zametkin et al. 1985), but their use also carries the risk of hypertensive crisis if dietary compliance cannot be guaranteed by the parents of the child.

Antipsychotics. Antipsychotics appear to be effective in controlling some manifestations of ADHD in children, but the risk of neurological side effects with long-term treatment precludes the use of these medications except in severely ill patients who have not responded to other interventions.

■ Psychosocial Interventions

Psychosocial treatments are also commonly used in the treatment of ADHD. Three main modalities of treatment are individual psychotherapeutic interventions with the child who has the disorder, strategic educational interventions, and family approaches to altering the child's disruptive behavior pattern.

Individual Psychotherapy

Targeting the child as the focus of attention through psychological intervention has some support from scientific studies (Whalen and Henker 1991). There have been empirical trials of behavior therapy and cognitive therapy (Abikoff and Gittelman 1984; Brown et al. 1986; Fehlings et al. 1991). In general, behavior therapy techniques seem to have a higher success rate than do cognitive interventions in the reduction of symptoms of ADHD. Controlled trials of psychodynamic psychotherapy are not available, although one series of studies reported that insight-oriented psychotherapy appears to be less effective as a treatment for children and adolescents with disruptive behavior disorders than for those with more emotionally based symptoms (Fonagy and Target 1994).

Behavior therapy attempts to deliver consistent targeted behavioral contingencies that reinforce desired positive behaviors and extinguish negative unwanted behaviors. Positive reinforcement is delivered when the child is attending appropriately, is keeping on task, and is maintaining some degree of control over hyperactivity and impulsivity. Some therapists recommend the judicious and consistent use of "response cost" and punishment techniques, including "time-out" and loss of positive reinforcements, as necessary to reduce ingrained disruptive behaviors, such as aggression and oppositional defiance. Behavior therapy techniques have been used both in children taking medication and in those not taking medication. One problem with applying behavioral techniques in an individual psychotherapy format is that the therapist generally will not be present in the contexts where the problematic behavior is most likely to occur—namely, at home or at school. Therefore, attempts have been made to educate teachers and parents to use behavior management with the child directly in the environment of the classroom and at home. In effect, the parent and teacher may become surrogate behavior therapists. The role of the professional psychotherapist in this situation is to teach and supervise the use of the techniques by the teacher and parent and to monitor the efficacy of the therapy in helping the child.

Educational Interventions

The academic risk for the child with ADHD is significant (Frick et al. 1991). School performance and achievement in children with ADHD are generally significantly worse than in nonaffected children (Faraone et al. 1993). Behavioral problems may cause poor academic performance and recurrent conflicts with teachers and school administrators. Learning disabilities also appear to co-occur with ADHD at an increased rate compared with children without ADHD (Semrud-

Clikeman et al. 1992). Psychological testing can be beneficial in determining learning potential and cognitive strengths, as well as in identifying specific learning disorders. With appropriate intervention, children with uncomplicated forms of ADHD can usually be educated in regular mainstream classrooms. Appropriate medication treatment may occasionally normalize the child's behavior to such a degree that no supplementary educational intervention may be necessary (Abikoff and Gittelman 1985b). Classroom behavior management techniques may be of additional benefit with children who have persistent symptoms, children who are not taking medications, or children who have comorbid oppositional behavior or conduct disturbances. Some children who cannot be educated in classrooms with a large student-to-teacher ratio may require special classrooms.

Intensive summer treatment programs (essentially summer day camps for children with ADHD) have been promoted as beneficial therapeutic interventions whereby focused treatment strategies can be applied over several weeks to modify the child's behavior (Pelham et al. 1993). Usually, these programs incorporate classroom time and structured recreational activities to create a school-like atmosphere in which the efficacy of the introduction of a behavior management program can be monitored and measured. The benefits of such a summer treatment program can presumably be enhanced if program personnel can directly link therapeutic strategies established in the summer to the child's educational setting in the following fall. In some programs, this is accomplished by having counselors from the summer program work directly in the classroom for a period during the following school year to help educational staff members work with the individual child in a therapeutic fashion.

Family Interventions

The parental relationships with children with ADHD are often negative and permeated with frustrations (Befera and Barkley 1985). This does not necessarily mean that the adults lack parenting skills, because their relationships with siblings who do not have ADHD may be more appropriate and positive (Tarver-Behring et al. 1985). Children with ADHD may require more specialized parenting skills than do nonaffected children. Although different family interventions have been used in the treatment of ADHD in children, parent training is the most common approach and, until the recent findings of the MTA study were made available, had received increasing support from the scientific literature (Anastopoulos et al. 1993) as an effective approach to intervention. Essentially, the parents are taught the techniques of sophisticated behavior therapy to be used with their children. The therapist arranges individual or group meetings with the parents, supplemented by readings and homework. Treatment plans are developed with child-oriented positive reinforcements and response cost contingencies.

▧ Multimodality Treatment and the NIMH MTA Study

Although it would seem logical that combined treatments would improve outcomes for the child with ADHD (Whalen and Henker 1991), this is not necessarily supported by the scientific literature. It appears that a subgroup of children treated with medication may actually normalize in terms of their observable behavior and functioning (Abikoff and Gittelman 1985b), and the additional benefit provided by psychosocial interventions with these children is minimal. Multimodality treatment has been theorized to be of particular benefit for children who do not normalize with medication or who have comorbid disorders.

The MTA study randomly assigned children ages 7–9 years with DSM-IV (American Psychiatric Association 1994) ADHD (combined subtype), with and without comorbid disorders, to either 1) algorithmic medication treatment (mainly relying on psychostimulants), 2) a comprehensive psychosocial treatment package (parent training, intensive summer treatment program, and school consultation), 3) the combined psychosocial package and algorithmic medication treatment, or 4) community referral as a control group. Treatments in the four study arms were delivered over the course of 14 months. Children randomized to the medication treatment arms overall had significantly improved outcomes compared with children receiving psychosocial treatment alone or those referred out for community care (MTA Cooperative Group 1999). The role of psychosocial interventions delivered in combination with medication treatment may be of questionable benefit, since the results of this study also suggest that subjects receiving the combination medication and psychosocial treatment fared little better in general than subjects receiving medication treatment alone. In secondary analyses of the MTA data, there was some evidence suggesting that using alternative definitions of treatment response may support a statistically significant better response to combination therapy than relying solely on medication treatment strategies (Conners et al. 2001; Swanson et al. 2001), but overall the advantage of combination therapy over medication treatment alone was small. This historic study provides important evidence of the strong treatment effect of well-delivered pharmacotherapy and some evidence that combination treatment may benefit some patients. Maintenance of benefits of MTA medication management has been demonstrated out to 24 months postrandomization, even though the controlled treatment component of the study ended at 14 months (MTA Cooperative Group 2004a). The results of this study refute any ideas that an intensive psychosocial treatment package provides therapeutic effects equivalent to medication treatment for children with the combined subtype of ADHD and suggests that medication treatment should be considered first-line therapy in these children. A recently published study, using a very different design from the MTA study, similarly suggested that intensive psychosocial treatment offered little additional long-term benefit to children with ADHD who benefited from short-term stimulant treatment and continued on stimulant therapy (Abikoff et al. 2004a, 2004b; Hechtman et al. 2004a, 2004b; Klein et al 2004).

■ General Rules for Successful Management

Practice parameters for children and adolescents with ADHD are currently available (American Academy of Child and Adolescent Psychiatry 1997). The best management of the many needs of children with ADHD is through the assembly of a multidisciplinary team, consisting of the child, the parents, a medical doctor, a psychologist, a social worker, and an educational specialist. The professionals on the team may be practitioners in separate offices, with referrals alternating among colleagues, or in group practice settings.

The use of medication intervention strategies for all patients with ADHD should be seriously considered as a first-line intervention and should be discussed with parents. If medications are incorporated into the treatment plan, then certain approaches can be helpful. On completion of the evaluation of the child, it is often best to set a meeting with parents to present the results of the evaluation and for psychoeducational counseling. An open discussion of the benefits and risks of the various treatment options, including medication strategies, should be included. If a medication trial is recommended and is agreed to by the parents, it is optimal to plan a trial that will allow for an eventual once-a-day dosing regimen. Regular contact with school personnel is absolutely essential to collect information about the child's behavior and academic progress as well as the evaluation by the school personnel of the child's response to the medication trial. Once a satisfactory acute response is obtained, medication treatment is best maintained as tolerated for several months to allow the child to consolidate gains made in terms of behavioral control and academic achievement. Intermittent drug holidays can be used once or twice a year to evaluate the need for continued medication treatment. Tutoring may be necessary to teach compensatory skills to children with learning difficulties. Clinicians should see children on a once-weekly (during titration) to once-monthly (during maintenance) schedule during treatment. The use of psychosocial interventions—such as parent training, school interventions, intensive summer treatment programs, and individual therapy—above and beyond common-sense parenting advice and communication with the educational system may best be held in reserve pending the outcome of the medication trial and may be of more benefit for children with comorbid externalizing or internalizing disorders.

Long-Term Outcome

The outcome studies available are, for the most part, based on follow-up of clinically referred samples, generally males, who may have a particularly severe form of the disorder and may have more associated comorbid conditions. Multiple studies have found that the disorder persists into adolescence and adulthood in a substantial proportion of patients, and conduct disorder develops in 25%–50% (Babinski et al. 1999; Barkley et al. 1991; Biederman et al. 1996; Gittelman et al. 1985; Hechtman 1991; Lie 1992; Mannuzza et al. 1998; McGee et al. 1991). Compared with control subjects without ADHD, children with ADHD followed up into adulthood show higher rates of antisocial behavior and residual symptoms of ADHD, although the percentage of patients meeting full criteria for ADHD may be low. An increased risk of substance use disorders has been reported in some studies, and the substance use will generally follow (not precede) the onset of antisocial behavior (Gittelman et al. 1985).

It can be expected that in a minority of children, after clinical referral and proper diagnosis, the disorder will remit by adolescence, but the majority of cases will remit at least partially by adulthood. As a group, children with ADHD can be expected to have a more negative outcome as they grow up than children without the disorder, showing higher rates of criminal activity, incarceration, and substance abuse, particularly in the subgroup who develop antisocial personality disorder (Mannuzza et al. 1993). On an individual basis, however, it is difficult to forecast the future for a child with ADHD. Clear predictors of negative outcome in children with the disorder, other than the onset of conduct disorder or antisocial personality disorder (Satterfield et al. 1994), have not been identified (Fischer et al. 1993). Little information about the course of the disorder specifically in females is available.

Conclusion

ADHD maintains its central position in psychiatry as a leading cause of problems for children and adolescents. It is a complex syndrome that is best understood, researched, and treated within a biopsychosocial model. Underlying biological abnormalities appear to exist at least in a subgroup of these patients, and with the application of more sophisticated functional neuroimaging and other technologies, the biology of the disorder likely will be better understood in the years to come. The psychological manifestations of the disorder cause major problems for patients and lead to difficulties with interpersonal relationships and academic and vocational performance and often a loss of self-worth and self-esteem. Socially, these children are often stigmatized by the symptoms of the disorder and ostracized by peers and family members. However, clinical and research experience with these patients continues to grow. A clinician can confidently state to a parent and the patient that effective treatments are now available. At this point, medication treatment is clearly established as effective in terms of suppressing the core symptoms of the disorder in the short and the middle term, and in general it appears that psychostimulant medication is safe and well tolerated by the majority of patients. What is necessary in the future is to better understand subgroups of patients, distinguished by associated conditions or various etiological subtypes of the disorder, and to learn to predict how these patients differ in terms of the natural history of their symptoms and associated morbidity.

Eventually it may be possible to understand the role of treatment interventions in affecting the long-term outcomes of large numbers of patients.

References

Abikoff H, Gittelman R: Does behavior therapy normalize the classroom behavior of hyperactive children? Arch Gen Psychiatry 41:449–454, 1984

Abikoff H, Gittelman R: Hyperactive children treated with stimulants: is cognitive training a useful adjunct? Arch Gen Psychiatry 42:953–961, 1985a

Abikoff H, Gittelman R: The normalizing effects of methylphenidate on the classroom behavior of ADHD children. J Abnorm Child Psychol 13:33–44, 1985b

Abikoff H, Courtney M, Pelham WEJ, et al: Teachers' ratings of disruptive behaviors: the influence of halo effects. J Abnorm Child Psychol 21:519–533, 1993

Abikoff H, Hechtman L, Klein RG, et al: Social functioning in children with ADHD treated with long-term methylphenidate and multimodal psychosocial treatment. J Am Acad Child Adolesc Psychiatry 43:820–829, 2004a

Abikoff H, Hechtman L, Klein RG et al: Symptomatic improvement in children with ADHD treated with long-term methylphenidate and multimodal psychosocial treatment. J Am Acad Child Adolesc Psychiatry 43:802–811, 2004b

Achenbach TM, Edelbrock CS: Manual of the Child Behavior Checklist and Revised Child Behavior Profile. Burlington, VT, University of Vermont, Department of Psychiatry, 1983

Adesman AR, Altshuler LA, Lipkin PH, et al: Otitis media in children with learning disabilities and in children with attention deficit disorder with hyperactivity. Pediatrics 85:442–446, 1990

Alon U, Naveh Y, Gardos M, et al: Neurological sequelae of septic meningitis: a follow-up study of 65 children. Isr J Med Sci 15:512–517, 1979

Altman J: Morphological and behavioral markers of environmentally induced retardation of brain development: an animal model. Environ Health Perspect 74:153–168, 1987

Aman MG, Marks RE, Turbott SH, et al: Clinical effects of methylphenidate and thioridazine in intellectually subaverage children. J Am Acad Child Adolesc Psychiatry 30:246–256, 1991

American Academy of Child and Adolescent Psychiatry (Dulcan M): Practice parameters for the assessment and treatment of children, adolescents, and adults with attention-deficit/hyperactivity disorder. J Am Acad Child Adolesc Psychiatry 36 (10 suppl):85S–121S, 1997

American Psychiatric Association: Diagnostic and Statistical Manual of Mental Disorders, 4th Edition. Washington, DC, American Psychiatric Association, 1994

American Psychiatric Association: Diagnostic and Statistical Manual of Mental Disorders, 4th Edition, Text Revision. Washington, DC, American Psychiatric Association, 2000

Anastopoulos AD, Shelton TL, DuPaul GJ, et al: Parent training for attention-deficit hyperactivity disorder: its impact on parent functioning. J Abnorm Child Psychol 21:581–596, 1993

Applegate B, Lahey BB, Hart EL, et al: Validity of the age-of-onset criterion for ADHD: a report from the DSM-IV field trials. J Am Acad Child Adolesc Psychiatry 36:1211–1221, 1997

Arcia E, Roberts JE: Otitis media in early childhood and its association with sustained attention in structured situations. J Dev Behav Pediatr 14:181–183, 1993

Babinski LM, Hartsough CS, Lambert NM: Childhood conduct problems, hyperactivity-impulsivity, and inattention as predictors of adult criminal activity. J Child Psychol Psychiatry 40:347–355, 1999

Barkley RA: Hyperactive Children: A Handbook for Diagnosis and Treatment. New York, Guilford, 1982

Barkley RA: The ecological validity of laboratory and analogue assessment methods of ADHD symptoms. J Abnorm Child Psychol 19:149–178, 1991

Barkley RA, Biederman J: Toward a broader definition of the age-of-onset criterion for attention-deficit hyperactivity disorder. J Am Acad Child Adolesc Psychiatry 36:1204–1210, 1997

Barkley RA, Fischer M, Edelbrock C, et al: The adolescent outcome of hyperactive children diagnosed by research criteria, III: mother-child interactions, family conflicts and maternal psychopathology. J Child Psychol Psychiatry 32:233–255, 1991

Barling J, Bullen G: Dietary factors and hyperactivity: a failure to replicate. J Genet Psychol 146:117–123, 1985

Barrickman LL, Perry PJ, Allen AJ, et al: Bupropion versus methylphenidate in the treatment of attention-deficit hyperactivity disorder. J Am Acad Child Adolesc Psychiatry 34:649–657, 1995

Befera MS, Barkley RA: Hyperactive and normal girls and boys: mother-child interaction, parent psychiatric status and child psychopathology. J Child Psychol Psychiatry 26:439–452, 1985

Biederman J, Baldessarini RJ, Wright V, et al: A double-blind placebo controlled study of desipramine in the treatment of ADD, I: efficacy. J Am Acad Child Adolesc Psychiatry 28:777–784, 1989a

Biederman J, Baldessarini RJ, Wright V, et al: A double-blind placebo controlled study of desipramine in the treatment of ADD, II: serum drug levels and cardiovascular findings. J Am Acad Child Adolesc Psychiatry 28:903–911, 1989b

Biederman J, Faraone SV, Keenan K, et al: Family genetic and psychosocial risk factors in DSM-III attention deficit disorder. J Am Acad Child Adolesc Psychiatry 29:526–533, 1990

Biederman J, Newcorn J, Sprich S: Comorbidity of attention deficit hyperactivity disorder with conduct, depressive, anxiety, and other disorders. Am J Psychiatry 148:564–577, 1991

Biederman J, Faraone SV, Milberger S, et al: Diagnoses of attention-deficit hyperactivity disorder from parent reports predict diagnoses based on teacher reports. J Am Acad Child Adolesc Psychiatry 32:315–317, 1993

Biederman J, Milberger S, Faraone SV, et al: Associations between childhood asthma and ADHD: issues of psychiatric comorbidity and familiality. J Am Acad Child Adolesc Psychiatry 33:842–848, 1994

Biederman J, Faraone SV, Mick E, et al: High risk for attention deficit hyperactivity disorder among children of parents with childhood onset of the disorder: a pilot study. Am J Psychiatry 152:431–435, 1995

Biederman J, Faraone S, Milberger S, et al: A prospective 4-year follow-up study of attention-deficit hyperactivity and related disorders. Arch Gen Psychiatry 53:437–446, 1996

Biederman J, Mick E, Faraone SV: Age-dependent decline of symptoms of attention deficit hyperactivity disorder: impact of remission definition and symptom type. Am J Psychiatry 157:816–818, 2000

Biederman J, Heiligenstein JH, Faries DE, et al: Atomoxetine ADHD Study Group. Efficacy of atomoxetine versus placebo in school-age girls with attention-deficit/hyperactivity disorder. Pediatrics 110:E75, 2002a

Biederman J, Lopez FA, Boellner SW, et al: A randomized, double-blind, placebo-controlled, parallel-group study of SLI381 (Adderall XR) in children with attention-deficit/hyperactivity disorder. Pediatrics 110:258–266, 2002b

Biederman J, Faraone SV, Monuteaux MC, et al: Growth deficits and attention-deficit/hyperactivity disorder revisited: impact of gender, development, and treatment. Pediatrics 111:1010–1016, 2003

Bird HR, Gould MS, Staghezza B: Aggregating data from multiple informants in child psychiatry epidemiological research. J Am Acad Child Adolesc Psychiatry 31:78–85, 1992

Bird HR, Gould MS, Staghezza BM: Patterns of diagnostic comorbidity in a community sample of children aged 9 through 16 years. J Am Acad Child Adolesc Psychiatry 32:361–368, 1993

Birmaher B, Greenhill LL, Cooper TB, et al: Sustained release methylphenidate: pharmacokinetic studies in ADHD males. J Am Acad Child Adolesc Psychiatry 28:768–772, 1989

Brown RT, Wynne ME, Borden KA, et al: Methylphenidate and cognitive therapy in children with attention deficit disorder: a double-blind trial. J Dev Behav Pediatr 7:163–174, 1986

Cantwell DP, Baker L: Association between attention deficit–hyperactivity disorder and learning disorders. J Learn Disabil 24:88–95, 1991

Carlson C, Lahey BB, Neeper R: Direct assessment of the cognitive correlates of attention deficit disorders with and without hyperactivity. Journal of Psychopathology and Behavioral Assessment 8:69–86, 1986

Casey BJ, Castellanos FX, Giedd JN, et al: Implication of right frontostriatal circuitry in response inhibition and attention-deficit/hyperactivity disorder. J Am Acad Child Adolesc Psychiatry 36:374–383, 1997

Castellanos FX, Giedd JN, Eckburg P, et al: Quantitative morphology of the caudate nucleus in attention deficit hyperactivity disorder. Am J Psychiatry 151:1791–1796, 1994

Castellanos FX, Giedd JN, Berquin PC, et al: Quantitative brain magnetic resonance imaging in girls with attention-deficit/hyperactivity disorder. Arch Gen Psychiatry 58:289–295, 2001

Castellanos FX, Lee PP, Sharp W, et al: Developmental trajectories of brain volume abnormalities in children and adolescents with attention-deficit/hyperactivity disorder. JAMA 288:1740–1748, 2002

Castellanos FX, Sharp WS, Gottesman RF, et al: Anatomic brain abnormalities in monozygotic twins discordant for attention deficit hyperactivity disorder. Am J Psychiatry 160:1693–1696, 2003

Chandola CA, Robling MR, Peters TJ, et al: Pre- and perinatal factors and the risk of subsequent referral for hyperactivity. J Child Psychol Psychiatry 33:1077–1090, 1992

Cohen DJ, Leckman JF: Commentary. J Am Acad Child Adolesc Psychiatry 28:580–582, 1989

Collett BR, Ohan JL, Myers KM. Ten-year review of rating scales, V: scales assessing attention-deficit/hyperactivity disorder. J Am Acad Child Adolesc Psychiatry 42:1015–1037, 2003

Comings DE, Comings BG: A controlled family history study of Tourette's syndrome, I: attention-deficit hyperactivity disorder and learning disorders. J Clin Psychiatry 51:275–280, 1990

Conners CK, Taylor E: Pemoline, methylphenidate, and placebo in children with minimal brain dysfunction. Arch Gen Psychiatry 37:922–930, 1980

Conners CK, Werry JL: Pharmacotherapy of psychopathology in children, in Psychopathological Disorders of Childhood, 2nd Edition. Edited by Quay H, Werry JL. New York, Wiley, 1979, pp 336–386

Conners CK, Casat CD, Gualtieri CT, et al: Bupropion hydrochloride in attention deficit disorder with hyperactivity. J Am Acad Child Adolesc Psychiatry 35:1314–1321, 1996

Conners CK, Epstein JN, March JS, et al: Multimodal treatment of ADHD in the MTA: an alternative outcome analysis. J Am Acad Child Adolesc Psychiatry 40:159–167, 2001

Connor DF, Fletcher KE, Swanson JM: A meta-analysis of clonidine for symptoms of attention-deficit hyperactivity disorder. J Am Acad Child Adolesc Psychiatry 38:1551–1559, 1999

Corkum PV, Siegel LS: Is the Continuous Performance Test a valuable research tool for use with children with attention-deficit-hyperactivity disorder? J Child Psychol Psychiatry 34:1217–1239, 1993

Cornblatt BA, Winters L, Maminski B, et al: Methylphenidate-SR: effect on sustained attention in ADHD males (abstract). Proceedings of the American Academy of Child and Adolescent Psychiatry 3:47, 1987

Cornblatt BA, Risch JJ, Faris G, et al: The Continuous Performance Test, Identical Pairs Version (CPT-IP), I: new findings about sustained attention in normal families. Psychiatry Res 26:223–238, 1988

Cox WHJ: An indication for use of imipramine in attention deficit disorder. Am J Psychiatry 139:1059–1060, 1982

Denckla MB: Attention deficit hyperactivity disorder—residual type. J Child Neurol 6 (suppl):S44–S50, 1991

Diaz-Granados JL, Greene PL, Amsel A: Selective activity enhancement and persistence in weanling rats after hippocampal X-irradiation in infancy: possible relevance for ADHD. Behav Neural Biol 61:251–259, 1994

DiBattista D, Shepherd ML: Primary school teachers' beliefs and advice to parents concerning sugar consumption and activity in children. Psychol Rep 72:47–55, 1993

Douglas VI: Attentional and cognitive problems, in Developmental Neuropsychiatry. Edited by Rutter M. New York, Guilford, 1983, pp 280–329

DuPaul GJ, Anastopoulos AD, Shelton TL, et al: Multimethod assessment of attention-deficit hyperactivity disorder: the diagnostic utility of clinic-based tests. J Clin Child Psychol 21:394–402, 1992

DuPaul GJ, McGoey KE, Eckert TL, et al: Preschool children with attention-deficit/hyperactivity disorder: impairments in behavioral, social, and school functioning. J Am Acad Child Adolesc Psychiatry 40:508–515, 2001

Egger J, Stolla A, McEwen LM: Controlled trial of hyposensitization in children with food-induced hyperkinetic syndrome. Lancet 339:1150–1153, 1992

Elia J, Borcherding BG, Rapoport JL, et al: Methylphenidate and dextroamphetamine treatments of hyperactivity: are there true nonresponders? Psychiatry Res 36:141–155, 1991

Elia J, Gulotta C, Rose SR, et al: Thyroid function and attention-deficit hyperactivity disorder. J Am Acad Child Adolesc Psychiatry 33:169–172, 1994

Ernst M, Cohen RM, Liebenauer LL, et al: Cerebral glucose metabolism in adolescent girls with attention-deficit/hyperactivity disorder. J Am Acad Child Adolesc Psychiatry 36:1399–1406, 1997

Ernst M, Zametkin AJ, Matochik JA, et al: High midbrain [18F]DOPA accumulation in children with attention deficit hyperactivity disorder. Am J Psychiatry 156:1209–1215, 1999

Faraone SV, Biederman J, Keenan K, et al: A family genetic study of girls with DSM-III attention deficit disorder. Am J Psychiatry 148:112–117, 1991

Faraone SV, Biederman J, Lehman BK, et al: Intellectual performance and school failure in children with attention deficit hyperactivity disorder and in their siblings. J Abnorm Psychol 102:616–623, 1993

Faraone SV, Doyle AE, Mick E, et al: Meta-analysis of the association between the 7-repeat allele of the dopamine D(4) receptor gene and attention deficit hyperactivity disorder. Am J Psychiatry 158:1052–1057, 2001

Fehlings DL, Roberts W, Humphries T, et al: Attention deficit hyperactivity disorder: does cognitive behavioral therapy improve home behavior? J Dev Behav Pediatr 12:223–228, 1991

Fergusson DM, Lynskey MT, Horwood LJ: The effect of maternal depression on maternal ratings of child behavior. J Abnorm Child Psychol 21:245–269, 1993

Fergusson DM, Horwood LJ, Lynskey MT: Structure of DSM-III-R criteria for disruptive childhood behaviors: confirmatory factor models. J Am Acad Child Adolesc Psychiatry 33:1145–1157, 1994

Fischer M, Barkley RA, Fletcher KE, et al: The adolescent outcome of hyperactive children: predictors of psychiatric, academic, social, and emotional adjustment. J Am Acad Child Adolesc Psychiatry 32:324–332, 1993

Fonagy P, Target M: The efficacy of psychoanalysis for children with disruptive disorders. J Am Acad Child Adolesc Psychiatry 33:45–55, 1994

Frick PJ, Kamphaus RW, Lahey BB, et al: Academic underachievement and the disruptive behavior disorders. J Consult Clin Psychol 59:289–294, 1991

Gainetdinov RR, Caron MG: Genetics of childhood disorders: XXIV. ADHD, part 8: hyperdopaminergic mice as an animal model of ADHD. J Am Acad Child Adolesc Psychiatry 40:380–382, 2001

Garfinkel BD, Brown WA, Klee SH, et al: Neuroendocrine and cognitive responses to amphetamine in adolescents with a history of attention deficit disorder. J Am Acad Child Adolesc Psychiatry 25:503–510, 1986

Giedd JN, Castellanos FX, Casey BJ, et al: Quantitative morphology of the corpus callosum in attention deficit hyperactivity disorder. Am J Psychiatry 151:665–669, 1994

Gittelman R, Mannuzza S, Shenker R, et al: Hyperactive boys almost grown up, I: psychiatric status. Arch Gen Psychiatry 42:937–947, 1985

Goodman R, Stevenson J: A twin study of hyperactivity, II: the aetiological role of genes, family relationships and perinatal adversity. J Child Psychol Psychiatry 30:691–709, 1989

Gordon M, Mettelman BB: The assessment of attention, I: standardization and reliability of a behavior-based measure. J Clin Psychol 44:682–690, 1988

Goyette CH, Conners CK, Ulrich RF: Normative data on Revised Conners' Parent and Teacher Rating Scales. J Abnorm Child Psychol 6:221–236, 1978

Green SM, Loeber R, Lahey BB: Stability of mothers' recall of the age of onset of their child's attention and hyperactivity problems. J Am Acad Child Adolesc Psychiatry 30:135–137, 1991

Greenhill LL, Halperin JM, Abikoff H: Stimulant medications. J Am Acad Child Adolesc Psychiatry 38:503–512, 1999

Greenhill LL, Findling RL, Swanson JM, et al: A double-blind, placebo-controlled study of modified-release methylphenidate in children with attention-deficit/hyperactivity disorder. Pediatrics 109:E39, 2002

Greenhill LL, Swanson JM, Steinhoff K, et al: A pharmacokinetic/pharmacodynamic study comparing a single morning dose of Adderall to twice-daily dosing in children with ADHD. J Am Acad Child Adolesc Psychiatry 42:1234–1241, 2003

Gross MD: Imipramine in the treatment of minimal brain dysfunction in children. Psychosomatics 14:283–285, 1973

Hagerman RJ, Falkenstein AR: An association between recurrent otitis media in infancy and later hyperactivity. Clin Pediatr (Phila) 26:253–257, 1987

Halperin JM, Newcorn JH, Matier K, et al: Discriminant validity of attention-deficit hyperactivity disorder. J Am Acad Child Adolesc Psychiatry 32:1038–1043, 1993

Hauser P, Zametkin AJ, Martinez P, et al: Attention deficit–hyperactivity disorder in people with generalized resistance to thyroid hormone. N Engl J Med 328:997–1001, 1993

Hechtman L: Resilience and vulnerability in long-term outcome of attention deficit hyperactive disorder. Can J Psychiatry 36:415–421, 1991

Hechtman L: Genetic and neurobiological aspects of attention deficit hyperactive disorder: a review. J Psychiatry Neurosci 19:193–201, 1994

Hechtman L, Abikoff H, Klein RG, et al: Academic achievement and emotional status of children with ADHD treated with long-term methylphenidate and multimodal psychosocial treatment. J Am Acad Child Adolesc Psychiatry 43:812–819, 2004a

Hechtman L, Abikoff H, Klein RG, et al: Children with ADHD treated with long-term methylphenidate and multimodal psychosocial treatment: impact on parental practices. J Am Acad Child Adolesc Psychiatry 43:830–838, 2004b

Hoagwood K, Kelleher KJ, Feil M, et al: Treatment services for children with ADHD: a national perspective. J Am Acad Child Adolesc Psychiatry 39:198–206, 2000

Hoegerman GS, Resnick RJ, Schnoll SH: Attention deficits in newly abstinent substance abusers: childhood recollections and attention performance in thirty-nine subjects. J Addict Dis 12:37–53, 1993

Hynd GW, Hern KL, Novey ES, et al: Attention deficit–hyperactivity disorder and asymmetry of the caudate nucleus. J Child Neurol 8:339–347, 1993

Jensen PS, Salzberg AD, Richters JE, et al: Scales, diagnoses, and child psychopathology, I: CBCL and DISC relationships. J Am Acad Child Adolesc Psychiatry 32:397–406, 1993a

Jensen PS, Shervette RE, Xenakis SN, et al: Anxiety and depressive disorders in attention deficit disorder with hyperactivity: new findings. Am J Psychiatry 150:1203–1209, 1993b

Keller MB, Lavori PW, Beardslee WR, et al: The disruptive behavioral disorder in children and adolescents: comorbidity and clinical course. J Am Acad Child Adolesc Psychiatry 31:204–209, 1992

Kelly DP, Kelly BJ, Jones ML, et al: Attention deficits in children and adolescents with hearing loss: a survey. Am J Dis Child 147:737–741, 1993

Kelsey DK, Sumner CR, Casat CD, et al: Once-daily atomoxetine treatment for children with attention-deficit/hyperactivity disorder, including an assessment of evening and morning behavior: a double-blind, placebo-controlled trial. Pediatrics 114:E1–E8, 2004

Klein RG, Mannuzza S: Hyperactive boys almost grown up, III: methylphenidate effects on ultimate height. Arch Gen Psychiatry 45:1131–1134, 1988

Klein RG, Mannuzza S: Long-term outcome of hyperactive children: a review. J Am Acad Child Adolesc Psychiatry 30:383–387, 1991

Klein RG, Abikoff H, Hechtman L, et al: Design and rationale of controlled study of long-term methylphenidate and multimodal psychosocial treatment in children with ADHD. J Am Acad Child Adolesc Psychiatry 43:792–801, 2004

Kupietz SS, Winsberg BG, Sverd J: Learning ability and methylphenidate (Ritalin) plasma concentration in hyperkinetic children. J Am Acad Child Psychiatry 21:27–30, 1982

Lahey BB, Pelham WE, Stein MA, et al: Validity of DSM-IV attention-deficit/hyperactivity disorder for younger children. J Am Acad Child Adolesc Psychiatry 37:695–702, 1998

Lapouse R, Monk M: An epidemiologic study of behavioral characteristics in children. Am J Public Health 48:1134–1144, 1953

Lie N: Follow-ups of children with attention deficit hyperactivity disorder (ADHD): review of literature. Acta Psychiatr Scand Suppl 368:1–40, 1992

Lowe TL, Cohen DJ, Detlor J, et al: Stimulant medications precipitate Tourette's syndrome. JAMA 247:1729–1731, 1982

Madras BK, Miller GM, Fischman AJ: The dopamine transporter: relevance to attention deficit hyperactivity disorder (ADHD). Behav Brain Res 130:57–63, 2002

Mann EM, Ikeda Y, Mueller CW, et al: Cross-cultural differences in rating hyperactive-disruptive behaviors in children. Am J Psychiatry 149:1539–1542, 1992

Mannuzza S, Klein RG, Bessler A, et al: Adult outcome of hyperactive boys: educational achievement, occupational rank, and psychiatric status. Arch Gen Psychiatry 50:565–576, 1993

Mannuzza S, Klein RG, Bessler A, et al: Adult psychiatric status of hyperactive boys grown up. Am J Psychiatry 155:493–498, 1998

Matochik JA, Nordahl TE, Gross M, et al: Effects of acute stimulant medication on cerebral metabolism in adults with hyperactivity. Neuropsychopharmacology 8:377–386, 1993

Mayes SD, Crites DL, Bixler EO, et al: Methylphenidate and ADHD: influence of age, IQ and neurodevelopmental status. Dev Med Child Neurol 36:1099–1107, 1994

McCracken JT, Biederman J, Greenhill LL, et al: Analog classroom assessment of a once-daily mixed amphetamine formulation, SLI381 (Adderall XR), in children with ADHD. J Am Acad Child Adolesc Psychiatry 42:673–683, 2003

McGee R, Feehan M, Williams S, et al: DSM-III disorders in a large sample of adolescents. J Am Acad Child Adolesc Psychiatry 29:611–619, 1990

McGee R, Partridge F, Williams S, et al: A twelve-year follow-up of preschool hyperactive children. J Am Acad Child Adolesc Psychiatry 30:224–232, 1991

McGee R, Williams S, Feehan M: Attention deficit disorder and age of onset of problem behaviors. J Abnorm Child Psychol 20:487–502, 1992

McGee R, Stanton WR, Sears MR: Allergic disorders and attention deficit disorder in children. J Abnorm Child Psychol 21:79–88, 1993

Mercugliano M, Hyman SL, Batshaw ML: Behavioral deficits in rats with minimal cortical hypoplasia induced by methylazoxymethanol acetate. Pediatrics 85:432–436, 1990

Michelson D, Faries D, Wernicke J, et al: Atomoxetine in the treatment of children and adolescents with attention-deficit/hyperactivity disorder: a randomized, placebo-controlled, dose-response study. Pediatrics 108:E83, 2001

Michelson D, Allen AJ, Busner J, et al: Once-daily atomoxetine treatment for children and adolescents with attention deficit hyperactivity disorder: a randomized, placebo-controlled study. Am J Psychiatry 159:1896–1901, 2002

Michelson D, Buitelaar JK, Danckaerts M, et al: Relapse prevention in pediatric patients with ADHD treated with atomoxetine: a randomized, double-blind, placebo-controlled study. J Am Acad Child Adolesc Psychiatry 43:896–904, 2004

Milberger S, Biederman J, Faraone SV, et al: ADHD is associated with early initiation of cigarette smoking in children and adolescents. J Am Acad Child Adolesc Psychiatry 36:37–44, 1997

Minder B, Das-Smaal EA, Brand EFJM, et al: Exposure to lead and specific attentional problems in schoolchildren. J Learn Disabil 27:393–399, 1994

MTA Cooperative Group: A 14-month randomized clinical trial of treatment strategies for attention-deficit/hyperactivity disorder: the MTA Cooperative Group. Multimodal Treatment Study of Children with ADHD. Arch Gen Psychiatry 56:1073–1086, 1999

MTA Cooperative Group: National Institute of Mental Health Multimodal Treatment Study of ADHD follow-up: 24-month outcomes of treatment strategies for attention-deficit/hyperactivity disorder. Pediatrics 113:754–761, 2004a

MTA Cooperative Group: National Institute of Mental Health Multimodal Treatment Study of ADHD follow-up: changes in effectiveness and growth after the end of treatment. Pediatrics 113:762–769, 2004b

National Institutes of Health Consensus Development Conference Statement: diagnosis and treatment of attention-deficit/hyperactivity disorder (ADHD). J Am Acad Child Adolesc Psychiatry 39:182–193, 2000

Ornoy A, Uriel L, Tennenbaum A: Inattention, hyperactivity and speech delay at 2–4 years of age as a predictor for ADD-ADHD syndrome. Isr J Psychiatry Relat Sci 30:155–163, 1993

Palfrey JS, Levine MD, Walker DK, et al: The emergence of attention deficits in early childhood: a prospective study. J Dev Behav Pediatr 6:339–348, 1985

Pelham WEJ, Gnagy EM, Greenslade KE, et al: Teacher ratings of DSM-III-R symptoms for the disruptive behavior disorders. J Am Acad Child Adolesc Psychiatry 31:210–218, 1992

Pelham WEJ, Carlson C, Sams SE, et al: Separate and combined effects of methylphenidate and behavior modification on boys with attention deficit-hyperactivity disorder in the classroom. J Consult Clin Psychol 61:506–515, 1993

Physicians' Desk Reference, 55th Edition. Montvale, NJ, Medical Economics, 2001

Pliszka SR: Tricyclic antidepressants in the treatment of children with attention deficit disorder. J Am Acad Child Adolesc Psychiatry 26:127–132, 1987

Porrino LJ, Rapoport JL, Behar D, et al: A naturalistic assessment of the motor activity of hyperactive boys, I: comparison with normal controls. Arch Gen Psychiatry 40:681–687, 1983

Pratt DS, Dubois RS: Hepatotoxicity due to pemoline (Cylert): a report of two cases. J Pediatr Gastroenterol Nutr 10:239–241, 1990

Prince JB, Wilens TE, Biederman J, et al: Clonidine for sleep disturbances associated with attention-deficit hyperactivity disorder: a systematic chart review of 62 cases. J Am Acad Child Adolesc Psychiatry 35:599–605, 1996

Rapport MD, Stoner G, DuPaul GJ, et al: Methylphenidate in hyperactive children: differential effects of dose on academic, learning, and social behavior. J Abnorm Child Psychol 13:227–243, 1985

Riddle MA, Geller B, Ryan N: Another sudden death in a child treated with desipramine. J Am Acad Child Adolesc Psychiatry 32:792–797, 1993

Roth N, Beyreiss J, Schlenzka K, et al: Coincidence of attention deficit disorder and atopic disorders in children: empirical findings and hypothetical background. J Abnorm Child Psychol 19:1–13, 1991

Rounsaville BJ, Anton SF, Carroll K, et al: Psychiatric diagnoses of treatment-seeking cocaine abusers. Arch Gen Psychiatry 48:43–51, 1991

Rowe KS, Rowe KJ: Synthetic food coloring and behavior: a dose response effect in a double-blind, placebo-controlled, repeated-measures study. J Pediatr 125:691–698, 1994

Rubia K, Overmeyer S, Taylor E, et al: Hypofrontality in attention deficit hyperactivity disorder during higher-order motor control: a study with functional MRI. Am J Psychiatry 156:891–896, 1999

Sallee FR, Stiller RL, Perel JM: Pharmacodynamics of pemoline in attention-deficit disorder with hyperactivity. J Am Acad Child Adolesc Psychiatry 31:244–251, 1992

Satterfield J, Swanson J, Schell A, et al: Prediction of antisocial behavior in attention-deficit hyperactivity disorder boys from aggression/defiance scores. J Am Acad Child Adolesc Psychiatry 33:185–190, 1994

Scahill L, Schwab-Stone M: Epidemiology of ADHD in school-age children. Child Adolesc Psychiatr Clin N Am 9:541–555, 2000

Scahill L, Chappell PB, Kim YS, et al: A placebo-controlled study of guanfacine in the treatment of children with tic disorders and attention deficit hyperactivity disorder. Am J Psychiatry 158:1067–1074, 2001

Schwab-Stone M, Fallon T, Briggs M, et al: Reliability of diagnostic reporting for children aged 6–11 years: a test-retest study of the Diagnostic Interview Schedule for Children–Revised. Am J Psychiatry 151:1048–1054, 1994

Sechzer JA, Faro MD, Windle WF: Studies of monkeys asphyxiated at birth: implications for minimal cerebral dysfunction. Semin Psychiatry 5:19–34, 1973

Semrud-Clikeman M, Biederman J, Sprich-Buckminster S, et al: Comorbidity between ADDH and learning disability: a review and report in a clinically referred sample. J Am Acad Child Adolesc Psychiatry 31:439–448, 1992

Semrud-Clikeman M, Steingard RJ, Filipek P, et al: Using MRI to examine brain-behavior relationships in males with attention deficit disorder with hyperactivity. J Am Acad Child Adolesc Psychiatry 39:477–484, 2000

Shaffer D: Attention deficit hyperactivity disorder in adults (editorial). Am J Psychiatry 151:633–688, 1994

Shaffer D, Greenhill LL: A critical note on the predictive validity of the hyperactive syndrome. J Child Psychol Psychiatry 20:61–72, 1979

Shaffer D, Schoenfeld I, O'Conner P, et al: Neurological soft signs. Arch Gen Psychiatry 42:329–335, 1985

Shaffer D, Fisher P, Lucas CP, et al: NIMH Diagnostic Interview Schedule for Children Version IV (NIMH DISC-IV): description, differences from previous versions, and reliability of some common diagnoses. J Am Acad Child Adolesc Psychiatry 39:28–38, 2000

Shastry BS: Molecular genetics of attention-deficit hyperactivity disorder (ADHD): an update. Neurochem Int 44:469–474, 2004

Shaywitz BA, Yager RD, Klopper JH: Selective brain dopamine depletion in developing rats: an experimental model of minimal brain dysfunction. Science 191:305–308, 1976

Shen YC, Wang YF, Yang XL: An epidemiological investigation of minimal brain dysfunction in six elementary schools in Beijing. J Child Psychol Psychiatry 26:777–787, 1985

Sobotka TJ, Cook MP: Postnatal lead acetate exposure in rats: possible relationship to minimal brain dysfunction. Am J Ment Defic 79:5–9, 1974

Solanto MV, Wender EH: Does methylphenidate constrict cognitive functioning? J Am Acad Child Adolesc Psychiatry 28:897–902, 1989

Speiser Z, Korczyn AD, Teplitzky I, et al: Hyperactivity in rats following postnatal anoxia. Behav Brain Res 7:379–382, 1983

Spencer TJ, Biederman J, Steingard R, et al: Bupropion exacerbates tics in children with attention-deficit hyperactivity disorder and Tourette's syndrome. J Am Acad Child Adolesc Psychiatry 32:211–214, 1993

Spencer T, Biederman J, Wilens T, et al: Pharmacotherapy of attention-deficit hyperactivity disorder across the life cycle. J Am Acad Child Adolesc Psychiatry 35:409–432, 1996

Sprague RL, Sleator EK: Methylphenidate in hyperkinetic children: differences in dose effects on learning and social behavior. Science 198:1274–1276, 1977

Sprich-Buckminster S, Biederman J, Milberger S, et al: Are perinatal complications relevant to the manifestation of ADD? issues of comorbidity and familiality. J Am Acad Child Adolesc Psychiatry 32:1032–1037, 1993

Srinivas NR, Hubbard JW, Quinn D, et al: Enantioselective pharmacokinetics and pharmacodynamics of dl-threo-methylphenidate in children with attention deficit hyperactivity disorder. Clin Pharmacol Ther 52:561–568, 1992

Stein MA, Sarampote CS, Waldman ID, et al: A dose-response study of OROS methylphenidate in children with attention-deficit/hyperactivity disorder. Pediatrics. 112:E404, 2003

Steingard R, Biederman J, Spencer T, et al: Comparison of clonidine response in the treatment of attention-deficit hyperactivity disorder with and without comorbid tic disorders. J Am Acad Child Adolesc Psychiatry 32:350–353, 1993

Strayhorn JM, Weidman CS: Reduction of attention deficit and internalizing symptoms in preschoolers through parent-child interaction training. J Am Acad Child Adolesc Psychiatry 28:888–896, 1989

Streissguth AP, Barr HM, Sampson PD, et al: Prenatal alcohol and offspring development: the first fourteen years. Drug Alcohol Depend 36:89–99, 1994

Sullivan A, Kelso J, Stewart M: Mothers' views on the ages of onset for four childhood disorders. Child Psychiatry Hum Dev 20:269–278, 1990

Swanson J, Cantwell D: Cognitive toxicity of methylphenidate: evidence from reaction times study of memory scanning. Proceedings of the Annual Meeting of the American Academy of Child and Adolescent Psychiatry 5:49–50, 1989

Swanson JM, Kraemer HC, Hinshaw SP, et al: Clinical relevance of the primary findings of the MTA: success rates based on severity of ADHD and ODD symptoms at the end of treatment. J Am Acad Child Adolesc Psychiatry 40:168–179, 2001

Swanson J, Gupta S, Lam A, et al: Development of a new once-a-day formulation of methylphenidate for the treatment of attention-deficit/hyperactivity disorder: proof-of-concept and proof-of-product studies. Arch Gen Psychiatry 60:204–211, 2003

Swanson JM, Wigal SB, Wigal T, et al: A comparison of once-daily extended-release methylphenidate formulations in children with attention-deficit/hyperactivity disorder in the laboratory school (the Comacs Study). Pediatrics 113:E206–E216, 2004

Sykes DH, Douglas VI, Morgenstern G: The effect of methylphenidate (Ritalin) on sustained attention in hyperactive children. Psychopharmacologia 25:262–274, 1972

Tarver-Behring S, Barkley RA, Karlsson J: The mother-child interactions of hyperactive boys and their normal siblings. Am J Orthopsychiatry 55:202–209, 1985

Verhulst FC, Achenbach TM, Ferdinand RF, et al: Epidemiological comparisons of American and Dutch adolescents' self-reports. J Am Acad Child Adolesc Psychiatry 32:1135–1144, 1993

Vitiello B, Stoff D, Atkins M, et al: Soft neurological signs and impulsivity in children. J Dev Behav Pediatr 11:112–115, 1990

Walsh BT, Giardina EG, Sloan RP, et al: Effects of desipramine on autonomic control of the heart. J Am Acad Child Adolesc Psychiatry 33:191–197, 1994

Ward MF, Wender PH, Reimherr FW: The Wender Utah Rating Scale: an aid in the retrospective diagnosis of childhood attention deficit hyperactivity disorder. Am J Psychiatry 150:885–890, 1993

Wechsler J: Wechsler Intelligence Scale for Children—Revised. New York, Psychological Corporation, 1974

Weingartner H, Rapoport JL, Buchsbaum MS, et al: Cognitive processes in normal and hyperactive children and their response to amphetamine treatment. J Abnorm Psychol 89:25–35, 1980

Wender PH, Reimherr FW: Bupropion treatment of attention-deficit hyperactivity disorder in adults. Am J Psychiatry 147:1018–1020, 1990

Werry JS, Elkind GS, Reeves JC: Attention deficit, conduct, oppositional, and anxiety disorders in children, III: laboratory differences. J Abnorm Child Psychol 15:409–428, 1987

Whalen CK, Henker B: Therapies for hyperactive children: comparisons, combinations, and compromises. J Consult Clin Psychol 59:126–137, 1991

Whalen CK, Henker B, Collins BE, et al: A social ecology of hyperactive boys: medication effects in structured classroom environments. J Appl Behav Anal 12:65–81, 1979

Whalen CK, Henker B, Castro J, et al: Peer perception of hyperactivity and medication effects. Child Dev 58:816–828, 1987

Whitaker AH, Van Rossem R, Feldman JF, et al: Psychiatric outcomes in low-birth-weight children at age 6 years: relation to neonatal cranial ultrasound abnormalities. Arch Gen Psychiatry 54:847–856, 1997

Wigal S. Swanson JM, Feifel D, et al: A double-blind, placebo-controlled trial of dexmethylphenidate hydrochloride and d,l-threo-methylphenidate hydrochloride in children with attention-deficit/hyperactivity disorder. J Am Acad Child Adolesc Psychiatry 43:1406–1414, 2004

Wilens TE, Biederman J, Geist DE, et al: Nortriptyline in the treatment of ADHD: a chart review of 58 cases. J Am Acad Child Adolesc Psychiatry 32:343–349, 1993a

Wilens TE, Biederman J, Spencer T, et al: A retrospective study of serum levels and electrocardiographic effects of nortriptyline in children and adolescents. J Am Acad Child Adolesc Psychiatry 32:270–277, 1993b

Wilens TE, Spencer TJ, Biederman J, et al: A controlled clinical trial of bupropion for attention deficit hyperactivity disorder in adults. Am J Psychiatry 158:282–288, 2001

Wilens T, Pelham W, Stein M, et al: ADHD treatment with once-daily OROS methylphenidate: interim 12-month results from a long-term open-label study. J Am Acad Child Adolesc Psychiatry 42:424–433, 2003

Willoughby MT, Curran PJ, Costello EJ, et al: Implications of early versus late onset of attention-deficit/hyperactivity disorder symptoms. J Am Acad Child Adolesc Psychiatry 39:1512–1519, 2000

Wolraich ML, Greenhill LL, Pelham W, et al: Randomized, controlled trial of oros methylphenidate once a day in children with attention-deficit/hyperactivity disorder. Pediatrics 108:883–892, 2001

Zahner GE, Jacobs JH, Freeman DHJ, et al: Rural-urban child psychopathology in a Northeastern U.S. state: 1986–1989. J Am Acad Child Adolesc Psychiatry 32:378–387, 1993

Zametkin A, Rapoport JL, Murphy DL, et al: Treatment of hyperactive children with monoamine oxidase inhibitors, I: clinical efficacy. Arch Gen Psychiatry 42:962–966, 1985

Zametkin AJ, Liebenauer LL, Fitzgerald GA, et al: Brain metabolism in teenagers with attention-deficit hyperactivity disorder. Arch Gen Psychiatry 50:333–340, 1993

Zentall SS, Meyer MJ: Self-regulation of stimulation of ADD-H children during reading and vigilance task performance. J Abnorm Child Psychol 15:519–536, 1987

Self-Assessment Questions

Select the single best response for each question.

15.1 Which of the following is *not* one of the core symptom clusters of attention-deficit/hyperactivity disorder (ADHD) as identified in DSM-IV-TR (American Psychiatric Association 2000)?

A. Hyperactivity.

B. Inattention.

C. Impulsivity.

D. Disruptive behavior.

E. Distractibility.

15.2 Which of the following is *not* one of the DSM-IV-TR diagnostic criteria for ADHD?

A. Symptoms must have persisted for at least 6 months.

B. Symptoms must be evident in at least two different environments.

C. Symptoms must have been present before age 5 years.

D. Symptoms must be maladaptive in terms of functioning.

E. Symptoms cannot be accounted for by another DSM-IV-TR diagnosis (e.g., a pervasive developmental disorder).

15.3 Which of the following comorbid psychiatric disorders has been reported to occur most frequently in children diagnosed with ADHD?

A. Schizophrenia.

B. Oppositional defiant disorder.

C. Autism.

D. Bipolar disorder.

E. Panic disorder.

15.4 Which of the following statements concerning the epidemiology of ADHD is *false*?

A. The disorder seems to be more common in boys than in girls.

B. The prevalence reported in DSM-IV-TR is 3%–7% of school-age children.

C. ADHD is more common in school-age populations than in older populations.

D. Prevalence rates show little variation across cultures, countries, and settings (urban, suburban, and rural).

E. None of the above.

15.5 Which of the following statements concerning research findings on the course and duration of ADHD is *correct?*

  A. At least some impairment from the disorder is present in most adolescents who were referred for clinical treatment as school-age children.
  B. The disorder is generally episodic rather than chronic.
  C. Inattention tends to remit over time, in contrast to hyperactivity, which is remarkably persistent.
  D. Inattention symptoms may place a child at greater risk for the development of antisocial behavior.
  E. None of the above.

15.6 The research literature supports the use of all of the following medications for ADHD *except*

  A. Tricyclic antidepressants.
  B. Psychostimulants.
  C. Clonidine.
  D. Bupropion.
  E. Benzodiazepines.

Conduct Disorder and Oppositional Defiant Disorder

Robert L. Hendren, D.O.

David J. Mullen, M.D.

Children with conduct disorder (CD) are a varied group because of the myriad manifestations of antisocial behavior and the numerous and complex factors that contribute to the evolution of antisocial behavior. First, the classification of conduct disorder is a controversial and unsettled issue in mental health (Cantwell and Baker 1988; Frick et al. 1994), and the relationship between conduct disorder and oppositional defiant disorder (ODD) remains unclear. Depending on the constellation of symptoms, conduct disorder might be diagnosed based predominantly on irresponsible, delinquent behaviors such as truancy and running away; covert violations of the rights of others such as nonconfrontative theft; or overt physical aggression such as assault or rape. These behaviors share an antisocial quality but differ significantly in other respects. In addition, the specific antisocial behaviors involved tend to vary

significantly with development. For example, oppositional defiant behaviors tend to precede more serious violations of age-appropriate behavioral norms. Second, the etiology of conduct disorder is manifold, with biological, psychological, and social factors having various degrees of significance. Some children may have a prominent family history of criminality, whereas in others histories of abuse and neglect or social chaos and the presence of neighborhood youth gangs may be more prominent. Or, not uncommonly, all of these and other factors may be present. In addition, children with conduct disorder and ODD frequently manifest other psychiatric symptoms, and many (if not most) will meet criteria for another psychiatric disorder, further complicating issues of assessment, diagnosis, and treatment. It is clear that a comprehensive assessment and treatment program depends not only on the knowledge of developmental signs and symptoms but also on a thorough exploration of the underlying biopsychosocial factors. Finally, as with many other psychiatric syndromes, conduct disorder and ODD may be conceptualized as stemming at least in part from disturbances in the self-regulation of affect and behavior. In the case of conduct disorder and ODD, problems with the regulation of anger and impulsivity may be the principal self-regulatory defects observed, and these defects may be initiated and maintained by a broad range of underlying biological, psychological, and social factors (Bradley 2000; Moeller et al. 2001).

Prevalence

The prevalence of conduct disorder is difficult to estimate because of the different definitions that have been used and the variations that occur in different age groups and between the sexes. In DSM-IV (American Psychiatric Association 1994) the prevalence of conduct disorder is estimated as approximately 9% for males and 2% for females younger than 18 years. In DSM-IV-TR (American Psychiatric Association 2000) the prevalence is estimated to be between 1% and 16%. The childhood-onset type of the disorder, defined by the presence of at least one criterion characteristic of conduct disorder before age 10 years, is clearly much more common in males; physical aggression is frequently displayed toward others, peer relationships are typically disturbed, and criteria for ODD are often met during early childhood. Individuals with childhood-onset conduct disorder appear to be more likely to develop adult antisocial personality disorder than are young people with onset of conduct disorder in adolescence. The preponderance of males also appears to be less prominent in the adolescent-onset type.

ODD occurs at a prevalence ranging from 2% to 16% according to both DSM-IV and DSM-IV-TR and is approximately twice as common in males as in females.

Diagnostic Classification

■ DSM-IV-TR Criteria

The essential feature of conduct disorder, according to DSM-IV-TR, is a persistent pattern of behavior that violates the basic rights of others and major age-appropriate social norms or rules. Diagnostic criteria are divided into four basic categories: 1) aggression to people and animals, which includes behaviors ranging from bullying or intimidating others to physical cruelty and forcing someone into sexual activity; 2) destruction of property, which includes fire setting or other deliberate property destruction; 3) deceitfulness or theft, which includes more surreptitious or covert antisocial behaviors such as lying or nonconfrontative theft; and 4) serious violations of rules, which includes truancy or socially irresponsible behaviors. Three or more of these criteria must have been present within 12 months of the assessment, with at least one criterion occurring within 6 months. Because the diagnosis is based on a broad range of behavioral criteria without reference to etiology, individuals who meet criteria for conduct disorder may have significantly different underlying psychopathology. Furthermore, the impact of social context may result in diagnostic variation (Angold and Costello 1996). Thus, individuals with a diagnosis of conduct disorder are a very heterogeneous group (Lavigne et al. 2001).

ODD is characterized by a pattern of hostile, negativistic, defiant, and disobedient attitudes and behaviors, especially toward authority figures, that is associated with impairment. This pattern is frequently seen in young people who meet the criteria for conduct disorder, and there is some controversy regarding the validity of ODD as a separate diagnosis. In DSM-IV-TR, conduct disorder and ODD are not allowed to be diagnosed together, given the extent of symptom overlap. However, the current consensus supports the idea that there is a valid distinction between symptoms of ODD and some of the symptoms of conduct disorder, especially the covert variety. In DSM-IV-TR it is also recognized that in many children increased negativity and hostility may occur as part of the course of a mood or psychotic disorder, and the diagnosis of ODD is not allowed when the symptoms occur exclusively during the course of a psychotic or mood disorder.

■ Subtypes of Conduct Disorder

Several approaches have been used in the classification of conduct disorder. In DSM-IV-TR two diagnostic subtypes—a childhood-onset type and an adolescent-onset type—are recognized. The value of this subtyping is clearly related to the prognostic significance of age at onset, with early onset being more ominous. Soderstrom et al. (2004) found in a forensic analysis of adult offenders that the most relevant psychiatric symptom cluster in relation to pervasive adult violent behavior was childhood onset social and behavioral problems while late-onset mental disorders were associated with single acts of violent or sexual aggression.

In a cluster analysis of the symptoms of disturbed children, Wolff (1971) found two groups of children with behavioral disturbance: aggressive-overactive and antisocial. Hospitalized children with conduct disorder and aggressive and destructive behavior have a particularly poor prognosis (Gabel and Shindledecker 1991).

Subtyping aggressive behavior into predatory and affective categories is another useful distinction (Blair 2001; Vi-

tiello et al. 1990). Predatory aggression is goal directed, with minimal associated autonomic arousal. Affective aggression is characterized by the presence of high levels of autonomic and emotional arousal with little apparent instrumental gain. Vitaro et al. (1998) found that children who manifested proactive aggression (similar conceptually to predatory aggression) were more delinquent than those whose problems with aggression tended to be more reactive (and affective) in nature.

In a review of the literature on delinquency, Rutter and Giller (1984) found that the categories of socialized and undersocialized conduct disorder were the most valid, with the socialized group having the better prognosis. However, at least one study found that group involvement is common in delinquent conduct and that no category of offense is predominantly solitary (Emler et al. 1987). Adolescent girls were especially likely to commit offenses in the company of others. In a 4-year follow-up study, Cantwell and Baker (1989) found that the conduct disorder diagnoses were not stable. At follow-up, many children with an initial diagnosis of conduct disorder had other diagnoses, and a few had no disorders. Thus, the research literature suggests that age at onset, degree of aggressivity, and extent of socialization are important variables to consider in conduct disorder; however, no system of subclassification is completely validated.

■ Other Classification Approaches

Other approaches to classification attempt to identify salient symptoms that yield reliable and clinically meaningful subgroups of children with antisocial behavior (Kazdin 1987). Patterson (1982) found two symptom clusters in children: a primary problem of aggression and a significant problem of theft. Family structure and treatment responsiveness differed between the two groups; the group who stole had the poorer prognosis. Children with both types of characteristics were likely to have been abused.

Recently, some attempt has been made to subtype youths with conduct disorder by the presence or absence of the trait of callousness—a central feature of the concept of psychopathy. The presence of this trait was indeed found to correlate with more police contacts and a greater number and variety of conduct problems, as well as with higher levels of aggressiveness and self-reported delinquency (Christian et al. 1997; Frick and Ellis 1999). Interestingly, in these studies, children and adolescents with high levels of callousness tended to have higher IQs than other children with conduct disorder.

Another classification method for antisocial behavior is based on the distinction between overt and covert behavior (Loeber and Schmaling 1985). Overt behaviors, such as physical and verbal aggression, are more direct and obvious. Covert behaviors, such as stealing and fire setting, are not as openly confrontational. Cluster analyses support the validity of these distinctions. Children with a mixture of the two types appear to be at greater risk for future dysfunction.

The 10th revision of the *International Classification of Diseases* (World Health Organization 1992) presents yet another method for the classification of conduct disorder, which includes a number of "combination categories" that represent commonly co-occurring conditions. For example, categories exist for depressive conduct disorder and hyperkinetic conduct disorder. Subdivisions of conduct disorder include conduct disorder confined to the family context, unsocialized conduct disorder, socialized conduct disorder, and conduct disorder not otherwise specified. In a study examining the

symptom patterns and correlates of the depressive conduct disorder subtype, Simic and Fombonne (2001) found that patients with the depressive subtype of conduct disorder had fewer biological depressive features, fewer anxiety symptoms, less guilt, and less overall depressive severity than patients with depressive disorder and less overt aggression and violence than patients with simple conduct disorder. The results of the study were believed to tentatively support the depressive conduct disorder construct.

All the classification systems proposed for antisocial behavior in childhood and adolescence contain some commonalities. Each approach identifies certain symptom clusters, such as aggression and delinquency, or the time course of symptoms as important subcategories. However, neither the category of conduct disorder nor the subcategories have been fully validated as to their developmental and predictive significance.

The principal subdivision to be made in ODD is between the variety that appears to progress to conduct disorder and the variety that does not. Greater severity and early onset of oppositional behavior, frequent physical fighting, parental substance abuse, and low socioeconomic status appear to increase the risk of progression to the more severe antisocial behaviors observed in conduct disorder (Loeber et al. 1995).

Comorbidity

Many children and adolescents who meet the criteria for a diagnosis of conduct disorder or ODD have coexisting psychiatric disorders that may have led to their antisocial behavior and will influence their responsiveness to treatment and their long-term prognosis (Woolston et al. 1989). For instance, depression-like symptoms have been noted in some patients with conduct disorder (Harrington et al. 1991; Kovacs et al. 1988). Puig-Antich (1982) reported that symptoms of conduct disorder may start and stop with the onset of and recovery from affective illness. Conduct disorder that is comorbid with depression is also found to have a variable course, which may or may not abate as the depression diminishes (Kovacs et al. 1988). Conduct disorder and major depression in adolescents were both found to be related to maternal major depression, paternal antisocial behavior and high parent-child conflict and thus share a number of risk factors (Marmorstein and Iacono 2004). Lavigne et al. (2001) found ODD in preschool children to be a moderate to highly stable diagnosis and that it displayed a pattern of increasing comorbidity with attention-deficit/hyperactivity disorder (ADHD), anxiety, or mood disorders over time.

Children and adolescents with bipolar mood disorder may also meet criteria for a comorbid conduct disorder. Some authors have considered the possibility that the combination presents a unique subtype of conduct disorder (Wozniak et al. 2001). Conceptually, the poor judgment, irritability, increased activity level, and impaired impulse control associated with mania might easily lead to repeated instances of antisocial behavior such that the criteria for conduct disorder are met.

Children and adolescents with conduct disorder or ODD frequently also have coexisting ADHD. Reeves et al. (1987) found that children with ADHD plus conduct disorder or ODD had many demographic and clinical variables that were very similar to those of children with ADHD alone. The combination of ADHD and conduct disorder is associated with more severe physical aggression and antisocial behavior than is conduct disorder alone (Walker et al. 1987). In addition, a significant number of chil-

dren who are first given a diagnosis of conduct disorder are found to have ADHD at follow-up (Cantwell and Baker 1989). Although it is clear that the comorbidity is common, the relationship between the conditions requires further clarification. Mannuzza et al. (2004) found that children with ADHD were at risk for the development of adolescent conduct disorder even in the absence of significant conduct disorder symptoms at the time of initial assessment. Other studies have found no evidence that children initially diagnosed with ADHD alone were more likely to develop antisocial behavior (Loeber et al. 2000). However, as noted above, when the two are found together, the severity of the conduct disorder is often worse.

Some children and adolescents may exhibit antisocial and aggressive behavior in the years preceding the onset of schizophrenia that could lead to a diagnosis of conduct disorder (Offord and Cross 1969; Watt et al. 1983). A clear familial link exists between antisocial behavior and schizophrenia (Silverton et al. 1988). The basis of this linkage is not clear, although paranoid ideation and other cognitive distortions in psychotic patients could well contribute to antisocial behavior.

Disturbances in conduct are also found in children with Tourette's disorder. In fact, associated behavioral disturbances often contribute substantially to the overall impairment observed in patients with Tourette's disorder. Of note, the basal ganglia are likely involved in the etiology of tics as well as obsessive-compulsive disorder, and this brain region also appears to be involved in impulse regulation (D.L. Clark and Boutros 1999)—as noted above, a common prominent area of impairment in children with conduct disorder. One study estimated that in children who are not economically disadvantaged, 10%–30% of cases of conduct disorder may be due to the presence of a Tourette's disorder gene (Comings and Comings 1987).

Substance use frequently co-occurs with conduct disorder. One study reported that more than 50% of youths with conduct disorder also met criteria for substance use disorder (Reebye et al. 1995). The comorbidity was higher in the younger (ages 10–13) group. Childhood aggression is a predictor of adolescent drug use and delinquency, and delinquency predicts later drug use (Brook et al. 1992). Substance abuse likely reflects the presence of temperamental risk factors—novelty seeking and impulsivity—but is also likely to directly promote antisocial behavior through adversely affecting judgment, further decreasing impulse control, and—in the presence of marked psychological or physiological dependence—leading to strenuous and illegal efforts to obtain the substance. Of course, antisocial behavior may be indirectly promoted through increasing affiliation with antisocial peers.

Although the majority of the literature on conduct disorder has focused on males, due to a previous assumption that the disorder is rare in females, an increasing recognition that the disorder is common among girls has led to a growing literature regarding the disorder in females. Relative to males, females may be more likely to develop internalizing disorders as comorbid conditions (Keenan et al. 1999). Females also appear less likely to engage in overt physical aggression and are more inclined to use verbal and relational aggression such as alienation and character defamation (Loeber et al. 2000).

This diagnostic comorbidity found in children and adolescents who meet criteria for conduct disorder or ODD demonstrates the heterogeneity of this patient group. Clinicians and researchers working with these young people must carefully examine all of the symptoms and background information to accurately identify factors to classify each child and adolescent.

Etiology

Conduct disorder and ODD have complex and multifactorial etiologies. Biological, psychological, social, and developmental factors each contribute in differing degrees to the development and clinical course of the disorders (Lewis et al. 1987). We delineate some of the known biopsychosocial factors, but it is the interaction of these variables that leads to a complete understanding of the etiology of the disorder. For instance, the presence of birth complications combined with early maternal rejection at age 1 year is associated with violent crime at age 18 years. This effect was specific to violence and was not associated with either risk factor alone (Raine et al. 1994). As noted above, numerous factors are likely to contribute to the observed impairments in affective and behavioral regulation in conduct disorder and ODD. Some factors may contribute through direct alterations in brain structure and function stemming from the actions of gene products; others, through adverse effects on intrauterine development; and still others, through postnatal damage impinging through mechanical, toxic, or psychological injury. Other factors are likely to relate to deviant learning acquired though exposure to chaotic and destructive family and peer environments.

■ Biological Factors

Genetics

The role of genetic vulnerability in developing conduct disorder has yet to be fully elucidated, although it is likely that genetic factors play at least some role either directly or through a mediating factor such as temperament. Genetic factors have been identified in a number of traits that are believed to contribute to conduct disorder, including inattention, hyperactivity, aggressiveness, and novelty seeking. The role of genetics in adult antisocial personality is fairly robust. It is likely that psychosocial factors play a stronger role in child and adolescent conduct disorder because children, unlike adults, are less able to self-select the social contexts in which they must live and develop. Most studies involving youths with disruptive behavior disorders suggest a significant role for psychosocial and environmental factors that, acting in concert with genetic factors, substantially increase the risk of psychopathology (Burt et al. 2001; Steiner and Wilson 1999). Cross-situational conduct problems in children and adolescence may have a particularly strong genetic component (Scourfield et al. 2004). Dick et al. (2004), in a genomewide linkage analysis, found that chromosomes 2 and 19 may have regions conferring a risk for conduct disorder. Chromosome 2 was also found to be linked to alcohol dependence in the same sample.

Children characterized as possessing a difficult temperament are more likely to show or develop behavioral problems (Rutter et al. 1964). When familial genetic factors predispose a child to conduct disorder and delinquency, it is also more likely that at least one parent is antisocial (Lahey et al. 1988b; Mednick et al. 1984; Moffitt 1987). Children with a difficult temperament may interact with their family and environment in such a way that the initial behavioral disturbance becomes even more problematic. For instance, self-regulation at age 4 years could be predicted by maternal ratings of the child's impulsivity and attention span, an objective measure of delay ability, and maternal negativity at age 24 months (Silverman and Ragusa 1993). In a study using the Junior Temperament and Char-

acter Inventory, adolescents who showed elevations in novelty seeking and reduced harm avoidance demonstrated increased rates of aggressive and delinquent behavior (Schmeck and Poustka 2001).

There have been some interesting findings of specific gene frequencies and genetic polymorphisms found to be associated with conduct disturbances. Enhanced rates of expression of the L/L variant of the serotonin transporter gene, the presence of which effectively increases the function of the serotonin transporter, were found in a sample of hyperactive children and adolescents both with and without conduct disorder (Seeger et al. 2001). Soyka et al. (2004) found an association between alcohol dependence and comorbid antisocial traits and a lower frequency of the 861 allele of the 5-HT$_{1B}$ receptor gene. In a multivariate regression analysis of 20 genes, Comings et al. (2000) found that adrenergic genes were strongly implicated in ADHD and that these same genes were often shared with patients with conduct disorder and ODD. In a study illustrating the interactive quality of genotype environmental relationships, Foley et al. (2004) found that low monoamine oxidase A activity did increase risk for conduct disorder, but only in the presence of an adverse childhood environment.

Hormonal Factors

It is commonly believed that hormonal changes have a direct influence on adolescent behavior. However, there are few scientific studies that demonstrate this influence as a direct effect. A few studies have found that hormone levels correlate with emotional and aggressive attributes in boys. Olweus et al. (1988) found high levels of testosterone in boys who were more impatient and irritable, resulting in an increased propensity to engage in aggressive-destructive behavior. Susman et al. (1987) found that higher levels of androstenedione were related to higher levels of act-ing-out problems in boys. Dmitrieva et al. (2001) found dehydroepiandrosterone (DHEAS) and corticotropin levels to be el-evated in boys with conduct disorder. van Goozen et al. (2000) found similar eleva-tions in DHEAS in boys with ODD. Rowe et al. (2004) found a biosocial interaction be-tween circulating testosterone levels and nonaggressive conduct symptoms. Boys who associated with deviant peers had in-creases in these symptoms but boys in non-deviant peer groups demonstrated greater degrees of leadership, suggesting a rela-tionship between testosterone levels and social dominance that varied in nature by social context. Buydens-Branchey and Branchey (2004) found that among a group of adult cocaine addicts, those who retrospectively qualified for a diagnosis of conduct disorder had increased levels of DHEAS and decreased cortisol reactivity.

There is also some evidence of dimin-ished salivary cortisol levels in aggressive boys. This finding was most robust, and was more indicative of persistent aggression, when a restricted range of cortisol levels was found on repeated measures than when a low concentration was identified at any particular point in time (McBurnett et al. 2000). Decreased plasma cortisol levels were also found in girls with conduct disor-der (Pajer et al. 2001).

Neurotransmitter Dysfunction

Evidence of potential monoamine neu-rotransmitter dysfunction or deviation has been identified in numerous studies of an-tisocial and aggressive adults, children, and adolescents. The systems studied have also been heavily implicated in expression and regulation of affect and in impulse control. Disturbed serotonergic function has been implicated in episodic aggression and ap-pears to be related to the capacity for be-havioral inhibition. The role of serotonin is likely to be that of a neuromodulator en-

suring that the motivational systems do not "overshoot" their targets through modify-ing the "signal-to-noise ratio" (Spoont 1992). Male monkeys with low cerebrospi-nal fluid levels of 5-hydroxyindoleacetic acid (5-HIAA) are at risk for violent, aggres-sive behavior and loss of impulse control (Mehlman et al. 1994) and have less social competence and sociality (Mehlman et al. 1995). Cloninger (1987) described a cen-tral role of serotonin in affecting the trait of harm avoidance—a characteristic observed to be low in antisocial patients. Measures of cerebrospinal fluid 5-HIAA have been found to be low in adult samples with vio-lent suicidal behavior and early-onset alco-holism (Steiner and Wilson 1999). Platelet serotonin measures have been found to be abnormal in adolescents with conduct dis-order (Unis et al. 1997). There is a strong suggestion that cerebrospinal fluid levels of 5-HIAA and homovanillic acid and auto-nomic measures can be used to predict risk for future problems (Kruesi et al. 1992). Disturbed platelet monoamine oxidase lev-els have been reported in disruptive behav-ior disorders (Stoff et al. 1989). Decreased levels of methoxyhydroxyphenyl glycol have been identified in aggressive patients (Steiner and Wilson 1999). van Goozen et al. (1999) found plasma 5-HIAA and homovanillic acid to be inversely related to aggression in a sample of boys with ODD.

Neurological and Autonomic Findings

Minor neurological abnormalities are found in some children and adolescents with delinquency (Lewis et al. 1987). Kruesi et al. (2004), using regional brain volumes derived from magnetic resonance imaging (MRI) scans, found reduced temporal lobe volumes in early-onset conduct disorder. In adolescents with conduct disorder, the fron-tal P300 event-related potential shows re-duced amplitude in association with deficits in executive function and inhibition (Kim et al. 2001). Bauer and Hesselbrock (2001) also found abnormalities in the frontal P300 event-related potential in a sample of adolescents with conduct disorder, suggesting frontal cortex dysfunction. However, it is not clear whether these abnormalities are related to conduct disorder per se or to comorbid ADHD-like symptoms and executive dysfunction. For example, Satterfield et al. (1987) followed up hyperactive children into adolescence and found that the nondelinquent hyperactive subjects had abnormal auditory evoked response potentials, whereas the delinquent hyperactive subjects had normal maturational changes in these same measures. In addition, because delinquent children are known to have had more head and face trauma (Lewis et al. 1979), early neurological signs may be the result of abuse or risk-taking behavior rather than constitutional abnormalities (Kazdin 1987).

Neuropsychological deficit is clearly associated with delinquency. A consistent association is found between low IQ and delinquency that persists when assessed prospectively and is independent of social class (Moffitt et al. 1981). Studies routinely cite impaired verbal and executive functions (attention, concentration, abstraction, planning, inhibition of inappropriate responses, and sequencing) (Moffitt and Silva 1988).

Young people with conduct disorder also may possess a degree of autonomic hypoactivity, which results in the individual being slow to respond to stressful stimuli with anticipatory anxiety (Mednick 1981). These individuals then tend to recover slowly once aroused. Such a pattern may result in impairment in the person's ability to learn to escape harm or punishment through passive avoidance. Higher levels of arousal may be protective. Fifteen-year-old males with antisocial behavior who had higher electrodermal and cardiovascular arousal were less likely to have engaged in criminal behavior by age 29 years than the group with lower arousal (Raine et al. 1995). Some work by Beauchaine et al. (2001) suggests that patients with conduct disorder may be differentiated from patients with ADHD by differential patterns of autonomic responsiveness. Herpertz et al. (2003) showed that children with CD showed decreased electrodermal responses and accelerated habituation in a pattern analogous to that seen in antisocial adults. However, the relationship between anxiety and conduct disorder needs further refining because some data suggest that the presence of anxiety may protect against the development of conduct disorder, whereas other data suggest an increased likelihood of developing anxiety symptoms after the establishment of conduct disorder. In a study seeking to clarify the genetic and environmental origins of covariance between anxiety and conduct disorder, Gregory et al. (2004) found that most of the phenotypic correlation between and anxiety and conduct symptoms was accounted for by shared environmental factors, especially for girls.

Prenatal Toxin Exposures

Wakschlag et al. (1997) demonstrated that maternal smoking during pregnancy is associated with a significant increase in the rate of conduct disorder even after controlling for previously identified risk factors. However, Maughan et al. (2004) found that this association may be largely accounted for by other known developmental and genetic risks. Mothers who smoke during pregnancy were more likely to be antisocial, to have children with more antisocial men, and to be raising their children in adverse, disadvantaged circumstances. Children with fetal alcohol exposure are frequently noted to manifest disruptive behavior disorders characterized by substantial inattention and hyperactivity as well as poor social judgment (Kelly et al. 2000).

Evolutionary Biology

A perspective derived from evolutionary biology suggests that antisocial behavior in some individuals belonging to a strongly prosocial but behaviorally flexible species is likely to persist at a relatively stable equilibrium given a substantial potential for a Darwinian advantage to be gained through cheating to obtain resources from more trusting persons. This model suggests that at least some antisocial individuals are likely to be present in any population, and their problems with self-regulation are most likely to be perceived as problems from the perspective of the victims, whereas the perpetrators themselves may be quite satisfied with themselves and their behavior. These individuals may be conceived as primary antisocials, whereas another group, who appear to adopt antisocial strategies secondary to difficulties achieving a more prosocial adaptation or in reaction to environmental constraints, may be described as secondary antisocials (Mealy 1997). In this model, the primary antisocials are likely to develop along the lines of the concept of psychopathy with high levels of callousness associated with low anxiety and minimal mood disturbances, whereas the secondary antisocials are likely to manifest more internalizing comorbidity and other evidence of adaptive dysfunction.

■ Psychological Factors

Cognitive Factors

Delinquent and aggressive children have distinctive cognitive and psychological profiles compared with children with other psychiatric disorders and control subjects. A group of delinquent males in a correctional facility displayed more immature modes of role taking, logical cognition, and moral reasoning (Lee and Prentice 1988). Compared with low-aggressive boys, high-aggressive boys 1) defined social problems based on the perception that others are hostilely motivated adversaries, 2) found fewer and less effective solutions, and 3) were less likely to get into trouble for exhibiting aggression (Guerra and Slaby 1989). Webster-Stratton and Lindsay (1999) found that boys with conduct disorder or ODD had significantly fewer social problem-solving strategies, more negative conflict management strategies, and delayed play skills relative to their peers without these disorders.

In addition, high-aggressive delinquent children were less able to perceive the viewpoints of other people than were low-aggressive delinquent children (Short and Simeonsson 1986). Aggressive children pay greater attention to aggressive environmental cues than do nonaggressive children and often misperceive cues. They quickly and impulsively think of nonverbal, action-oriented solutions to social situations (Kendall 1993). In a large longitudinal study that explored Cloninger's suggestion that boys who were high in impulsivity, low in anxiety (harm avoidance), and low in reward dependence would be at greater risk for delinquency, Tremblay et al. (1994) demonstrated that boys in kindergarten with this combination of traits were more likely to develop a stable pattern of antisocial behavior. Increased reward dependence decreased delinquency. Exposure to violence as both witness and victim has also been associated with the development of behavioral problems. Moss (2003) found that witnessing violence was predictive of overt aggression in both boys and girls and of increased anxiety in girls.

Although some studies have identified the presence of executive dysfunction in patients with conduct disorder, the extent to which executive function impairments are related to conduct disorder per se versus comorbid conditions such as ADHD remains unclear. In one study examining the issue specifically, marked impairments in executive function seemed to be principally related to the presence of comorbid ADHD rather than primarily associated with conduct disorder or ODD (C. Clark et al. 2000).

Steiner and co-workers identified different patterns of antisocial behavior related to the extent of psychic distress reported by a group of delinquent youths compared with their respective levels of restraint (Steiner and Wilson 1999; Steiner et al. 1997). Those characterized by low restraint had longer courses of antisocial behavior. However, adolescents who appeared to be overcontrolled (high restraint) often presented with short but dramatic criminal careers. A particularly interesting finding here is that restraint, typically considered to be a protective factor in conduct disorder, may under some circumstances be associated with episodes of severe antisocial behavior. This suggests that significant potential variability in specific delinquency presentation may be generated by the interaction between issues related to subjective affective distress and degree of inhibition. It also suggests that the relationship between inhibition and acting out is not a simple one.

Familial Factors

Parental psychopathology and seriously disadvantaged, dysfunctional, and disorganized home environments are common in children who have or who eventually develop conduct disorder (Fergusson et al. 1994). Antisocial personality disorder, criminal behavior, and alcoholism—particularly in the father—are the stronger and more consistently reported familial factors that increase the child's risk for conduct disorder (Robins 1966; Rutter and Giller 1984). In addition, mothers of children with a diagnosis of conduct disorder often have antisocial personality, somatization, or alcohol abuse (Lahey et al. 1988b). Lahey et al. (1988b) found evidence of parental psychopathology among children with conduct disorder but not among children with ADHD.

An accepted theory is that children who are aggressive have parents who are also aggressive, especially toward the children. However, a critical review of the studies supporting this association (Widom 1989) concluded that convincing evidence is lacking that this linkage is simple or direct. Further refinement of the study of the association between parental and child violence reveals that certain processes transmit aggressiveness to children (McCord 1988). Such processes include messages that expressive behavior (including injurious actions) is normal and justified and that egocentrism is both normal and virtuous.

Learning theorists have posited that oppositional defiant behaviors may be promoted through a negative reinforcement model. In this model the child learns to escape unpleasant tasks such as chores by becoming hostile and negativistic. Repeated parental requests for compliance are met with escalating negativity until the parent eventually relents and the child escapes the demand situation. Failure of parental follow-through with consequences is also a factor in this model. However, what is not addressed is, of course, why some children seem willing very early to escalate hostility and negativity to a marked extent despite frequently very negative relationship repercussions (Forehand et al. 1975; Wells and Egan 1988).

Familial, peer, and attentional variables interact to predict delinquency (Hoge et al. 1994). Family interactions that are characterized as unsupportive and lacking in the ability to cope with transitions and stress may lead to delinquency (Tolan 1988). The families of delinquent children also tend to emphasize personal growth dimensions, such as achievement, and cultural and ethical interests less than families of nondelinquent children (LeFlore 1988). In addition, the mother–child dyad is characterized by more conflict when adolescents have behavioral problems (Forehand et al. 1987).

Families of children and adolescents with conduct disorder have several other characteristics in common that have emerged from descriptive studies. Parental divorce is correlated with the development of conduct disorder in the children (Rutter 1971). However, this association is found between parental antisocial personality disorder, divorce, and conduct disorder but not directly between divorce and conduct disorder (Lahey et al. 1988a). Also, it appears that regardless of whether the parents are separated, it is the extent of the parental discord that is associated with the high risk for childhood dysfunction (Hetherington and Stanley-Hagan 1999). Other family variables related to offspring with conduct disorder include large family size and greater risk for conduct disorder in the middle child, especially when separated by several years from older brothers (Wadsworth 1979). The absence of the biological father has also been identified as a risk factor for antisocial behavior in any family member (Pfiffner et al. 2001). In a study assessing intergenerational continuities across three generations, Smith and Farrington (2004) found that authoritarian parenting and parental conflict were related to childhood conduct problems in two successive generations. Prominent assortative mating effects were also found, with antisocial males tending to partner antisocial females.

■ Social Factors

The contribution of general social factors is another unsettled issue in the literature on disruptive behavior disorders. Loeber et al.

(1995) found low socioeconomic status to be a risk factor for the progression of ODD to conduct disorder, and others have also found associations between low socioeconomic status and conduct disorder (Rutter and Giller 1984). However, when factors associated with social class—such as family size, overcrowding, and supervision—are controlled for, social class shows very little relation to antisocial behavior (Wadsworth 1979). These data suggest that the influence of low socioeconomic status on the risk of conduct disorder and ODD is primarily indirect and is mediated by a variety of other factors. Early antisocial behavior and peer group rejection are important factors that have been found to precede delinquent behavior (Snyder et al. 1986). However, the ability for deviant peer affiliation to predict delinquent outcome is related to the amount of parental supervision. Heinze et al. (2004) examined associations among gender, antisocial behavior, and peer group affiliation. They found that for both boys and girls, having many deviant peers was associated with more antisocial behavior and that the effect was somewhat more pronounced for boys. Cultural variables are also associated with antisocial behavior. Culturally derived beliefs—such as acceptance of aggression, respect for authority, role of the parent, and the value of independence—are noted to be significant factors in the expression of aggression and antisocial behaviors (Ekblad 1988). It also appears that minority children are more likely to be incarcerated—and thereby identified as delinquent—than are nonminority youths, given a similar degree of disturbance (R. Cohen et al. 1990).

Assessment

The assessment of the signs, symptoms, and risk factors of conduct disorder in children should include information from multiple sources. This information should focus on current behavior as well as developmental signs and symptoms. Diagnostic interviews, rating scales, and a review of pertinent records from the school and clinics (health care, mental health, juvenile court) are useful ways to gather information. Jewell et al. (2004) found that youth diagnosed with CD using the Diagnostic Interview Schedule for Children displayed significantly more CD behaviors in the first 6 months of participation in a treatment program than did youth diagnosed with CD by clinician only. This study suggests that structured interviews may be a more effective diagnostic tool than reliance on clinician interview alone.

The assessment is guided by knowledge of the biopsychosocial model of etiology. This model includes information about cognitive style, family structure and functioning, and physical signs and symptoms. This information should include the presence or absence of symptoms necessary to make a DSM-IV-TR diagnosis. However, as discussed above, the symptoms are not specific to one particular disorder and do not guide treatment or predict outcome. Additional biopsychosocial and developmental information may help determine treatment and prognosis.

A number of rating scales are available to help identify disturbed behavior. The Child Behavior Checklist (Achenbach 1991a, 1991b, 1991c, 1992) is designed for teachers and parents to complete and yields a scale score on symptom clusters such as delinquency, aggression, hyperactivity, and depression. Self-report measures have proved effective in identifying antisocial behavior, especially in adolescents. Specific scales for rating aggression include the Iowa Conners Aggression Factor (Loney and Milich 1985), derived from the Conners Teacher Questionnaire (Conners 1969), and the Modified Overt Aggression Scale (Kay et al. 1988). Peer and teacher ratings of behavior and likeability in ele-

mentary school are significant predictive factors for delinquent behavior in adolescence (Tremblay et al. 1988). Halperin et al. (2003) provided preliminary psychometric data on the Children's Aggression Rating Scale—Teacher Version, reporting that as a whole it had excellent reliability and distinguished among various types and severity of aggression as distinct from oppositional defiant behaviors.

One of the most important factors in the assessment of antisocial behavior in children and adolescents is the attitude of the clinician making the assessment. Clinical judgment is significantly affected by contextual factors such as resource availability and agency setting in the assessment of amenability to treatment (Mulvey and Reppucci 1988). The setting in which one works, as well as one's own biases, can in part determine the adequacy of the assessment and treatment recommendations. For this reason, the clinician must know the etiology, treatment approaches, resources, and outcome variables to assess antisocial behavior in a youth.

Working with an impulsive patient requires regular monitoring and management of feelings aroused in the therapist by the patient. Some of these feelings are expected reactions to undependable behavior such as missed appointments, dangerous risk-taking behavior, impulsive and thoughtless comments, and potential legal issues raised in working with these high-risk patients. At times, these patients also may arouse countertransference feelings in the therapist. These feelings might range from envy and vicarious pleasure derived from exciting, unrestricted behavior to anger, revulsion, indignation, and even hatred for thoughtless, destructive acts with consequences that go far beyond the patient and the therapist. The first and most important step is for the therapist to recognize and acknowledge these feelings, which often prevents the feelings from becoming counter-productive or destructive. When the feelings significantly interfere with the therapy or the well-being of the patient or therapist, outside consultation should be sought.

Treatment

Treatment of youths with conduct disorder takes place in a variety of settings, including short- and long-term inpatient psychiatric units, residential and day treatment centers, correctional facilities, and outpatient settings. Treatment approaches also differ greatly. Behavior therapy, family therapy, individual and group therapy, parent management training, cognitive therapy, systems theory–based approaches, and pharmacotherapy are all used to a greater or lesser extent, depending on the treatment setting and the clinician's orientation. One of the major problems facing researchers in this area is the nonspecificity of the diagnosis of conduct disorder. In addition, clinicians may approach this group of children with a sense of therapeutic nihilism that clearly does not promote therapeutic success. Fortunately there are now a number of empirically well-supported approaches to the treatment of these often challenging patients and families. In general, the effective treatment of conduct disorder requires a multimodal approach that addresses multiple areas of impairment and continues over an extensive period of time (Steiner 1997).

As discussed above, children and adolescents with antisocial behavior have extremely varied psychopathology. Some may have depression, some may have psychosis, and others may have ADHD. Others may not have any psychiatric disorder other than conduct disorder. Their behavior may be the result of their culture or a history of abuse or neglect. Most treatment studies do not differentiate the associated psychopathology. As a result, an approach believed to be successful for certain patients with conduct disorder in a particular setting cannot be generalized to all children and adolescents with a diagnosis of conduct disorder. Keeping this caveat in mind, we briefly describe the more successful approaches.

■ Problem-Solving Skills Training

Cognitive-behavioral approaches with youths who have conduct disorder focus on modifying cognitive deficiencies (e.g., communication skills, problem-solving skills, impulse control, and anger management) that are believed to underlie antisocial behavior (Faulstich et al. 1988). Generally, these are step-by-step approaches to interpersonal situations that use modeling, rehearsal, role playing, and development of an internal dialogue for self-evaluation (Kazdin 1987). Most studies of this approach provide anecdotal evidence attesting to its success (Englander-Golden et al. 1989; Haggerty et al. 1989; Hains and Hains 1987). In a controlled study, Kazdin et al. (1989) randomly assigned 112 children with severe antisocial behavior to one of three treatments: problem-solving skills training, problem-solving skills training with therapeutic practice activities, or client-centered relationship therapy. Both problem-solving skills training interventions showed significantly greater reductions in antisocial behavior and greater increases in prosocial behavior than did relationship therapy. These effects were evident at the end of treatment and at 1-year follow-up.

■ Family-Focused Treatments

Dysfunctional family structure and interactions have an important role in the development of antisocial behavior. Family therapy, using a wide variety of techniques, attempts to alter the family system. Many studies of the efficacy of family therapy in alleviating antisocial behavior in children rely on weak or questionable methodologies. However, in a review of the extensive literature, Tolan et al. (1986) found consistently positive results from family therapy. In many cases, family therapy was more effective than other therapeutic modalities. Behavioral, structural, strategic, and communication techniques appeared to be the most effective. Future research needs to delineate the family systems variables that are associated with childhood antisocial behavior, verify which techniques are effective with particular family dysfunctions, and evaluate the long-term effectiveness of family therapy compared with other treatment modalities. Functional family therapy (Alexander and Parsons 1982) is a family-based technique that has clear empirical support for its effectiveness (Kazdin 1998). The main goals of this treatment approach are to increase reciprocity and positive reinforcement among family members, improve communication, promote effective negotiation, and improve interpersonal problem solving.

Parent management training attempts to alter coercive parent–child interactions that foster antisocial behavior in the child (Patterson 1982). The major intervention is the direct training of parents to interact differently with their child, so that prosocial behavior is rewarded. Outcome studies of this technique demonstrate consistently positive results (Kazdin 1987; Kazdin et al. 1992). Outcome is affected by the duration of treatment, the severity of family dysfunction, and social supports outside the home. Preliminary evidence suggests that parent management training is more effective with aggressive children with conduct disorder than with non-

aggressive youths with conduct disorder (Patterson 1982). Further research is needed to delineate parent and child characteristics that respond best to parent management training. Nevertheless, parent management training is currently one of the best-researched and most promising treatment interventions for children and adolescents with conduct disorder.

Multisystemic therapy is another empirically well-supported treatment methodology that uses a systems theory perspective. This approach assumes that antisocial behavior becomes embedded within the life space of the patient such that the individual has been increasingly rewarded for engaging in antisocial conduct at the expense of more prosocial behaviors. The treatment involves extensive contact between the therapist and the multiple actual living contexts of the patient, especially those of the family and peer group. More individually focused elements may be used as appropriate to target specific issues (e.g., depression), but the majority of the treatment focuses on enabling the family to more successfully and positively shape the behavior of the child (Henggeller et al. 1998).

■ Peer Relationship and School-Based Interventions

Although disturbed parent–child interactions are clearly implicated in the developmental etiology of conduct disorder, problematic peer relationships and poor school performance are also significant factors, particularly in middle childhood (Offord and Bennett 1994). Peer rejection has been correlated with aggression, and school failure has been correlated with the development of behavioral problems. A variety of interventions have targeted these two areas. Social skills training programs have aimed to improve the peer relationships of children at high risk for antisocial behavior (Bierman and Furman 1984), and specific academic skills programs have sought to reduce rates of school failure (Kellam et al. 1991). Preliminary data are promising, but further study is indicated.

■ Pharmacotherapy

Because the range of psychopathology in conduct disorder is extensive and comorbidity is likely the rule rather than the exception, if another psychiatric syndrome is identified clearly, aggressive pharmacotherapy is probably warranted and may significantly diminish the behavioral morbidity. Psychotropic drugs have not yet shown specific effectiveness in the treatment of conduct disorder. However, several drugs are used to treat symptoms associated with conduct disorder, especially aggression.

Antipsychotic drugs have been extensively used in the treatment of acute and chronic aggression in a variety of clinical populations. For instance, haloperidol was effective in reducing aggressiveness, temper tantrums, and explosiveness in children with behavior disorder (Werry and Aman 1975). However, concerns about the potential for serious side effects associated with traditional antipsychotic agents have increasingly limited their use. With the advent of atypical antipsychotics and their greater tolerability and reduced liability for producing extrapyramidal side effects and tardive dyskinesia, these drugs may be used more frequently for the treatment of serious aggression. Risperidone was shown to be superior to placebo for the treatment of aggression in a small double-blind study of youths with conduct disorder (Findling et al. 2000), a large open-label study of children with disruptive behavior and subaverage IQ (Croonenberghs et al. 2005), and a study of children with disruptive behaviors with subaverage IQ with and without stimulant medication (Aman et al. 2004).

Psychostimulants have also been used to treat conduct disorder, but the results do not provide definite conclusions about effectiveness because of equivocal findings or methodological problems. In a recent meta-analysis, Connor et al. (2002) found psychostimulants to be as effective for aggressive symptoms within the context of ADHD as they are for the core symptoms of inattention, impulsivity, and hyperactivity. However, the effect sizes for overt aggression were noted to diminish in the presence of conduct disorder.

The number of studies examining the efficacy of antidepressants in the treatment of conduct disorder is surprisingly small, considering the degree of comorbidity with depression. Puig-Antich (1982) found that conduct disorder symptoms abated after imipramine treatment in a group of boys with comorbid major depressive disorder and conduct disorder. In a small open trial, trazodone was found to be effective for the treatment of aggressive children (Ghaziuddin and Alessi 1992). In boys with chronic conduct disorder and attention-deficit disorder, treatment with bupropion resulted in improvements in behavior, affect, and anxiety (Simeon et al. 1986). An open-label trial of bupropion was positive in a sample of adolescents with ADHD and substance use plus conduct disorder (Riggs et al. 1998). Theoretically, selective serotonin reuptake inhibitors (SSRIs) may be of benefit in conduct disorder given the evidence of serotonergic dysfunction in disorders of impulse control, and several adult studies have suggested that the SSRIs may have antiaggressive effects. However, in an open trial of SSRIs for aggression in hospitalized adolescents, no beneficial effects were demonstrated and the SSRIs may have contributed to an observed increase in verbal aggression (Constantino et al. 1997). Furthermore, the recent "black box" warning regarding suicidal ideation placed on antidepressants when used for the treatment of youth further complicates the potential treatment of youths with these agents, particularly when off-label uses are being contemplated. Methodologically sound studies are necessary to delineate the subgroup of youths with conduct disorder who respond to antidepressants.

When comorbid bipolar disorder is suspected, trials of lithium or anticonvulsants are indicated (Arredondo and Butler 1994). Lithium was also effective in reducing aggressive and explosive behavior in a subgroup of children with behavior disorder who had symptoms of an affective disorder (DeLong and Aldershof 1987). In the same study, another subgroup of children who had behavior disorder and neurological and medical disease also had decreased rage and aggressive outbursts after lithium treatment. Both haloperidol and lithium carbonate have been found to be effective in decreasing behavioral symptoms in hospitalized children with treatment-resistant conduct disorder (Campbell et al. 1984, 1995). In blind trials, carbamazepine has also been shown to be useful in the treatment of aggressive behavior (Kafantaris et al. 1992; Rosenberg et al. 1994). However, in a double-blind, placebo-controlled study in children with conduct disorder, carbamazepine was found not to be superior to placebo in reducing aggressive behavior, and untoward effects were common (Cueva et al. 1996). Valproate was shown to be efficacious in a double-blind, placebo-controlled cross-over study of youths with explosive temper and mood lability (Donovan et al. 2000) and in a controlled trial of youths

with conduct disorder (Steiner et al. 2003).

A small randomized, blinded group comparison study of methylphenidate and clonidine both alone and in combination suggested that clonidine had potential efficacy for aggression in ADHD comorbid with either ODD or conduct disorder (Connor et al. 2000). Propranolol has been proved to be effective in the treatment of aggressive behavior in children and adolescents with chronic brain dysfunction and in a few youths with conduct disorder that was refractory to other pharmacological approaches (Kuperman and Stewart 1987). Additional studies are needed to delineate effective psychotropic medications for youths with severe behavior disorders.

Prognosis

The clinical course of conduct disorder in children is variable: mild forms show improvement over time, whereas more severe forms tend to be chronic (American Psychiatric Association 1994). The difficulty in developing a definite subclassification system of conduct disorder has hindered outcome research, and researchers have developed their own subtypes to classify outcome. Aggressive conduct disorder is a commonly used subtype and has a worse prognosis. Outcome studies of aggressive boys with conduct disorder found that about half continued to have conduct disorder at follow-up 2 years later (Stewart and Kelso 1987). Persistence of conduct disorder was predicted by various antisocial and aggressive symptoms, fire setting, early age at onset, family deviance, and inattention (Kelso and Stewart 1986). Data are mixed regarding the stability of symptoms in males versus females; some studies suggest that externalizing symptoms are more stable in males (McGee et al.

1992), whereas others suggest an approximately equal degree of stability in both sexes (Tremblay et al. 1992). In either case, severity of symptoms tends to be positively correlated with persistence of symptoms (P. Cohen et al. 1993). However, girls with conduct disorder may subsequently develop more internalizing disorders, as noted above, and may have more general health problems as adults than males (Bardone et al. 1998). Mason et al. (2004), in a study examining the relationship between childhood behavioral problems and psychopathology in young adults of both sexes, found that children reporting higher levels of conduct problems were nearly four times more likely to report a depressive episode in early adulthood than children who reported lower levels.

It appears that children's neuropsychological problems interact cumulatively with their environment across development to determine the outcome of early antisocial behavior (Moffitt 1993). Lewis et al. (1989) found that the interaction of intrinsic vulnerabilities such as cognitive, psychiatric, and neurological impairment and a history of abuse or family violence was a better predictor of adult violent crime than was a history of violence. Longer-term outcome studies (Robins and Ratcliff 1979) found that 23%–41% of highly antisocial children became antisocial adults, 17%–28% did not become clearly antisocial, and the remainder did not fall clearly into either group. Factors that predicted adult antisocial behavior included a variety of antisocial behaviors in childhood, drug use before age 15, placement out of the home, and growing up in extreme poverty (Robins and Ratcliff 1979). When young people with antisocial behavior were followed up, the most frequent explanations for death were found to be uncertain causes and suicides (Rydelius 1988).

Early age at onset is the factor most consistently found to be associated with poor outcome (Tolan and Lorion 1988). Tolan (1987) found that a combination of demographic, individual, school, and family variables predicted age at onset. In a longitudinal study of high-risk children in Hawaii, certain factors were frequently found in adult men with a criminal record (Werner 1989). These factors included 1) having a younger sibling born less than 2 years after the subject, 2) being raised by an unmarried mother, 3) not having a father present during infancy and early childhood, 4) experiencing prolonged disruptions in family life, and 5) having a working mother without suitable caregivers during the first year of life.

Not all children with antisocial behavior become antisocial adults. Results of the long-term follow-up study in Hawaii found that "resilient" high-risk children who did not develop serious behavior disorders were more likely to be first-born children with high intelligence from smaller families with low discord (Werner 1989). In a longitudinal study of children from families judged to be at high risk for producing a delinquent child, it was found that boys who were characterized as neurotic at age 10 years, who had few or no friends at age 8 years, and who did not spend leisure time with their fathers demonstrated satisfactory social adjustment as men (Farrington et al. 1988). Shyness appeared to act as a protective factor for nonaggressive boys, but it was found to be an aggravating factor for aggressive boys.

In summary, the most consistent factors that predict poor prognosis for children with antisocial behavior are early age at onset; high rates of antisocial behavior; antisocial acts across multiple settings, such as the home, school, and community; and diverse antisocial behaviors (Rutter and Giller 1984). Further research is needed to identify prognostic factors associated with disorders comorbid with conduct disorder, such as ADHD, psychosis, and depression.

Prevention

Conduct disorder and the eventual outcome of this disorder appear to have a developmental etiology. Identifying children at neurodevelopmental risk and intervening early may therefore be helpful (Moffitt and Caspi 2001). Symptoms such as impaired executive function, poor impulse control, and autonomic underreactivity suggest increased risk. Patterson et al. (1989) proposed that a reliable developmental sequence of experiences leads to antisocial behavior. This sequence starts with ineffective parenting practices and is followed by academic failure and peer rejection, which lead to depressed mood and involvement in a deviant peer group. Prevention efforts that intervene early in this sequence have greater success than those that intervene later. Parent training interventions have been successful when applied to younger antisocial children (Kazdin 1987). Reid et al. (2004), in a study designed to assess parent and child moderators of treatment outcome in a parent training intervention involving head start children with conduct problems, found that children with the highest levels of baseline conduct problems and mothers with high levels of critical parenting benefited the most. Maternal engagement in program and the mother's success at reducing critical parenting was also positively associated with reduction in problem behaviors.

As noted above in the section "Peer-Related and School-Based Interventions," academic skills training has also shown promise as an intervention with predelinquent children (Johnson and Brekenridge 1982), especially when a learning disability is associated (Grande 1988; Meltzer et al. 1986). School-based interventions with the parent, teacher, and child have significantly decreased short- and long-term behavioral problems at school and in the community (Bry 1982). Finally, community-based interventions that involve activity and skill training programs have shown some promise (Offord and Reitsma-Street 1983), although they have not yet demonstrated broad-based and long-lasting results.

Juvenile Delinquency

Delinquency is a legal term that refers to the commission of an act by a juvenile that, if committed by an adult, would be considered a crime and therefore punishable by law (e.g., rape, murder, theft). Delinquent acts are usually differentiated from behaviors that may be forbidden by law by virtue of the immaturity of the youth such as truancy or running away. These are referred to as status offences as they are prohibited only by virtue of the minor child status of the offender and if committed by an adult would not be considered illegal. The literature on incarcerated delinquents is rather extensive and, as with youth meeting criteria for the clinical concept of conduct disorder, suggests that there is an extensive pattern of comorbidity for delinquent youth and a range of risk factors that are very similar to those for conduct disorder. Surveys assessing the extent of psychopathology among delinquents have identified markedly elevated rates of mental disorders with rates as high as 77% being reported (Thomas and Penn 2002). In addition to elevated levels of psychopathology generally, there is also evidence of elevated rates of suicidal ideation and suicide attempts among juvenile delinquents (Ruchkin et al. 2003). Female delinquents may be at particularly high risk, as most have a history of physical and/or sexual abuse and manifest significant other psychopathology at higher rates than males. Abram et al. (2003), in a study estimating the 6-month prevalence of comorbid psychiatric disorders in juvenile detainees by demographic group, found that significantly more males than females met criteria for two or more psychiatric disorders (56.5% vs. 45.9%). Dixon et al. (2004) found a strongly elevated rate of psychopathology in female juvenile offenders relative to controls; the number of psychiatric diagnoses was the most significant factor associated with offender status. The treatment of delinquency, like the treatment of conduct disorder, is most effective when multiple risk factors are addressed by the intervention. Some interventions that have been specifically targeted toward adjudicated youth include boot camps, "Scared Straight" programs, "Wilderness" programs, and for youths whose offenses involve substances, juvenile drug court programs have been implemented that are similar to adult-oriented programming. The effectiveness of some of these programs—in particular, the "Scared Straight" and boot camp programs—has been called into question by systematic research, although boot camp programs remain popular in some states. For delinquents who have been incarcerated, effective reintegration into the community is an important component of efforts to normalize the functioning of the youth (DePrato and Hammer 2002).

Research Issues

It is clear that additional and better quality research is necessary. More specific diagnostic criteria will help to delineate subcategories within the currently heterogeneous group of children with conduct disorders. Research should focus on comorbidity and etiological factors, such as family dysfunction and cognitive and neurological dysfunction, as well as cultural and environmental influences. Neuroimaging and neuropsychobiological testing will advance the understanding of the biological basis of impulse-control disorders and may help distinguish subcategories of conduct disorder. Outcome studies will be more meaningful when a specific subclassification system delineates particular aspects of the disorder that make an individual more vulnerable or resilient. Greater diagnostic specificity will also help to assess the effectiveness of various treatment interventions with particular symptom constellations. This exciting area for research has far-reaching implications not only for the prevention and treatment of serious mental disorders but also for the healthy functioning of society.

References

Abram KM, Teplin LA, McClelland GM, et al: Comorbid psychiatric disorders in juvenile detention. Arch Gen Psychiatry 60:1097–1108, 2003

Achenbach TM: Manual for the Child Behavior Checklist/4–18 and 1991 Profile. Burlington, VT, University of Vermont, 1991a

Achenbach TM: Manual for the Teacher's Report Form and 1991 Profile. Burlington, VT, University of Vermont, 1991b

Achenbach TM: Manual for the Youth Self-Report and 1991 Profile. Burlington, VT, University of Vermont, 1991c

Achenbach TM: Manual for the Child Behavior Checklist/2–3 and 1992 Profile. Burlington, VT, University of Vermont, 1992

Alexander JF, Parsons BV: Functional Family Therapy. Monterey, CA, Brooks/Cole, 1982

Aman MG, Binder C, Turgay A:. Risperidone effects in the presence/absence of psychostimulant medicine in children with ADHD, other disruptive behavior disorders, and subaverage IQ. J Child Adolesc Psychopharmacol 14:243–254, 2004

American Psychiatric Association: Diagnostic and Statistical Manual of Mental Disorders, 4th Edition. Washington, DC, American Psychiatric Association, 1994

American Psychiatric Association: Diagnostic and Statistical Manual of Mental Disorders, 4th Edition, Text Revision. Washington, DC, American Psychiatric Association, 2000

Angold A, Costello EJ: Toward establishing an empirical basis for the diagnosis of oppositional defiant disorder. J Am Acad Child Adolesc Psychiatry 35:1205–1212, 1996

Arredondo DE, Butler SF: Affective comorbidity in psychiatrically hospitalized adolescents with conduct disorder or oppositional defiant disorder: should conduct disorder be treated with mood stabilizers? J Child Adolesc Psychopharmacol 4:151–158, 1994

Bardone AM, Moffitt TE, Caspi A, et al: Adult physical health outcomes of adolescent girls with conduct disorder, depression, and anxiety. J Am Acad Child Adolesc Psychiatry 37:594–601, 1998

Bauer LO, Hesselbrock VM: CSD/BEM localization of P300 sources in adolescents "at-risk": evidence of frontal cortex dysfunction in conduct disorder. Biol Psychiatry 50:600–608, 2001

Beauchaine TP, Katkin ES, Strassburg Z, et al: Disinhibitory psychopathology in male adolescents discriminating conduct disorder from attention deficit/hyperactivity disorder through assessment of multiple autonomic states. J Abnorm Psychol 110:610–624, 2001

Bierman KL, Furman W: The effects of social skills training and peer involvement on the social adjustment of pre-adolescents, in Primary Prevention of Psychopathology, Vol 10: Prevention of Delinquent Behavior. Edited by Burchard JD, Burchard SN. Newbury Park, CA, Sage, 1984, pp 220–240

Blair RJ: Neurocognitive models of aggression, the antisocial personality, and psychopathy. J Neurol Neurosurg Psychiatry 71:727–731, 2001

Bradley S: Affect Regulation and the Development of Psychopathology. New York, Guilford, 2000

Brook JS, Whiteman NM, Finch S: Childhood aggression, adolescent delinquency, and drug use: a longitudinal study. J Genet Psychol 153:369–383, 1992

Bry BH: Reducing the incidence of adolescent problems through preventive intervention: one- and five-year follow-up. Am J Community Psychol 10:265–276, 1982

Burt SA, Krueger RF, McGue M, et al: Sources of covariation among attention deficit/hyperactivity disorder, oppositional defiant disorder, and conduct disorder: the importance of shared environment. J Abnorm Psychol 110:516–525, 2001

Buydens-Branchey L, Branchey M: Cocaine addicts with conduct disorder are typified by decreased cortisol responsivity and high plasma levels of DHEA-S. Neuropsychobiology 50:161–166, 2004

Campbell M, Small AM, Green WH, et al: Behavioral efficacy of haloperidol and lithium carbonate. Arch Gen Psychiatry 41:650–656, 1984

Campbell M, Adams PB, Small AM, et al: Lithium in hospitalized aggressive children with conduct disorder: a double-blind and placebo-controlled study. J Am Acad Child Adolesc Psychiatry 34:445–453, 1995

Cantwell DP, Baker L: Issues in the classification of child and adolescent psychopathology. J Am Acad Child Adolesc Psychiatry 27:521–533, 1988

Cantwell DP, Baker L: Stability and natural history of DSM-III childhood diagnoses. J Am Acad Child Adolesc Psychiatry 28:691–700, 1989

Christian RE, Frick PJ, Hill NL, et al: Psychopathy and conduct problems in children, II: implications for subtyping children with conduct problems. J Am Acad Child Adolesc Psychiatry 36:233–241, 1997

Clark C, Prior M, Kinsella GJ: Do executive function deficits differentiate between adolescents with AD/HD and oppositional defiant/conduct disorder? A neuropsychological study using the Six Elements Test and Hayling Sentence Completion Test. J Abnorm Psychol 28:403–414, 2000

Clark DL, Boutros NN: The Brain and Behavior: An Introduction to Behavioral Neuroanatomy. Malden, MA, Blackwell Science, 1999

Cloninger CR: A systematic method for clinical description and classification of personality variants: a proposal. Arch Gen Psychiatry 44:573–588, 1987

Cohen P, Cohen J, Brook J: An epidemiological study of disorder in late childhood and adolescence, II: persistence of disorders. J Child Psychol Psychiatry 34:869–877, 1993

Cohen R, Parmelee DX, Irwin L, et al: Characteristics of children and adolescents in a psychiatric hospital and a corrections facility. J Am Acad Child Adolesc Psychiatry 29:909–913, 1990

Comings DE, Comings BG: A controlled study of Tourette syndrome, II: conduct. Am J Hum Genet 41:742–760, 1987

Comings DE, Gade-Andavolu R, Gonzales N, et al: Comparison of the role of dopamine, serotonin, and noradrenaline genes in ADHD, ODD and conduct disorder: multivariate regression analysis of 20 genes. Clin Genet 57:178–196, 2000

Conners CK: A teacher rating scale for use in drug studies with children. Am J Psychiatry 126:884–888, 1969

Connor DF, Barkley RA, Davis HT: A pilot study of methylphenidate, clonidine, or the combination in ADHD comorbid with aggressive oppositional defiant or conduct disorder. Clin Pediatr (Phila) 39:15–25, 2000

Connor DF, Glatt SJ, Lopez ID, et al: Psychopharmacology and aggression, I: a meta-analysis of stimulant effects on overt/covert aggression—related behaviors in ADHD. J Am Acad Child Adolesc Psychiatry 41:253–261, 2002

Constantino JN, Liberman M, Kincaid M: Effects of serotonin reuptake inhibitors on aggressive behavior in psychiatrically hospitalized adolescents: results of an open trial. J Child Adolesc Psychopharmacol 7:31–44, 1997

Croonenberghs J, Fegert JM, Findling RL, et al: Risperidone Disruptive Behavior Study Group: Risperidone in children with disruptive behavior disorders and subaverage intelligence: a 1-year, open-label study of 504 patients. J Am Acad Child Adolesc Psychiatry 44:64–72, 2005

Cueva JE, Overall JE, Small AM, et al: Carbamazepine in aggressive children with conduct disorder: a double blind and placebo-controlled study. J Am Acad Child Adolesc Psychiatry 35:480–490, 1996

DeLong GR, Aldershof AL: Long-term experience with lithium treatment in childhood: correlation with clinical diagnosis. J Am Acad Child Adolesc Psychiatry 26:389–394, 1987

DePrato DK, Hammer JH: Assessment and treatment of juvenile offenders, in Principles and Practice of Child and Adolescent Forensic Psychiatry. Edited by Schetky DH, Benedek EP. Washington, DC, American Psychiatric Publishing, 2002, pp 267–278

Dick DM, Li TK, Edenberg HJ, et al: A genome-wide screen for genes influencing conduct disorder. Mol Psychiatry 9:81–86, 2004

Dixon A, Howie P, Starling J: Psychopathology in female juvenile offenders. J Child Psychol Psychiatry 45:1150–1158, 2004

Dmitrieva TN, Oades RD, Hauffa BP, et al: Dehydroepiandrosterone sulphate and corticotropin levels are high in young male patients with conduct disorder: comparisons for growth factors, thyroid, and gonadal hormones. Neuropsychobiology 43:134–140, 2001

Donovan SJ, Stewart JW, Nunes EV, et al: Divalproex treatment for youth with explosive temper and mood lability: a double-blind, placebo-controlled crossover design. Am J Psychiatry 157:818–820, 2000

Ekblad S: Influence of child-rearing on aggressive behavior in a transcultural perspective. Acta Psychiatr Scand Suppl 344:133–139, 1988

Emler N, Reicher S, Ross A: The social context of delinquent conduct. J Child Psychol Psychiatry 28:99–109, 1987

Englander-Golden P, Jackson JE, Crane K, et al: Communication skills and self-esteem in prevention of destructive behaviors. Adolescence 24:481–502, 1989

Farrington DP, Gallagher B, Morley L, et al: Are there any successful men from criminogenic backgrounds? Psychiatry 51:116–130, 1988

Faulstich ME, Moore JR, Roberts RW, et al: A behavioral perspective on conduct disorders. Psychiatry 51:398–416, 1988

Fergusson DM, Horwood LJ, Lynskey M: The childhoods of multiple problem adolescents: a 15-year longitudinal study. J Child Psychol Psychiatry 35:1123–1140, 1994

Findling RL, McNamara WK, Branicky MA, et al: Pilot study of risperidone in the treatment of conduct disorder. J Am Acad Child Adolesc Psychiatry 39:509–516, 2000

Foley DL, Eaves LJ, Wormley B et al: Childhood adversity, monoamine oxidase a genotype, and risk for conduct disorder. Arch Gen Psychiatry 61:738–744, 2004

Forehand R, King H, Peed S, et al: Mother-child interactions: comparison of a non-compliant clinic group and a non-clinic group. Behav Res Ther 13:79–84, 1975

Forehand R, Long N, Hedrick M: Family characteristics of adolescents who display overt and covert behavior problems. J Behav Ther Exp Psychiatry 18:325–328, 1987

Frick PJ, Ellis M: Callous-unemotional traits and subtypes of conduct disorder. Clin Child Fam Psychol Rev 2:149–168, 1999

Frick PJ, Lahey BB, Applegate B, et al: DSM-IV field trials for the disruptive behavior disorders: symptom utility estimates. J Am Acad Child Adolesc Psychiatry 33:529–539, 1994

Gabel S, Shindledecker R: Aggressive behavior in youth: characteristics, outcome, and psychiatric diagnoses. J Am Acad Child Adolesc Psychiatry 30:982–988, 1991

Ghaziuddin N, Alessi N: An open clinical trial of trazodone in aggressive children. J Child Adolesc Psychopharmacol 2:291–297, 1992

Grande CG: Delinquency: the learning disabled student's reaction to academic school failure? Adolescence 23:209–219, 1988

Gregory AM, Eley TC, Plomin R: Exploring the association between anxiety and conduct problems n a large sample of twins aged 2–4. J Abnorm Child Psychol 32:111–122, 2004

Guerra NG, Slaby RG: Evaluative factors in social problem solving by aggressive boys. J Abnorm Child Psychol 17:277–289, 1989

Haggerty KP, Wells EA, Jenson JM, et al: Delinquents and drug use: a model program for community reintegration. Adolescence 24: 439–456, 1989

Hains AA, Hains AH: The effects of a cognitive strategy intervention on the problem-solving abilities of delinquent youths. J Adolesc 10:399–413, 1987

Halperin JM, McKay KE, Grayson RH, et al: Reliability, validity, and preliminary normative data for the Children's Aggression Scale—Teacher Version. J Am Acad Child Adolesc Psychiatry 42:965–971, 2003

Harrington R, Fudge H, Rutter M, et al: Adult outcomes of childhood and adolescent depression, II: links with antisocial disorders. J Am Acad Child Adolesc Psychiatry 30:434–439, 1991

Heinze HJ, Toro PA, Urberg KA: Antisocial behavior and affiliation with deviant peers. J Clin Child Adolesc Psychol 33:336–346, 2004

Henggeller SW, Schoenwald SK, Borduin CM, et al: Multi-systemic Treatment of Anti-social Behavior in Children and Adolescents. New York, Guilford, 1998

Herpertz SC, Mueller B, Wenning B, et al: Autonomic responses in boys with externalizing disorders. J Neural Transm 110:1181–1195, 2003

Hetherington EM, Stanley-Hagan M: The adjustment of children with divorced parents: a risk and resiliency perspective. J Child Psychol Psychiatry 40:129–140, 1999

Hoge RD, Andrews DA, Leschied AW: Tests of three hypotheses regarding the predictors of delinquency. J Abnorm Child Psychol 22:547–559, 1994

Jewell J, Handwerk M, Almquist J, et al: Comparing the validity of clinician generated diagnosis of conduct disorder to the diagnostic interview schedule for children. J Clin Child Adolesc Psychology 33:536–546, 2004

Johnson DL, Brekenridge JN: The Houston Parent-Child Development Center and the primary prevention of behavior problems in young children. Am J Community Psychol 10:305–316, 1982

Kafantaris V, Campbell M, Padron-Gayol MV, et al: Carbamazepine in hospitalized aggressive conduct disorder children: an open pilot study. Psychopharmacol Bull 28:193–199, 1992

Kay SR, Wolkenfield F, Murrill LM: Profiles of aggression among psychiatric patients, I: nature and prevalence. J Nerv Ment Dis 176:539–546, 1988

Kazdin AE: Conduct Disorders in Childhood and Adolescence (Developmental Clinical Psychology and Psychiatry Series, Vol 9). Newbury Park, CA, Sage, 1987

Kazdin AE: Psychosocial treatments for conduct disorder in children, in Treatments That Work. Edited by Nathan PE, Gorman JM. New York, Oxford University Press, 1998, pp 85–91

Kazdin AE, Bass D, Siegel T, et al: Cognitive-behavior therapy and relationship therapy in the treatment of children referred for antisocial behavior. J Consult Clin Psychol 57:522–535, 1989

Kazdin AE, Siegel TC, Bass D: Cognitive problem-solving skills training and parent management training in the treatment of antisocial behavior in children. J Consult Clin Psychol 60:733–747, 1992

Keenan K, Loeber R, Green S: Conduct disorder in girls: a review of the literature. Clin Child Fam Psychol Rev 2:3–19, 1999

Kellam SG, Werthamer-Larsson L, Dolan LF, et al: Developmental epidemiologically based preventative trials: baseline modeling of early target behaviors and depressive symptoms. Am J Community Psychol 4:563–584, 1991

Kelly SJ, Day N, Streissguth AP: Effects of pre-natal alcohol exposure on social behavior in humans and other species. Neurotoxicol Teratol 22:143–149, 2000

Kelso J, Stewart MA: Factors which predict the persistence of aggressive conduct disorder. J Child Psychol Psychiatry 27:77–86, 1986

Kendall PC: Cognitive-behavioral therapies with youth: guiding theory, current status, and emerging development. J Consult Clin Psychol 61:235–247, 1993

Kim MS, Kim JJ, Kwon JS: Frontal P300 decrement and executive dysfunction in adolescents with conduct problems. Child Psychiatry Hum Dev 32:93–106, 2001

Kovacs M, Paulauskas S, Gatsonis C, et al: Depressive disorders in childhood, III: a longitudinal study of comorbidity with and risk for conduct disorders. J Affect Disord 15:205–217, 1988

Kruesi MJP, Hibbs ED, Zahn TP, et al: A 2-year prospective follow-up of children and adolescents with disruptive behavior disorders. Arch Gen Psychiatry 49:429–435, 1992

Kruesi MJ, Casanova MF, Mannheim G, et al: Reduced temporal lobe volume in early onset conduct disorder. Psychiatry Res 132:1–11, 2004

Kuperman S, Stewart M: Use of propranolol to decrease aggressive outbursts in younger patients. Psychosomatics 28:315–319, 1987

Lahey BB, Hartdagen SE, Frick PJ, et al: Conduct disorder: parsing the confounded relation to parental divorce and antisocial personality. J Abnorm Psychol 97:334–337, 1988a

Lahey BB, Piacentini JC, McBurnett K, et al: Psychopathology in the parents of children with conduct disorder and hyperactivity. J Am Acad Child Adolesc Psychiatry 27:163–170, 1988b

Lavigne JV, Cicchetti C, Gibbons RD, et al: Oppositional defiant disorder with onset in preschool years: longitudinal stability and pathways to other disorders. J Am Acad Child Adolesc Psychiatry 40:1393–1400, 2001

Lee M, Prentice NM: Interrelations of empathy, cognition, and moral reasoning with dimensions of juvenile delinquency. J Abnorm Child Psychol 16:127–139, 1988

LeFlore L: Delinquent youths and family. Adolescence 23:629–642, 1988

Lewis DO, Shanok SS, Balla DA: Perinatal difficulties, head and face trauma, and child abuse in the medical histories of seriously delinquent children. Am J Psychiatry 136:419–423, 1979

Lewis DO, Pincus JH, Lovely R, et al: Biopsycho-social characteristics of matched samples of delinquents and nondelinquents. J Am Acad Child Adolesc Psychiatry 26:744–752, 1987

Lewis DO, Lovely R, Yeager C, et al: Toward a theory of the genesis of violence: a follow-up study of delinquents. J Am Acad Child Adolesc Psychiatry 28:431–436, 1989

Loeber R, Schmaling KB: Empirical evidence for overt and covert patterns of antisocial conduct problems: a meta-analysis. J Abnorm Child Psychol 13:315–335, 1985

Loeber R, Green SM, Keenan K, et al: Which boys will fare worse? Early predictors for the onset of conduct disorder in a six-year longitudinal study. J Am Acad Child Adolesc Psychiatry 34:499–509, 1995

Loeber R, Burke JD, Lahey BB, et al: Oppositional defiant disorder and conduct disorder: a review of the last 10 years, I. J Am Acad Child Adolesc Psychiatry 39:1468–1484, 2000

Loney J, Milich R: Hyperactivity, aggression, and inattention in clinical practice, in Advances in Developmental and Behavioral Pediatrics. Edited by Wollrach M, Routh D. New York, JAI Press, 1985, pp 113–147

Mannuzza S, Klein RG, Abikoff H, et al: Significance of childhood conduct problems to later development of conduct disorder among children with ADHD: a prospective follow-up study. J Abnorm Child Psychol 32:565–573, 2004

Marmorstein NR, Iacono WG: Major depression and conduct disorder in youth: associations with parental psychopathology and parent–child conflict. J Child Psychol Psychiatry 45:377–386, 2004

Mason WA, Kosterman R, Hawkins JD, et al: Predicting depression, social phobia, and violence in early adulthood from childhood behavior problems. J Am Acad Child Adolesc Psychiatry 43:307–315, 2004

Maughan B, Taylor A, Caspi A, et al: Prenatal smoking and early childhood conduct problems: testing genetic and environmental explanations of the association. Arch Gen Psychiatry 31:836–843, 2004

McBurnett K, Lahey BB, Rathouz PJ, et al: Low salivary cortisol and persistent aggression in boys referred for disruptive behavior. Arch Gen Psychiatry 57:38–43, 2000

McCord J: Parental behavior in the cycle of aggression. Psychiatry 51:14–23, 1988

McGee R, Williams S, Feehan M: Attention deficit disorder and age of onset of problem behaviors. J Abnorm Child Psychol 20:487–502, 1992

Mealy L: The sociobiology of sociopathy: an integrated evolutionary model, in The Maladapted Mind: Classic Readings in Evolutionary Psychopathology. Edited by Baron-Cohen S. Sussex, United Kingdom, Psychology Press, 1997, pp 133–173

Mednick SA: The learning of morality: biosocial bases, in Vulnerabilities to Delinquency. Edited by Lewis DO. New York, Spectrum, 1981, pp 187–204

Mednick SA, Gabrielli WF, Hutchings B: Genetic factors in criminal behavior: evidence from an adoption cohort. Science 224:891–893, 1984

Mehlman PT, Higley JD, Faucher I, et al: Low CSF 5-HIAA concentrations and severe aggression and impaired impulse control in nonhuman primates. Am J Psychiatry 151:1485–1491, 1994

Mehlman PT, Higley JD, Faucher I, et al: Correlation of CSF 5-HIAA concentration with sociality and the timing of emigration in free-ranging primates. Am J Psychiatry 152:907–913, 1995

Meltzer LJ, Roditi BN, Fenton T: Cognitive and learning profiles of delinquent and disabled adolescents. Adolescence 21:581–591, 1986

Moeller FG, Barratt ES, Dougherty DM, et al: Psychiatric aspects of impulsivity. Am J Psychiatry 158:1783–1793, 2001

Moffitt TE: Parental mental disorder and offspring criminal behavior: an adoption study. Psychiatry 50:346–360, 1987

Moffitt TE: Adolescence-limited and life-course-persistent antisocial behavior: a developmental taxonomy. Psychol Rev 100:674–701, 1993

Moffitt TE, Caspi A: Childhood predictors differentiate life-course persistent and adolescence-limited antisocial pathways among males and females. Dev Psychopathol 13:355–375, 2001

Moffitt TE, Silva PA: Neuropsychological deficit and self-reported delinquency in an unselected birth cohort. J Am Acad Child Adolesc Psychiatry 27:233–240, 1988

Moffitt TE, Gabrielli WF, Mednick SA: Socioeconomic status, IQ, and delinquency. J Abnorm Psychol 90:152–156, 1981

Moss K: Witnessing violence—aggression and anxiety in young children. Health Rep 14 (suppl):53–66, 2003

Mulvey EP, Reppucci ND: The context of clinical judgement: the effect of resource availability on judgements of amenability to treatment in juvenile offenders. Am J Community Psychol 16:525–545, 1988

Offord DR, Bennett KJ: Conduct disorder: long-term outcomes and intervention effectiveness. J Am Acad Child Adolesc Psychiatry 33:1069–1078, 1994

Offord DR, Cross LA: Behavioral antecedents of adult schizophrenia. Arch Gen Psychiatry 21:267–283, 1969

Offord DR, Reitsma-Street M: Problems of studying antisocial behavior. Psychiatr Dev 1:207–224, 1983

Olweus D, Mattsson A, Schalling D, et al: Circulating testosterone levels and aggression in adolescent males: a causal analysis. Psychosom Med 50:261–272, 1988

Pajer K, Gardner W, Rubin RT, et al: Decreased salivary cortisol levels in adolescent girls with conduct disorder. Arch Gen Psychiatry 58:297–302, 2001

Patterson GR: Coercive Family Process. Eugene, OR, Castalia, 1982

Patterson GR, DeBaryshe BD, Ramsey E: A developmental perspective on antisocial behavior. Am Psychol 44:329–355, 1989

Pfiffner LJ, McBurnett K, Rathouz PJ: Father absence and familial anti-social characteristics. J Abnorm Psychol 29:347–367, 2001

Puig-Antich J: Major depression and conduct disorder in prepuberty. J Am Acad Child Psychiatry 2:118–128, 1982

Raine A, Brennan P, Sarnoff A, et al: Birth complications combined with early maternal rejection at age 1 year predispose to violent crime at age 18 years. Arch Gen Psychiatry 51:984–988, 1994

Raine A, Venables PH, Williams M: High autonomic arousal and electrodermal orientating at age 15 years as protective factors against criminal behavior at age 29 years. Am J Psychiatry 152:1595–1600, 1995

Reebye P, Moretti MM, Lessard JC: Conduct disorder and substance use disorder: comorbidity in a clinical sample of preadolescents and adolescents. Can J Psychiatry 40:313–319, 1995

Reeves JC, Werry JS, Elkind GS, et al: Attention deficit, conduct oppositional, and anxiety disorders in children, II: clinical characteristics. J Am Acad Child Adolesc Psychiatry 26:144–155, 1987

Reid MJ, Webster-Stratton C, Baydar N: Halting the development of conduct problems in head start children: the effects of parent training. J Clin Child Adolesc Psychol 33:279–291, 2004

Riggs PD, Leon SL, Mikulich SK, et al: An open label trial of bupropion for ADHD in adolescents with substance use disorders and conduct disorder. J Am Acad Child Adolesc Psychiatry 37:1271–1278, 1998

Robins LN: Deviant Children Grown Up. Baltimore, MD, Williams & Wilkins, 1966

Robins LN, Ratcliff KS: Risk factors in the continuation of childhood antisocial behavior into adulthood. Int J Ment Health 7:96–111, 1979

Rosenberg D, Holltum J, Gershon S: Textbook of Child and Adolescent Psychiatric Disorders. New York, Brunner/Mazel, 1994

Rowe R, Maughan B, Worthman CM, et al: Testosterone, antisocial behavior, and social dominance in boys: pubertal development and biosocial interaction. Biol Psychiatry 55:546–552, 2004

Ruchkin VV, Schwab-Stone M, Koposov RA, et al: Suicidal ideations and attempts in juvenile delinquents. J Child Psychol Psychiatry 44:1058–1066, 2003

Rutter M: Parent-child separation: psychological effects on the child. J Child Psychol Psychiatry 12:233–260, 1971

Rutter M, Giller H: Juvenile Delinquency: Trends and Perspectives. New York, Penguin, 1984

Rutter M, Birch HG, Thomas A, et al: Temperamental characteristics in infancy and the later development of behavior disorders. Br J Psychiatry 110:651–661, 1964

Rydelius A: The development of antisocial behavior and sudden violent death. Acta Psychiatr Scand 77:398–403, 1988

Satterfield JH, Schell AM, Backs RW: Longitudinal study of AERP's in hyperactive and normal children: relationship to antisocial behavior. Electroencephalogr Clin Neurophysiol 67:531–536, 1987

Schmeck K, Poustka F: Temperament and disruptive behavior disorders. Psychopathology 34:159–163, 2001

Scourfield J, Van den Bree M, Martin N, et al: Conduct problems in children and adolescents: a twin study. Arch Gen Psychiatry 61:489–496, 2004

Seeger G, Schloss P, Schmidt MH: Functional polymorphism within the promoter of the serotonin transporter gene is associated with severe hyperkinetic disorders. Mol Psychiatry 6:235–238, 2001

Short RJ, Simeonsson RJ: Social cognition and aggression in delinquent adolescent males. Adolescence 21:159–176, 1986

Silverman IW, Ragusa DM: A short-term longitudinal study of the early development of self-regulation. J Abnorm Psychol 20:415–435, 1993

Silverton L, Harrington ME, Mednick SA: Motor impairment and antisocial behavior in adolescent males at high risk for schizophrenia. J Abnorm Child Psychol 16:177–186, 1988

Simeon JG, Ferguson HB, Fleet JVW: Bupropion effects in attention deficit and conduct disorders. Can J Psychiatry 31:581–585, 1986

Simic M, Fombonne E: Depressive conduct disorder: symptom patterns and correlates in referred children and adolescents. J Affect Disord 62:175–185, 2001

Smith CA, Farrington DP: Continuities in antisocial behavior and parenting across three generations. J Child Psychol Psychiatry 45:230–247, 2004

Snyder JJ, Dishian TJ, Petterson GR: Determinants and consequences of associating with deviant peers during preadolescence. Journal of Early Adolescence 61:20–43, 1986

Soderstrom H, Sjodin AK, Carlstedt A, et al: Adult psychopathic personality with childhood-onset hyperactivity and conduct disorder: a central problem constellation in forensic psychiatry. Psychiatry Res 121:271–280, 2004

Soyka M, Preuss UW, Koller G, et al: Association of 5-HT$_{1B}$ receptor gene and antisocial behavior in alcoholism. J Neural Transm 111:101–109, 2004

Spoont MR: Modulatory role of serotonin in neural information processing: implications for human psychopathology. Psychol Bull 112:330–350, 1992

Steiner H: Practice parameters for the assessment and treatment of children and adolescents with conduct disorder. J Am Acad Child Adolesc Psychiatry 36:122S–139S, 1997

Steiner H, Wilson J: Conduct disorder, in Disruptive Behavior Disorders in Children and Adolescents. Edited by Hendren RL. Washington, DC, American Psychiatric Press, 1999, pp 47–92

Steiner H, Garcia IG, Matthews Z: Posttraumatic stress disorder in incarcerated juvenile delinquents. J Am Acad Child Adolesc Psychiatry 36:357–365, 1997

Steiner H, Petersen ML, Saxena K, et al: Divalproex sodium for the treatment of conduct disorder: a randomized controlled clinical trial. J Clin Psychiatry. 64:1183–1191, 2003

Stewart M, Kelso J: A two-year follow-up of boys with aggressive conduct. Psychopathology 20:296–304, 1987

Stoff DM, Friedman E, Pollack L, et al: Elevated platelet MAO is related to impulsivity in disruptive behavior disorders. J Am Acad Child Adolesc Psychiatry 28:754–760, 1989

Susman EJ, Inoff-Germain G, Nottelmann ED, et al: Hormones, emotional dispositions and aggressive attributes in young adolescents. Child Dev 58:1114–1134, 1987

Thomas CR, Penn JV: Juvenile justice mental health services. Child Adolesc Psychiatr Clin N Am 11:731–748, 2002

Tolan PH: Implications of age of onset for delinquency risk. J Abnorm Child Psychol 15:45–63, 1987

Tolan PH: Socioeconomic, family, and social stress correlates of adolescent antisocial and delinquent behavior. J Abnorm Child Psychol 16:317–331, 1988

Tolan PH, Lorion RP: Multivariate approaches to the identification of delinquency proneness in adolescent males. Am J Community Psychol 16:547–561, 1988

Tolan PH, Cromwell RE, Brasswell M: Family therapy with delinquents: a critical review of the literature. Fam Process 25:619–650, 1986

Tremblay RE, LeBlanc M, Schwartzman AE: The pediatric power of first-grade peer and teacher ratings of behavior: sex differences in antisocial behavior and personality at adolescence. J Abnorm Child Psychol 16:571–583, 1988

Tremblay RE, Masse B, Perron D, et al: Early disruptive behavior, poor school achievement, delinquent behavior, and delinquent personality: longitudinal analyses. J Consult Clin Psychol 60:64–72, 1992

Tremblay RE, Pihl RO, Vitaro F, et al: Predicting early onset of male antisocial behavior from preschool behavior. Arch Gen Psychiatry 51:732–739, 1994

Unis AS, Cook EH, Vincent JG, et al: Platelet serotonin measures in adolescents with conduct disorder. Biol Psychiatry 42:553–559, 1997

van Goozen SH, Matthys W, Cohen-Kettenis PT, et al: Plasma monoamine metabolites and aggression: two studies of normal and oppositional defiant disorder children. Eur Neuropsychopharmacol 9:141–147, 1999

van Goozen SH, van den Ban E, Matthys W, et al: Increased adrenal androgen functioning in children with oppositional defiant disorder: a comparison with psychiatric and normal controls. J Am Acad Child Adolesc Psychiatry 39:1446–1451, 2000

Vitaro F, Gendreau PL, Tremblay RE, et al: Reactive and proactive aggression differentially predict later conduct problems. J Child Psychol Psychiatry 39:377–385, 1998

Vitiello B, Behar D, Hunt J, et al: Subtyping aggression in children and adolescents. J Neuropsychiatry Clin Neurosci 2:189–192, 1990

Wadsworth MEJ: Roots of Delinquency: Infancy, Adolescence, and Crime. New York, Barnes & Noble Books, 1979

Wakschlag LS, Lahey B, Loeber R, et al: Maternal smoking during pregnancy and the risk of conduct disorder in boys. Arch Gen Psychiatry 54:670–676, 1997

Walker JL, Lahey BB, Hynd GW, et al: Comparison of specific patterns of antisocial behavior in children with conduct disorder with or without coexisting hyperactivity. J Consult Clin Psychol 55:910–913, 1987

Watt NF, Grup TW, Erlenmeyer-Kimling L: Social, emotional, and intellectual behavior at school among children at high risk for schizophrenia. J Consult Clin Psychol 50:171–181, 1983

Webster-Stratton LC, Lindsay DW: Social competence and conduct disorder problems in young children: issues in assessment. J Clin Child Psychol 28:25–43, 1999

Wells KC, Egan J: Social learning and systems family therapy for childhood oppositional disorder: comparative treatment outcome. Compr Psychiatry 29:138–146, 1988

Werner EE: High risk children in young adulthood: a longitudinal study from birth to 32 years. Am J Orthopsychiatry 59:72–81, 1989

Werry JS, Aman MG: Methylphenidate and haloperidol in children: effects on attention, memory and activity. Arch Gen Psychiatry 32:790–795, 1975

Widom CSA: Does violence beget violence? a critical examination of the literature. Psychol Bull 106:3–28, 1989

Wolff S: Dimensions and clusters of symptoms in disturbed children. Br J Psychiatry 118:421–427, 1971

Woolston JL, Rosenthal SL, Riddle MA, et al: Childhood comorbidity of anxiety/affective disorders and behavior disorders. J Am Acad Child Adolesc Psychiatry 28:707–713, 1989

World Health Organization: The ICD-10 Classification of Mental and Behavioural Disorders: Clinical Descriptions and Diagnostic Guidelines. Geneva, World Health Organization, 1992

Wozniak J, Biederman J, Faraone SV, et al: Heterogeneity of childhood conduct disorder: further evidence of a subtype of conduct disorder linked to bipolar disorder. J Affect Disord 64:121–131, 2001

Self-Assessment Questions

Select the single best response for each question.

16.1 Which of the following statements regarding the diagnoses of conduct disorder and oppositional defiant disorder (ODD) is *true?*

     A. Children with these disorders are a distinct group that presents in a uniform and narrow fashion.

     B. The relationship between conduct disorder and ODD is clearly defined.

     C. The diagnosis of conduct disorder is controversial in child psychiatry.

     D. ODD behaviors typically are preceded by more serious violations of age-appropriate behavioral norms.

     E. Conduct disorder has been determined to be a biological condition.

16.2 All of the following statements regarding the prevalence of conduct disorder are correct *except*

     A. The prevalence of conduct disorder is difficult to estimate because of variations in definition.

     B. The prevalence is estimated as approximately 9% for males and 2% for females younger than 18 years.

     C. The childhood-onset type of the disorder (onset before 10 years of age) is clearly much more common in males.

     D. Individuals with adolescent-onset conduct disorder are much more likely to develop adult antisocial personality disorder than are those with childhood-onset conduct disorder.

     E. Adolescent-onset conduct disorder is less likely than childhood-onset conduct disorder to involve a preponderance of males.

16.3 Which of the following statements regarding subtypes of conduct disorder is *true?*

     A. Subtyping aggressive behavior into predatory and affective categories is not a useful distinction.

     B. Predatory aggression is characterized by the presence of high levels of autonomic and emotional arousal with little apparent instrumental gain.

     C. Children who demonstrate reactive aggression tend to be more delinquent than those demonstrating proactive aggression.

     D. The process of subclassifying conduct disorder according to age at onset, degree of aggressivity, and extent of socialization has been completely validated.

     E. The value of subtyping conduct disorder into childhood-onset and adolescent-onset variants is related to the prognostic significance of age at onset.

16.4 A biological factor associated with conduct disorder is

     A. Reduced novelty-seeking trait.

     B. A history of maternal smoking during pregnancy.

     C. Anxious temperament.

     D. Reduced rates of expression of the L/L variant of the serotonin transporter gene.

     E. Elevated harm-avoidance trait.

16.5 All of the following statements concerning treatment of youngsters with conduct disorder are correct *except*

A. Treatment may take place in a variety of different long-term and short-term programs in outpatient, inpatient, and residential settings.

B. Cognitive-behavioral approaches include improvement in problem-solving skills, impulse control, and anger management.

C. Family therapy is not an effective treatment modality in conduct disorder patients.

D. Parent management training focuses on modifying coercive parent–child interactions that encourage child antisocial behaviors.

E. When used, pharmacotherapy commonly targets aggression in the conduct disorder population.

Substance Abuse Disorders

Steven L. Jaffe, M.D.

Ramon Solhkhah, M.D.

Substance use and abuse continue to constitute an epidemic in the adolescent population. Most teenagers use drugs or alcohol occasionally without negative consequences (71% of high school seniors drank alcohol during 2001), which gives parents and adolescents the impression that alcohol and drug use is normal. The reality is that half of these alcohol-using adolescents (35% of the seniors) have had a binge episode (five or more drinks at one time) in the past month, and 3.6% drink daily (Johnston et al. 2001). These adolescents become the group in which high-risk behaviors (e.g., driving after drinking, unprotected sex, and violence) will occur, with their associated morbidity and mortality. Whereas 13% of high school students drive a car after drinking, another 33% ride in cars in which the driver has been drinking (Levy et al. 2002). Homicides, suicides, and injuries account for 80% of teenage deaths, and more than half of these are associated with alcohol (Rogers and Adger 1993).

Substance abuse disorder and substance dependence disorder are specific DSM-IV-TR diagnoses defined by essential clinical criteria (American Psychiatric Association 2000). (Note: the DSM-IV-TR terminology has been modified for use in this chapter, as explained below under "Diagnostic Criteria.") Substance abuse disorder involves alcohol or drug usage that causes recurrent school, legal, and social failures and other high-risk behavior. A recent survey of 31,000 high school seniors (Harrison et al. 1998) reported that 15% met criteria for substance abuse disorder. Substance dependence disorder involves compulsive seeking and using alcohol or drugs despite negative physical or psychological problems. In the community survey of high school seniors, 7% met criteria for substance dependence disorder. Thus, more than 20% of seniors in high school are significantly involved with using alcohol and drugs and are in need of an intervention.

Significant substance abuse is a major or complicating factor in adolescents with severe psychiatric problems. Grunebaum et al. (1991) found that 40% of adolescents treated in psychiatric day or residential pro-

389

grams were comorbid for substance abuse disorder or substance dependence disorder related to alcohol or marijuana. In a study of adolescents admitted to an acute psychiatric impatient unit, Deas-Nesmith et al. (1998) found that 33% met criteria for substance abuse or dependence disorder that had not been identified during the hospitalization. Even higher rates, up to 80%, are found in adolescents in the juvenile justice system (Neighbors et al. 1992). These studies demonstrate that mental health professionals treating adolescents need to be knowledgeable and proficient in the assessment and treatment of adolescent substance use disorder.

Adolescents with psychiatric disorders also frequently have substance abuse disorders, and because 40%–90% of adolescents with substance use disorders have comorbid psychiatric disorders—specifically attention-deficit/hyperactivity disorder (ADHD), conduct disorders, anxiety disorders, and affective disorders (Jaffe 1996a)—the common practice of separating community psychiatric services from alcohol and drug services is inappropriate for adolescents. Substance abuse assessment and treatment services for adolescents need to be integrated with psychiatric services so that a higher level of therapeutic success can be attained.

Diagnostic Criteria

Adolescent substance abuse is a general nonspecific term that includes any use of alcohol or drugs by teenagers. This includes the entire range from occasional recreational use without negative consequences to the full syndrome of substance dependence disorder. The term *substance use* is rarely employed because all use by minors is illegal and therefore fits under *substance abuse.* In DSM-IV-TR under "Substance Use Disorders," *substance dependence* and *substance abuse* are listed. We recommend

that the word *disorder* be appended to these terms (as we have done in this chapter) because it defines specific criteria and differentiates the DSM-IV-TR diagnosis from the general meaning of *substance abuse.* Tables 17–1 and 17–2 list the DSM-IV-TR diagnostic criteria for substance abuse disorder and substance dependence disorder.

Table 17–1.   DSM-IV-TR diagnostic criteria for substance abuse

---

A.   A maladaptive pattern of substance use leading to clinically significant impairment or distress, as manifested by one (or more) of the following, occurring within a 12-month period:

   (1)   recurrent substance use resulting in a failure to fulfill major role obligations at work, school, or home (e.g., repeated absences or poor work performance related to substance use; substance-related absences, suspensions, or expulsions from school; neglect of children or household)

   (2)   recurrent substance use in situations in which it is physically hazardous (e.g., driving an automobile or operating a machine when impaired by substance use)

   (3)   recurrent substance-related legal problems (e.g., arrests for substance-related disorderly conduct)

   (4)   continued substance use despite having persistent or recurrent social or interpersonal problems caused or exacerbated by the effects of the substance (e.g., arguments with spouse about consequences of intoxication, physical fights)

B.   The symptoms have never met the criteria for substance dependence for this class of substance.

Source. From American Psychiatric Association: *Diagnostic and Statistical Manual of Mental Disorders,* 4th Edition, Text Revision. Washington, DC, American Psychiatric Association, 2000. Copyright 2000, American Psychiatric Association. Used with permission.

Table 17–2.   DSM-IV-TR diagnostic criteria for substance dependence

A maladaptive pattern of substance use, leading to clinically significant impairment or distress, as manifested by three (or more) of the following, occurring at any time in the same 12-month period:

(1) tolerance, as defined by either of the following:

    (a) a need for markedly increased amounts of the substance to achieve intoxication or desired effect

    (b) markedly diminished effect with continued use of the same amount of the substance

(2) withdrawal, as manifested by either of the following:

    (a) the characteristic withdrawal syndrome for the substance (refer to criteria A and B of the criteria sets for withdrawal from the specific substances)

    (b) the same (or a closely related) substance is taken to relieve or avoid withdrawal symptoms

(3) the substance is often taken in larger amounts or over a longer period than was intended

(4) there is a persistent desire or unsuccessful efforts to cut down or control substance use

(5) a great deal of time is spent in activities necessary to obtain the substance (e.g., visiting multiple doctors or driving long distances), use the substance (e.g., chain-smoking), or recover from its effects

(6) important social, occupational, or recreational activities are given up or reduced because of substance use

(7) the substance use is continued despite knowledge of having a persistent or recurrent physical or psychological problem that is likely to have been caused or exacerbated by the substance (e.g., current cocaine use despite recognition of cocaine-induced depression, or continued drinking despite recognition that an ulcer was made worse by alcohol consumption)

Specify if:

With physiological dependence: evidence of tolerance or withdrawal (i.e., either Item 1 or 2 is present)

Without physiological dependence: no evidence of tolerance or withdrawal (i.e., neither Item 1 nor 2 is present)

Source.   From American Psychiatric Association: *Diagnostic and Statistical Manual of Mental Disorders,* 4th Edition, Text Revision. Washington, DC, American Psychiatric Association, 2000. Copyright 2000, American Psychiatric Association. Used with permission.

These diagnostic categories were developed from adult studies, and their validity in adolescents has not been demonstrated. Winters (2001) summarizes the problems in applying DSM-IV-TR criteria to adolescents: 1) withdrawal and drug-related medical problems are rare; 2) one abuse symptom yields a diagnosis; 3) abuse symptoms often do not precede dependence symptoms; and 4) two dependence symptoms with no abuse symptoms yields no diagnosis, but these "diagnostic orphans" do need

therapeutic intervention. Substance dependence disorder that corresponds to addiction results from induced neurological changes in brain functioning in the reward circuitry (Roberts and Koob 1997). This results in the inability to moderate substance use despite severe harmful consequences even when the person tries to regulate use. This is often problematic to apply to adolescents who are heavily involved with substances but have made no acknowledged effort to control their use. Despite these problems, DSM-IV-TR does define clinically useful categories that require intensive treatment with the goals of abstinence, decreasing risks, and minimizing impairment.

Epidemiology

There are two major population-based surveys of substance abuse in adolescents. The Monitoring the Future Survey (Johnston et al. 2001, 2004) is school based and surveys about 50,000 students in grades 8, 10, and 12. The National Household Survey (Office of Applied Studies 2000) involves face-to-face interviewers and may include school dropouts but will still miss adolescents in juvenile justice and psychiatric residential settings. Data from these settings are used to demonstrate past and current general trends. Because overall abuse varies directly with availability and inversely with perceived risk of harm, these factors have recently been surveyed.

Information from the Monitoring the Future Survey reveals the following data and trends. Use of alcohol, the most commonly abused drug, has been fairly consistent over the past 25 years. (An apparent decrease in 1993 resulted from a change in the wording of the question defining a drink to "more than a few sips.") (Harrison 2001). Annual use by seniors has remained at about 73% since 1994. Use of marijuana in the previous year by seniors peaked in 1979 at 50.8% and reached a low of 21.8% in 1992, but it has increased rapidly with a recent high of 38.5% in 1997 and 37% in 2001. A decline to 34.9% occurred in 2003. The perceived harmfulness of marijuana use significantly decreased in the 1990s.

Cigarette smoking by adolescents peaked in the late 1970s, dropped in the 1980s, and remained just below the 1980s level in the 1990s. After a relative increase in 1997, the rate returned to the low of 1992. Of course the rate of 24.4% of seniors who smoked cigarettes in the past month in 2003 is much too high. Nonprescription amphetamine use peaked in 1981, reached a low in 1992, and has shown a small increase recently. Methamphetamine use has increased in recent years. LSD use peaked in 1975 and reached a low between 1988 and 1990, but returned to almost peak use in 1997. By 2003, however, it had significantly decreased, to 1.9%. Inhalant use, which peaks in early adolescence, has slowly decreased in the 1990s, with the annual rate for eighth-graders decreasing to 8.1% in 2003. This steady decline appears to be related to increased perception of the high risk of harm. Heroin use has recently declined after some years of growth, and cocaine use moderately decreased after a high in 1999.

The increase in the use of 3,4-methylenedioxymethamphetamine (MDMA; "ecstasy") has halted. The annual rate for seniors increased from 3.6% in 1998 to 9.2% in 2001 but then decreased to 4.5% in 2003. An area of significant concern is the continued increase in the use of anabolic steroids, with the 1.3% annual rate of use among seniors in 1994 increasing to 2.1% in 2003. These statistics indicate that although there is some variability in extent and drug of choice, during the past 25 years adolescents have continued to abuse substances at frightening levels.

Assessment

■ Domains and Stages to Be Assessed

All adolescents presenting with mental health problems should be screened for substance abuse. Any change in behavior, mood, or cognitive functioning may indicate that substance abuse is a major or contributing factor. Tarter (1990) presents the importance of exploring problems in all the domains of the adolescent's life. These include physical health status, aggressive-behavior problems, psychiatric disorders, social skills, family relationships, school adjustment, peer relationships, work adjustment, and recreation.

In terms of these domains, the severity of substance use and the consequences for the adolescent (including physical, emotional, and cognitive areas as well as school, peer, and family functioning) need to be defined. Patterns of use—including age at onset, amount, frequency, types of agents, and negative consequences—should be explored. Adolescents tend to move along a specific progression, with fewer individuals using each agent in the sequence (Kandel 1975). Thus many adolescents begin with cigarettes, beer, and wine; some progress to marijuana; some of those progress to problem drinking; and fewer still move on to hallucinogens, stimulants, and opiates. Adolescents tend not to stop using the substances used earlier in the sequence, which results in the characteristic that adolescents are multiple drug users. Assessment involves defining the times, places, peer use, antecedents, consequences, and attempts and failures to control use for each type of substance used. Because the adolescent may not be fully honest in what is revealed, information from the family, school, peers, and legal authorities is essential.

In addition to a progression of specific substances used, there is a progression of stages that describes increased involvement, effects, and consequences of substances on the life of the adolescent (Chatlos 1996; Macdonald 1984; Nowinski 1990). These stages are outlined below. Assessing the stage of substance involvement helps in specific treatment planning.

1. *Experimental or social stage.* This is the beginning stage of use, in which the important factors are curiosity and doing what one's peers may be doing. Teenagers are often told that drugs are fun, and they seek the thrill of doing something they are not supposed to be doing. They often find that drug use helps them gain acceptance by specific peers. As they become somewhat more involved in using alcohol and drugs they may then enter the second stage.

2. *Substance misuse.* In this stage the teenager is actively seeking the pleasurable experiences of using alcohol and drugs. Often he or she has also learned that the misuse helps him or her to escape from feelings of frustration, anger, depression, and inadequacy. At this stage the teenager tends to use substances primarily on weekends, and there will be some deterioration in grades and in conforming with rules. Increased usage and involvement may then lead to the third stage.

3. *Substance abuse disorder.* At this stage the teenager is clearly harmfully involved and preoccupied with using alcohol and drugs. Drugs and alcohol are now being used during the week. The peer group is primarily a drug- and alcohol-using group. The adolescent knows where and how to obtain alcohol and drugs and is increasingly involved in these activities. Alcohol and drugs are now significantly taking over the teenager's life, and there are significant impairments in functioning at school and at home. The teenager has become secretive, deceptive, and dishonest. DSM-IV-TR criteria of substance abuse disorder will be met. This involves a maladaptive pattern of failure of major role obligations at work, school, or home because of substance use; recurrent use in physically hazardous situations; recurrent substance-related legal problems; or continued use despite recurrent social or interpersonal problems. Further involvement in the progression may lead to the fourth stage of substance dependence disorder.

4. *Substance or chemical dependence disorder (also described as addiction).* This is the stage of harmful dependence. DSM-IV-TR criteria of substance dependence will be met. Usually tolerance has developed. Withdrawal symptoms, which tend to be infrequent in the adolescent population, may be present. Attempts to control usage have been unsuccessful. Use of larger amounts than were intended and failure in attempts to stop or reduce usage have occurred. Obtaining, using, and dealing with the consequences of use of alcohol and drugs have taken over most of the teenager's life, and he or she continues to use despite knowledge of the severe consequences. Addiction involves an inability to use alcohol and drugs in moderation. An adolescent at this stage of drug involvement might be able to have some periods of not using drugs at all, but when or if he or she begins to use, the use rapidly goes out of control, with return of severe negative consequences.

■ **Standardized Assessment Instruments**

The well-known CAGE screening questions were developed for adults and are not very useful for adolescents. During the past several years, a number of screening and evaluation instruments have been developed that specifically assess adolescent substance abuse. These include the following:

• *The CRAFFT.* This screening instrument, developed in a medical office setting, consists of the following questions:

> C—Have you ever ridden in a **Car** driven by someone (including yourself) who was high or had been using alcohol or drugs?
> R—Do you ever use alcohol/drugs to **R**elax, feel better about yourself, or fit in?

> A—Do you ever use alcohol/drugs while you are by yourself or **A**lone?
> F—Do you ever **F**orget things you did while using alcohol/drugs?
> F—Do your **F**amily or **F**riends ever tell you that you should cut down on your drinking or drug use?
> T—Have you ever gotten into **T**rouble while you were using alcohol or drugs?

Two or more "yes" answers suggest serious problems with substances and indicate that further evaluation is needed (Knight et al. 1999).

• *Drug Use Screening Inventory (DUSI).* This self-report instrument, which consists of 149 yes/no questions, identifies specific problem areas in the 10 domains that need further evaluation (Tarter 1990).

• *Problem Oriented Screening Instrument for Teenagers (POSIT).* This self-report questionnaire, consisting of 139 true/false questions, identifies problems in 10 domains. It is available at no charge from the National Institute on Drug Abuse.

• *Personal Experience Screening Questionnaire (PESQ).* An initial screening instrument, the self-report PESQ consists of 38 questions. It measures problem severity and drug use history and includes a validity scale for lying (Center for Substance Abuse Treatment 1999a; Winters 2001).

• *Personal Experience Inventory (PEI).* A self-report questionnaire with 300 items, the PEI measures problem severity of substance use and personal risk factors; it includes a validity scale (Center for Substance Abuse Treatment 1999a; Winters 2001).

• *Adolescent Diagnostic Interview (ADI).* The ADI is a structured interview to evaluate DSM-III-R (American Psychiatric Association 1987) substance abuse diagnosis, school and interpersonal functioning, and psychosocial stresses

(Center for Substance Abuse Treatment 1999a; Winters 2001).

- *Teen-Addiction Severity Index.* This is a semistructured interview that rates severity in seven domains. It is intended for use in follow-up studies (Kaminer et al. 1991).
- *Global Appraisal of Individual Needs (GAIN).* A standardized semistructured interview, GAIN measures patient characteristics and is used for diagnosis and outcome monitoring. This is the instrument currently being used in most National Institute on Drug Abuse– and Substance Abuse and Mental Health Services Administration–sponsored adolescent studies (Dennis et al. 2004).
- *Urine drug screens.* Urine drug tests are commonly used to detect recent use of illegal drugs. Mental health professionals and parents need to be aware of the uses and limitations of the urine drug screen. The urine must be obtained under observed conditions to make sure that it is the test subject's sample, that a foreign substance such as apple juice has not been substituted, and that it has not been adulterated. The accuracy of the urine drug test is limited to the length of time the specific drug stays in the body and will therefore be present in the urine. Stimulants may be detected up to 48 hours after the last use; cocaine and its metabolite benzoylecgonine may be detected up to 3 days; and opiates (morphine, codeine) may be detected up to 2 days after last use. Short-acting barbiturates can be detected for 1 day, diazepam, up to 4 days, and methaqualone, up to 2 weeks. Marijuana, which is stored in fatty tissue, may be detected in the urine up to 4 days in recreational users and up to a month in daily users (Schwartz 1993). A negative urine test result does not prove that the adolescent does not use

drugs, although many parents use a negative test to confirm their denial. A positive test result should be confirmed by more specific testing. A positive test result only demonstrates use and not a substance use disorder. Results of the urine drug screen need to be integrated into the entire assessment of the adolescent and the family and should be used as important but not conclusive data.

Etiology

Certain factors put children and adolescents at risk for the development of a substance use disorder. These factors are summarized in Table 17–3.

No one risk factor leads to substance abuse. In fact, the more risk factors an individual has, the greater the risk of developing the disorder. Different combinations of risk factors can lead to different potentials for negative outcomes, based on the strength and nature of the individual risk factors. Some protective factors, however, may cushion the effect of the risk factor and modify the severity or prevent negative outcome. Some researchers have begun to identify the interaction between risk factors and protective factors (Newcomb 1995; Pandina et al. 1992).

Some studies highlight the complexity of these interacting factors with biopsychosocial development. Certain genetic factors may not come into play until after substances have begun to be used. In adoption studies on 485 monozygotic and 335 dizygotic female twins, Kendler and Prescott (1998a) demonstrated that cannabis use was influenced by genetic and familial environmental factors, whereas cannabis abuse and dependence were solely related to genetic factors. The same was also true for cocaine use versus abuse and dependence (Kendler and

Table 17–3.   Risk factors for development of substance abuse disorders

Genetic factors
- Presence of a substance abuse problem in one or both parents

Constitutional and psychological factors
- Psychiatric comorbidity
- History of physical, sexual, or emotional abuse
- History of attempted suicide

Sociocultural factors

Family
- Parental experiences and positive attitudes toward drug use
- History of parental divorce (or separation)
- Low expectations for the child

Peers
- Friends who use drugs
- Friends' positive attitudes toward drug use
- Antisocial or delinquent behavior

School
- School failure or dropping out

Community
- Positive attitudes toward drug use
- Economic and social deprivation
- Availability of drugs and alcohol (including cigarettes)

Prescott 1998b). Inherited susceptibility can be explained by the neurobiological research conducted by Nestler (1994, 1995). Individuals who have a greater genetic predisposition to develop substance abuse may be more susceptible to the influence of alcohol on gene expression. Consistent exposure of the ventral tegmentum and nucleus accumbens to alcohol and other drugs may form permanent changes in the second messenger system inside the cell. This may influence the turning on of genes, which may in turn influence the drive mechanism to use substances.

The age and developmental level at which substance use begins are important factors. Rapid progression of alcohol and drug disorders occurred often with earlier age at onset and with greater frequency, not longer duration, of use (DeWitt et al. 2000; Kandel 1992). Individuals with earlier onset had a shorter time span from first exposure to dependence than did individuals in adult-onset groups (Clark et al. 1998). Age at onset of heavy drinking also predicted alcohol-related problems (Lee and DiClimente 1985).

Peer issues are some of the strongest factors of risk. Peer attitudes about use of substances predicted initiation of use of alcohol and other substances (Bauman and Ennett 1994; Kandel 1975). In fact, strong peer attachment rather than parent attachment has been shown to be more influential during adolescence in predicting susceptibility to substance abuse (Brook et al. 1980; Kandel 1975). Peer influence also plays a strong role in predicting relapse. Ninety percent of teenagers who relapse do so because of peer pressure (Brown 1993).

Treatment

After careful evaluation, the clinician should make a determination of the stage of substance abuse involvement. In the framework outlined below, each stage of substance abuse involvement is described along with the corresponding treatment approaches. This framework provides an initial strategy for relating treatment to the degree of involvement in substance abuse (Chatlos 1996; Jaffe 1996b) (Figure 17–1).

■ Treatment Strategies for Experimental or Social Use

For adolescents at the stage of experimental or social use, education and counseling

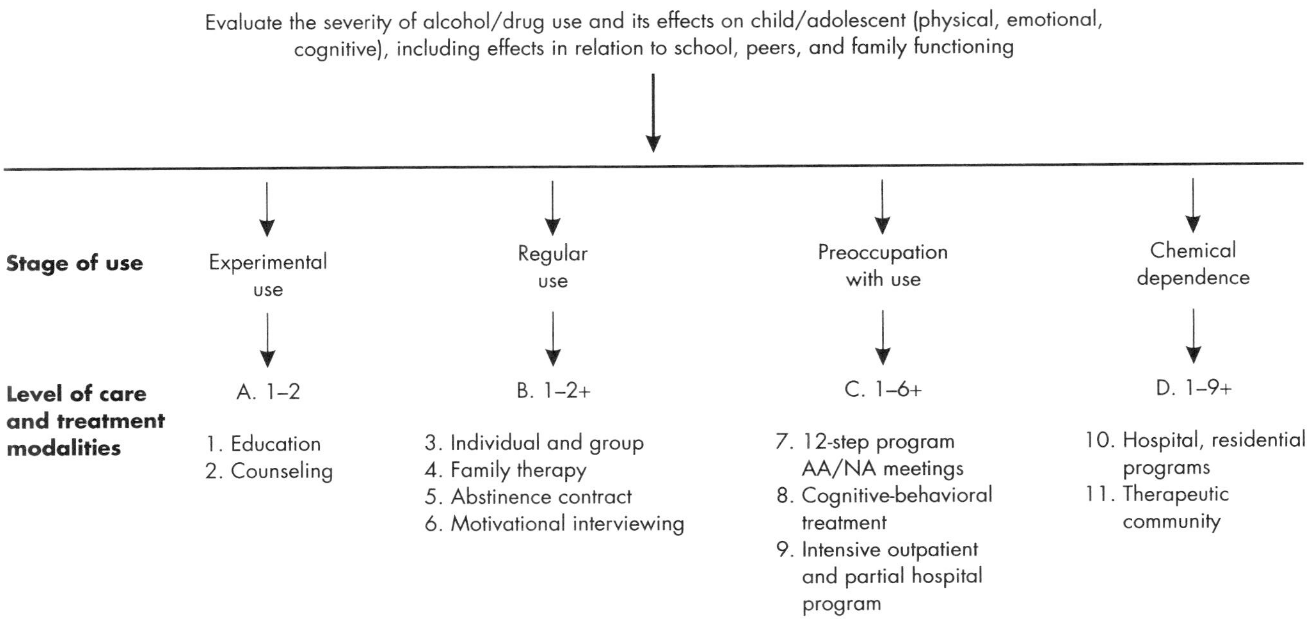

Evaluate the severity of alcohol/drug use and its effects on child/adolescent (physical, emotional, cognitive), including effects in relation to school, peers, and family functioning

Stage of use	Experimental use	Regular use	Preoccupation with use	Chemical dependence
Level of care and treatment modalities	A. 1–2	B. 1–2+	C. 1–6+	D. 1–9+
	1. Education 2. Counseling	3. Individual and group therapy 4. Family therapy 5. Abstinence contract 6. Motivational interviewing	7. 12-step program AA/NA meetings 8. Cognitive-behavioral treatment 9. Intensive outpatient and partial hospital program	10. Hospital, residential programs 11. Therapeutic community

Figure 17–1. Substance abuse decision tree.

Note. AA=Alcoholics Anonymous; NA=Narcotics Anonymous.

are appropriate. Teenagers use drugs in direct proportion to the availability and perceived safety of the drug. Learning about the realistic dangers of drugs and alcohol is helpful. For example, although adolescents tend to view marijuana as a benign drug, they should be taught that marijuana use poses a serious threat to brain functioning. Marijuana has been clearly demonstrated to cause loss of short-term memory, decreased concentration, and decreased motivation (Schwartz et al. 1989). Marijuana has been demonstrated to be addictive (Budney et al. 1999), but this information is usually not helpful in discussions with teenagers. More meaningful is the fact that as teenagers increase their consumption of marijuana to two or three times a week, their school work declines; their motivation decreases; and they spend more time being preoccupied with obtaining, smoking, and thinking about marijuana and tend to lose goals and productivity. Impairment, such as reduced ability to drive after smoking marijuana, may last up to 24 hours and is often not recognized by the adolescent (Leirer et al. 1991).

In addition to education, counseling is needed for adjustment issues, and parents may need help regarding how to set appropriate limits with rewards and consequences. Much educational material appropriate for teenagers may be obtained from the National Institute on Drug Abuse (http://www.drugabuse. gov; 1-888-644-6432) and the National Clearinghouse for Alcohol and Drug Information (http://www.health.org; 1-888-729-6686) of the Substance Abuse and Mental Health Services Administration.

■ Treatment Strategies for Substance Misuse

At the substance misuse stage, individual and group therapies, family treatments,

and an abstinence contract may be needed in addition to education and counseling. At this stage family therapies—such as strategic, structural, systemic, and behavioral therapy—will be important interventions. Behavioral family therapy involves parent management training as well as contingency contracting. Specific, clear rules are established between parents and adolescents so that there are negative consequences for any drug use. Positive reinforcement is given for going to school, doing homework, avoiding peers who use drugs, and developing other recreational activities that are incompatible with drug use.

The abstinence or "honest look" contract is often helpful (Bailey 1996). In this situation, the teenager expresses a willingness to stop using drugs and alcohol and to stop "druggie" types of behavior. Specific rewards and punishments are contracted between the adolescent and the parents. Unannounced urine drug screens are included. If the teenager is unable to abide by the contract, specific consequences are dictated; these can include undergoing treatment at a more intense level of care.

Brief interventions using a combination of motivational interviewing, education, and development of coping skills have been developed as a harm reduction approach for the prevention and treatment of heavy alcohol use at college (Dimeff et al. 1999).

■ Treatment Strategies for Substance Abuse Disorder and Substance Dependence Disorder

In 1990, Catalano et al. (1990–1991) extensively reviewed the literature on adolescent drug abuse treatment and found that in residential programs, time in treatment was related to reduced alcohol and drug use. Family participation was associated with better outcome. No treatment modality was significantly better than any other, leading the researchers to conclude that some treatment was better than no treatment.

During the past several years, significant progress has been made. The National Institute on Drug Abuse has specifically increased support and direction for controlled studies on adolescent drug abuse treatment. Standards for clinical assessment and treatment, called *practice parameters,* have been published (Bukstein 1997). Deas and Thomas (2001) reviewed controlled studies on adolescent substance abuse and concluded that no treatment modality had been demonstrated as being more effective than any other. They recommended increased use of standardized assessment instruments and improved adolescent-specific outcome measures. A number of different treatment approaches have been used alone or in various combinations for the treatment of adolescent substance abuse and dependence disorders. The three most commonly used modalities are family therapy, 12-Step–based programs, and therapeutic communities (Center for Substance Abuse Treatment 1999b). These and other treatment modalities are reviewed in the following sections.

Family Treatment

Treatment studies have demonstrated strong empirical support for the efficacy of family therapy (Stanton and Shadish 1997). Classic family therapy is based on the hypothesis that there is a connection between family relationships and the development and maintenance of drug abuse. Family therapy targets these specific interpersonal family processes. With structural-strategic family therapy, the emphasis is on establishing a coherent family hierarchy with appropriate rules and authority. Lewis et al. (1990) com-

bined a number of different family therapy models to develop a 12-session treatment called the Purdue model. The goals included redefining substance use as a family problem, reestablishing parental influence, interrupting dysfunctional sequences of family behavior, and assessing the interpersonal function of the drug abuse. Families receiving this treatment model significantly decreased adolescent drug abuse compared with families receiving parent skill training.

Azrin et al. (1994) combined family therapy with behavior therapy techniques. The most important treatment component was the social–family contract, in which parents reinforced drug-incompatible activities, supervised home urge-control assignments, and employed written specification of desired behavior with contingent reinforcers. The control group received only supportive counseling. Significant results were demonstrated, with abstinence rates after 6 months of treatment being 73% for the treatment group and only 9% for the supportive-counseling group. Treated youths also had improved schoolwork and family relationships.

Multisystemic and Multidimensional Family Therapy

Henggeler's multisystemic therapy integrates family therapy with direct interventions in the multiple interacting systems involving the individual, school, peer group, and community (Henggeler et al. 1993). Responsible behavior among all family members is promoted, and individuals develop the capacity to manage their own problems. Therapists work intensively with each adolescent and family and see them within their home, school, and even neighborhood peer group. Randomized studies in which multisystemic therapy was compared with individual counseling or probation for chronic juvenile offenders demonstrated reduced criminal activity continuing through a 4-year follow-up period. Preliminary data from a current study on multisystemic therapy for substance-abusing delinquents demonstrate excellent retention rates and favorable outcomes (Pickrel and Henggeler 1996).

Multidimensional family therapy integrates substance abuse treatment with family therapy to provide multiple interventions involving families, peers, and the school and welfare systems (Liddle 2002).

Twelve-Step–Based Programs

Treatment based on the 12-Step program is the treatment model that has been most commonly applied in adolescents. There are many misunderstandings about this treatment modality. The mental health professional who wishes to use and understand it not only needs to read the important literature but also needs to attend Alcoholics Anonymous (AA) or Narcotics Anonymous meetings, participate in adolescent substance abuse groups, and learn from counselors in recovery. Working the 12 Steps is a very concrete process that does not require abstract thinking.

In the development of AA, Bill Wilson set up clear guidelines that enable AA to avoid problematic issues of money, politics, and powerful leaders. AA owns no property, does no fund-raising, accepts no outside contributions, and is open and free to anyone who wants to stop drinking. The 12 Steps, conceived by Wilson and other early members, were first published in *Alcoholics Anonymous* in 1939 (Alcoholics Anonymous 1976). The 12 Steps are the guide for the changes in actions, thoughts, feelings, and belief that an individual addict slowly undergoes so that he or she can establish a stage of recovery and abstain from drinking. Be-

cause an addict cannot use alcohol and drugs in moderation, abstinence is the necessary goal.

Presented below are the first five steps and descriptions of ways they can be modified to make them meaningful for adolescents. Jaffe (1990) uses a workbook format whereby the adolescent writes answers to specific questions, which are reviewed by counselors and may be presented to a group.

1. *We admitted we were powerless over alcohol—that our lives had become unmanageable.* The workbook instructs the adolescents to examine in detail the negative consequences of their alcohol and drug use. Various issues are explored, such as the ways that drug and alcohol use puts their own and others' lives in danger and the effects it has on family, school, work, mood, and self-esteem. The major issue is whether drugs and alcohol are destroying their lives such that they need to stop using to make their lives better. Because adolescents desire to become more powerful, the workbook emphasizes that by abstaining from alcohol and drugs the individual becomes powerful to have a life. Although many adult programs emphasize the concept of "surrendering" and admitting one is an addict, these are not useful for adolescents. Rather, enhancing power by doing what one needs to do (i.e., stop using alcohol and drugs) instead of what one wants to do (i.e., use alcohol and drugs) is emphasized.

2. *We came to believe that a power greater than ourselves could restore us to sanity.* This step is approached in the adolescent workbook by recognizing that the first higher power in a child's life is the person that raised him or her. For many drug-abusing or drug-addicted adolescents, their parental figures were ne-

glectful or abusive. Mourning—eliciting the pain and sadness caused by the disappointments of their childhood higher powers—enables them to begin to develop a sense of something positive in the universe that they can turn to for help. The concept of a higher power is not a religious belief but a spiritual feeling that one can trust something positive (i.e., the group, another person, nature, etc.) to take care of those aspects of one's life that one cannot control. One needs to have trust in the stability of the world and realize one controls one's own behavior but not what others say or do. For many adolescents, the concrete positive feelings of their relationships with other members becomes their 12-Step higher power.

3. *We made a decision to turn our will and our lives over to the care of God as we understood Him.* The adolescent workbook presents an interpretation of this step that involves having the adolescents make a decision to commit themselves to working the steps and having a positive spiritual power. The teenagers are helped to recognize that they had turned over their lives to alcohol and drugs. Now they are being asked to turn their lives over to a positive program.

4. *We made a searching and fearless moral inventory of ourselves.* The workbook instructs the adolescents to answer numerous detailed questions covering all aspects of their childhood and present life.

5. *We admitted to God, to ourselves, and to another human being the exact nature of our wrongs.* At this point the adolescents verbalize their inventories to a counselor or to their sponsor.

Twelve-Step programs provide the opportunity to attend free AA or Narcotics Anonymous meetings, which are conducted several times a day in almost every city and town in the United States and most other countries. It is well recognized that adolescents will return to using alcohol and drugs if they return to contact with their alcohol- and drug-using friends (Jaffe 1992). Twelve-Step programs provide the opportunity to meet other recovering peers and to provide "big brother" or "big sister" relationships in the form of sponsors. In this relationship, an older member with at least a year of sobriety provides a relationship and guidance on how to work the program toward sobriety. For many adolescents, it can be helpful for them to view themselves as being "on the way to becoming an addict" if they do not see themselves as already being one.

Although research on 12-Step programs for adolescents has been sparse, the Chemical Abuse Treatment Outcome Registry (CATOR) (Harrison and Hoffman 1989) residential treatment follow-up program indicated that teenagers who attend two or more meetings per week were almost six times more likely to report abstinence at 1 year than were those who never attended. A more recent follow-up study by Winters (Center for Substance Abuse Treatment 1999b) used improved methodology with a high follow-up contact rate and meaningful comparison groups. At 12-month follow-up, adolescents who completed 12-Step–based treatment had an abstinence/minor relapse rate of 53% compared with 27% of those who needed but did not receive treatment.

Therapeutic Communities

The therapeutic community involves long-term treatment (12–18 months) for youths with the most severe problems. Under this model, the community itself becomes the treatment process. Residents move through stages of increasing responsibility and privileges. Work, education, group activities, seminars, meals, job functions, and formal and informal interactions with peers and staff become the experiences of self-development. Staff members who are recovering and family members have important functions. Outcome studies indicated that 31% completed the residential phase of treatment and 52% dropped out. Treatment completers at 1 year after treatment had more positive outcomes, with reduction in substance use and decreased criminal activity (Center for Substance Abuse Treatment 1999b).

Cognitive-Behavioral Therapy

Cognitive-behavioral therapy (CBT) uses the learning principles of classical and operant conditioning along with approaches to correct cognitive distortions and underlying negative belief systems. This treatment includes having the adolescent learn specific techniques to deal with drugs and alcohol. Skills to refuse alcohol and drugs are taught and practiced through role-playing exercises. For example, adolescents are taught to immediately say "no" in a firm manner, making direct eye contact with the person offering them alcohol or drugs. They are then to suggest an alternative activity, or if that is not successful, to simply tell the person to stop asking. Cognitive-behavioral coping skills to deal with urges, to manage using thoughts, and to handle emergencies and lapses are taught and practiced. Because deficits in coping skills for negative feelings and life stresses contribute to continued substance abuse, more general coping skills—such as communication skills, problem-solving strategies, anger, and mood management—as well as relaxation training are taught and practiced. CBT is being studied in random clinical trials (e.g., Botvin et al. 1990). Kaminer and Burleson (1999)

compared CBT group therapy with interactional group therapy in adolescents with dual disorders. CBT demonstrated a decrease in severity of substance use but was not shown to be superior to interactional therapy at the 15-month follow-up evaluation.

Motivational Treatment

According to Prochaska and DiClemente (1982), in stopping an addictive behavior an individual goes through a series of stages of change: 1) precontemplation, in which the person is not even thinking about stopping and does not recognize any problem with alcohol or drug use; 2) contemplation, which is the stage of ambivalence wherein the person goes back and forth between reasons to change and reasons not to change; 3) preparation, in which the person increases his or her commitment to change; 4) action, in which the person stops using alcohol and drugs; and 5) maintenance, in which the person develops a lifestyle to avoid relapse. Individuals have different levels of motivation, depending on their stage of change.

Therapeutic intervention involves helping the patient in an empathetic, nonconfrontational manner to move along the stages. Brief motivational interventions consist of one to four sessions in which, after an assessment, direct feedback and advice are given in a nonconfrontational manner respecting the person's personal responsibility for making a decision. Monti et al. (2001) studied the use of a single brief 45-minute emergency room motivational interview for adolescents with accidents related to alcohol use. Follow-up revealed fewer alcohol-related problems. Jaffe's (2001) *Adolescent Substance Abuse Intervention Workbook* instructs the adolescent to concretely explore how 12 areas of his or her life have been negatively affected by substances in an effort to move them from precontemplation into contemplation.

The Community-Reinforcement Approach

The community-reinforcement approach is an adult alcohol treatment approach with strong empirical research support whereby the person's life is rearranged so that abstinence is more rewarding than drinking. The community-reinforcement approach for adolescents, as defined in the Cannabis Youth Treatment Study, incorporates elements of operant conditioning, skills training, and social systems and uses individual sessions, family sessions, and case management (Dennis et al. 2004).

Level of Care

Adolescents rarely need medical detoxification. Reasons for this seem to be related to the fact that adolescents tend to use multiple drugs in an episodic time course. Also, adolescents are usually in better general physical health than adults. Despite this, physical addiction to alcohol, sedatives, or minor tranquilizers may occur with life-threatening withdrawal symptoms that necessitate detoxification in an inpatient setting. Adolescents are usually not very honest about the types, amounts, and frequency of their alcohol or drug use. The physician needs to clarify the importance of honesty in relation to the use of these physically addictive substances, especially the benzodiazepines (i.e., diazepam, clonazepam, and alprazolam), because this could be a life-and-death issue. Other indications for inpatient hospitalization include danger to self or others, psychotic symptoms, and high-risk behavior that could be life-threatening.

Adolescents with substance abuse disorder or substance dependence disorder often need a short period of inpatient hospitalization so that they can be fully evaluated and stabilized. Then they may be stepped down to a day patient or intensive outpatient program. Within these programs family therapy, 12-Step facilitation therapy, CBT, and motivational interviewing may be used. Full biopsychosocial evaluation is needed, because comorbid disorders are present in 40%–90% of these patients (Bukstein et al. 1989). These comorbid affective, behavioral, and anxiety disorders should be defined and considered for concurrent treatment. The major issue for adolescents with substance abuse disorder or substance dependence disorder who are to be treated in day or intensive outpatient program is whether they can resist returning to contact with their peers who are using drugs.

The American Society of Addiction Medicine has developed treatment levels of care for adolescents, which include the dimensions of treatment resistance, relapse potential, and recovery environment (Fishman 2003).

Comorbid Psychiatric Disorders

In this section, the terms *dual diagnosis* and *comorbidity* are used as general terms to refer to patients who meet the criteria for a psychoactive substance use disorder and for another psychiatric diagnosis on Axis I or II using DSM-IV-TR (American Psychiatric Association 2000).

■ Prevalence

In different patients with the same two comorbid disorders, the course and treatment may vary depending on which disorder is primary (i.e., which one preceded the other) (Miller and Fine 1993) and on their relative severity (Bukstein 1997; Caton et al. 1989; King et al. 1996; Ries et al. 1994; Schuckit 1985; Weiss et al. 1992). It is unhelpful to assume that all patients with dual diagnoses are the same and require the same treatment (Weiss et al. 1992). Although a high prevalence of comorbidity has been reported among adolescent inpatients with drug use disorders (Clark et al. 1995, 1997; Grilo et al. 1995; Hovens et al. 1994; Kaminer et al. 1991), it is unclear how many exhibit psychiatric symptoms secondary to the substance abuse disorder and how many have a primary or coexisting psychiatric diagnosis. Miller and Fine (1993) argue that methodological considerations—including the length of abstinence required before the diagnosis is made, the population sampled, and the perspective of the examiner—affect prevalence rates for psychiatric disorders in individuals who abuse substances and that these considerations account for the variability. These authors see the prevalence rates for psychiatric disorders as being artificially elevated by the tendency to make a diagnosis before abatement of some of the psychiatric symptoms that are secondary to substance use.

Until very recently, studies involving adolescents were smaller and involved clinical populations. Stowell and Estroff (1992) studied 226 adolescents receiving inpatient treatment in private psychiatric hospitals for a primary substance abuse disorder. Psychiatric diagnoses were made 4 weeks into treatment by using a semistructured diagnostic interview. Of the total, 82% of the patients met DSM-III-R criteria for an Axis I psychiatric disorder; 61% had mood disorders; 54% had conduct disorders; 43% had anxiety disorders; and 16% had substance-induced organic disorder. Seventy-four percent of the patients had two or more psychiatric disorders. Westermeyer and colleagues (1994) studied 100 adolescents ages 12–20 years who sought care at two university-based outpatient substance abuse treatment programs; the researchers found

similar high rates of comorbidity and multiple diagnoses.

Burke and colleagues (1990) studied data from the Epidemiologic Catchment Area Study of the National Institute of Mental Health to determine hazard rates for the development of disorders. They concluded that 15–19 years were the peak ages for the onset of depressive disorders in females and for the onset of substance use disorders and bipolar disorders in both sexes. The National Comorbidity Study included a large noninstitutional sample of persons ages 15–24 years, although adolescents were not studied separately from young adults (Kessler et al. 1996). Compared with older adults, 15- to 24-year-olds had the highest prevalence of three or more disorders occurring together and of any disorders, including substance use disorders. The Methods for the Epidemiology of Child and Adolescent Mental Disorders Study obtained data for 401 subjects ages 14–17 years (Kandel et al. 1999). Adolescents with substance use disorders had much higher rates of mood and conduct disorders than did those without substance use disorders.

■ Major Diagnostic Categories

Depressive Disorders

Studies of adults who abused substances showed that the substance-induced mood disorder dissipated with abstinence, but the primary depressive disorder did not, and if left untreated it could interfere with treatment and recovery (Burke et al. 1990; Miller 1993; Miller and Fine 1993; Schuckit 1985). Deykin and colleagues (1992) interviewed 223 adolescents in residential treatment for substance abuse and found that almost 25% met the DSM-III-R (American Psychiatric Association 1987) criteria for depression. Of these, 8% met the criteria for primary depression; the remaining 16% had a secondary mood disorder. Bukstein et al. (1992) studied adolescent inpatients on a dual-diagnosis unit and reported that almost 31% had comorbid major depression, with secondary depressive disorder much more common than primary depressive disorder. Unlike findings reported for adults, Bukstein et al. (1992) found that the secondary depression did not remit with abstinence.

Depression interferes with treatment, owing to the lack of concentration, motivation, and hope and the tendency toward isolation. Kempton and colleagues (1994) found cognitive distortions, including magnification (all-or-nothing thinking) and personalizing, to be particularly prominent among adolescents with the multiple diagnoses of conduct disorder, depressive disorder, and substance abuse. A depressed adolescent may benefit from a specific cognitive intervention for depression (Beck et al. 1979; Kaminer 1994).

If the adolescent has a depressive disorder that predates the substance abuse, has a family history of depression, and has a mood disorder that interferes with treatment several weeks into abstinence despite cognitive interventions, pharmacotherapy is indicated. Serotonergic agents such as fluoxetine have a relatively safe profile for side effects and may be most appropriate for youth, considering reports suggesting that young substance abusers have a preexisting serotonin deficit (Crowley and Riggs 1995; Horowitz et al. 1992; Riggs et al. 1997).

Bipolar Disorder

The diagnosis of bipolar disorder may be among the hardest to make in children and adolescents, and it is even more difficult in teenagers with substance abuse. Issues such as change in sleeping patterns and mood swings can be symptoms of bipolar disorder, substance abuse, or even normal adolescence. The diagnosis of bipolar disorder should certainly be considered in substance-abusing youths, particularly those with a binge pattern.

Wilens and colleagues (1999) found an increased risk of substance use disorders in adolescents with bipolar disorder. Children who were diagnosed and received appropriate treatment at a younger age had a lower risk of substance abuse. Some patients use substances, particularly alcohol, to calm themselves during a manic phase. Clearly, some of these symptoms are also seen with substance intoxication. If a patient exhibits these symptoms after a period of abstinence, the diagnosis of bipolar disorder should be considered. Bipolar disorders are most often treated with mood stabilizers, the most common of which is lithium carbonate (Geller et al. 1998).

Anxiety Disorders and Posttraumatic Stress Disorder

Anxiety disorders are among the most common psychiatric conditions coexisting in adolescents and adults with substance use disorders. Anxiety disorders are often not detected or treated, especially when they are present with depression or psychoactive substance use disorders (Burke et al. 1990; Clark and Bukstein 1998). Because some of the symptoms of panic attacks might be seen in substance intoxication or withdrawal, it is important to establish abstinence before making a diagnosis. Patients with social phobia may isolate themselves on an inpatient unit or within a group. Behavioral treatment, including relaxation training, is often helpful for anxiety disorders (Kaminer 1994). The issue of pharmacotherapy is controversial. Buspirone hydrochloride and serotonin reuptake inhibitors have been recommended as nonaddictive antianxiety agents (Wilens et al. 1998).

In clinical reports on adolescents, the incidences of severe trauma and symptoms of posttraumatic stress disorder are surprisingly high (Clark et al. 1995, 1997; Deykin and Buka 1997; Kandel et al. 1999). An adolescent who has been acting out and abusing substances may not have dealt with previous trauma, such as physical and sexual abuse or exposure to violence, or with the trauma that may be incurred when abusing substances (Clark et al. 1997). Symptoms and memories of trauma may manifest themselves only during abstinence.

Care should be taken to acknowledge the trauma without arousing anxiety that will interfere with abstinence and substance abuse treatment. Groups that support self-care and a first-things-first attitude may be the best approach; the patient needs to learn to stay safe, and treatment for substance abuse is a most important aspect of safety.

Organic Mental Disorders

The abuse of substances—including alcohol, marijuana, cocaine, ecstasy, hallucinogens, and inhalants—is associated in some patients with acute and residual cognitive damage (American Psychiatric Association 2000; Kempton et al. 1994; Stowell and Estroff 1992). Acute symptoms may include impaired concentration and receptive and expressive language abilities, as well as irritability. Long-term interference with memory and other executive functions occurs. The possibility of substance-induced dementia should be considered in adolescents who have difficulty coping with the cognitive and organizational demands of a structured and supportive program. Some of the adolescents will be able to use the program if instructions are simplified and if they comprehend information accurately. There may be rapid improvement in cognitive func-

tioning, but the cognitive functioning of some patients continues to improve for as long as a year or more after cessation of the chemical assault to the brain. Some may be left with residual impairment.

Schizophrenia

Because the late adolescent years are a time when many schizophrenic disorders begin, and the use of substances may precipitate incipient psychosis, patients with this disorder may seek treatment during early stages of schizophrenia (Kaminer et al. 1991; Miller and Fine 1993; Ries 1993a). Increasingly, younger schizophrenic patients abuse substances (Buckley 1999; Minkoff 1989; Ries 1993b), sometimes in an attempt to manage or deny their psychotic symptoms. Their abuse of substances often interferes with treatment for their psychotic disorder. These patients are best managed in special dual-diagnosis programs for psychotic patients (Buckley 1999; Caton et al. 1989; Mason and Siris 1992; Ries 1993a; Ries et al. 1994).

Attention-Deficit/Hyperactivity Disorder

Many involved in the treatment of adolescents who abuse substances have noted the large numbers of adolescents who also have ADHD (Bukstein 1997; Bukstein et al. 1989; Riggs 1998; Wilens et al. 1996). Treatment should include behavioral and educational intervention. Pharmacotherapy for adolescents has been controversial, particularly because some have argued that the use of psychostimulants might predispose adolescents to abuse other substances (Riggs 1998). Riggs and colleagues (1998) reported some success with the use of bupropion. Wilens and colleagues (1996) suggested that the successful treatment of adolescents with ADHD with stimulants may actually lower the probability that they will develop a substance use disorder. Because the successful treatment of substance abuse involves teaching patients to plan and to delay impulses, the effective treatment of ADHD is necessary in an integrated plan. The Concerta formulation of methylphenidate is the safest to use because it cannot be abused by intranasal route (Jaffe 2002).

Conduct Disorder and Antisocial Personality Disorder

Conduct disorder and antisocial personality disorder are the most common comorbid diagnoses in substance abuse, particularly among males (Bukstein 1997; Crowley and Riggs 1995; Kandel et al. 1999; King et al. 1996; Rao et al. 1999; Schuckit 1985; Stowell and Estroff 1992; Westermeyer et al. 1994; Wilens et al. 1996). Cloninger (1987) presented an interesting scheme of hereditary factors on three axes that may help account for many psychiatric diagnoses and their interrelationships. The three axes are reward dependence, harm avoidance, and novelty seeking. Based on these axes, Cloninger (1987) distinguished type 1 and type 2 alcoholic patients. Type 2 alcoholic patients score low on reward dependence and harm avoidance and high on novelty seeking. Younger alcoholic patients with antisocial personality disorder fit the type 2 classification. The higher prevalence of antisocial personality disorder and conduct disorder among younger alcoholic patients may explain why many clinicians find adolescent substance abusers more difficult to treat. Adolescents with conduct disorders and antisocial personality disorder need a strong behavioral program with clear limits. If there is a comorbid disorder (such as a mood or attention disorder) that can be treated successfully, the adolescents are more likely to do well (Crowley and Riggs 1995; Riggs 1998; Wilens et al. 1996).

Eating Disorders

Because the incidences of eating disorders and substance abuse have increased in the adolescent population (Katz 1990; Ross and Ivis 1999; Westermeyer and Specker 1999; Westermeyer et al. 1994), it is not uncommon to find them together. In fact, one-quarter of all patients with an eating disorder have a history of substance abuse or are currently abusing substances (Katz 1990). Anorexia nervosa is not as prevalent as bulimia in the general population and among persons who abuse substances (Westermeyer and Specker 1999).

Psychiatric disorders and substance abuse frequently occur together. This leads to difficulty in both assessment and treatment. An awareness of the prevalence and manifestations of psychiatric diagnoses is essential for the quality treatment of adolescents who abuse substances. Frequently, the use of psychiatric medications such as antidepressants, mood stabilizers, psychostimulants, and others is of benefit. However, care must be taken to avoid potential interactions between the illicit drugs and the prescribed medications (Wilens et al. 1997).

Prevention

Prevention of substance abuse in adolescents has proved to be a complex problem. Reducing availability—for example, by increasing the drinking age or increasing the cost of cigarettes—has had some positive effect in decreasing substance use in adolescents. The widely used prevention strategy of increasing the knowledge of consequences (as in the DARE [Drug Abuse Resistance Education] program) was shown in a controlled study to result in no short-term or long-term effects (Ennett et al. 1994). In a review of the effectiveness of program components, Hansen (1996) demonstrated that programs with an informational or affective component had little effect. Programs that enhanced social skills and drug refusal skills were more successful. The life skills training developed by Botvin et al. (1995) used an intervention in the seventh grade and booster sessions during the following 2 years. Significant decreases in drug use were found when these students reached the twelfth grade. Prevention programs that target high-risk youth (e.g., those with poor academic achievement) are being developed and studied.

Research Issues

In the future, research should continue to build on the foundations laid in the past decade. Much still needs to be done in the areas of etiology, diagnostic and nosological issues, and, of course, treatment. The Cannabis Youth Treatment Study demonstrated the effectiveness of five different treatments; however, the limited long-term results indicate a need for further development of treatment and aftercare strategies (Dennis et al. 2004).

Perhaps the greatest need for research is in prevention. Stopping substance use before it begins may perhaps be the most effective strategy in the "war on drugs." A better understanding of the progression from experimentation to recreational use to abuse and ultimately to dependence may help tailor interventions specific to each stage. Lastly, a developmentally appropriate understanding of treatment also needs to be refined with future research endeavors. How does a substance abusing 12-year-old differ from a substance abusing 18-year-old? Are different genetic factors at play? Different psychiatric comorbidities? Different sociocultural factors? It can be hoped that future research will begin to find answers for these and other questions.

References

Alcoholics Anonymous: The Story of How Many Thousands of Men and Women Have Recovered From Alcoholism, 3rd Edition. New York, Alcoholics Anonymous World Services, 1976

American Psychiatric Association: Diagnostic and Statistical Manual of Mental Disorders, 3rd Edition, Revised. American Psychiatric Association, Washington, DC, 1987

American Psychiatric Association: Diagnostic and Statistical Manual of Mental Disorders, 4th Edition, Text Revision. Washington, DC, American Psychiatric Association, 2000

Azrin NH, Donohue B, Besale VA, et al: Youth drug abuse treatment: a controlled outcome study. Journal of Child and Adolescent Substance Abuse 3:1–16, 1994

Bailey GW: Helping the resistant adolescent enter substance abuse treatment: the office intervention. Child Adolesc Psychiatr Clin N Am 5:149–164, 1996

Bauman KE, Ennett S: Peer influence on adolescent drug use. Am Psychol 49:820–822, 1994

Beck AT, Rush AJ, Shaw BF, et al: Cognitive Therapy of Depression. New York, Guilford, 1979

Botvin GJ, Baker E, Dusenbury L, et al: Preventing adolescent drug abuse through multimodal cognitive behavioral approach: results of a three year study. J Consult Clin Psychol 58:437–446, 1990

Botvin GJ, Baker E, Dusenbury L, et al: Long-term follow-up of randomized drug abuse prevention trial in a white middle-class population. JAMA 273:1106–1112, 1995

Brook JS, Lukoff IF, Whiteman M: Initiation into adolescent marijuana use. J Genet Psychol 137:133–142, 1980

Brown SA: Recovery patterns in adolescent substance abusers, in Addictive Behavior Across the Life Span: Prevention, Treatment and Policy Issues. Edited by Baer JS, Marlatt, GA, McMahon, RJ. Beverly Hills, CA, Sage, 1993, pp 161–163

Buckley PF: Substance abuse in schizophrenia: a review. J Clin Psychiatry 59 (suppl 3): 26–30, 1999

Budney AJ, Novy PL, Hughes JR: Marijuana withdrawal among adults seeking treatment for marijuana dependence. Addiction 94:1311–1322, 1999

Bukstein O: Practice parameters for the assessment and treatment of children and adolescents with substance use disorders. J Am Acad Child Adolesc Psychiatry 36 (10 suppl): 140S–156S, 1997

Bukstein OG, Brent DA, Kaminer Y: Comorbidity of substance abuse and other psychiatric disorders in adolescents. Am J Psychiatry 146:1131–1141, 1989

Bukstein OG, Glancy LJ, Kaminer Y: Patterns of affective comorbidity in a clinical population of dually diagnosed adolescent substance abusers. J Am Acad Child Adolesc Psychiatry 31:1041–1045, 1992

Burke KC, Burke JD Jr, Regier DA, et al: Age at onset of selected mental disorders in five community populations. Arch Gen Psychiatry 47:511–518, 1990

Catalano RF, Hankins JD, Wells EA, et al: Evaluation of the effectiveness of adolescent drug abuse treatment, assessment of risk for relapse, and promising approaches for relapse prevention. Int J Addict 25:1085–1140, 1990–1991

Caton CL, Gralnick A, Bender S, et al: Young chronic patients and substance abuse. Hosp Community Psychiatry 40:1037–1040, 1989

Center for Substance Abuse Treatment: Screening and assessing adolescents for substance use disorders (Treatment Improvement Protocol Series, No 31). Rockville, MD, Substance Abuse and Mental Health Services Administration, 1999a

Center for Substance Abuse Treatment: Treatment of adolescents with substance abuse disorder (Treatment Improvement Protocol Series, No 32). Rockville, MD, Substance Abuse and Mental Health Services Administration, 1999b

Chatlos JC: Recent trends and a developmental approach to substance abuse in adolescents. Child Adolesc Psychiatr Clin North Am 5:1–28, 1996

Clark DB, Bukstein OG: Psychopathology in adolescent alcohol abuse and dependence. Alcohol Health Res World 22:117–126, 1998

Clark DB, Bukstein O, Smith MG, et al: Identifying anxiety disorders in adolescents hospitalized for alcohol abuse and dependence. Psychiatr Serv 46:618–620, 1995

Clark DB, Lesnick L, Hegedus AM: Traumas and other adverse life events in adolescents with alcohol use and dependence. J Am Acad Child Adolesc Psychiatry 36:1744–1751, 1997

Clark DB, Kirisci L, Tarter RE: Adolescent versus adult onset and the development of substance use disorders in males. Drug Alcohol Depend 49:115–121, 1998

Cloninger CR: Neurogenetic adaptive mechanisms in alcoholism. Science 236:410–416, 1987

Crowley TJ, Riggs PD: Adolescent substance use disorder with conduct disorder and comorbid conditions. NIDA Res Monogr 156:49–111, 1995

Deas D, Thomas SE: An overview of controlled studies of adolescent substance abuse treatment. Am J Addict 10:178–189, 2001

Deas-Nesmith D, Campbell S, Brady KT: Substance use disorders in an adolescent inpatient psychiatric population. J Natl Med Assoc 90:233–238, 1998

Dennis M, Godley SH, Diamond G, et al: The Cannabis Youth Treatment (CYT) Study: main findings from two randomized trials. J Subst Abuse Treat 27:197–213, 2004

DeWitt DJ, Adlaf EM, Offord DR, et al: Age of first alcohol use: a risk factor for the development of alcohol disorders. Am J Psychiatry 157:745–750, 2000

Deykin EY, Buka SL: Prevalence and risk factors for posttraumatic stress disorder among chemically dependent adolescents. Am J Psychiatry 154:752–757, 1997

Deykin EY, Buka SL, Zeena TH: Depressive illness among chemically dependent adolescents. Am J Psychiatry 149:1341–1347, 1992

Dimeff LA, Baer JS, Kivlahan DR, et al: Brief Alcohol Screening and Intervention for College Students. New York, Guilford, 1999

Ennett ST, Rigwatt C, Flewelling RL: How effective is drug abuse resistance education? A meta-analysis of project DARE evaluations. Am J Public Health 84:1394–1401, 1994

Fishman M: Placement criteria and strategies for adolescent treatment matching, in Principles of Addiction Medicine, 3rd Edition. Edited by Graham AW, Schultz TK, Mayo-Smith M, et al. Chevy Chase, MD, American Society of Addiction Medicine, 2003, pp 1559–1572

Geller B, Cooper TB, Sun K, et al: Double-blind and placebo-controlled study of lithium for adolescent bipolar disorders with secondary substance dependency. J Am Acad Child Adolesc Psychiatry 37:171–178, 1998

Grilo CM, Becker DF, Walker ML, et al: Psychiatric comorbidity in adolescent inpatients with substance use disorders. J Am Acad Child Adolesc Psychiatry 34:1085–1091, 1995

Grunebaum PE, Prange ME, Friedman RM, et al: Substance abuse prevalence and comorbidity with other psychiatric disorders among adolescents with severe emotional disturbances. J Am Acad Child Adolesc Psychiatry 30:575–583, 1991

Hansen WB: Pilot test results comparing the All Stars program with seventh grade DARE: program integrity and mediating variable analysis. Subst Use Misuse 31:1359–1377, 1996

Harrison PA: Epidemiology, in Manual of Substance Abuse Treatment. Edited by Estroff TW. Washington, DC, American Psychiatric Publishing, 2001, pp 1–12

Harrison PA, Hoffman NC: CATOR Report: Adolescent Treatment Completion One Year Later. St. Paul, MN, Ramsey Clinic, 1989

Harrison PA, Fullerson JA, Beebe TJ: DSM-IV substance use disorder criteria for adolescents: a critical examination based on a statewide school survey. Am J Psychiatry 155:486–492, 1998

Henggeler SW, Melton GB, Smith LA, et al: Family preservation using multisystemic treatment: long-term follow-up to a clinical trial with serious juvenile offenders. Journal of Child and Family Studies 2:283–293, 1993

Horowitz HA, Overton WF, Rosenstein D, et al: Comorbid adolescent substance abuse: a maladaptive pattern of self-regulation. Adolesc Psychiatry 18:465–483, 1992

Hovens JG, Cantwell DP, Kiriakos R: Psychiatric comorbidity in hospitalized adolescent substance abusers. J Am Acad Child Adolesc Psychiatry 33:476–483, 1994

Jaffe SL: Step Workbook for Adolescent Chemical Dependency Recovery: A Guide to the First Five Steps. Washington, DC, American Psychiatric Press, 1990

Jaffe SL: Pathways to relapse in chemically dependent adolescents. Adolescent Counselor 55:42–44, 1992

Jaffe SL (ed): Adolescent Substance Abuse and Dual Disorders. Child Adolesc Psychiatr Clin N Am 5:1–261, 1996a

Jaffe SL: The substance abusing youth, in Child and Adolescent Psychiatry. Edited by Parmelee DX. St. Louis, MO, Mosby, 1996b, pp 237–244

Jaffe SL: Adolescent Substance Abuse Intervention Workbook: Taking a First Step. Washington, DC, American Psychiatric Press, 2001

Jaffe SL: Failed attempts at intranasal abuse of Concerta. J Am Acad Child Adolesc Psychiatry 41:5, 2002

Johnston LD, O'Malley PM, Bachman JG: National Survey Results on Drug Use From the Monitoring the Future Study, 1975–2000, Vol 1: Secondary School Students (NIH Publ No 01-4924). Rockville, MD, National Institute on Drug Abuse, 2001

Johnston LD, O'Malley PM, Bachman JG, et al: Monitoring the Future national survey results on drug use, 1975–2003. Bethesda, MD, National Institute on Drug Abuse, 2004

Kaminer Y: Adolescent Substance Abuse: A Comprehensive Guide to Theory and Practice. New York, Plenum, 1994

Kaminer Y, Burleson J: Psychotherapies for adolescent substance abusers: 15-month follow-up of a pilot study. Am J Addict 8:114–119, 1999

Kaminer Y, Bukstein OG, Tarter RE: The Teen Addiction Severity Index: rationale and reliability. Int J Addict 26:219–226, 1991

Kandel D: Stages in adolescent involvement in drug use. Science 190:912–914, 1975

Kandel DB, Yamaguchi K, Chen K: Stages of progression in drug involvement from adolescence to adulthood: further evidence for the gateway theory. J Stud Alcohol 53:447–457, 1992

Kandel DB, Johnson JG, Bird HR, et al: Psychiatric comorbidity among adolescents with substance use disorders: findings from the MECA study. J Am Acad Child Adolesc Psychiatry 38:693–699, 1999

Katz JL: Eating disorders: a primer for the substance abuse specialist, I: clinical features. J Subst Abuse Treat 7:143–149, 1990

Kempton T, Van Hasselt VB, Bukstein OG, et al: Cognitive distortions and psychiatric diagnosis in dually diagnosed adolescents. J Am Acad Child Adolesc Psychiatry 33:217–222, 1994

Kendler KS, Prescott CA: Cannabis use, abuse, and dependence in a population-based sample of female twins. Am J Psychiatry 155:1016–1022, 1998a

Kendler KS, Prescott CA: Cocaine use, abuse and dependence in a population-based sample of female twins. Br J Psychiatry 173:345–350, 1998b

Kessler RC, Nelson CB, McGonagle KA, et al: The epidemiology of co-occurring addictive and mental disorders: implications for prevention and service utilization. Am J Orthopsychiatry 66:17–31, 1996

King C, Ghaziuddin N, McGovern L, et al: Predictors of comorbid alcohol and substance abuse in depressed adolescents. J Am Acad Child Adolesc Psychiatry 35:743–751, 1996

Knight JR, Shrier LA, Bravender TD, et al: A new brief screen for adolescent substance abuse. Arch Pediatr Adolesc Med 153:591–596, 1999

Lee GP, DiClimente CC: Age of onset versus duration of problem drinking on the Alcohol Use Inventory. J Stud Alcohol 46:298–402, 1985

Leirer VO, Yesavage JA, Morrow DG: Marijuana carry-over effects on aircraft pilot performance. Aviat Space Environ Med 62:221–227, 1991

Levy S, Vaughan BL, Knight JR: Office-based intervention for adolescent substance abuse. Pediatr Clin North Am 49:329–343, 2002

Lewis RA, Piercy FP, Sprenkle DH, et al: Family based interventions for helping drug abusing adolescents. J Adolesc Res 5:82–95, 1990

Liddle HA: Multidimensional Family Therapy Treatment (MDFT) for Adolescent Cannabis Users (Vol 5 of Cannabis Youth Treatment [CYT] manual series). Rockville, MD, Center for Substance Abuse Treatment, 2002

Macdonald DI: Drugs, drinking and adolescence. Am J Dis Child 138:117–125, 1984

Mason SE, Siris SG: Dual diagnosis: the case for case management. Am J Addict 1:77–82, 1992

Miller NS: Comorbidity of psychiatric and alcohol/drug disorders: interactions and independent status. J Addict Dis 12:5–16, 1993

Miller NS, Fine J: Current epidemiology of comorbidity of psychiatric and addictive disorders. Psychiatr Clin North Am 16:1–10, 1993

Minkoff K: An integrated treatment model for dual diagnosis of psychosis and addiction. Hosp Community Psychiatry 40:1031–1036, 1989

Monti PM, Barnett NP, O'Leary JA, et al: Motivational enhancement for school-involved adolescents, in Adolescents, Alcohol, and Substance Abuse. Edited by Monti PM, Colby SM, O'Leary TA. New York, Guilford, 2001, pp 145–182

Neighbors B, Kempton D, Forehand R: Co-occurrence of substance abuse with conduct, anxiety and depressive disorders in juvenile delinquents. Addict Behav 17:379–386, 1992

Nestler EJ: Molecular neurobiology of drug addiction. Neuroscientist 11:77–87, 1994

Nestler EJ: Molecular basis of addiction states. Neuroscientist 1:212–220, 1995

Newcomb MD: Identifying high-risk youth: prevalence and patterns of adolescent drug abuse. NIDA Res Monogr 156:7–38, 1995

Nowinski J: Substance Abuse in Adolescents and Young Adults: A Guide to Treatment. New York, WW Norton, 1990 pp 38–65

Office of Applied Studies: Summary of Findings From the 1999 National Household Survey on Drug Abuse (DHHS Publ No [SMA] 00-3466). Rockville, MD, Substance Abuse and Mental Health Services Administration, 2000

Pandina RJ, Johnson V, Labouvie EW, et al: Affectivity: a central mechanism in the development of drug dependence, in Vulnerability to Drug Abuse. Edited by Glantz M, Pickens R. Washington, DC, American Psychological Association, 1992, pp 179–209

Pickrel SG, Henggeler SW: Multisystemic therapy for adolescent substance abuse and dependence. Child Adolesc Psychiatr Clin N Am 5:201–211, 1996

Prochaska JO, DiClemente CC: Transtheoretical therapy: toward a more integrated model of change. Psychotherapy: Theory, Research and Practice 19:276–288, 1982

Rao U, Ryan N, Dahl DE, et al: Factors associated with the development of substance use disorders in depressed adolescents. J Am Acad Child Adolesc Psychiatry 38:1109–1117, 1999

Ries RK: Clinical treatment matching models for dually diagnosed patients. Psychiatr Clin North Am 16:167–175, 1993a

Ries RK: The dually diagnosed patient with psychotic symptoms. J Addict Dis 12:103–122, 1993b

Ries R, Mullen M, Cox G: Symptom severity and utilization of treatment resources among dually diagnosed inpatients. Hosp Community Psychiatry 45:562–568, 1994

Riggs PD: Clinical approach to treatment of ADHD in adolescents with substance use disorders and conduct disorder. J Am Acad Child Adolesc Psychiatry 37:331–332, 1998

Riggs PD, Mikulich SC, Coffman L, et al: Fluoxetine in drug-dependent delinquents with major depression: an open trial. J Child Adolesc Psychopharmacol 7:87–95, 1997

Riggs PD, Mikulich SC, Pottle LC: An open trial of bupropion for ADHD in adolescents with substance use disorder and conduct disorder. J Am Acad Child Adolesc Psychiatry 37:1271–1278, 1998

Roberts AJ, Koob GF: The neurobiology of addiction. Alcohol Health Res World 21:101–106, 1997

Rogers PD, Adger H Jr: Alcohol and adolescents. Adolesc Med 4:295–304, 1993

Ross HE, Ivis F: Binge eating and substance abuse among male and female adolescents. Int J Eat Disord 26:245–260, 1999

Schuckit MA: The clinical implications of primary diagnostic groups among alcoholics. Arch Gen Psychiatry 42:1043–1049, 1985

Schwartz RH: Testing for drugs of abuse: controversies and techniques. Adolesc Med 4:353–370, 1993

Schwartz RH, Gruenwald PJ, Klitzner M, et al: Short-term memory impairment in cannabis-dependent adolescents. Am J Dis Child 143:1214–1219, 1989

Stanton MD, Shadish WR: Outcome, attrition and family-couples treatment for drug abuse: a meta-analysis and review of the controlled, comparative studies. Psychol Bull 122:170–191, 1997

Stowell JA, Estroff TW: Psychiatric disorders in substance-abusing adolescent inpatients: a pilot study. J Am Acad Child Adolesc Psychiatry 31:1036–1040, 1992

Tarter RE: Evaluation and treatment of adolescent substance abuse: a decision tree method. Am J Drug Alcohol Abuse 16:1–46, 1990

Weiss RD, Mirin SM, Frances RJ: Alcohol and drug abuse: the myth of the typical dual diagnosis patient. Hosp Community Psychiatry 43:107–108, 1992

Westermeyer J, Specker S: Social resources and social function in comorbid eating and substance disorder: a matched-pairs study. Am J Addict 8:332–336, 1999

Westermeyer J, Specker S, Neider J, et al: Substance abuse and associated psychiatric disorder among 100 adolescents. J Addict Dis 13:67–89, 1994

Wilens TE, Biederman J, Spencer TJ: Attention deficit hyperactivity disorder and psychoactive substance use disorders. Child Adolesc Psychiatr Clin N Am 5:73–91, 1996

Wilens TE, Biederman J, Spencer TJ: Case study: adverse effects of smoking marijuana while receiving tricyclic antidepressants. J Am Acad Child Adolesc Psychiatry 36:45–48, 1997

Wilens T, Spencer T, Frazier J, et al: Psychopharmacology in children and adolescents, in Handbook of Child Psychopathology. Edited by Ollendick T, Hersen M. New York, Plenum, 1998, pp 603–636

Wilens TE, Biederman J, Millstein RB, et al: Risk for substance use disorders in youths with child- and adolescent-onset bipolar disorder. J Am Acad Child Adolesc Psychiatry 38:680–685, 1999

Winters KC: Assessing adolescent substance use problems and other areas of functioning: state of the art, in Adolescents, Alcohol, and Substance Abuse. Edited by Monti PM, Colby SM, O'Leary TA. New York, Guilford, 2001, pp 80–108

Self-Assessment Questions

Select the single best response for each question.

17.1 Which of the following has been reported to be a problem in applying DSM-IV-TR (American Psychiatric Association 2000) criteria to adolescents?

　　A. Withdrawal and drug-related medical problems are common.
　　B. One abuse symptom yields a diagnosis.
　　C. Abuse symptoms frequently precede dependence symptoms.
　　D. Two dependence symptoms with no abuse symptoms yields a diagnosis.
　　E. None of the above.

17.2 In the 2001 Monitoring the Future Survey (Johnston et al. 2001), epidemiological findings concerning substance abuse in high school seniors included all of the following *except*

　　A. Marijuana use by about 37%.
　　B. Cigarette smoking during the past month by 29.5%.
　　C. MDMA (3,4-methylenedioxymethamphetamine; "ecstasy") use by 9.2%.
　　D. Anabolic steroid use by 12.4%.
　　E. Alcohol use by about 73%.

17.3 The well-known CAGE screening questions developed for adults are not useful for adolescents. The CRAFFT, a screening instrument developed for adolescents, includes all of the following questions *except*

　　A. "Have you ever ridden in a **C**ar driven by someone (including yourself) who was high or had been using alcohol or drugs?"
　　B. "Do you ever use alcohol/drugs to **R**elax, feel better about yourself, or fit in?"
　　C. "Do you get **A**ngry when you are told that you have a problem?"
　　D. "Do you ever **F**orget things you did while using alcohol/drugs?"
　　E. "Have you ever gotten into **T**rouble while you were using alcohol/drugs?"

17.4 Risk factors for the development of substance abuse disorders include all of the following *except*

　　A. Economic and social advantage.
　　B. School failure.
　　C. Friends who use drugs.
　　D. Psychiatric comorbidity.
　　E. History of parental divorce.

17.5 A common comorbid diagnosis in male adolescents with substance abuse is

　　A. Conduct disorder.
　　B. Attention-deficit/hyperactivity disorder.
　　C. Avoidant personality disorder.
　　D. Oppositional defiant disorder.
　　E. None of the above.

Separation Anxiety Disorder and Generalized Anxiety Disorder

Gail A. Bernstein, M.D.

Ann E. Layne, Ph.D.

In DSM-IV-TR (American Psychiatric Association 2000), separation anxiety disorder (SAD) is characterized by developmentally inappropriate and excessive anxiety about being apart from the individuals to whom a child is most attached. Frequently, the individual worries excessively that harm may come to either a parent (or attachment figure) or himself or herself, which would result in their separation.

Generalized anxiety disorder (GAD) is characterized by marked worry and anxiety that the individual finds difficult to control and that causes impairment in functioning. Before the publication of DSM-IV (American Psychiatric Association 1994), children with excessive worry were diagnosed with overanxious disorder (OAD) rather than GAD. Reasons for the change from OAD to GAD included concern that the criteria for OAD were vague and nonspecific and a recognition that the symptoms overlapped with those of other disorders, including social phobia (Beidel 1991; Werry 1991). Because the previous research on children with generalized anxiety was done using DSM-III-R (American Psychiatric Association 1987) criteria for OAD, some data on OAD are included in this chapter.

Diagnostic Criteria

Separation anxiety is a normative part of development, typically beginning around 6 or 7 months, peaking around 18 months, and decreasing after 30 months. Features of separation anxiety may persist into childhood and early adolescence while remaining subclinical. In a study of 62 children without any psychiatric diagnoses, isolated subclinical SAD symptoms were reasonably common

(Bell-Dolan et al. 1990). For example, fear of harm to attachment figures was present in 16.1% of the sample, and fear of harm to self was endorsed by 9.7% of the sample. Each of these symptoms was present at a clinical level in 1.6% of the sample. However, when separation anxiety develops outside these normative parameters, is persistent and excessive, and is associated with significant distress or impairment, a diagnosis of SAD should be considered. The child must have three of the eight symptoms listed in Table 18–1 to meet DSM-IV-TR diagnostic criteria. The individual must have the symptoms for at least 4 weeks and an onset before age 18 years.

Worry, like separation anxiety, can also be a normative part of development. Muris et. al. (1998) found that 69% of children and adolescents worry every now and then. Unlike normative worry, GAD is characterized by excessive and uncontrollable worry that results in significant impairment or distress. In addition, the worry is associated with feelings of restlessness, fatigability, difficulty concentrating, irritability, muscle tension, and sleep disturbance. Three of these six symptoms are required for adults; only one is needed in children. Symptoms must be present for at least 6 months. DSM-IV-TR diagnostic criteria for GAD are presented in Table 18–2.

Table 18–1.   DSM-IV-TR criteria for separation anxiety disorder

A. Developmentally inappropriate and excessive anxiety concerning separation from home or from those to whom the individual is attached, as evidenced by three (or more) of the following:

   (1) recurrent excessive distress when separation from home or major attachment figures occurs or is anticipated

   (2) persistent and excessive worry about losing, or about possible harm befalling, major attachment figures

   (3) persistent and excessive worry that an untoward event will lead to separation from a major attachment figure (e.g., getting lost or being kidnapped)

   (4) persistent reluctance or refusal to go to school or elsewhere because of fear of separation

   (5) persistently and excessively fearful or reluctant to be alone or without major attachment figures at home or without significant adults in other settings

   (6) persistent reluctance or refusal to go to sleep without being near a major attachment figure or to sleep away from home

   (7) repeated nightmares involving the theme of separation

   (8) repeated complaints of physical symptoms (such as headaches, stomachaches, nausea, or vomiting) when separation from major attachment figures occurs or is anticipated

B. The duration of the disturbance is at least 4 weeks.

C. The onset is before age 18 years.

D. The disturbance causes clinically significant distress or impairment in social, academic (occupational), or other important areas of functioning.

E. The disturbance does not occur exclusively during the course of a pervasive developmental disorder, schizophrenia, or other psychotic disorder and, in adolescents and adults, is not better accounted for by panic disorder with agoraphobia.

Source.   Reprinted from American Psychiatric Association: *Diagnostic and Statistical Manual of Mental Disorders*, 4th Edition, Text Revision. Washington, DC, American Psychiatric Association, 2000. Copyright 2000, American Psychiatric Association. Used with permission.

Table 18–2. DSM-IV-TR criteria for generalized anxiety disorder

---

A. Excessive anxiety and worry (apprehensive expectation), occurring more days than not for at least 6 months, about a number of events or activities (such as work or school performance).

B. The person finds it difficult to control the worry.

C. The anxiety and worry are associated with three (or more) of the following six symptoms (with at least some symptoms present for more days than not for the past 6 months). **Note:** Only one item is required in children.

  (1) restlessness or feeling keyed up or on edge

  (2) being easily fatigued

  (3) difficulty concentrating or mind going blank

  (4) irritability

  (5) muscle tension

  (6) sleep disturbance (difficulty falling or staying asleep, or restless unsatisfying sleep)

D. The focus of the anxiety and worry is not confined to features of an Axis I disorder, e.g., the anxiety or worry is not about having a panic attack (as in panic disorder), being embarrassed in public (as in social phobia), being contaminated (as in obsessive-compulsive disorder), being away from home or close relatives (as in separation anxiety disorder), gaining weight (as in anorexia nervosa), having multiple physical complaints (as in somatization disorder), or having a serious illness (as in hypochondriasis), and the anxiety and worry do not occur exclusively during posttraumatic stress disorder.

E. The anxiety, worry, or physical symptoms cause clinically significant distress or impairment in social, occupational, or other important areas of functioning.

F. The disturbance is not due to the direct physiological effects of a substance (e.g., a drug of abuse, a medication) or a general medical condition (e.g., hyperthyroidism) and does not occur exclusively during a mood disorder, a psychotic disorder, or a pervasive developmental disorder.

Source. Reprinted from American Psychiatric Association: *Diagnostic and Statistical Manual of Mental Disorders,* 4th Edition, Text Revision. Washington, DC, American Psychiatric Association, 2000. Copyright 2000, American Psychiatric Association. Used with permission.

Clinical Findings

■ Separation Anxiety Disorder

In SAD, there is an overwhelming fear of losing or becoming separated from a parent. Typically, the child fears that separation or loss will occur as the result of a catastrophic event such as death, kidnapping, or serious accident (Albano et al. 1996). Frequently the manifestations of the underlying fear of separation include the reluctance to be apart or nightmares about separation. Thus, children with SAD display a range of avoidance behaviors from procrastination during the morning routine before school to refusing to leave the side of their parent (e.g., refusing to attend school or to sleep alone). Individuals with SAD often have multiple somatic complaints (e.g., stomachaches, headaches). These complaints can be the result of anxiety or can be designed to support the individual's avoidance of separation (e.g., complaining of a stomachache so that he or she can stay home from school).

SAD can interfere with normative development in a number of ways. Children and adolescents with SAD often have difficulty attending school, participating in extracurricular activities, and attending sleepovers. As a result, academic achievement, peer relationships, and overall maturation are often compromised. School refusal, although not a separate DSM-IV-TR diagnosis, is a childhood symptom commonly presumed to be the behavioral manifestation of SAD. However, "not all children with school refusal or fear of school suffer from SAD, and not all children with SAD manifest school refusal" (Black 1995, p. 217). School refusal can be associated with many different diagnoses, including SAD, specific phobia of school, and depression.

The prevalence of SAD decreases with increasing age (Anderson et al. 1987; McGee et al. 1990). In a study of community ($n=2,384$) and clinical ($n=217$) samples, Compton et al. (2000) found that preadolescents were significantly more likely than adolescents to endorse symptoms of separation anxiety on the Multidimensional Anxiety Scale for Children (March et al. 1997). Results also indicated that females were more likely to endorse symptoms of separation anxiety than were males. Sociodemographic assessment of a large clinic sample ($N=188$) of children with anxiety disorders showed that those with SAD had the earliest age at onset (7.5 years) and the earliest age at intake (10.3 years) (Last et al. 1992). The gender ratio of those with SAD was approximately equal.

■ Generalized Anxiety Disorder

The primary symptom of GAD is excessive worry for at least 6 months. Children with GAD worry a great deal about things such as future events, peer relationships, social acceptability, competency, and pleasing others. Unlike children with social phobia, SAD, or specific phobia, children with GAD have numerous and diffuse worries that are not limited to a specific stimulus or environment. They are often described by their parents as "worry warts" and as overly conscientious. Children with GAD tend to overestimate the likelihood of negative consequences, predict catastrophic outcomes for future events, and underestimate their ability to cope with unfavorable situations (Albano et al. 1996).

As mentioned above, worry and anxiety can be a normative part of development and are experienced throughout life. Fears, worries, and scary dreams are common in healthy children, occurring at rates of 76%, 68%, 81%, respectively ($N=190$) (Muris et al. 2000). Muris et al. (1998) compared children with OAD and GAD with children not meeting criteria for an anxiety disorder. Children with OAD or GAD reported, on average, six specific worries, whereas control children identified, on average, one topic of worry. Children with OAD or GAD endorsed a higher frequency of their main worry, stronger interference associated with their worry, more anxiety linked to their worry, and increased difficulty controlling their worry. Although 31% of the control children reported that their worry had some positive aspects, none of the children with OAD or GAD identified their worry as having positive aspects. Finally, children with OAD or GAD less frequently engaged in activities that distracted them from their worried thoughts and more frequently discussed their worries with others.

Masi et al. (2004) investigated the symptoms most commonly associated with GAD in 157 children and adolescents. Results indicated that feelings of tension (100%), apprehension (94%), negative self-image (90%), need for reassurance (86%), irritability (77%), physical complaints (75%), difficulty concentrating (69%), brooding (i.e., ruminating) (67%), and fatigue (65%) were the most common symptoms co-occurring with GAD. Less common symptoms included psychomotor agitation (54%) and sleep disturbance (51%).

Kendall and Pimentel (2003) examined physiological symptoms associated with GAD in 47 children ages 9–13 years. Results indicated that children endorse, on average, one physiological symptom, which is consistent with the DSM-IV-TR requirement. Parents, on the other hand, endorsed an average of three symptoms in their children. Not surprisingly, there was low concordance between parent and child report of associated symptoms. Results also indicated that the number of physiological symptoms endorsed by children with GAD increased with age. The most common associated symptom endorsed by children was "unable to sit still or relax" (34.8%); least common was muscle aches (28.3%).

A number of studies have demonstrated that girls tend to worry more and have more numerous worries than boys (e.g., Muris et al. 1998; Silverman et al. 1995). Therefore, it is not surprising that higher prevalence rates for GAD have been reported for females (9%) than for males (3.8%) (N=193) (Muris et al. 1998). Among those diagnosed with GAD, the total number of symptoms associated with GAD did not differ based on age or gender (Masi et al. 2004).

Comorbidity

Children and adolescents with anxiety disorders often present with comorbid disorders. In a recent study of children and adolescents ages 7–18 with GAD, only 7% had GAD as a unique disorder (Masi et al. 2004). More than half of the sample had a comorbid depressive disorder (56%). SAD was commonly comorbid among the child participants (52%) but was less common among adolescents (22%). Forty-two percent of the sample had comorbid specific phobia, 28% had

social phobia, and 20% had comorbid obsessive-compulsive disorder. Comorbid externalizing disorders were present in 21%. In addition, children with anxiety disorders are at risk for developing alcohol abuse in adolescence (Manassis and Monga 2001).

In a study of 199 8- to 13-year-old children with SAD, GAD, and/or social phobia, children with SAD had a greater mean number of comorbid diagnoses than either the GAD or the social phobia groups (Verduin and Kendall 2003). However, the likelihood of comorbid mood disorders was significantly lower in children with a primary diagnosis of SAD than in children with a primary diagnosis of GAD or social phobia.

A poorer prognosis has been found in children with anxiety disorders and comorbid behavioral problems (Manassis and Hood 1998), comorbid depression (Last et al. 1997; Masi et al. 1999), and comorbid anxiety disorders (Woodward and Fergusson 2001) than in children with anxiety disorders without comorbid disorders. Manassis and Hood (1998) found that of a number of significant predictors (child depression, maternal phobic anxiety, developmental problems, and psychosocial adversity), maternal reporting of child conduct problems was most predictive of functional impairment in children with a primary anxiety disorder. Woodward and Fergusson (2001) conducted a 21-year longitudinal study of 1,265 New Zealand children. They found that among those with anxiety disorders there existed a significant association between a greater number of anxiety disorders reported in adolescence and later risks of additional anxiety disorders, major depression, illicit drug dependence, and failure to attend college. Finally, studies have reported that children and adolescents with comorbid anxiety and depressive disorders present with greater symptom severity (Bernstein 1991; Last et al. 1996), have a poorer response to treatment (Berman et al. 2000; Brent et al. 1998), and have more anxiety disorders (Masi et al. 1999).

Kendall et al. (2001) investigated the relationship between comorbidity in childhood anxiety disorders and treatment outcome. In their sample, 79% of children with a primary diagnosis of an anxiety disorder had at least one comorbid diagnosis. The most frequent comorbid diagnoses were simple phobia (46%), social phobia (34%), and GAD (29%). The study found that participants with comorbid diagnoses displayed more severe internalizing symptoms than participants with only a single anxiety disorder. However, comorbid diagnoses (i.e., anxiety and externalizing behavior disorders) did not affect treatment outcome; children with comorbid diagnoses at pretreatment were not significantly less likely to respond to treatment, as evidenced by remission of the primary diagnoses.

Differential Diagnosis

Because anxiety disorders share some common features, distinguishing among them requires that the primary focus of the anxiety be carefully delineated. In GAD, the anxiety is generalized and is not specifically focused on separation (as in SAD) and not specifically focused on social situations (as in social phobia). In panic disorder, the anxiety is focused on the fear of having a panic attack rather than on being separated from parental figures (as in SAD) and is not diffuse (as in GAD). Furthermore, whereas children with SAD and GAD may become extremely anxious and have accompanying sympathetic arousal (i.e., sweating, shaking, racing heart) when faced with separation or a focus of their worry (e.g., tak-

ing a test), panic attacks associated with panic disorder are most often out of the blue and in situations in which escape would be difficult. In obsessive-compulsive disorder, the child has specific, recurrent, intrusive thoughts that he or she attempts to ignore or neutralize with another thought or action. Although children with GAD describe their worry as difficult to control and may be ruminative, these worries can be differentiated from obsessions related to obsessive-compulsive disorder based on the content of the worry (i.e., they are usually related to daily stressors rather than a specific domain such as contamination) and because of the absence of rituals. All the symptoms of an adjustment disorder with anxiety would be related to the onset of a *specific* psychosocial stressor and occur within 3 months of the onset of the stressor. After the stressor remits, the anxiety symptoms in an adjustment disorder do not continue for longer than 6 months.

Epidemiology

The Great Smoky Mountains Study (GSMS) sampled 4,500 children ages 9, 11, and 13 years and produced the following 3-month prevalence rates for SAD and GAD: females with SAD, 4.3%; males with SAD, 2.7%; total with SAD, 3.5%; females with GAD, 2.4%; males with GAD, 1%; and total with GAD, 1.7% (Costello et al. 1996). In a more recent GSMS sample of 1,420 children ages 9–13 years, the 3-month prevalence rates for both disorders were lower: female SAD, 1%; male SAD, 1%; total SAD, 1%; female GAD, 0.9%; male GAD, 0.6%; total GAD, 0.8% (Costello et al. 2003). Higher rates for GAD in a sample of 8- to 13-year-olds were reported by Muris et al. (1998), with 9% of females and 3.8% of males meeting criteria for GAD. Rates for males and females with SAD in an epidemiological sample of twins (N=2,061) were 10.1% and 5.3%, respectively (Foley et al. 2004).

Rates of SAD and GAD vary by age, with SAD being more prevalent among younger children and OAD/GAD being more prevalent among older children and adolescents (Masi et al. 1999). Although rates of SAD decrease with age, rates of OAD/GAD increase with age (Anderson et al. 1987; McGee et al. 1990). Westenberg and colleagues (1999) found that participants with SAD (mean age, 10.3) were significantly younger than those with OAD (mean age, 14.5). Interestingly, the results indicate that the difference in prevalence could be attributed to differences in psychosocial maturity, with greater maturity being associated with OAD. The study found that level of ego development was the strongest predictor of having either SAD or OAD and that adding age, gender, IQ, or socioeconomic status did not improve the regression equation. The results also indicated that even within the same age cohort, the presence of SAD or OAD could be attributed to psychosocial maturity. These findings suggest that changes in the prevalence rates associated with SAD and OAD may represent changes in developmental maturity rather than age.

Etiology

The development of anxiety disorders in children is the result of interactions between a variety of factors. There are generally five domains recognized as being the most significant for consideration in the etiology of childhood anxiety disorders: genetics/temperament, attachment to caregivers, parental anxiety, parenting style, and life experiences (e.g., traumatic events, negative experiences).

■ Temperament

Temperament of the child is an important factor in the development of anxiety symptoms in children and adolescents. It has been found that approximately 20% of healthy infants are born with temperamental traits that predispose them to being highly reactive in novel or unfamiliar situations (Kagan and Snidman 1999). It appears that the crying and vigorous motor activity seen in highly reactive infants may be continuous with shy and fearful reactions in toddlers and with cautious, introverted, and avoidant behavior in school-age children in response to new situations (Kagan 1994; Kagan and Snidman 1999). The opposite of shy, inhibited, introverted children are those who are sociable, uninhibited, outgoing, extroverted, or fearless in response to unfamiliar people, objects, or events (Rosenbaum et al. 1988). Kagan (1994) described the temperamental characteristic of behavioral inhibition as a child's tendency to approach unfamiliar or novel situations with distress, restraint, and avoidance. Behavioral inhibition has been measured in the laboratory beginning at age 9 months (Kagan 1994). This area of study is of interest because temperament characteristics, such as behavioral inhibition, are thought to have a genetic basis (Daniels and Plomin 1985; Hirshfeld-Becker et al. 2004; Robinson et al. 1992).

Two independent samples of children identified as being either behaviorally inhibited or uninhibited at 21 or 31 months have been studied prospectively by Kagan et al. (1988). It was found that the tendency to approach or avoid new situations is often an enduring temperamental trait. Children with behavioral inhibition are differentiated from those without behavioral inhibition based on neurophysiological markers, including increased, less variable heart rates; elevated urinary cate-cholamine levels; increased salivary corti-sol levels; and increased tension in the lar-ynx and vocal cords (Kagan et al. 1988).

A 3-year follow-up study of children with behavioral inhibition showed in-creased rates of avoidant disorder, SAD, agoraphobia, and two or more anxiety disorders per child (Biederman et al. 1993). Subsequently it was found that be-havioral inhibition was linked specifically to an increased risk of social phobia in adolescence, with about one-third of the inhibited toddlers showing symptoms of social phobia as adolescents (Kagan and Snidman 1999). In a review by Bieder-man et al. (1995), it was emphasized that the increased risk for anxiety disorders was primarily in children with a history of persistent shyness and inhibition from 21 months to 7.5 years. Furthermore, risk for developing anxiety disorders was greater if the parents had anxiety disor-ders (Biederman et al. 1995).

In a recent study, Hirshfeld-Becker et al. (2004) examined whether the rela-tionship between parental anxiety and child behavioral inhibition was mediated by environmental factors. These factors included family conflict, parental pathol-ogy, and indicators of adversity such as low social class and large family size. Re-sults indicated no significant associations between behavioral inhibition and any of the factors examined. The authors con-cluded that their findings support the moderate to high heritability of behav-ioral inhibition.

A large community sample of chil-dren in Australia (N=2,443) was studied from infancy to adolescence to evaluate the role of shy-inhibited temperament in the development of anxiety disorders (Prior et al. 2000). Children were as-sessed every 18 months with parent, teacher, and self-report ratings from questionnaires based on the models of

temperament developed by Thomas and Chess (1977). No observational data were obtained. Logistic regression analy-ses showed that shy temperament was as-sociated with increased risk of later anxi-ety symptoms, especially at ages 9–10 years and 12–13 years. Children who were rated as shy at multiple time points were at greater risk for anxiety symptoms compared with children who were de-scribed as never shy or only occasionally rated as shy. Highly reactive tempera-ment, in combination with shy tempera-ment, did not confer additional risk for developing anxiety symptoms. It is also important to note that many very shy children did not develop anxiety prob-lems.

■ Attachment

An insecure attachment pattern between mother and child appears to be another factor contributing to the development of childhood anxiety disorders. Attach-ment theory suggests that a tendency to-ward anxiety can be exacerbated or alle-viated in the context of the child's interactions with primary attachment fig-ures (Manassis and Bradley 1994). A study evaluated attachment patterns of 18 mothers with anxiety disorders and their 20 preschool-age children (Manas-sis et al. 1994). All mothers were classi-fied as insecure in their current and past relationships. Similarly, 80% of the pre-schoolers were identified as having inse-cure attachments with their mothers. Of the 3 children with a diagnosis of an anx-iety disorder (2 with SAD and 1 with avoidant disorder), all were classified as insecurely attached.

Infants with anxious-resistant attach-ment (i.e., type of insecure attachment) are at risk for anxiety disorders in child-hood and adolescence compared with se-curely attached infants (Warren et al. 1997). In the longitudinal study by Warren et al. (1997), beginning in the third trimester of pregnancy, mothers and their offspring were studied prospectively. At 12 months, attachment was assessed with Ainsworth's Strange Situation Procedure, and at age 17.5 years anxiety disorders were evaluated with a semistructured psychiatric interview. It was found that anxious-resistant attachment significantly predicted anxiety disorders in adolescence. In the regression analyses, this finding accounted for a larger percentage of the variance than the role of maternal anxiety and the role of the child's temperament in predicting the later onset of anxiety disorders.

■ Parental Anxiety

Children of parents with anxiety disorders are at greater risk of developing anxiety disorders themselves. Biederman et al. (2001) reported that children of parents with major depression or panic disorder were at increased risk for developing SAD. In a study of children with anxiety-based school refusal, Martin et al. (1999) found that 81% of the parents had a history of psychiatric illness, with anxiety and depressive disorders being most common. Merikangas et al. (1998) examined psychopathology among offspring (ages 7–18) of parents with substance abuse or anxiety disorders. The study showed that there was a twofold increased risk of anxiety disorders among offspring of parents with anxiety disorders compared with offspring of substance abusers or control subjects. SAD and GAD/OAD were the most common diagnoses, both occurring in 12% of the children of parents with anxiety disorders. Beidel and Turner (1997) examined the risk for anxiety among children of a parent with an anxiety disorder, major depressive disorder, comorbid anxiety and depressive disorders, and children of

psychiatrically healthy control subjects. Anxiety disorders were significantly more common among children of parents with anxiety or depression (33%). The offspring of parents with anxiety disorders primarily had anxiety disorders, whereas the offspring of parents with depression with or without anxiety had many different disorders. Merikangas et al. (1999) found that children with one parent with an anxiety disorder had a threefold increased risk of OAD and an additional threefold risk when both parents had an anxiety disorder. Donovan and Spence (2000) state that parental anxiety is a risk factor that is not independently causal but is mediated or moderated through another mechanism (e.g., parenting style).

■ Parenting Style

Two main factors in parenting style have emerged as most relevant to the development of anxiety disorders: parental warmth/rejection and parental control (Rapee 1997). Parental warmth/rejection is conceptualized as positive (warm) versus negative (hostile) feelings the parent has toward the child. Parental control refers to the degree to which parental behaviors are designed to protect the child from possible harm. Siqueland et al. (1996) observed 17 families of children with SAD and OAD (and 27 control families) during discussion of issues of disagreement. The parents of children with anxiety disorders were rated by the independent observers as less granting of autonomy than the parents of control children, and children with anxiety disorders rated their mothers and fathers as significantly less accepting than did control children.

Similar results were found by Hudson and Rapee (2001) in an observational study in which children were asked to complete two difficult cognitive tasks while their mothers were told to sit nearby and provide support. The study found that mothers of anxious children were more involved, more intrusive, and more negative than mothers of control children. In discussing ambiguous hypothetical situations, parents of anxious children have also been significantly more likely to agree with and encourage their child's avoidance than were parents of control or aggressive children (Dadds et al. 1996). Muris et al. (1998) found anxious parenting style and parental control to be significantly correlated with GAD and SAD symptomatology occurring in a population of psychiatrically healthy school children. Based on a review of the literature, Rapee (1997) comments that excessive parental control and overprotection may suggest to the child that the world is a dangerous place and may interfere with the child's ability to learn otherwise.

■ Life Experiences

Anxiety in children can be related to exposure to negative life events (Dadds and Barrett 2001). Furthermore, these events need not be traumatic to play a role in the development of anxiety disorders. In a study of the development of worries and fears in healthy children, Muris et al. (2000) found that 54% of children attributed the origin of their main worry to a conditioning experience (e.g., the death of a grandmother), 33% reported an information pathway (e.g., the evening news), and 13% reported a modeling experience (e.g., seeing parents worried). The authors concluded that these experiences contribute to common anxiety phenomena in children. However, Muris et al. (1998) reported that threatening or aversive life events were *not* critical in the development of worry in children with OAD/GAD. They reported that only 7.7% of children with GAD/OAD recalled their worry as being related to a negative conditioning experience.

Poulton et al. (2001) conducted a longitudinal study of the relationship between separation experiences and the development of separation anxiety at ages 3, 11, and 18 years. The results failed to provide strong evidence for a relationship between environmental events (e.g., separation experiences) and separation anxiety at any of the ages. The variable most strongly related to separation anxiety in 11-year-old children was the mother's fear of going out alone. The results regarding the development of GAD and SAD are consistent with the following conclusion: "On their own, stressful life events do not provide a full explanation for the development of anxiety disorders" (Dadds and Barrett 2001, p. 1001).

Manassis and Bradley (1994) presented an integrated model for the development of childhood anxiety disorders. In this model, temperament, attachment, social systems (e.g., access to other family members, peers, and community support systems) and the interplay between them are incorporated as important factors contributing to anxiety disorders. The literature reviewed in this chapter supports the notion that temperament, attachment, parental anxiety, and parenting style all play a part in the development of anxiety in children and adolescents.

Treatment

A complete diagnostic assessment of the child with an anxiety disorder would include interviewing the child and parents, both individually and together, and considering whether other important adults and siblings in the child's life should also be included. Reports from the school, previous or current psychotherapists, and the pediatrician may be important. In addition to collecting a complete description of the current symptoms, the clinician should review the developmental, medical, and family psychiatric history. It is important to conduct an assessment of the family to evaluate possible problems such as family discord, marital difficulties, difficulties of an individual family member, inappropriate roles or boundaries, and abuse. In general, a multimodal approach is designed to integrate psychosocial and psychopharmacological treatments for the child (Bernstein and Shaw 1993).

■ Psychopharmacotherapy

Several classes of psychopharmacological medication have been used in the treatment of childhood anxiety disorders (see reviews by Rosenberg et al. 2003; Velosa and Riddle 2000). The first-line choice is a selective serotonin reuptake inhibitor (SSRI), and a second choice is a tricyclic antidepressant (TCA). Benzodiazepines can be considered on a short-term basis, alone or in combination with an SSRI or a TCA while waiting for the SSRI or TCA to reach therapeutic level.

Selective Serotonin Reuptake Inhibitors

The first choice for the pharmacological treatment of SAD or GAD is an SSRI. This approach is supported by controlled studies (Birmaher et al. 2003; Research Unit on Pediatric Psychopharmacology 2001; Rynn et al. 2001) that demonstrate the efficacy and short-term safety of SSRIs for children and adolescents with anxiety disorders.

Three randomized, controlled trials provide solid support for the efficacy of the SSRIs in treating childhood anxiety disorders. A relatively large multicenter treatment study compared fluvoxamine with pill placebo for 128 youths with GAD, SAD, or social phobia (Research Unit on Pediatric Psychopharmacology 2001). All participants had had no response to 3 weeks of psychosocial intervention for their anxiety symptoms before being randomized to 8 weeks of fluvoxamine or placebo. Medication was given in combination with supportive psychotherapy. Primary outcome measures included the Pediatric Anxiety Rating Scale (PARS) (Research Units on Pediatric Psychopharmacology 2002a) and the Clinical Global Impressions (CGI) scale (Guy 1976). After 8 weeks, children in the active medication group showed a significant decrease in clinician-rated anxiety on the PARS compared with the placebo group. In addition, 76% (48 of 63) of the fluvoxamine group versus 29% (19 of 65) in the placebo group were rated at or above "improved" on the CGI. The medication was generally well tolerated, with only 5 children receiving fluvoxamine and 1 child receiving placebo discontinuing due to side effects. With respect to specific side effects, significantly more children in the fluvoxamine group reported stomachaches, and more children receiving fluvoxamine experienced increased motor activity.

Rynn et al. (2001) studied sertraline in the treatment of 22 children and adolescents with a primary diagnosis of GAD. A 2–3 week assessment period was followed by random assignment to 9 weeks of sertraline (up to 50 mg/day) or placebo. At the end of treatment, youths receiving sertraline showed significant improvement on the Hamilton Anxiety Scale (Hamilton 1959), a clinician rating scale, compared with those taking placebo. Self-report measures also showed significant decreases in anxiety symptoms for participants in the active medication group versus the placebo group. Significant differences in anxiety between conditions were noted initially at 4 weeks. The anxiolytic effect was independent of the antidepressant effect of the medication. Of note, there was minimal response to placebo. Side effects were mild and not substantially different between groups.

In a controlled study of 74 children and adolescents with GAD, SAD, and/or social phobia, participants were randomly assigned to fluoxetine 20 mg/day or placebo (Birmaher et al. 2003). After 12 weeks of treatment, 61% of the children who received fluoxetine versus 35% of those on placebo were rated as much improved or very much improved on the CGI improvement scale. Other outcome measures also supported the benefit of fluoxetine in decreasing anxiety symptoms and enhancing functioning. Side effects of fluoxetine included transient stomachaches and headaches in the first 2 weeks. Abdominal pain was the only adverse effect that was more common throughout the study in the active medication group compared with the placebo group. With these studies, child and adolescent psychiatrists have scientific evidence that SSRIs are beneficial for targeting anxiety symptoms in youth.

In a 6-month open-label extension of the Research Units on Pediatric Psychopharmacology fluvoxamine study (Research Units on Pediatric Psychopharmacology 2002b), participants who had been treated in the 8-week study were offered the opportunity to enter an open-label phase. Subjects who responded to fluvoxamine were maintained on the same medication; placebo nonresponders were given fluvoxamine; and participants who did not respond to fluvoxamine were changed to fluoxetine. During the open-label treatment, 94% (33 of 35) of the original fluvoxamine responders continued to show low levels of anxiety symptoms. Of those who were switched to

fluoxetine, 71% (10 of 14) showed significant improvement in their anxiety symptoms. In the placebo nonresponders, 56% (27 of 48) had a significant improvement in anxiety symptoms with fluvoxamine. Thus, it appears that beneficial response to fluvoxamine in a short-term trial is likely to be maintained with continuation of treatment, that some fluvoxamine nonresponders will respond to a different SSRI (fluoxetine), and that placebo nonresponders have a reasonable likelihood of responding to fluvoxamine.

In a review of studies employing SSRIs in the short-term treatment of children and adolescents with anxiety disorders or major depression, it was suggested that after remission of target symptoms, a drug-free trial should be considered (Pine 2002). It was further recommended that the medication-free trial should occur during the first period of low stress, after a year of SSRI treatment. If a youth relapses during the period without medication, the SSRI should be restarted (Pine 2002).

Tricyclic Antidepressants

Five controlled studies of TCA trials for SAD or school refusal have reported contrasting findings. Gittelman-Klein and Klein (1973) reported that imipramine, 100–200 mg/day (mean, 152 mg/day), was superior to placebo in a 6-week study of 35 children with school refusal. The imipramine group was significantly more successful in returning to school (81% taking imipramine returned to school versus 47% taking placebo). Furthermore, those taking imipramine were rated by mothers, clinicians, and self-report as having a significant decrease in somatic and anxiety symptoms compared with those taking placebo. Berney et al. (1981) reported that low-dose clomipramine was not superior to placebo in a 12-week double-blind trial for school refusers. The study included 51 anxious children and adolescents; 44% had comorbid depression. A shortcoming of this study was the probably subtherapeutic medication dosage.

Bernstein et al. (1990) compared imipramine, alprazolam, and placebo in an 8-week double-blind trial of 24 school refusers (ages 7–17 years). Mean dosages were 164.3 mg/day for imipramine and 1.8 mg/day for alprazolam. Concurrent treatments consisted of individual psychotherapy and returning the child to school. Trends suggested that the active medications were superior to placebo, but it was unclear whether the trends were due to medication effects or baseline difference in severity of symptoms among groups. Klein et al. (1992) reported on a 6-week double-blind study of imipramine compared with placebo in 20 children with SAD (ages 6–15 years). All subjects had had no response to a 1-month trial of behavior therapy. The mean dosage of imipramine was 153 mg/day. At the end of the treatment, no differences were found between the imipramine and placebo groups, with 50% in each group showing improvement. Therefore, this study did not replicate the earlier findings of Gittelman-Klein and Klein (1973).

Bernstein et al. (2000) compared 8 weeks of imipramine versus placebo, each in combination with individual cognitive-behavioral therapy (CBT) for 63 school-refusing teenagers with comorbid anxiety and major depressive disorders. The average school attendance rate was 31% before entering the study. The mean dosage of imipramine at the end of the study was 182.3 mg/day. School attendance improved significantly for the imipramine plus CBT group but not for the placebo plus CBT group. At the end of 8 weeks, the imipramine group was attending 70% of the time and the placebo group was attending only 28% of the time. In addition, the imipramine group showed a faster rate of improvement in clinician-rated symptoms of depression. Overall, the study demonstrated the efficacy of imipramine in combination with CBT for treating anxious and depressed adolescent school refusers. The findings support a multimodal approach in the treatment of severe school refusal in adolescents.

In summary, one study supports the use of TCAs to treat SAD with or without school refusal (Gittelman-Klein and Klein 1973) and another supports combining a TCA with CBT for anxious, depressed teenagers with severe, refractory symptoms (Bernstein et al. 2000). The other three studies are hampered by either small sample sizes (Bernstein et al. 1990; Klein et al. 1992) or low medication dosage (Berney et al. 1981). Overall, these studies suggest that a TCA may be considered for anxiety symptoms in children and adolescents. However, the first choice is typically an SSRI, both because of that class's safety in overdose and because recent controlled clinical trials demonstrate the efficacy of SSRIs in children with anxiety disorders (Birmaher et al. 2003; Research Unit on Pediatric Psychopharmacology 2001; Rynn et al. 2001).

Benzodiazepines

There are limited data on the efficacy of benzodiazepines in the treatment of GAD or SAD in children and adolescents. The existing studies are limited by small sample sizes and short duration of treatment. In a 4-week double-blind, placebo-controlled study of 30 children with OAD ($n=21$) or avoidant disorder ($n=9$), participants in the alprazolam group (0.5–3.5 mg/day) showed no significant difference on global ratings of improvement compared with the placebo group (Simeon et al. 1992). A double-blind crossover study of 15 children with anxiety disorders (primarily SAD) evaluated 4 weeks of clonazepam (0.5–2.0 mg/day) versus 4 weeks of placebo (Graae et al. 1994). There was no significant difference in improvement between the two treatment conditions.

Side effects of the benzodiazepines may include sedation, incoordination, slurred speech, and tremor (Kutcher et al. 1995). Behavioral disinhibition has been reported in children and adolescents taking clonazepam (Graae et al. 1994; Reiter and Kutcher 1991). The risk of tolerance and dependence in children has not been adequately studied (Velosa and Riddle 2000). However, because of the theoretical potential for dependence in youth (Riddle et al. 1999), trials in children and adolescents should be short, and benzodiazepines should be avoided in youth with a history of chemical dependence.

Further studies are needed to evaluate the role of benzodiazepines in children with GAD or SAD.

■ Cognitive-Behavioral Therapy

Although a number of psychosocial approaches exist for treating anxiety disorders in children (e.g., CBT, psychodynamic psychotherapy, play therapy, supportive therapy), CBT is the only one whose efficacy is supported by data from randomized controlled studies (Compton et al. 2004). Velting et al. (2004) list the following as the six essential components of CBT for child anxiety: psychoeducation, somatic management, cognitive restructuring, problem solving, exposure, and relapse prevention. In the past 10 years, a number of treatment programs have been developed and evaluated for use in individual, group, and family therapy that include various combinations of these components. Research

has demonstrated the superiority of both individual and group CBT to waiting-list control condition (i.e., no treatment) (Flannery-Schroeder and Kendall 2000; Kendall 1994; Kendall et al. 1997).

Kendall (1994) compared a 16-week cognitive-behavioral treatment package with a waiting-list control group for 47 children ages 9–13 years with anxiety disorders. Of the subjects, 30 had a primary diagnosis of OAD, 8 had SAD, and 9 had avoidant disorder; in addition, 32% of the subjects had comorbid depressive disorder. The treatment program used was based on *The Coping Cat* (Kendall 1990). The CBT included cognitive components of recognizing anxious feelings and thoughts, identifying somatic reactions to anxiety, and developing a plan to cope with these symptoms. Behavioral techniques included modeling, exposure, role playing, relaxation training, and reinforcement. At the end of treatment, subjects who received the cognitive-behavioral package showed significant reductions in anxiety and depressive symptoms compared with those on the waiting list. Of the subjects who received the CBT, 64% no longer met criteria for anxiety disorder after the intervention, whereas only 1 participant in the waiting-list condition no longer met criteria after the wait period. At 1-year follow-up and 3-year follow-up, treatment gains were maintained (Kendall and Southam-Gerow 1996). Furthermore, at 7.4-year follow-up, Kendall et al. (2004) reported that the majority of anxiety-disordered youth maintained their gains. They also found that children who had a successful treatment response to CBT were less likely to develop problems with substance abuse. The authors concluded that "interventions for child mental health problems can have an ameliorative effect not only on the target disorder but also on the sequelae" (p. 283).

Kendall et al. (1997) conducted a second randomized trial with 94 participants with OAD (n=55), SAD (n=22), or avoidant disorder (n=17). Treatment was the same as that described above. Results indicated that 50% of the treated patients were free of their primary anxiety disorder compared with 6% in the waiting-list control group when evaluated at posttreatment. Furthermore, those who continued to have an anxiety disorder had significant decreases in ratings of severity. Maintenance of treatment gains was demonstrated at 1-year follow-up.

Flannery-Schroeder and Kendall (2000) compared the efficacy of individual CBT and group CBT based on *The Coping Cat* treatment protocol (Kendall 1990) to waiting-list control condition. Treatment consisted of 18 weeks of 50- to 60-minute sessions for the individual treatment (n=13) and 18 weeks of 90-minute sessions for the group treatment (n=12). Results indicated that after treatment, 73% of children who had received individual CBT and 50% of children who had received group CBT no longer met diagnostic criteria for their primary anxiety disorder, whereas only 8% of children in the waiting-list control group no longer met criteria. Results indicate that the treatment gains associated with individual CBT versus group CBT were not significantly different. Treatment gains were maintained at 3-month follow-up. Berman et al. (2000) also reported no significant difference between treatment outcome for anxious children treated with individual versus group CBT.

Silverman et al. (1999) conducted a randomized clinical trial (N=56) to evaluate the benefits of group CBT versus a waiting-list control condition for treating anxious children. In this study, children and parents met in separate, concurrent groups. Results supported the superiority of group CBT over waiting-list control

condition: 64% of children receiving treatment no longer met criteria for their primary diagnosis compared with only 13% of the children in the waiting-list control group.

Studies have also been conducted to evaluate the role of parental involvement in the treatment of child anxiety disorders (e.g., Barrett 1998; Barrett et al. 1996; Cobham et al. 1998; Mendlowitz et al. 1999; Nauta et al. 2003). Barrett et al. (1996) found that significantly more children who participated in a CBT intervention that included a family therapy component were free of their anxiety diagnosis at posttreatment and at 12-month follow-up than children who participated in CBT that did not include parental involvement. However, at 6-year follow-up the superiority of the CBT plus family therapy was no longer present (Barrett et al. 2001). Nauta et al. (2003) compared CBT for children, CBT for children plus a parent training program, and a wait-list control. Results indicated that both CBT groups were superior to wait-list control, but no additional benefit of parent training was identified.

Mendlowitz et al. (1999) reported that child-only group CBT, parent-only group CBT, and child-plus-parent group CBT all resulted in a significant decrease in anxiety and depression symptoms. However, children in the child-plus-parent intervention used coping strategies that had been taught in therapy more often than children in the other treatment groups. In addition, parents in the child-plus-parent intervention rated their children as significantly more improved than did parents of children in the other two treatment conditions. Cobham et al. (1998) compared the efficacy of child-focused CBT and child-focused CBT plus parental anxiety management for children with anxiety disorders. Results indicated that the parental anxiety management component increased the efficacy of the CBT component only for children with at least one anxious parent.

Dadds et al. (1997, 1999) evaluated the potential benefits of prevention and early intervention with children demonstrating symptoms of anxiety. Almost 2,000 Australian children ages 7–14 years were screened for anxiety symptoms in their classrooms. After screening and diagnostic interviewing, 128 children were selected for inclusion. Children selected for inclusion either had subclinical features of an anxiety disorder or met criteria but had low severity ratings. Participants were assigned to either a 10-week child and parent intervention or a monitoring group. After 10 weeks, both groups showed improvement. At 6-month follow-up, the benefit was maintained in the treatment group only, with a decrease in number of baseline anxiety diagnoses and a lower rate of new anxiety disorders. Only 16% of children who received the preventive intervention developed a new anxiety disorder compared with 54% in the monitoring condition. At 2-year follow-up, only the treatment group showed gains with a durable reduction in anxiety symptoms and decreased likelihood of developing new anxiety disorders (Dadds et al. 1999).

CBT for children with anxiety offers clinicians an efficacious, time-limited, and structured approach to treatment. Individual and group CBT appear equally efficacious. Findings also suggest that for children with anxiety who also have a parent with anxiety, parental involvement in therapy may improve treatment outcome. Additional research comparing CBT with other therapeutic interventions is needed. Two studies have compared CBT for child anxiety with a control therapy. Last et al. (1998) compared CBT and educational support for children with anxiety-based school re-

fusal. Results indicated that CBT and educational support have comparable success in reducing anxiety symptoms and facilitating return to school. Muris et al. (2002) compared group CBT, emotional disclosure, and a no-treatment control condition. Results indicated that CBT was superior to both emotional disclosure and no treatment. The limited studies and mixed results highlight the need for additional research comparing CBT with alternative therapeutic interventions.

Prognosis

Last et al. (1996) evaluated children with anxiety disorders every 12 months for 3–4 years. The results suggest a "generally favorable course and outcome" for children with anxiety disorders (Last et al. 1996, p. 1508). The vast majority of primary anxiety disorders (82%) had remitted by the end of the follow-up period, with only 8% experiencing relapse after initial remission. SAD and OAD both had high rates of recovery: 96% for SAD and 80% for OAD. Over the course of follow-up, one-third of participants developed new psychiatric disorders. Children with OAD had the highest rate of new disorders during follow-up. The authors concluded that children with OAD are at increased risk for developing additional psychiatric disorders over time. Cohen et al. (1993) found that greater severity of OAD symptoms at baseline interview predicted greater likelihood of continuation of the disorder. At follow-up 2.5 years later, OAD was still present in almost half of the patients with severe symptoms at baseline.

In an epidemiological study of 2,067 8- to 17-year-old twins, 161 were found to meet criteria for SAD (Foley et al. 2004). Results indicated that over an 18-month span, 80% of SAD cases remitted. The cases of SAD that did not remit were associated with a higher prevalence of oppositional defiant disorder, more impairment due to attention-deficit/hyperactivity disorder, and mothers with lower marital satisfaction. In a study of young children with SAD, Kearney et al. (2003) found that at 3.5-year follow-up, the majority of cases no longer met criteria. Results indicated that cases not in remission at follow-up were associated with greater parental psychopathology and greater internalizing symptoms at baseline.

Last et al. (1997) also conducted an 8-year follow-up study with young adults who had been evaluated as children and adolescents (see Last et al. 1996 sample described above). The participants had a history of either anxiety and depressive disorders, anxiety disorder only, or no psychiatric illness. The results indicated that participants with anxiety disorders were functioning similarly to control subjects with one exception: young adults with a childhood history of an anxiety disorder (without comorbid depression) were less likely than control subjects to be living independently. The outcome was less positive for young adults with a history of anxiety and comorbid depression. These individuals were 1) less likely than control subjects to be employed or in school, 2) more likely than purely anxious participants to utilize mental health services, and 3) more likely than both groups to report psychological problems (e.g., difficulty with depression, anxiety, drugs, or alcohol).

Pine et al. (1998) conducted a prospective epidemiological study of 776 children and adolescents with follow-ups 2 and 9 years later. At initial assessment, 111 participants had OAD or GAD; at the 9-year follow-up (N=716) only 36 participants met criteria. However, the study found that having OAD/GAD at initial assessment was significantly predictive of

having social phobia, major depression, GAD, or panic disorder at the 9-year follow-up. These results are consistent with the finding reported by Last et al. (1996) that children with OAD are especially at risk for new disorders over time. The overall findings indicate that most adolescent disorders are no longer present in adulthood; however, most adult disorders are preceded by an internalizing disorder in adolescence.

Compelling questions pertain to which childhood anxiety disorders are the "equivalents" of or precursors to those in adults. It has been suggested that SAD may be a precursor to panic disorder in adulthood. Manicavasagar et al. (1998), using adults' retrospective recall of symptoms of SAD in childhood, found that panic disorder with agoraphobia was likely to be associated with high levels of SAD symptoms in childhood. However, half of adult participants with panic disorder with agoraphobia did not report heightened levels of early separation anxiety. Furthermore, when studied prospectively, children with SAD were not significantly more likely to develop panic disorder (Pine et al. 1998). Children with SAD, GAD, and/or social phobia (N=85) who had previously completed treatment at an anxiety disorders clinic were reevaluated with diagnostic interviews 7.4 years later (Aschenbrand et al. 2003). In comparison with participants who had a childhood diagnosis of GAD or social phobia, participants with SAD as children were not more likely to meet criteria for panic disorder and agoraphobia in young adulthood. These findings do not support a specific link between SAD in childhood and panic disorder in adulthood. Additional research is needed to determine whether significant relationships exist between specific childhood anxiety disorders and specific adult anxiety disorders.

Research Issues

There are solid data supporting the short-term efficacy of CBT (e.g., Kendall et al. 1997) and SSRIs (Birmaher et al. 2003; Research Unit on Pediatric Psychopharmacology 2001; Rynn et al. 2001) for children and adolescents with anxiety disorders. Direct comparison of CBT, SSRI, CBT plus SSRI, and pill placebo is in progress through the National Institute of Mental Health (i.e., Child/Adolescent Anxiety Multimodal Treatment Study Collaborative Group). In practice, combined treatments are commonly used for children and adolescents with severe impairing anxiety disorders. Therefore, it is important to delineate whether combined treatments provide additional benefit above and beyond CBT alone or medication alone. Analyses of mediators and moderators of treatment response will help identify which participants are more likely to benefit from a multimodal intervention versus single treatment.

Future research should determine the optimal duration of acute treatments. In addition, studies should be designed to evaluate the type, duration, and safety of maintenance treatments. With the increasing use of pharmacotherapy, additional data on the short-term and long-term safety of SSRIs are needed. Assessing the potential benefit of booster sessions for maintenance of CBT efficacy is also an important goal.

The interaction of temperament, attachment, parental anxiety, and parenting style in contributing to the onset of anxiety disorders is a fertile area of research to pursue. For example, parenting characteristics (e.g., high maternal expressed emotion) may moderate the child's temperament in determining risk for anxiety disorders (Hirshfeld et al. 1997; Spence 2001). Similarly, attachment pattern may interact with temperament in establishing risk for later

onset of anxiety (Spence 2001). The examination of the interplay of multiple risk and protective factors will help identify which children will develop anxiety disorders (Kazdin and Kagan 1994).

Another important avenue for research is early intervention. Early identification and intervention for children with subthreshold anxiety symptoms may serve to prevent the onset of full-criteria anxiety disorders, and for children with mild to moderate anxiety disorders it appears to decrease the likelihood of continuing to manifest an anxiety disorder (Dadds et al. 1999). It is likely that early intervention will help to avert negative outcomes associated with untreated anxiety disorders. Longitudinal follow-up of treated and untreated children will support or refute this prediction.

References

Albano AN, Chorpita BF, Barlow DH: Childhood anxiety disorders, in Child Psychopathology. Edited by Mash EJ, Barkley RA. New York, Guilford, 1996, pp 196–241

American Psychiatric Association: Diagnostic and Statistical Manual of Mental Disorders, 3rd Edition—Revised. Washington, DC, American Psychiatric Association, 1987

American Psychiatric Association: Diagnostic and Statistical Manual of Mental Disorders, 4th Edition. Washington, DC, American Psychiatric Association, 1994

American Psychiatric Association: Diagnostic and Statistical Manual of Mental Disorders, 4th Edition, Text Revision. Washington, DC, American Psychiatric Association, 2000

Anderson JC, Williams S, McGee R, et al: DSM-III disorders in preadolescent children. Arch Gen Psychiatry 44:69–76, 1987

Aschenbrand SG, Kendall PC, Webb A, et al: Is childhood separation anxiety disorder a predictor of adult panic disorder and agoraphobia? A seven-year longitudinal study. J Am Acad Child Adolesc Psychiatry 42:1478–1485, 2003

Barrett PM: Evaluation of cognitive-behavioral group treatments for childhood anxiety disorders. J Clin Child Psychol 27:459–468, 1998

Barrett PM, Dadds MR, Rapee RM: Family treatment of childhood anxiety: a controlled trial. J Consult Clin Psychol 64:333–342, 1996

Barrett PM, Duffy AL, Dadds MR, et al: Cognitive-behavioral treatment of anxiety disorders in children: long-term (6-year) follow-up. J Consult Clin Psychol 69:135–141, 2001

Beidel DC: Social phobia and overanxious disorder in school-age children. J Am Acad Child Adolesc Psychiatry 30:545–552, 1991

Beidel DC, Turner SM: At risk for anxiety, I: psychopathology in the offspring of anxious parents. J Am Acad Child Adolesc Psychiatry 36:918–924, 1997

Bell-Dolan DJ, Last CG, Strauss CC: Symptoms of anxiety disorders in normal children. J Am Acad Child Adolesc Psychiatry 29:759–765, 1990

Berman SL, Weems CF, Silverman WK, et al: Predictors of outcome in exposure-based cognitive and behavioral treatments for phobic and anxiety disorders in children. Behav Ther 31:713–731, 2000

Berney T, Kolvin I, Bhate SR, et al: School phobia: a therapeutic trial with clomipramine and short-term outcome. Br J Psychiatry 138:110–118, 1981

Bernstein GA: Comorbidity and severity of anxiety and depressive disorders in a clinic sample. J Am Acad Child Adolesc Psychiatry 30:43–50, 1991

Bernstein GA, Shaw K: Practice parameters for the assessment and treatment of anxiety disorders. American Academy of Child and Adolescent Psychiatry. J Am Acad Child Adolesc Psychiatry 32:1089–1098, 1993

Bernstein GA, Garfinkel BD, Borchardt CM: Comparative studies of pharmacotherapy for school refusal. J Am Acad Child Adolesc Psychiatry 29:773–781, 1990

Bernstein GA, Borchardt CM, Perwien AR, et al: Imipramine plus cognitive-behavioral therapy in the treatment of school refusal. J Am Acad Child Adolesc Psychiatry 39:276–283, 2000

Biederman J, Rosenbaum JF, Bolduc-Murphy EA, et al: A 3-year follow-up of children with and without behavioral inhibition. J Am Acad Child Adolesc Psychiatry 32:814–821, 1993

Biederman J, Rosenbaum JF, Chaloff J, et al: Behavioral inhibition as a risk factor for anxiety disorders, in Anxiety Disorders in Children and Adolescents. Edited by March JS. New York, Guilford, 1995, pp 61–81

Biederman J, Faraone SV, Hirshfeld-Becker DR, et al: Patterns of psychopathology and dysfunction in high-risk children of parents with panic disorder and major depression. Am J Psychiatry 158:49–57, 2001

Birmaher B, Axelson DA, Monk K, et al; Fluoxetine for the treatment of childhood anxiety disorders. J Am Acad Child Adolesc Psychiatry 42:415–423, 2003

Black B: Separation anxiety disorder and panic disorder, in Anxiety Disorders in Children and Adolescents. Edited by March JS. New York, Guilford, 1995, pp 212–234

Brent DA, Kolko DJ, Birmaher B, et al: Predictors of treatment efficacy in a clinical trial of three psychosocial treatments for adolescent depression. J Am Acad Child Adolesc Psychiatry 37:906–914, 1998

Cobham VE, Dadds MR, Spence SH: The role of parental anxiety in the treatment of childhood anxiety. J Consult Clin Psychol 66:893–905, 1998

Cohen P, Cohen J, Brook J: An epidemiological study of disorders in late childhood and adolescence, II: persistence of disorders. J Child Psychol Psychiatry 34:869–877, 1993

Compton SN, Nelson AH, March JS: Social phobia and separation anxiety symptoms in community and clinical samples of children and adolescents. J Am Acad Child Adolesc Psychiatry 39:1040–1046, 2000

Compton SN, March JS, Brent D, et al: Cognitive-behavioral psychotherapy for anxiety and depressive disorders in children and adolescents: an evidence-based medicine review. J Am Acad Child Adolesc Psychiatry 43:930–959, 2004

Costello EJ, Angold A, Burns BJ, et al: The Great Smoky Mountains study of youth: goals, design, methods, and the prevalence of DSM-III-R disorders. Arch Gen Psychiatry 53:1129–1136, 1996

Costello EJ, Mustillo S, Erkanli A, et al: Prevalence and development of psychiatric disorders in childhood and adolescence. Arch Gen Psychiatry 60:837–844, 2003

Dadds MR, Barrett PM: Practitioner review: psychological management of anxiety disorders in childhood. J Child Psychol Psychiatry 42:999–1011, 2001

Dadds MR, Barrett PM, Rapee RM: Family process and child anxiety and aggression: an observational analysis. J Abnorm Child Psychol 24:715–734, 1996

Dadds MR, Spence SH, Holland DE, et al: Prevention and early intervention for anxiety disorders: a controlled trial. J Consul Clin Psychol 65:627–635, 1997

Dadds MR, Holland DE, Spence SH, et al: Early intervention and prevention of anxiety disorders in children: results at 2-year follow-up. J Consult Clin Psychol 67:145–150, 1999

Daniels D, Plomin RL: Origins of individual differences in shyness. Dev Psychol 21:118–121, 1985

Donovan CL, Spence SH: Prevention of childhood anxiety disorders. Clin Psychol Rev 20:509–531, 2000

Flannery-Schroeder EC, Kendall PC: Group and individual cognitive-behavioral treatments for youth with anxiety disorders: a randomized clinical trial. Cognit Ther Res 24:251–278, 2000

Foley DL, Pickles A, Maes HM, et al: Course and short-term outcomes of separation anxiety disorder in a community sample of twins. J Am Acad Child Adolesc Psychiatry 43:1107–1114, 2004

Gittelman-Klein R, Klein DF: School phobia: diagnostic considerations in the light of imipramine effects. J Nerv Ment Dis 156:199–215, 1973

Graae F, Milner J, Rizzotto L, et al: Clonazepam in childhood anxiety disorders. J Am Acad Child Adolesc Psychiatry 33:372–376, 1994

Guy W: ECDEU Assessment Manual for Psychopharmacology (DHEW Publ No ADM 76-338). Rockville, MD, National Institute of Mental Health, Psychopharmacology Research Branch, 1976

Hamilton M: The assessment of anxiety states by rating. Br J Med Psychol 32:50–55, 1959

Hirshfeld DR, Biederman J, Brody L, et al: Associations between expressed emotion and child behavioral inhibition and psychopathology: a pilot study. J Am Acad Child Adolesc Psychiatry 36:205–213, 1997

Hirshfeld-Becker DR, Biederman J, Faraone SV, et al: Lack of association between behavioral inhibition and psychosocial adversity factors in children at risk for anxiety disorders. Am J Psychiatry 161:547–555, 2004

Hudson JL, Rapee RM: Parent-child interactions and anxiety disorders: an observational study. Behav Res Ther 39:1411–1427, 2001

Kagan J: Galen's Prophecy. New York, Basic Books, 1994

Kagan J, Reznick JS, Snidman N: Biological bases of childhood shyness. Science 240:167–171, 1988

Kagan J, Snidman N: Early childhood predictors of adult anxiety disorders. Biol Psychiatry 46:1536–1541, 1999

Kazdin AE, Kagan J: Models of dysfunction in developmental psychopathology. Clinical Psychology: Science and Practice 1:35–52, 1994

Kearney CA, Sims KE, Pursell CR, et al: Separation anxiety disorder in young children: a longitudinal and family analysis. J Clin Child Adolesc Psychol 32:593–598, 2003

Kendall PC: Coping Cat Workbook. Ardmore, PA, Workbook Publishing, 1990

Kendall PC: Treating anxiety disorders in children: results of a randomized clinical trial. J Consult Clin Psychol 62:100–110, 1994

Kendall PC, Pimentel SS: On the physiological symptom constellation in youth with generalized anxiety disorder (GAD). J Anxiety Disord 17:211–221, 2003

Kendall PC, Southam-Gerow MA: Long-term follow-up of a cognitive-behavioral therapy for anxiety-disordered youth. J Consult Clin Psychol 64:724–730, 1996

Kendall PC, Flannery-Schroeder E, Panich-elli-Mindel SM, et al: Therapy for youths with anxiety disorders: a second randomized clinical trial. J Consult Clin Psychol 65:366–380, 1997

Kendall PC, Brady EU, Verduin TL: Comorbidity in childhood anxiety disorders and treatment outcome. J Am Acad Child Adolesc Psychiatry 40:787–794, 2001

Kendall PC, Safford S, Flannery-Schroeder E, et al: Child anxiety treatment: outcomes in adolescence and impact on substance use and depression at 7.4-year follow-up. J Consult Clin Psychol 72:276–287, 2004

Klein RG, Koplewicz HS, Kanner A: Imipramine treatment of children with separation anxiety disorder. J Am Acad Child Adolesc Psychiatry 31:21–28, 1992

Kutcher S, Reiter S, Gardner D: Pharmacotherapy: approaches and applications, in Anxiety Disorders in Children and Adolescents. Edited by March JS. New York, Guilford, 1995, pp 341–385

Last CG, Perrin S, Hersen M, et al: DSM-III-R anxiety disorders in children: sociodemographic and clinical characteristics. J Am Acad Child Adolesc Psychiatry 31:1070–1076, 1992

Last CG, Perrin S, Hersen M, et al: A prospective study of childhood anxiety disorders. J Am Acad Child Adolesc Psychiatry 35:1502–1510, 1996

Last CG, Hansen C, Franco N: Anxious children in adulthood: a prospective study of adjustment. J Am Acad Child Adolesc Psychiatry 36:645–652, 1997

Last CG, Hansen C, Franco N: Cognitive-behavioral treatment of school phobia. J Am Acad Child Adolesc Psychiatry 37:404–411, 1998

Manassis K, Bradley S: The development of childhood anxiety disorders: toward an integrated model. J Appl Dev Psychol 15:345–366, 1994

Manassis K, Hood J: Individual and familial predictors of impairment in childhood anxiety disorders. J Am Acad Child Adolesc Psychiatry 37:428–434, 1998

Manassis K, Monga S: A therapeutic approach to children and adolescents with anxiety disorders and associated comorbid conditions. J Am Acad Child Adolesc Psychiatry 40:115–117, 2001

Manassis K, Bradley S, Goldberg S, et al: Attachment in mothers with anxiety disorders and their children. J Am Acad Child Adolesc Psychiatry 33:1106–1113, 1994

Manicavasagar V, Silove D, Hadzi-Pavlovic D: Subpopulations of early separation anxiety: relevance to risk of adult anxiety disorders. J Affect Disord 48:181–190, 1998

March JS, Parker JDA, Sullivan K: The Multidimensional Anxiety Scale for Children (MASC): factor structure, reliability, and validity. J Am Acad Child Adolesc Psychiatry 36:554–565, 1997

Martin C, Cabrol S, Bouvard MP, et al: Anxiety and depressive disorders in fathers and mothers of anxious school-refusing children. J Am Acad Child Adolesc Psychiatry 38:916–922, 1999

Masi G, Mucci M, Favilla L, et al: Symptomatology and comorbidity of generalized anxiety disorder in children and adolescents. Compr Psychiatry 40:210–215, 1999

Masi G, Millepiedi S, Mucci M, et al: Generalized anxiety disorder in referred children and adolescents. J Am Acad Child Adolesc Psychiatry 43:752–760, 2004

McGee R, Feehan M, Williams S, et al: DSM-III disorders in a large sample of adolescents. J Am Acad Child Adolesc Psychiatry 29:611–619, 1990

Mendlowitz SL, Manassis K, Bradley S, et al: Cognitive-behavioral group treatments in childhood anxiety disorders: the role of parental involvement. J Am Acad Child Adolesc Psychiatry 38:1223–1229, 1999

Merikangas KR, Dierker LC, Szatmari P: Psychopathology among offspring of parents with substance abuse and/or anxiety disorders: a high-risk study. J Child Psychol Psychiatry 39:711–720, 1998

Merikangas KR, Avenevoli S, Dierker L, et al: Vulnerability factors among children at risk for anxiety disorders. Biol Psychiatry 46:1523–1535, 1999

Muris P, Meesters C, Merckelbach H, et al: Worry in normal children. J Am Acad Child Adolesc Psychiatry 37:703–720, 1998

Muris P, Merckelbach H, Gadet B, et al: Fears, worries, and scary dreams in 4- to 12-year-old children: their content, developmental pattern, and origins. J Clin Child Psychol 29:43–52, 2000

Muris P, Meesters C, van Melick M: Treatment of childhood anxiety disorders: a preliminary comparison between cognitive-behavioral group therapy and a psychological placebo intervention. J Behav Ther Exp Psychiatry 33:143–158, 2002

Nauta MH, Scholing A, Emmelkamp PMG, et al: Cognitive-behavioral therapy for children with anxiety disorders in a clinical setting: no additional effect of a cognitive parent training. J Am Acad Child Adolesc Psychiatry 42:1270–1278, 2003

Pine DS: Treating children and adolescents with selective serotonin reuptake inhibitors: how long is appropriate? J Child Adolesc Psychopharmacol 12:189–203, 2002

Pine DS, Cohen P, Gurley D, et al: The risk for early adulthood anxiety and depressive disorders in adolescents with anxiety and depressive disorders. Arch Gen Psychiatry 55:56–64, 1998

Poulton R, Milne BJ, Craske MG, et al: A longitudinal study of the etiology of separation anxiety. Behav Res Ther 39:1395–1410, 2001

Prior M, Smart D, Sanson A, et al: Does shy-inhibited temperament in childhood lead to anxiety problems in adolescence? J Am Acad Child Adolesc Psychiatry 39:461–468, 2000

Rapee RM: Potential role of childrearing practices in the development of anxiety and depression. Clin Psychol Rev 17:47–67, 1997

Reiter S, Kutcher S: Disinhibition and anger outbursts in adolescents treated with clonazepam (letter). J Clin Psychopharmacol 11:268, 1991

Research Unit on Pediatric Psychopharmacology Anxiety Study Group: Fluvoxamine for the treatment of anxiety disorders in children and adolescents. N Engl J Med 344:1279–1285, 2001

Research Units on Pediatric Psychopharmacology Anxiety Study Group: The Pediatric Anxiety Rating Scale (PARS): development and psychometric properties. J Am Acad Child Adolesc Psychiatry 41:1061–1069, 2002a

Research Units on Pediatric Psychopharmacology Anxiety Study Group: Treatment of pediatric anxiety disorders: an open-label extension of the research units on pediatric psychopharmacology anxiety study. J Child Adolesc Psychopharmacol 12:175–188, 2002b

Riddle MA, Bernstein GA, Cook EH, et al: Anxiolytics, adrenergic agents, and naltrexone. J Am Acad Child Adolesc Psychiatry 38:546–556, 1999

Robinson JL, Kagan J, Reznick JS, et al: The heritability of inhibited and uninhibited behavior: a twin study. Dev Psychol 28:1030–1037, 1992

Rosenbaum JF, Biederman J, Gersten M, et al: Behavioral inhibition in children of parents with panic disorder and agoraphobia. Arch Gen Psychiatry 45:463–470, 1988

Rosenberg DR, Banerjee S, Ivey JL, et al: Psychopharmacology of child and adolescent anxiety disorders. Psychiatric Annals 33:273–278, 2003

Rynn MA, Sigueland L, Rickels K: Placebo-controlled trial of sertraline in the treatment of children with generalized anxiety disorder. Am J Psychiatry 158:2008–2014, 2001

Silverman WK, La Greca AM, Wasserstein S: What do children worry about? Worries and their relation to anxiety. Child Dev 66:671–686, 1995

Silverman WK, Kurtines WM, Ginsburg GS, et al: Treating anxiety disorders in children with group cognitive-behavioral therapy: a randomized clinical trial. J Consult Clin Psychol 67:995–1003, 1999

Simeon JG, Ferguson HB, Knott V, et al: Clinical, cognitive, and neurophysiological effects of alprazolam in children and adolescents with overanxious and avoidant disorders. J Am Acad Child Adolesc Psychiatry 31:29–33, 1992

Siqueland L, Kendall PC, Steinberg L: Anxiety in children: perceived family environments and observed family interaction. J Clin Child Psychol 25:225–237, 1996

Spence SH: Prevention strategies, in The Developmental Psychopathology of Anxiety. Edited by Vasey M, Dadds MR. New York, Oxford University Press, 2001, pp 325–351

Thomas A, Chess S: Temperament and Development. New York, Brunner/Mazel, 1977

Velosa JF, Riddle MA: Pharmacological treatment of anxiety disorders in children and adolescents. Child Adolesc Psychiatr Clin N Am 9:119–133, 2000

Velting ON, Setzer NJ, Albano AM: Update on and advances in assessment and cognitive-behavioral treatment of anxiety disorders in children and adolescents. Professional Psychology: Research and Practice 35:42–54, 2004

Verduin TL, Kendall PC: Differential occurrence of comorbidity within childhood anxiety disorders. J Clin Child Adolesc Psychol 32:290–295, 2003

Warren SL, Huston L, Egeland B, et al: Child and adolescent anxiety disorders and early attachment. J Am Acad Child Adolesc Psychiatry 36:637–644, 1997

Werry JS: Overanxious disorder: a review of its taxonomic properties. J Am Acad Child Adolesc Psychiatry 30:533–544, 1991

Westenberg PM, Siebelink BM, Warmenhoven NJC, et al: Separation anxiety and overanxious disorders: relations to age and level of psychosocial maturity. J Am Acad Child Adolesc Psychiatry 38:1000–1007, 1999

Woodward LJ, Fergusson DM: Life course outcomes of young people with anxiety disorders in adolescence. J Am Acad Child Adolesc Psychiatry 40:1086–1093, 2001

Self-Assessment Questions

Select the single best response for each question.

18.1 Separation anxiety

- A. Begins at age 18 months and peaks at age 30 months.
- B. Is a normative part of development.
- C. Usually indicates the presence of a disorder.
- D. Symptoms are seldom subclinically present in the pediatric population.
- E. Is rarely persistent and excessive.

18.2 Which of the following DSM-IV-TR (American Psychiatric Association 2000) criteria is not required in order to make a diagnosis of generalized anxiety disorder (GAD) in children?

- A. Excessive anxiety and worry for at least a 6-month period.
- B. Difficulty controlling the worry.
- C. Three or more associated physiological symptoms (restlessness, fatigue, difficulty concentrating, irritability, muscle tension, or sleep disturbance).
- D. The focus of the worry is not related to another Axis I condition.
- E. Presence of clinically significant distress or impairment.

18.3 Which of the following statements regarding the epidemiology of GAD and SAD is *true?*

- A. SAD is more prevalent among older children.
- B. GAD is more prevalent among younger children.
- C. Rates of SAD increase with age.
- D. Rates of SAD and GAD do not vary with age.
- E. Rates of GAD increase with age.

18.4 Which of the following statements about temperament and its contributing role to childhood anxiety is *false?*

- A. Approximately 20% of healthy infants are born with traits that predispose them to become highly reactive in novel environments (Kagan and Snidman 1999).
- B. Kagan (1994) described the temperamental characteristic of behavioral inhibition as a child's tendency to approach unfamiliar or novel situations with distress, restraint, or avoidance.
- C. Behavioral inhibition appears to be a highly unstable temperamental trait.
- D. Children with behavioral inhibition may be differentiated from non–behaviorally inhibited children through neurophysiological markers (Kagan et al. 1988).
- E. Children who are identified as shy may be more prone to anxiety symptoms than those who are not (Biederman et al. 1995).

18.5 The use of selective serotonin reuptake inhibitors (SSRIs) in the treatment of childhood anxiety disorders

    A. Is considered a second-line choice (after benzodiazepines).

    B. Has been supported by the results of several recent randomized, placebo-controlled trials.

    C. Should usually continue indefinitely once initiated.

    D. Has resulted in no documented side effects.

    E. Has resulted in minimal clinical benefit over placebo.

Obsessive-Compulsive Disorder

Jennifer B. Freeman, Ph.D.

Abbe M. Garcia, Ph.D.

Susan E. Swedo, M.D.

Judith L. Rapoport, M.D.

Janet S. Ng, B.A.

Henrietta L. Leonard, M.D.

Obsessive-compulsive disorder (OCD) is characterized in DSM-IV-TR (American Psychiatric Association 2000) by recurrent obsessions or compulsions that are severe enough to cause distress or to interfere in one's life. *Obsessions* are defined as persistent thoughts, images, or impulses that are ego-dystonic, intrusive, and, for the most part, senseless. *Compulsions* are "repetitive behaviors...or mental acts...that the person feels driven to perform in response to an obsession" (American Psychiatric Association 2000, p. 462). A change in the diagnostic criteria from DSM-III-R (American Psychiatric Association 1987) to DSM-IV (American Psychiatric Association 1994) and DSM-IV-TR was that younger children do not always recognize their obsessions and compulsions as being excessive or unreasonable.

Diagnostic Criteria

A person with OCD may have either obsessions or compulsions, or both. An individual typically attempts to ignore, suppress, or neutralize the intrusive obsessive thoughts. The specific content of the obsession should not be related to another Axis I diagnosis, such as thoughts about food resulting from an eating disorder or guilty thoughts (ruminations) from depression. Generally, compulsions are performed to dispel anxiety or in response to an obsession (e.g., to ward off harm to someone). An adult recognizes that the behavior is excessive or unreasonable, although this may not always hold true for young children. Obsessions and compulsions must be severe enough to "cause marked distress" or to "significantly interfere with the person's normal routine" (American Psychiatric Association 2000, p. 463).

Clinical Findings

Reports as early as 1903 described salient features of what is now called OCD (Janet 1903). These were observational reports of OCD in children, and it was not until the mid-1980s that OCD was systematically studied in children.

At the National Institute of Mental Health (NIMH), 70 consecutive child and adolescent patients were prospectively examined (Swedo et al. 1989b). These 47 boys and 23 girls met diagnostic criteria for primary severe OCD and had a mean age at onset of 10 years. Boys tended to have an earlier (prepubertal) age at onset, around age 9, whereas girls were more likely to have an onset around puberty, such as age 11. The children with early-onset OCD were also more likely to have a family member with OCD or a tic disorder. Subsequent studies have noted the male predominance in young children, and in adolescence the gender distribution becomes more equal (Geller et al. 1998).

The clinical presentation of OCD in children is generally similar to that in adults (Hanna 1995; Rapoport 1986). One of the first studies to examine OCD in children found that common rituals included excessive cleaning (e.g., hand washing, showering), repeating rituals (e.g., restating phrases, rereading), and checking behaviors (e.g., making sure that doors and windows are locked) (Swedo et al. 1989b). Other common rituals included counting, ordering/arranging, and hoarding. More unusual obsessions included scrupulosity, the preoccupying fear that one might harm oneself or others, and having a tune in the head (Swedo et al. 1989b). Some of the obsessions and rituals involved an internal sense that "it didn't feel right" until the thought or action was completed.

In young children, compulsions without obsessions are common (Geller et al. 1998). Although their symptoms still meet DSM-IV diagnostic criteria, some very young children deny any anxiety or distress in association with their rituals. Children often disguise their rituals until they become so extreme as to be discovered.

The less severely ill patients, and those attempting to hide their symptoms, may be difficult to recognize. Behaviors that suggest a diagnosis of OCD include spending unproductive hours doing homework, erasing excessively (until there are holes in the paper), retracing, and rereading. OCD may also manifest itself in a dramatic increase in laundry volume or toilets becoming clogged from the use of too much paper. Other suspicious behaviors include long, rigid bedtime rituals; an exaggerated need for reassurance; and requests for family members to repeat phrases. Hoarding of useless objects may also be a symptom of OCD. The reader is referred to the practice parameters of the American Academy of Child and Adolescent Psychiatry (1998) as a general guideline for the assessment of children with OCD. The Children's Yale-Brown Obsessive Compulsive Scale (CY-BOCS) (Scahill et al. 1997) symptom checklist is a particularly useful tool for detecting baseline symptoms and studying them over time.

Subtypes

Retrospective analysis has indicated that specific symptom content (e.g., washing vs. checking) is unlikely to provide clues about pediatric subgroups of OCD (Rettew et al. 1992). Current research focuses on whether early-onset or juvenile OCD is a unique subtype of the disorder. Some proposed subtypes, which are neither necessarily distinct nor mutually exclusive, include early-onset, tic-related, and streptococcal-precipitated OCD. Early-onset OCD is associated with male preponderance, comorbidity with attention-deficit/hyperactivity disorder (ADHD) and other disorders, frequent absence of insight, and increased family loading for OCD (Geller et al. 1998). Age at onset may help identify meaningful developmental subtypes of the disorder beyond chronological age (Geller et al. 2001a). Patients with onset of OCD before age 9 are more likely to have the familial subtype of OCD and also are likely to have related tic disorders (Pauls et al. 1995). Adult patients with early onset of symptoms (before age 10) had a higher rate of tic-like compulsions and comorbid tic disorders than did adults with onset of OCD after age 17, suggesting that age at onset may be an important factor in subtyping OCD and that the phenotypical differences were not restricted to childhood (Rosario-Campos et al. 2001). Research in OCD and comorbid tics suggests that such comorbidity may represent a subtype. Patients with OCD and a comorbid tic disorder may be more likely to have compulsions with more sensory phenomena and may need to perform the compulsions until they are "just right" (Leckman et al. 1994).

A different subgroup of children with pediatric onset of either OCD or a tic disorder have been described as having pediatric autoimmune neuropsychiatric disorders associated with streptococcal infection (PANDAS). These children have an abrupt onset of symptoms after becoming infected with group A β-hemolytic streptococcus (GABHS), and their course of illness is characterized by dramatic acute worsening of symptoms with periods of remission (Swedo 1994; Swedo et al. 1998).

The PANDAS subgroup is defined by five clinical characteristics: 1) the presence of OCD or a tic disorder (or both); 2) pre-pubertal symptom onset; 3) dramatic onset and acute exacerbations with an episodic course of symptom severity; 4) temporal association between symptom exacerbations and GABHS infections; and 5) associated neurological abnormalities (Swedo et al. 1998). In a prospective study of school-age children, Murphy and Pichichero (2002) found that a notable feature of the tonsillopharyngitis episode was the lack of severity (sore throats were mild), and none of the patients displayed the typical features of classic severe GABHS tonsillopharyngitis. In follow-up, when recurrence of behavioral symptoms occurred, this sometimes preceded a positive throat culture by 3 days. Delineation of subtypes is important because these children may require a different assessment and treatment (Leckman et al. 1993; Leonard and Swedo 2001; Scahill et al. 2003). When a child has acute onset of OCD or tics or has had a dramatic deterioration, medical illnesses (including seemingly benign upper-respiratory infections) in the previous months should be carefully considered.

Differential Diagnosis

Disorders of depression, anxiety, and eating (anorexia or bulimia) may initially resemble the obsessional behavior of OCD. However, specific obsessions in OCD usually result in a compulsive ritual, and there is no body image disturbance in OCD. Persons with specific phobia are usually fearful only when confronted with the stimuli, unlike people with OCD.

The repetitive stereotypies seen in children with autism, mental retardation, pervasive developmental disorders, or organic brain damage syndromes may superficially resemble rituals in children with OCD; however, unlike stereotypies, the OCD rituals are well organized, complex, and ego-dystonic. In addition, the clinical picture and the accompanying symptoms can help to differentiate between stereotypies and compulsive rituals.

It is sometimes difficult to categorize a behavior as a ritual or a tic. Patients with Tourette's disorder may have associated obsessive-compulsive symptoms or a diagnosis of OCD (Cohen and Leckman 1994; Frankel et al. 1986; Leckman et al. 1993; Leonard et al. 1992). Generally, if an action is preceded by a specific cognition, then it is considered to be a compulsive ritual; however, some complex motor tics may be preceded by a sensation or "urge." Sensory tics are usually not accompanied by anxiety. It may be impossible to distinguish a complex motor tic from a compulsive ritual, especially in patients with both OCD and Tourette's disorder. However, it is important to attempt to make the distinction, because each responds to different treatments. For a more detailed discussion, refer to Leckman et al. (1993).

Epidemiology

One in 200 young people suffers from OCD (Flament et al. 1988). Among adults with OCD, one-third to one-half developed the disorder during childhood or adolescence (Black 1974; Rasmussen and Eisen 1990). These figures suggest that OCD is a relatively common psychiatric disorder in adolescents, perhaps as common as 3% (lifetime) in late adolescence (Zohar et al. 1992). This rate is compatible with the estimated prevalence in the general population (Karno et al. 1988).

In a cross-sectional and longitudinal epidemiological study, Peterson et al. (2001) found that tics and ADHD symptoms were associated with OCD symptoms in late adolescence and early adulthood. In prospective analyses, tics in childhood and early adolescence predicted an increase in OCD in late adolescence and early adulthood.

Etiology

The etiology of OCD is unknown, but several lines of research suggest that it may be the result of a frontal lobe–limbic–basal ganglia dysfunction (Insel 1992; Wise and Rapoport 1989). Evidence supporting neurobiological etiologies include neuroanatomical, neurophysiological, and neuroimmunological associations and metabolic abnormalities. Neurotransmitter dysregulation, genetic susceptibility, and environmental triggers appear to play a role in developing illness. The serotonin hypothesis of OCD is primarily based on the results of treatment studies, which report that the serotonin reuptake inhibitors (SRIs) are specifically efficacious for the treatment of OCD. It is unlikely that the neurotransmitter dysregulation can be attributed to just one system, and others (e.g., dopamine) have also been implicated.

Numerous brain insults that result in basal ganglia damage (e.g., head injury, brain tumors) have been reported to be related to the onset of OCD. Neuroimaging studies reveal that adult patients with OCD who have a history of childhood onset of their illness have decreased size of the caudate nucleus (a principal structure in the basal ganglia) on computed tomographic scans (Luxenberg et al. 1988) and have abnormal patterns of regional glucose metabolism on positron emission tomographic scans compared with a group of control subjects without OCD (Swedo et al. 1989c, 1992).

Perhaps the most exciting work in the field of OCD has been that describing the relationship between OCD and Sydenham's chorea (the neurological variant of rheumatic fever). The incidence of OCD is increased in pediatric patients with Sydenham's chorea. Sydenham's chorea is an autoimmune response in the basal ganglia region caused by misdirected antibodies from a streptococcal infection (Swedo et al.

1989a, 1993). Children with PANDAS may have an underlying pathophysiology similar to that of Sydenham's chorea, although they do not have Sydenham's chorea and the diagnoses are mutually exclusive. This group of children with PANDAS likely represents a genetic vulnerability different from that of later-onset OCD.

It has been hypothesized that tics and OCD may be different manifestations of the same gene or genes (Grados et al. 2001; Pauls et al. 1986). More recently, a mixed model of inheritance has been proposed (Walkup et al. 1995). Family studies of OCD probands have reported that 20% of first-degree relatives (i.e., parents and siblings) of the OCD probands met diagnostic criteria for OCD (Lenane et al. 1990). Interestingly, the OCD symptoms of the relatives usually differed from those of the proband. Pauls et al. (1995) found that children with an onset between ages 5 and 9 years had a much higher rate of family members with tics (suggesting a genetic association).

Treatment

■ Selection of Treatment

The choice of a treatment plan will depend on the individual symptoms and issues of the child and his or her family. Issues of comorbidity and psychosocial stressors will also need to be considered. The expert consensus guidelines (March et al. 1997) and the practice parameters of the American Academy of Child and Adolescent Psychiatry (1998) provide an excellent framework from which to develop the treatment intervention. In general, both guidelines favor cognitive-behavioral therapy (CBT) as the initial treatment, particularly for younger children and for those with milder OCD symptoms and no significant comorbidity. CBT may have more durability than other treatments (although this premise has not been tested in systematic studies),

and obviously it does not have the risks associated with medication. Some suggest that pharmacotherapy could be selected as the initial treatment because of severity of illness, the child's inability to participate in CBT, or the absence of skilled CBT therapists. At this point, the treatment guidelines mentioned above are used, and treatment is often individualized. Only one randomized controlled trial has investigated the relative efficacy of CBT, medication, and combination treatment in OCD (POTS Team 2004). Results suggest that the first line of treatment should be CBT or combined CBT and medication.

■ Behavioral Treatment

Cognitive-behavioral treatments are used clinically with much success (March 1995). Early pediatric case reports suggested that the techniques used with adults (Marks 1987) appeared to be appropriate for children (March et al. 1994; Wolfe and Wolfe 1991). For an excellent review of CBT see Piacentini (1999). Exposure with response prevention (ERP) is the most frequently implemented treatment and may be used in addition to other specific behavioral treatment techniques (e.g., anxiety management training) (March et al. 1994). Habit reversal may play a role in the treatment of the more repetitive complex tic-like rituals (Vitulano et al. 1992).

A structured treatment protocol for children with OCD has been developed as a manual, "How I Ran OCD Off My Land: A Cognitive-Behavioral Program for the Treatment of Obsessive Compulsive Disorder in Children and Adolescents" (March and Mulle 1998; March et al. 1994). This protocol appears to be practical to implement and effective for treatment. Behavior modification therapy may be less successful for patients who have obsessions only (as opposed to both obsessions and compulsions), who are very young, and who are uncooperative.

Small trials treating children and adolescents with CBT with ERP reported 61%–67% improvement at the end of treatment and 51%–62% at follow-up (Franklin et al. 1998; Scahill et al. 1996). The Pediatric OCD Treatment Study (POTS Team 2004) found that CBT with ERP was a more effective treatment for children and adolescents than medication alone. The superiority of CBT to medication monotherapy demonstrates the appropriateness of behavioral treatment for children and adolescents. Thus, CBT should be considered as one of the treatments of choice.

■ Pharmacological Treatment

An increasing body of literature supports the short-term efficacy of the SRI clomipramine and of the selective serotonin reuptake inhibitors (SSRIs) in the treatment of children and adolescents with OCD. Early double-blind, placebo-controlled studies of clomipramine (a tricyclic and an SRI) found that clomipramine was significantly more effect than placebo in decreasing OCD symptoms in children with OCD (Flament et al. 1985; Leonard et al. 1989). To address whether the specificity of the medication was important, a double-blind crossover comparison of clomipramine and desipramine (a selective noradrenergic reuptake blocker) found that clomipramine was significantly better than desipramine in ameliorating the OCD symptoms (Leonard et al. 1989). Similarly, in the large multicenter trial, DeVeaugh-Geiss et al. (1992) reported that clomipramine was superior to placebo for the treatment of OCD in adolescents, and this finding led to the first approval by the U.S. Food and Drug Administration (FDA) of an SRI in pediatric OCD (in children age 10 years and older).

Clomipramine has not been directly compared with an SSRI, and therefore it is not known whether it is more effective than any of the SSRIs. Expert consensus guidelines and clinical experience suggest that clomipramine may be more cost-effective, although it may have a higher rate of discontinuation based on side effects and necessitates periodic administration of electrocardiograms during treatment. It is sometimes used for patients with more treatment-refractory OCD (March et al. 1997, 1998).

With the development and availability of the SSRIs (citalopram, escitalopram, fluoxetine, fluvoxamine, paroxetine, and sertraline), these agents have become popular because of their more tolerable side-effect profile (fewer anticholinergic effects), their relative safety profile in overdoses (in comparison to the tricyclic antidepressants), and the fact that electrocardiographic monitoring is not required. In large systematic trials, fluvoxamine, fluoxetine, and sertraline have each been shown to be superior to placebo for children and adolescents with OCD (Geller et al. 2001b; March 1999; March et al. 1998; Riddle et al. 2001). Sertraline has an FDA-approved indication for the treatment of OCD in children ages 6 years and older, fluoxetine in children ages 7 and older, and fluvoxamine has such approval for children ages 8 years and older. The SSRIs have had only limited pharmacokinetic study in the pediatric age group. A study of sertraline (Alderman et al. 1998) and another study of paroxetine (Findling et al. 1999) found wide intraindividual and interindividual pharmacokinetic variability but generally similar results as those reported in adults.

Fluoxetine and other SSRIs have fewer anticholinergic side effects than the tricyclic antidepressants; however, activation (or agitation) and insomnia may be more common. Generally, the most common side effects seen with the SSRIs include sedation, nausea, diarrhea, insomnia, anorexia, tremor, sexual dysfunction, and hyperstimulation (March et al. 1998; Riddle et al. 2001). It is not known whether children may be more vulnerable to agitation or activation while taking an SSRI than are adults.

Generally, a 12-week trial of an SSRI with adequate dosage is considered necessary. Many patients do not have symptom relief until 6–12 weeks after a trial begins. Evidence has shown that an individual who does not respond to one SRI may respond to another, although a decreasing rate of success with successive trials has been described in the adult literature (March 1999). Most experts would recommend clomipramine after two or three failed SSRI trials (March et al. 1997).

For patients who partially respond to an SSRI, augmentation strategies may be considered. CBT would be a logical choice for augmentation if the patient has not already undergone such treatment. Limited availability in certain areas, severity of illness, and motivation are also factors to consider when recommending CBT. In medication augmentation, clonazepam is occasionally added, but disinhibition, dependence, and tolerance to the medication limit its use (Leonard et al. 1994). An increasing adult literature supports the role of augmentation with a neuroleptic in patients who do not respond or have partial response to SRIs (McDougle et al. 1994). A controlled trial of an SRI demonstrated that the addition of risperidone was superior to placebo in reducing OCD symptoms. Contrary to earlier studies, no differences in response were found between patients with and without comorbid tic or schizotypal personality disorders (McDougle et al. 2000). In one case series, children who did not respond to SRI therapy improved significantly after risperidone was added, and the authors called for controlled trials in this age group (Fitzgerald et al. 1999).

For how long should patients who respond to medication continue to take it? Although periodically decreasing the dosage should be considered, many patients require long-term maintenance therapy. A double-blind study of desipramine substitution in adolescents taking long-term clomipramine therapy found that 8 of 9 patients relapsed when switched to desipramine compared with 2 of 11 who continued taking clomipramine (Leonard et al. 1991). The limited durability of pharmacotherapy, although not well studied, argues for the role of CBT in the treatment of children with OCD.

■ Combined Treatments

On the basis of small trials, March et al. (1994) reported that patients treated with both medications and CBT seemed to have greater improvement and lower relapse rates. The Pediatric OCD Treatment Study (POTS Team 2004) was the first large, systematic trial of combined treatment in children and adolescents. The study investigated the relative efficacy of medication (sertraline) alone, CBT alone, combined CBT and medication, and placebo. The primary outcome measure (percentage change on CY-BOCS) found that combined treatment was superior to both CBT alone and medication alone. Comparing treatments using the rate of clinical remission (CY-BOCS ≥10), combined treatment did not differ from CBT alone, and was significantly better than medication alone and placebo. The remission rate of medication alone did not differ from that for placebo. Results demonstrate that children and adolescents with OCD should begin treatment with CBT alone or the combination of CBT plus an SSRI.

■ Psychodynamic and Psychosocial Treatments

Jenike (1990) reviewed the psychotherapeutic interventions that are available for the treatment of OCD and concluded that "traditional psychodynamic psychotherapy is not an effective treatment for obsessions or rituals in patients meeting criteria for OCD as defined in the DSM-III-R; there are no reports in the modern psychiatric literature of patients who stopped ritualizing when treated with this method alone" (p. 295). Psychodynamic psychotherapy can play an important role by addressing both general and specific issues in the patient's life—such as how OCD affects the individual's self-esteem, personal relationships, and outlook—and by encouraging compliance with the behavior or psychopharmacological therapies that focus more directly on the OCD symptoms. OCD clearly cannot be understood out of context of an individual's feelings, relationships, and past and current experiences. Character styles consistent with "obsessional defenses" and obsessive-compulsive personality are amenable to psychotherapy (for reviews, see Jenike 1990).

Family therapy is an important treatment for pediatric patients with OCD. Family discord, parental marital difficulties, problems of a specific family member, and inappropriate roles or boundaries will interfere with the family's and each member's successful functioning and, ultimately, with the long-term outcome of the identified patient (Hafner et al. 1981; Hoover and Insel 1984; Lenane 1991). A complete family assessment is a necessary part of the initial diagnostic evaluation of every child who has OCD. Lenane (1989) described the goals of family therapy as 1) involving the whole family in treatment, 2) getting all behaviors out in the open, 3) obtaining full and accurate understanding of how everyone participates in the OCD behavior, and 4) reframing of less-than-positive behavior. By dealing with the specific family dynamic issues, the family can participate in the OCD treatment plan of the identified patient in constructive and positive ways. A family-based treatment manual for young children with OCD is currently under development.

■ Investigational Treatments

Children with PANDAS merit a careful assessment of recent medical illnesses, including upper-respiratory infections. Garvey et al. (1999) found that there were no significant differences in severity of OCD or tic symptoms in children with PANDAS treated with penicillin versus those treated with placebo. However, oral penicillin did not provide adequate prophylaxis, and 14 of 35 GABHS infections were diagnosed during active penicillin treatment. The authors concluded that the study did not provide justification for penicillin prophylaxis in children with PANDAS, but they noted that because prophylaxis was not achieved, no conclusion about the efficacy of penicillin prophylaxis for PANDAS could be drawn. Further studies are needed.

Plasma exchange and intravenous immunoglobulin (IVIG) were effective in reducing symptom severity in children with the most severe cases of PANDAS (Perlmutter et al. 1999). However, the authors cautioned that these treatments are investigational and should be considered only in severely ill children with clear evidence of immune dysfunction and in the context of an institutional review board–approved research protocol. Further study of immune dysfunction may help clarify the role of these novel treatments.

Prognosis

In the only follow-up study of an epidemiological sample, Berg et al. (1989) reported that of the 16 adolescents with an initial diagnosis of OCD, 5 (31%) still met criteria at 2-year follow-up, and 4 (25%) had "subclinical" OCD. Interestingly, 2 (13%) of the original patients who had OCD no longer met criteria for OCD but did meet criteria for obsessive-compulsive personality disorder. The relationship between OCD and obsessive-compulsive personality disorder definitely requires additional study.

Follow-up studies of pediatric patients with OCD indicated that at least half of the patients remained symptomatic as adults (Hollingsworth et al. 1980; Warren 1965). Flament et al. (1990) found that of 25 patients seen 2–7 years after initial presentation, 17 (68%) still met diagnostic criteria for OCD, and 12 (48%) had an additional diagnosis (most often depression or anxiety). Only 7 (28%) no longer met DSM-III (American Psychiatric Association 1980) diagnostic criteria for any disorder. Surprisingly, neither baseline measures nor a positive response to clomipramine treatment could predict long-term outcome. These poor results could be explained in part by the fact that this group had not been actively treated during the 2- to 5-year interim period, and only 12 subjects had been taking clomipramine for more than a few months.

The largest and most recent systematic follow-up study of children with OCD took place when the patients had access to the SRIs and to behavior therapy. The 2- to 7-year follow-up study by Leonard et al. (1993) of 54 consecutively admitted children and adolescents with OCD reported that this group seemed to have a somewhat more improved outcome than did the group studied by Flament et al. (1990). Of the 54 subjects, 38 (70%) were taking psychoactive medication at follow-up; 23 patients (43%) still met diagnostic criteria for OCD, and 43 (80%) were improved from baseline. This study suggests that most patients can expect improvement with the new treatments available, but a small group of patients continue to have a chronic and debilitating course.

Research Issues

Several research issues for childhood-onset OCD are important. It is unknown which children respond better to behav-ioral treatment and which respond to drug treatment. It is presumed, but not yet proven, that the availability of these two treatment modalities may improve the long-term prognosis. A long-term comparison is needed to determine relative efficacy and long-term durability.

The identification of a new subtype of pediatric-onset OCD with abrupt onset and dramatic exacerbations (PANDAS group) may lead to new assessment and treatment techniques. It is unknown what percentage of children with OCD may be part of this subgroup. One treatment trial of penicillin prophylaxis for those with exacerbations of GABHS infection has been completed, and large controlled studies are needed. It will be important to determine the percentage of cases of pediatric-onset OCD that are precipitated by streptococcal infection.

The identification, through genetic or biological studies, of children who are at risk for developing OCD is a research priority. If a true subtype is validated, new avenues for genetic studies will emerge. Integrating neuroanatomical and neurological hypotheses with genetic susceptibility and environmental stressor hypotheses remains an important research goal.

References

Alderman J, Wolkow R, Chung M, et al: Sertraline treatment of children and adolescents with obsessive compulsive disorder or depression: pharmacokinetics, tolerability, and efficacy. J Am Acad Child Adolesc Psychiatry 37:386–394, 1998

American Academy of Child and Adolescent Psychiatry: Practice parameters for the assessment and treatment of children and adolescents with obsessive-compulsive disorder. J Am Acad Child Adolesc Psychiatry 37(10, suppl):27S–45S, 1998

American Psychiatric Association: Diagnostic and Statistical Manual of Mental Disorders, 3rd Edition. Washington, DC, American Psychiatric Association, 1980

American Psychiatric Association: Diagnostic and Statistical Manual of Mental Disorders, 3rd Edition, Revised. Washington, DC, American Psychiatric Association, 1987

American Psychiatric Association: Diagnostic and Statistical Manual of Mental Disorders, 4th Edition. Washington, DC, American Psychiatric Association, 1994

American Psychiatric Association: Diagnostic and Statistical Manual of Mental Disorders, 4th Edition, Text Revision. Washington, DC, American Psychiatric Association, 2000

Berg CZ, Rapoport JL, Whitaker A, et al: Childhood obsessive-compulsive disorder: a two-year prospective follow-up of a community sample. J Am Acad Child Adolesc Psychiatry 28:528–533, 1989

Black A: The natural history of obsessional neurosis, in Obsessional States. Edited by Beech HR. London, Methuen, 1974, pp 1–23

Cohen DJ, Leckman JF: Developmental psychopathology and neurobiology of Tourette's syndrome. J Am Acad Child Adolesc Psychiatry 33:2–15, 1994

DeVeaugh-Geiss J, Moroz G, Biederman J, et al: Clomipramine hydrochloride in childhood and adolescent obsessive-compulsive disorder: a multicenter trial. J Am Acad Child Adolesc Psychiatry 31:45–49, 1992

Findling RL, Reed MD, Myers C, et al: Paroxetine pharmacokinetics in depressed children and adolescents. J Am Acad Child Adolesc Psychiatry 38:952–959, 1999

Fitzgerald KD, Stewart CM, Tawile V, et al: Risperidone augmentation of serotonin reuptake inhibitor treatment of pediatric obsessive compulsive disorder. J Child Adolesc Psychopharmacol 9:115–123, 1999

Flament MF, Rapoport JL, Berg CJ, et al: Clomipramine treatment of childhood obsessive-compulsive disorder. Arch Gen Psychiatry 42:977–983, 1985

Flament MF, Whitaker A, Rapoport JL, et al: Obsessive compulsive disorder in adolescence: an epidemiological study. J Am Acad Child Adolesc Psychiatry 27:764–771, 1988

Flament MF, Koby E, Rapoport JL, et al: Childhood obsessive compulsive disorder: a prospective follow-up study. J Child Psychol Psychiatry 31:363–380, 1990

Frankel M, Cummings JL, Robertson MM, et al: Obsessions and compulsions in Gilles de la Tourette's syndrome. Neurology 36:378–382, 1986

Franklin ME, Kozak MJ, Cashman LA, et al: Cognitive-behavioral treatment of pediatric obsessive-compulsive disorder: an open clinical trial. J Am Acad Child Adolesc Psychiatry 37:412–419, 1998

Garvey MA, Perlmutter SJ, Allen AJ, et al: A pilot study of penicillin prophylaxis for neuropsychiatric exacerbations triggered by streptococcal infections. Biol Psychiatry 45:1564–1571, 1999

Geller DA, Biederman J, Jones J, et al: Is juvenile obsessive-compulsive disorder a developmental subtype of the disorder? A review of the pediatric literature. J Am Acad Child Adolesc Psychiatry 37:420–427, 1998

Geller DA, Biederman J, Faraone SV, et al: Disentangling chronological age from age of onset in children and adolescents with obsessive-compulsive disorder. Int J Neuropsychopharmacol 4:169–178, 2001a

Geller DA, Hoog SL, Heiligenstein JH, et al: Fluoxetine treatment for obsessive-compulsive disorder in children and adolescents: a placebo-controlled clinical trial. J Am Acad Child Adolesc Psychiatry 40:773–779, 2001b

Grados MA, Riddle MA, Samuels JF, et al: The familial phenotype of obsessive-compulsive disorder in relation to tic disorders: the Hopkins OCD family study. Biol Psychiatry 50:559–565, 2001

Hafner RJ, Gilchrist P, Bowling J, et al: The treatment of obsessional neurosis in a family setting. Aust N Z J Psychiatry 15:145–151, 1981

Hanna GL: Demographic and clinical features of obsessive-compulsive disorder in children and adolescents. J Am Acad Child Adolesc Psychiatry 34:19–27, 1995

Hollingsworth CE, Tanguey PE, Grossman L, et al: Long-term outcome of obsessive compulsive disorder in children. J Am Acad Child Psychiatry 19:134–144, 1980

Hoover CF, Insel TR: Families of origin in obsessive compulsive disorder. J Nerv Ment Dis 172:207–215, 1984

Insel TR: Toward a neuroanatomy of obsessive-compulsive disorder. Arch Gen Psychiatry 49:739–744, 1992

Janet P: Les Obsessions et la Psychasthenie [Obsessions and Psychasthenia], Vol 1. Paris, Felix Alan, 1903

Jenike MA: Psychotherapy of obsessive-compulsive personality disorder, in Obsessive-Compulsive Disorders: Theory and Management. Edited by Jenike MA, Baer L, Minichiello WE. Chicago, IL, Year Book Medical, 1990, pp 295–305

Karno B, Golding J, Sorenson S, et al: The epidemiology of obsessive compulsive disorder in five U.S. communities. Arch Gen Psychiatry 45:1094–1099, 1988

Leckman JF, Walker DE, Cohen DJ: Premonitory urges in Tourette's syndrome. Am J Psychiatry 150:98–102, 1993

Leckman JF, Walker DE, Goodman WK, et al: "Just right" perceptions associated with compulsive behavior in Tourette's syndrome. Am J Psychiatry 151:675–680, 1994

Lenane M: Families and obsessive-compulsive disorder, in Obsessive-Compulsive Disorder in Children and Adolescents. Edited by Rapoport JL. Washington, DC, American Psychiatric Press, 1989, pp 237–249

Lenane M: Family therapy for children with obsessive compulsive disorder, in Current Treatments of Obsessive-Compulsive Disorder. Edited by Pato MT, Zohar M. Washington, DC, American Psychiatric Press, 1991, pp 103–113

Lenane MC, Swedo SE, Leonard HL, et al: Psychiatric disorders in first degree relatives of children and adolescents with obsessive compulsive disorder. J Am Acad Child Adolesc Psychiatry 29:407–412, 1990

Leonard HL, Swedo SE: Paediatric autoimmune neuropsychiatric disorders associated with streptococcal infection (PANDAS). Int J Neuropsychopharmacol 4:191–198, 2001

Leonard HL, Swedo S, Rapoport JL, et al: Treatment of obsessive compulsive disorder with clomipramine and desipramine in children and adolescents: a double-blind crossover comparison. Arch Gen Psychiatry 46:1088–1092, 1989

Leonard HL, Swedo SE, Lenane MC, et al: A double-blind desipramine substitution during long-term clomipramine treatment in children and adolescents with obsessive compulsive disorder. Arch Gen Psychiatry 48:922–926, 1991

Leonard HL, Lenane MC, Swedo SE, et al: Tics and Tourette's syndrome: a 2- to 7-year follow-up of 54 obsessive compulsive children. Am J Psychiatry 149:1244–1251, 1992

Leonard HL, Swedo SE, Lenane MC, et al: A 2- to 7-year follow-up study of 54 obsessive compulsive children and adolescents. Arch Gen Psychiatry 50:429–439, 1993

Leonard HL, Topol D, Bukstein O, et al: Clonazepam as an augmenting agent in the treatment of childhood onset obsessive compulsive disorder. J Am Acad Child Adolesc Psychiatry 33:792–794, 1994

Luxenberg JS, Swedo SE, Flament MF, et al: Neuroanatomical abnormalities in obsessive-compulsive disorder detected with quantitative X-ray computed tomography. Am J Psychiatry 145:1089–1093, 1988

March J: Cognitive-behavioral psychotherapy for children and adolescents with obsessive-compulsive disorder: a review and recommendations for treatment. J Am Acad Child Adolesc Psychiatry 1:7–18, 1995

March J: Current status of pharmacotherapy for pediatric anxiety disorders, in Treating Anxiety Disorders in Youth: Current Problems and Future Solutions (ADAA/NIMH). Edited by Beidel D. Washington, DC, Anxiety Disorders Association of America, 1999, pp 42–62

March JS, Mulle K: OCD in Children and Adolescents: A Cognitive-Behavioral Treatment Manual. New York, Guilford, 1998

March J, Mulle K, Herbel B: Behavioral psychotherapy for children and adolescents with obsessive-compulsive disorder: an open trial of a new protocol driven treatment package. J Am Acad Child Adolesc Psychiatry 33:333–341, 1994

March J, Frances A, Kahn D, et al: Expert consensus guidelines: treatment of obsessive-compulsive disorder. J Clin Psychiatry 58 (suppl 4):1–72, 1997

March JS, Biederman J, Wolkow R, et al: Sertraline in children and adolescents with obsessive-compulsive disorder: a multicenter randomized controlled trial. JAMA 280:1752–1756, 1998

Marks IM: Fears, Phobias and Rituals: Panic Anxiety and Their Disorders. New York, Oxford University Press, 1987

McDougle C, Goodman W, Leckman J, et al: Haloperidol addition in fluvoxamine-refractory obsessive-compulsive disorder: a double-blind, placebo-controlled study in patients with and without tics. Arch Gen Psychiatry 5:302–308, 1994

McDougle CJ, Naylor ST, Cohen CJ, et al; A double-blind, placebo-controlled study of risperidone addition to serotonin re-uptake inhibitor-refractory obsessive-compulsive disorder. Arch Gen Psychiatry 57:794–801, 2000

Murphy ML, Pichichero ME: Prospective identification and treatment of children with pediatric autoimmune neuropsychiatric disorder associated with group A streptococcal infection (PANDAS). Arch Pediatr Adolesc Med 156:356–361, 2002

Pauls DL, Towbin K, Leckman J, et al: Gilles de la Tourette syndrome and obsessive compulsive disorder: evidence supporting a genetic relationship. Arch Gen Psychiatry 43:1180–1182, 1986

Pauls DL, Alsobrook JP, Goodman W, et al: A family study of obsessive compulsive disorder. Am J Psychiatry 1:76–84, 1995

Perlmutter SJ, Leitman SF, Garvey MA, et al: Therapeutic plasma exchange and intravenous immunoglobulin for obsessive compulsive disorder and tic disorders in childhood. Lancet 354:1153–1158, 1999

Peterson BS, Pine DS, Cohen P, et al: Prospective, longitudinal study of tic, obsessive-compulsive, and attention-deficit/hyperactivity disorders in an epidemiological sample. J Am Acad Child Adolesc Psychiatry 40:685–695, 2001

Piacentini J: Cognitive behavioral therapy of childhood OCD. Child Adolesc Psychiatr Clin N Am 8:599–616, 1999

POTS Team: Cognitive-behavior therapy, sertraline, and their combination for children and adolescents with obsessive-compulsive disorder. JAMA 292:1969–1976, 2004

Rapoport JL: Annotation, child obsessive-compulsive disorder. J Child Psychol Psychiatry 27:285–289, 1986

Rasmussen S, Eisen J: Epidemiology of obsessive compulsive diosrder. J Clin Psychiatry 51:10–13, 1990

Rettew DC, Swedo SE, Leonard HL, et al: Obsessions and compulsions across time in 79 children and adolescents with obsessive-compulsive disorder. J Am Acad Child Adolesc Psychiatry 31:1050–1056, 1992

Riddle M, Reeve E, Yaryura-Tobias J, et al: Fluvoxamine for children and adolescents with obsessive compulsive disorder: a randomized controlled multicenter trial. J Am Acad Child Adolesc Psychiatry, 40:222–229, 2001

Rosario-Campos MC, Leckman JF, Mercadante MT, et al: Adults with early onset obsessive-compulsive disorder. Am J Psychiatry 158:1899–1903, 2001

Scahill L, Vitulano LA, Brenner EM, et al: Behavioral therapy in children and adolescents with obsessive-compulsive disorder: a pilot study. J Child Adolesc Psychopharmacol 6:191–202, 1996

Scahill L, Riddle MA, McSwiggin-Hardin M, et al: Children's Yale-Brown Obsessive Compulsive Scale: reliability and validity. J Am Acad Child Adolesc Psychiatry 36:844–852, 1997

Scahill L, Kano Y, King R, et al: Influences of age and tic disorders on obsessive-compulsive disorder in a pediatric sample. J Child Adolesc Psychopharmcol 13:S7–S17, 2003

Swedo SE: Sydenham's chorea: a model for childhood autoimmune neuropsychiatric disorders. JAMA 272:1788–1791, 1994

Swedo SE, Rapoport JL, Cheslow DL, et al: High prevalence of obsessive-compulsive symptoms in patients with Sydenham's chorea. Am J Psychiatry 146:246–249, 1989a

Swedo S, Rapoport JL, Leonard HL, et al: Obsessive-compulsive disorder in children and adolescents: clinical phenomenology of 70 consecutive cases. Arch Gen Psychiatry 46:335–341, 1989b

Swedo SE, Schapiro MB, Grady CL, et al: Cerebral glucose metabolism in childhood-onset obsessive compulsive disorder. Arch Gen Psychiatry 46:518–523, 1989c

Swedo SE, Pietrini P, Leonard HL, et al: Cerebral glucose metabolism in childhood-onset obsessive compulsive disorder: revisualization during pharmacotherapy. Arch Gen Psychiatry 49:690–694, 1992

Swedo SE, Leonard HL, Schapiro MB, et al: Sydenham's chorea: physical and psychological symptoms of St. Vitus's dance. Pediatrics 91:706–713, 1993

Swedo SE, Leonard HL, Garvey M, et al: Pediatric autoimmune neuropsychiatric disorders associated with streptococcal infections: clinical description of the first 50 cases. Am J Psychiatry 155:264–271, 1998

Vitulano LA, King RA, Scahill L, et al: Behavioral treatment of children and adolescents with trichotillomania. J Am Acad Child Adolesc Psychiatry 31:139–146, 1992

Walkup JT, LaBuda MJ, Hurko O, et al: Evidence for a mixed model of inheritance in Tourette's syndrome. Paper presented at the 42nd annual meeting of the American Academy of Child and Adolescent Psychiatry, New Orleans, LA, October 21, 1995

Warren W: A study of adolescent psychiatric inpatients and the outcome six or more years later. J Child Psychol Psychiatry 6:141–160, 1965

Wise SP, Rapoport JL: Obsessive-compulsive disorder: is it basal ganglia dysfunction? in Obsessive-Compulsive Disorder in Children and Adolescents. Edited by Rapoport JL. Washington, DC, American Psychiatric Press, 1989, pp 327–344

Wolfe RP, Wolfe LS: Assessment and treatment of obsessive compulsive disorder in children. Behav Modif 15:372–393, 1991

Zohar AH, Ratzoni G, Pauls DL, et al: An epidemiological study of obsessive-compulsive disorder and related disorders in Israeli adolescents. J Am Acad Child Adolesc Psychiatry 31:1057–1061, 1992

Self-Assessment Questions

Select the single best response for each question.

19.1 According to studies conducted by Geller et al. (1998) and Swedo et al. (1989), which of the following epidemiological findings related to obsessive-compulsive disorder (OCD) is *false?*

A. Girls tended to have an earlier age at onset.

B. In young children, there was a male predominance (male-to-female ratio: 3 to 2).

C. The mean age at onset was 10 years.

D. Children with early-onset OCD were more likely to have a family member with OCD.

E. In adolescence, the gender distribution between girls and boys with OCD was about equal.

19.2 Which of the following is *not* a proposed subtype of OCD in children?

A. Early-onset OCD.

B. Late-onset OCD.

C. Tic-related OCD.

D. Streptococcal-precipitated OCD.

E. None of the above.

19.3 Several lines of neuroscience research have implicated, as a cause for OCD, a dysfunction in which brain structure?

A. Hippocampus.

B. Amygdala.

C. Basal ganglia.

D. Dorsal lateral prefrontal cortex.

E. Substantia nigra.

19.4 Recent research supports the addition of which of the following pharmacological agents as an appropriate augmentation to a selective serotonin reuptake inhibitor (SSRI)?

A. Lithium.

B. Imipramine.

C. Lamotrigine.

D. Bupropion.

E. Risperidone.

19.5 In the largest and most recent systematic follow-up study of children with OCD being treated with SSRIs and behavior therapy (Leonard et al. 1993), what percentage still met diagnostic criteria for OCD 2–7 years after initial presentation?

A. 17%.

B. 28%.

C. 43%.

D. 68%.

E. 82%.

Specific Phobia, Panic Disorder, Social Phobia, and Selective Mutism

Abbe M. Garcia, Ph.D.

Jennifer B. Freeman, Ph.D.

Chelsea M. Ale, A.B.

Bruce Black, M.D.

Henrietta L. Leonard, M.D.

Definitions

According to DSM-IV-TR (American Psychiatric Association 2000), specific phobia is a marked and persistent fear of circumscribed objects or situations (phobic stimuli), such as animals, blood, heights, closed spaces, or flying. The fear is excessive or unreasonable. Exposure to the phobic stimuli provokes an immediate anxiety response.

Panic disorder is characterized by recurrent, unexpected panic attacks, which are discrete periods of "intense fear or discomfort" accompanied by specific somatic symptoms and associated with characteristic sequelae such as fear and worry (American Psychiatric Association 2000).

Social phobia (or social anxiety disorder) involves a persistent fear of one or more social situations in which a person is exposed to unfamiliar persons or to scrutiny by others. Exposure to the feared social situations provokes marked anxiety (American Psychiatric Association 2000).

Selective mutism is characterized by persistent failure to speak in one or more major social situations in which speaking is expected, despite speaking in other situations. Although selective mutism is not classified as an anxiety disorder in DSM-IV-TR, a growing body of research has demonstrated that it is primarily a manifestation of social anxiety.

Diagnostic Criteria

Specific phobia is a "marked and persistent fear that is excessive or unreasonable, cued by the presence or anticipation of a specific object or situation" (American Psychiatric Association 2000, p. 449) that provokes immediate anxiety. The anxiety response may be accompanied by a variety of somatic symptoms or, in children, may be expressed by crying, tantrums, freezing, or clinging. To meet DSM-IV-TR criteria, the avoidance, anxious anticipation, or distress in the feared situation must interfere with a person's normal routine, social relationships, or academic (or occupational) functioning, or there must be marked distress about having the fear. The stimulus is either avoided or endured with intense anxiety. By definition, adults recognize that the fear is excessive or unreasonable, although children may not.

To meet the DSM-IV-TR criteria for *panic disorder,* an individual must have recurrent, unexpected panic attacks, as well as at least a month of persistent concern about having additional attacks, worry about the implications of the attacks (e.g., somatic preoccupations), or other behavioral changes related to the attacks.

Panic attacks are the hallmark of panic disorder, but they are also associated with other anxiety disorders (including specific phobia, social phobia, obsessive-compulsive disorder, and posttraumatic stress disorder). Panic attacks are discrete periods of fear or discomfort that develop abruptly and reach a peak rapidly and are associated with specific somatic and psychic symptoms. Panic attacks may be unexpected or uncued, situationally bound (cued), or situationally predisposed. Unexpected panic attacks are required for the diagnosis of panic disorder. Situationally bound panic attacks are more characteristic of specific phobia and social pho-

bia. Situationally predisposed panic attacks are common in panic disorder but also occur in individuals with specific phobia and social phobia.

Panic disorder may occur either with or without agoraphobia. Agoraphobia is characterized by "anxiety about being in places or situations from which escape might be difficult (or embarrassing) or in which help may not be available in the event of having a panic attack or panic-like symptoms" (American Psychiatric Association 2000, p. 432), as well as pervasive avoidance of the feared situations. Agoraphobia may also occur without a history of panic disorder.

To meet DSM-IV-TR diagnostic criteria for *social phobia,* the feared social situation or situations must elicit marked anxiety, resulting in interference with functioning or marked distress about experiencing the fear. Commonly feared situations include speaking in front of others, attending social gatherings, dealing with authority figures, performing in public, and speaking to strangers. As with specific phobia, adults recognize that the fear is excessive or unreasonable, but children may not.

Selective mutism is diagnosed in children who fail to speak in specific social situations for at least 1 month (not limited to the first month of school) and when the disturbance significantly interferes with educational or social functioning.

Clinical Findings

■ Specific Phobia

Many children have fears and anxieties; determining at what point the anxiety becomes "clinical" can be a fine distinction. Lapouse and Monk (1959) reported that 43% of interviewed mothers acknowledged that their children had seven or more fears. Ollendick (1983) reported that in 217 children, ages 3–11 years, the average number of extreme fears ranged from 9 to 13. The numerous general fears and anxieties of children decrease with age, and the specific focus of the fears changes (Evans et al. 1997; Graziano et al. 1979; Gullone 2000).

In examining the fears of children and adolescents, it is important to maintain a developmental perspective, because some fears are common and appropriate at young ages. (An excellent review of the development of fears in children and adolescents is available in Marks 1987.) Infants' fears diminish during the preschool years. Preschool children are typically afraid of strangers, the dark, animals, or imaginary creatures. Children of elementary school age are more likely to be afraid of animals, darkness, threats to their own safety, or thunder and lightning. Older children are more concerned with health, social, and school fears. Adolescent fears may focus more on failure, sex, or agoraphobia (Marks 1987). If the fears persist into older ages or if there is significant and persistent distress or functional impairment, then clinical evaluation is indicated.

Specified in DSM-IV-TR are five subtypes of specific phobia: 1) animal type, 2) natural environment type (e.g., fears of storms, heights, or water), 3) blood-injection-injury type, 4) situational type (fear cued by specific situations such as tunnels, bridges, flying, or driving), and 5) other type. Animal type, natural environment type, and blood-injection-injury type all usually begin in childhood. Situational type has a bimodal onset, with one peak in childhood and another in early adulthood. Situational type appears to be closely related to panic disorder with agoraphobia (Verburg et al. 1994).

School phobia is sometimes used broadly with reference to children who refuse or resist going to school for any reason. In fact, children may resist going to school for a variety of reasons, including specific phobia, another anxiety disorder, depression, conduct disorder (truancy), substance abuse, or family psychopathology. A more precise use of the term *school phobia* would be restricted to describing a child's fear of something specific about the school situation, such as a specific teacher or peer, taking a shower after physical education class, or something encountered on the way to school (Black 1995).

■ Panic Disorder

Panic disorder with or without agoraphobia most often begins in adolescence or early adult life but may develop at any age (Abelson and Alessi 1992; Nelles and Barlow 1988). Many cases of both prepubertal and adolescent-onset panic disorder have now been described in the clinical literature (Biederman et al. 1997; Black 1995; Black and Robbins 1990; Black et al. 1990; Diler et al. 2004; King et al. 1993, 1997; Moreau and Weissman 1992). Likewise, several studies of adults with panic disorder have reported that many patients recalled the onset to be in childhood or adolescence (Thyer et al. 1985; von Korff et al. 1985).

The symptoms, course, and associated complications and comorbid conditions (agoraphobia, depression) in children and adolescents with panic disorder appear to be very similar to those observed in adults with panic disorder. The most commonly reported symptoms among adolescents with panic attacks are trembling, dizziness or faintness, pounding heart, nausea, shortness of breath, and sweating (Kearney et al. 1997). Cognitive symptoms are reported less frequently than somatic ones (King et al. 1997).

Panic attacks are associated with an increased likelihood of a range of affective and anxiety disorders (Diler et al. 2004; Goodwin and Gotlib 2004). Comorbid separation anxiety disorder is an important and common feature in children and adolescents (Black 1995). It is not uncommon for individuals with panic disorder at any age to fear and avoid separation from attachment figures. For adults, these attachment figures are most commonly spouses, parents, or close friends, whereas for children the figure is usually a parent. As suggested by Black et al. (1990), symptoms of separation anxiety disorder may develop in response to panic attacks and may be viewed as "manifestations of agoraphobia, with specific features (e.g., fear of school, fear of not being able to contact a parent *in the event of a panic attack*) that one might expect to see in an agoraphobic child" (p. 835). In fact, it is difficult to imagine how a child could experience recurrent panic attacks and not develop full-blown symptoms of separation anxiety disorder. The extreme distress that the child manifests when separation is threatened or imminent may be seen as a situationally predisposed panic attack.

Children with early development of separation anxiety disorder are at increased risk for later development of panic disorder (Biederman et al. 1993b). Most children described in the clinical literature with prepubertal onset of panic disorder—as well as many adolescents with panic disorder—also manifest symptoms of separation anxiety disorder, which are commonly the primary presenting symptoms (Black 1995). An association between adult-onset panic disorder and childhood anxiety, specifically separation anxiety disorder, has also been noted (Gittelman and Klein 1984). Klein (1964) stated that half of a sample of female adult patients with panic and agoraphobia had a history of separation anxiety or school phobia. The agoraphobic adults with a history of school phobia had an earlier age at onset for the agoraphobia than did those without this history. Offspring of parents with panic disorder have a more than threefold increased risk for separation anxiety disorder (Leckman et al. 1985; Weissman et al. 1984).

The exact explanation for the relationship between panic disorder and separation anxiety disorder is not clear. The childhood anxiety and avoidance symptoms might represent early manifestations of the same disorder, might predispose the adult to develop agoraphobia, or might reflect some more common anxiety symptomatology (Klein 1964). Several investigators have suggested that panic disorder and separation anxiety disorder may be different clinical manifestations of a common underlying disorder (Abelson and Alessi 1992; Black and Robbins 1990; Klein 1981). For individuals with childhood separation anxiety disorder, the vulnerability to develop excessive distress when attachments are disrupted or threatened may be a stable personality trait throughout childhood and adolescence and into adulthood (Black 1995). Both anxiety symptoms (as manifested by separation anxiety and panic attacks) and depressive symptoms are expressed only when the separation or threat of separation actually occurs. Several studies have found an increased incidence of death or severe illness of a loved one preceding the onset of panic disorder in adults (Roy-Byrne et al. 1986) and adolescents (Black and Robbins 1990; Bradley and Hood 1993), as well as in children with separation anxiety disorder (Costello 1989). A heightened vulnerability to behavioral manifestations of separation distress has also been shown to be a relatively stable trait in nonhuman primates (Suomi et al. 1981). Recent work using a carbon dioxide inhalation procedure with children and adolescents suggests that child anxiety disorders in general and separation anxiety disorder in particular may share pathophysiological features with adult panic disorder (Pine et al. 2000).

■ Social Phobia

The primary features of social phobia are fearful apprehension, distress, and somatic symptoms in social situations in which the individual must interact with new or unfamiliar persons; fears of being evaluated or of being the center of attention; or fears that he or she might be embarrassed in some way. Individuals with social phobia commonly fear that others will find some fault with them; that others will consider them weird, unattractive, or stupid; or that they will do or say something foolish or embarrassing. Somatic symptoms are common and include racing heart, sweating, blushing, tremulousness, light-headedness, and diarrhea. These symptoms may be indistinguishable from a full-blown panic attack. Individuals with social phobia may fear that others will notice the somatic manifestations of their anxiety—such as tremulousness, sweating, or blushing—and that this will cause further embarrassment or ridicule.

Individuals with social phobia may fear one, several, or a wide variety of specific social situations. The most commonly feared situations are public speaking or performing, attending social gatherings, dealing with authority figures, and social interactions such as speaking to strangers or asking directions. Although some individuals with social phobia have very circumscribed fears, such as eating or writing in public or using public restrooms, most fear or avoid many different types of social situations. This clinical finding is part of the rationale that underlies the current trend in the field to refer to this set of symptoms as social anxiety disorder rather than as social phobia (Liebowitz et al. 2000).

Avoidant personality disorder is a closely related diagnostic category that is characterized by "a pervasive pattern of social inhibition, feelings of inadequacy, and hypersensitivity to negative evaluation" (American Psychiatric Association 2000, p. 721). There have been fewer empirical studies of avoidant personality disorder, and the validity of avoidant personality disorder as a distinct diagnostic category has been debated (Turner et al. 1992). The DSM-IV-TR diagnostic criteria for avoidant personality disorder include a pattern of enduring personality characteristics, whereas the DSM-IV-TR criteria for social phobia are more symptom focused. Empirical studies have shown considerable overlap between the two disorders; that is, many individuals meet criteria for both disorders.

An increasing number of studies are documenting the characteristics of children and adolescents with social phobia (Beidel 1991; Beidel et al. 1999; Black 1996; Francis et al. 1992; Last et al. 1987, 1992; Spence et al. 1999; Strauss and Last 1993). These studies have found that the disorder is valid, is not uncommon in clinic populations, and is associated with significant impairment. Significant comorbidity with other anxiety disorders and a high incidence of fear and avoidance of school have also been reported. More in-depth coverage of these issues can be found in the excellent review of the literature on the phenomenology, etiology, and treatment of social anxiety disorder in children and adolescents by Kashdan and Herbert (2001).

Young children with social phobia may cry, have a tantrum, or cling to or hide behind their mothers when confronted with a feared social situation, and they may be reluctant to attend school. Adolescents with social phobia may have great difficulty with dating or establishing any relationships with members of the opposite sex. Children and adolescents with social phobia may avoid participation in classroom activities, avoid class presentations, do poorly on tests or in presentations, and avoid physical education class. Generalized anxiety, multiple specific fears, somatization, school avoidance, and minor obsessive-compulsive symptoms are not uncommon (Beidel and Morris 1995; Black 1996; Francis et al. 1992). Children and adolescents with social phobia have significantly poorer social skills than psychiatrically healthy children (Beidel et al. 1999). Adolescents and young adults with social phobia may drop out of school or college or avoid classes in which classroom participation or presentation would be required. Occupational development may be impaired because of an inability to tolerate or to do well in job interviews or in social interactions at work. Individuals with social phobia have an increased incidence of alcohol abuse in adolescence and early adulthood, more suicidal ideation and suicide attempts, more physical and mental health problems, and greater use of health services than do individuals without social phobia (DeWit et al. 1999; Schneier et al. 1992; Uhde et al. 1991). Alcohol abuse seems to develop after the youth with social phobia discovers (accurately) that alcohol greatly reduces anxiety and facilitates peer interactions such as dating and attending parties (Clark et al. 1995).

■ Selective Mutism

The defining feature of selective mutism is the absence of speech (or an extreme reluctance to speak) in specific social situations in a child who is able to and does so in other situations (Dow et al. 1995). However, social situations are not easily dichotomized into mute and nonmute situations. Rather, the severity of mutism varies across a spectrum from situations in which speech is completely avoided to situations in which speech is completely uninhibited, not unlike the spectrum of social anxiety reported by persons with social phobia.

In a study of 30 school-referred children with selective mutism, Black and Uhde (1995) found that the severity of mutism varies among different types of social interactions, ranging from no reluctance to speak to siblings in the home to an almost complete avoidance of speech with unfamiliar adults at school. The children studied were significantly more reluctant to speak when away from home than at home (and most reluctant to speak at school), were more reluctant to speak to adults than to children, were more reluctant to speak to familiar nonfamily persons than to immediate family members, and were most reluctant to speak to unfamiliar nonfamily individuals. Although most children with selective mutism are markedly reluctant to speak with clinicians, the severity of mutism shown by the child in the clinician's office is not an accurate measure of the child's mutism severity in other settings or of his or her degree of improvement during the course of treatment (Black and Uhde 1995).

Some children with selective mutism will not communicate at all in their mute situations, whereas others may use gestures, head nodding or shaking, or whispering (Steinhausen and Juzi 1996). As children with selective mutism improve, many progress through stages, from virtually no social communication, to communicative facial gestures (e.g., communicative smiling), to gestures such as head-nodding, to limited whispering to more widespread whispering, and finally to normal social speech. Others make more abrupt jumps. Because social communication is intrinsically rewarding, once a mute, noncommunicative child starts to communicate more, his or her improvement is strongly reinforced. Therefore, it is not uncommon that a child will make no progress or very limited progress for very extended periods and then progress to normal social speech in a matter of days, as if a dam had finally broken.

Shyness, fear of embarrassment, and social withdrawal have been commonly mentioned as characteristics of children with selective mutism (Black and Uhde 1992; Kolvin and Fundudis 1981; Tancer 1992). Systematic assessment of children with selective mutism has revealed that nearly every child with selective mutism also meets criteria for either social phobia or avoidant disorder (Black and Uhde 1995; Dummit et al. 1997). In these investigations, social anxiety was the only behavioral feature (other than failure to speak) that stood out as an abnormal behavioral characteristic of the group as a whole. Social anxiety and selective mutism were generally reported to have developed at the same early age. Both parent and teacher behavioral ratings showed that social anxiety symptoms were significantly greater than all other symptom clusters and that only anxiety ratings (anxiety, separation anxiety, and social/performance anxiety) were significantly correlated with mutism severity, suggesting that the severity of the child's anxiety is a key factor determining the severity of mutism. Black and Uhde (1995) concluded that "the failure to speak in specific situations, which is the defining symptom of selective mutism, is a symptom of excessive social anxiety, specifically a fear of public speaking" and that "selective mutism is more appropriately viewed as a symptom or subtype of social phobia in children rather than as a distinct psychiatric disorder" (p. 854).

It has been widely suggested that early trauma is common among children with selective mutism and that selective mutism is often a posttraumatic disorder (Hayden 1980). However, empirical studies have failed to support this concept (Black and Uhde 1995). It has also been reported that children with selective mutism often demonstrate oppositional, stubborn, and negative personality traits and that their refusal to speak is primarily a manifestation of this oppositional and stubborn behavior (i.e., a struggle for control between the child and adults). Other reports have suggested that children with selective mutism often have a history of delayed speech and language development and high incidence rates of enuresis, encopresis, depression, and separation anxiety (Tancer 1992). However, none of these reported associations has been empirically validated, and the data reported by Black and Uhde (1995) did not confirm these associations.

Differential Diagnosis

There is considerable overlap among the different anxiety disorders in children and adolescents, as well as comorbidity with other anxiety disorders, depression, attention-deficit/hyperactivity disorder, and substance abuse (Clark et al. 1995; Curry and Murphy 1995). Anxious children seen in clinical settings often have multiple anxiety symptoms, including generalized anxiety and worry, somatic preoccupations, social anxiety, current or past separation anxiety, specific fears, mild obsessions or compulsions, and spontaneous panic attacks (often developing during early adolescence). The task of differentiating among the anxiety disorders and between anxiety symptoms and other disorders is often complicated in children because they are not yet able to report on the motivation behind their behaviors due to developmental differences in metacognitive awareness (Kashdan and Herbert 2001).

Situationally bound or situationally predisposed panic attacks are common in specific phobia, social phobia, obsessive-compulsive disorder, and posttraumatic stress disorder, but they may also occur in panic disorder. When generalized anxiety or panic attacks are related to another medical condition (such as pheochromocytoma, hyperthyroidism, asthma, or encephalitis), the diagnosis of *anxiety disorder due to a general medical condition* should be made. *Substance-induced anxiety disorder* is diagnosed when anxiety or panic attacks occur in association with substance intoxication (e.g., caffeine or cocaine) or withdrawal (e.g., alcohol or sedative-hypnotics).

Epidemiology

■ Prevalence

Prevalence estimates for anxiety disorders vary widely among studies and are influenced by differences in diagnostic ascertainment, survey methodology, and sample characteristics (Costello and Angold 1995). Epidemiological studies have generally reported that anxiety disorders are common at all ages (Anderson et al. 1987; Bird et al. 1989; Kessler et al. 1994; Regier et al. 1988). Estimates of the prevalence of any anxiety disorder in studies with exclusively child and adolescent subjects range from 7.5% to nearly 26% (Anderson et al. 1987; Bird et al. 1989; Costello et al. 1988; Kashani and Orvaschel 1988, 1990).

For simple (specific) phobia, reported prevalence rates range from less than 1% to as high as 9.2%, and rates for social phobia range from 0% to 1.4%. Only one study has reported a prevalence estimate for panic disorder in young people. Whitaker et al. (1990) surveyed a large community sample of 14- to 17-year-olds and estimated the prevalence of panic disorder to be 0.6%. The incidence of panic attacks is much higher than the incidence of full-blown panic disorder and increases greatly with the onset of puberty (Hayward et al. 1992).

Social phobia has been estimated to occur in approximately 1% of children and adolescents (Anderson et al. 1987; Costello et al. 1988; Kashani and Orvaschel 1988, 1990). However, studies of the prevalence

of social phobia among adults have reported rates from as low as 1.9% to as high as 18.7% (Schneier et al. 1992; Stein et al. 1994) depending on the cutoff criteria used to determine when an individual who reports significant social anxiety qualifies for a diagnosis of social phobia. Other studies have shown that up to 50%–60% of the population consider themselves to be shy or more anxious than others in social performance situations (Stein et al. 1994; Zimbardo 1977). These studies clearly indicate that social anxiety and the perception that one is more socially anxious than others are very common and that it is difficult to determine valid cutoff criteria for a disorder with common and continuously distributed traits. Recent research with adolescents suggests that lifetime prevalence rates for this age group are between 5% and 15% in the United States (Heimberg et al. 2000; Lewinsohn et al. 1993) and in Germany (Wittchen et al. 1999). Based on these figures and the reported early onset of social phobia in adults, it seems likely that the prevalence of 1% reported for social phobia in children may be a significant underestimate.

For selective mutism, two large-scale community-based epidemiological studies have reported prevalence rates. The Newcastle Epidemiologic Study reported a prevalence of 0.8 per 1,000 in a cohort of 7-year-old children (Fundudis et al. 1979). Brown and Lloyd (1975) reported the prevalence of selective mutism in young children: 8 weeks after the beginning of school the rate was 7 per 1,000, and 64 weeks after the beginning of school the rate was 0.17 per 1,000 (1 of 6,000). Thus, many more children appear to manifest selective mutism transiently after starting school rather than having more persistent selective mutism. More recently, two studies from Scandinavia reported higher prevalence rates among slightly older populations of children: 20 per 1,000 among second-graders in Finland (Kumpulainen et al. 1998), and 1.8 per 1,000 among school-age children (ages 7–15 years) in Sweden (Kopp and Gillberg 1997). A survey of teachers of kindergarten, first grade, and second grade in a Los Angeles school district revealed a prevalence of 7.1 per 1,000 (Bergman et al. 2002). Thus, prevalence estimates range from 0.03% to 2%. The variability in these estimates may be a function of the age of the children sampled, differences in the applications of the diagnostic criteria (i.e., differences in the threshold for considering a child mute), and vagueness of the DSM criteria in terms of the degree of impairment required.

■ Age at Onset

Solyom et al. (1986) compared 47 adults with social phobia, 80 adults with agoraphobia, and 72 adults with simple phobia. The subjects with social phobia experienced their first phobic symptoms earlier than the subjects with agoraphobia but later than those with simple phobia. The patients with simple phobia recalled the age at onset of their first symptoms to be 12.8 years on average, with onset of illness at 16.0 years; the patients with social phobia reported their age at onset to be 16.6 years for symptoms and 23.5 years for illness on average. Patients with agoraphobia had the latest age at onset at 24.5 years for symptoms and 26.0 years for illness on average.

The prevalence of panic attacks and panic disorder before puberty is unknown. However, numerous case reports have verified that the disorder does occur before puberty (Black and Robbins 1990; Black et al. 1990; Moreau and Weissman 1992), whereas retrospective studies of adults with panic disorder have shown that onset during adolescence is common. In 3,000 adults questioned retrospectively regarding age at onset of their panic disorder, the peak age at onset was between 15 and 20 years (von Ko-

rff et al. 1985). In a retrospective chart review of 62 adult patients with panic disorder without agoraphobia, the mean age at onset was 26.6 years, with 39% of patients reporting onset of symptoms before age 20 and 13% before age 10 years (Thyer et al. 1985). Among 95 patients with panic disorder with agoraphobia, the mean age at onset was 26.3 years, with 29% of these patients having onset before age 20 and 4% before age 10. In another study, 30 of 100 patients with panic disorder with agoraphobia reported that their first panic attack occurred before age 20, and 6 reported onset before age 10 (Sheehan et al. 1981b).

Social phobia has generally been shown to have an early age at onset, with a mean of 15 years and a bimodal distribution with peaks before age 5 years and at about age 13 years (Schneier et al. 1992). Of adult subjects with social phobia, 77% reported onset before age 20.

Onset for selective mutism is often insidious, with parents reporting that the child has "always been this way" (Leonard and Topol 1993). Data from recent studies document age at onset as early as 2.7–4.13 years (Black and Uhde 1995; Dummit et al. 1997; Kristensen 2000; Steinhausen and Juzi 1996).

Etiology

The development of phobias to specific objects or situations clearly is not random among either humans or animals. Rather, both humans and animals are predisposed to develop phobias of specific objects or situations. Controversy has existed regarding whether learning or conditioning is necessary or whether specific phobias may develop in some genetically predisposed individuals without learning ever taking place (Gray 1982; Marks 1987). Research suggests that both genetic (innate) and environmental factors play a role (Kendler et al. 1992).

Family genetic studies have provided substantial evidence that risk for development of an anxiety disorder is strongly influenced by genetic factors. These studies include the following types:

- *Top-down* studies evaluating the prevalence of anxiety disorders in the offspring of adult probands
- *Bottom-up* studies evaluating the prevalence of anxiety disorders in adult relatives of child and adolescent probands
- *High-risk* longitudinal studies examining young offspring of adult probands with anxiety disorders
- *Twin* studies comparing rates of co-occurrence of anxiety disorders in monozygotic and dizygotic twin pairs (Last and Beidel 1991)

Lifetime morbidity risk for first-degree relatives of individuals with specific phobia, panic disorder, and social phobia is threefold to sixfold higher than for first-degree relatives of control subjects without anxiety disorders (Fyer et al. 1990, 1993; Last and Beidel 1991). Twin studies have found significantly greater proband-wise concordance rates among monozygotic twins than among dizygotic twins for specific phobias, panic disorder, and social phobia (Kendler et al. 1992). Black and Uhde (1995) found a high familial prevalence of selective mutism and social phobia among first-degree relatives of subjects with selective mutism. Because the prevalence of social phobia among family members was actually much higher than that of selective mutism, the researchers concluded that social phobia is transmitted familially to children with selective mutism and that selective mutism is merely a symptomatic expression of social phobia. One study, examining age at onset of panic disorder

in families with multiple affected individuals in different generations, found a significant decrease in the time before the first episode of panic and onset of panic disorder in the younger generation relative to the older generation (Battaglia et al. 1998).

Although very little work has been done with children or adolescents, neurobiological and neurochemical abnormalities have been detected in individuals with anxiety disorders (see Pine 2002 for a comprehensive review of this literature). For example, panic attacks can be provoked in individuals with panic disorder by administering chemical agents, including sodium lactate, caffeine, cholecystokinin, and carbon dioxide (through inhalation). These responses are specific to patients with panic disorder. Control subjects without anxiety disorder and patients with other anxiety disorders do not have the same responses, and patients with panic disorder do not have panic attacks in response to placebo infusions. Pretreatment with specific pharmacological agents before chemical challenge blocks induction of anxiety symptoms. The differences in responses of individuals with and without panic disorder suggest that the neurobiological mechanisms controlling anxiety are abnormal in the individuals with panic disorder. Recent work examining the pathophysiological mechanism underlying carbon dioxide–induced panic attacks suggests that spontaneous panic is different from anticipatory anxiety because the hypothalamic–pituitary axis is not activated in the former condition, whereas it is in the latter (Sinha et al. 1999). This work has been replicated in children and adolescents (Coplan et al. 2002). Unique associations with respiratory dysregulation have also been found in patients with panic disorder and their asymptomatic first-degree relatives (Klein 1994; Papp et al. 1989; Pine et al. 1998). Asymptomatic first-degree relatives of patients with panic disorder have also demonstrated heightened sensitivity to carbon dioxide inhalation (Coryell et al. 2001).

However, more recent research has failed to support the hypothesis of carbon dioxide as a familial vulnerability marker (Pine et al. 2005). Neurochemically, regulatory dysfunction in brain monamine and γ-aminobutyric acid systems have been implicated in anxiety disorders (Crestani et al. 1999; Malizia et al. 1998; Roy-Byrne et al. 1996). In adults with panic disorder and social phobia, neuroendocrine abnormalities have been found, including a hyporesponsive hypothalamic growth hormone axis, as indicated by blunted growth hormone responses to pharmacological or physiological challenge (Uhde et al. 1992).

Conditioning or learning models postulate that anxiety is a learned response to noxious stimuli and that the acquisition of anxious or fearful reactions occurs as a result of conditioning or the linking of a previously benign conditioned stimulus to a noxious unconditioned stimulus. Biological and conditioning models are increasingly being integrated; the biological models illustrate how some individuals are either more or less predisposed or vulnerable to the development of anxiety disorders, whereas conditioning models illustrate how environmental or psychological factors may precipitate the development of an anxiety disorder in a vulnerable individual and can influence the course of the disorder and the development of complications (Barlow 1988). Recent evidence suggests that fear learning may be different in adults with anxiety disorders and in their children compared with unaffected individuals (Grillon et al. 1991, 1997a, 1997b, 1998a, 1998b; Merikangas et al. 1999; Pine and Grun 1999).

Children with panic disorder, social phobia, and selective mutism may have much in common with behaviorally inhibited children. *Behavioral inhibition* refers to an enduring temperamental trait characterized by quiet, withdrawing, and timid behavior; reluctance to speak; and a state of neurophysiological arousal in response to novel situations, including interaction with unfamiliar adults (Biederman et al. 1993a; Kagan et al. 1987). Defined laboratory paradigms have been developed to classify young children as either more or less behaviorally inhibited. Longitudinal studies assessing the stability of behavioral inhibition and risk for development of psychiatric disorder have found that children identified as behaviorally inhibited during early childhood remain inhibited at follow-up in middle childhood, are markedly reluctant to speak to unfamiliar persons in unfamiliar environments, and are at increased risk for the development of anxiety disorders (Biederman et al. 1993b). Schwartz et al. (1999) reported some specificity in terms of the risk conveyed by behavioral inhibition. They reported that 13-year-olds who had been classified as behaviorally inhibited when they were toddlers were more likely to have generalized social anxiety compared with their uninhibited peers. In this study, 34% of the adolescents who were originally classified as behaviorally inhibited met criteria for social phobia at age 13. Family studies have shown a high familial prevalence of social phobia and childhood anxiety disorders among first-degree relatives of inhibited children. Likewise, studies of offspring of adults with panic disorder with agoraphobia have found that 85% are behaviorally inhibited compared with 15% of the offspring of psychiatrically healthy control parents (Rosenbaum et al. 1988).

Treatment

■ Specific Phobia

The most successful treatment approach for children with specific phobia appears to be graduated in vivo exposure in combination with contingency management and self-control strategies (Morris and Kratochwill 1998; Silverman et al. 1999a). In vivo exposure involves gradually bringing the child into contact with progressively more distressing variations on phobic stimuli. Habituation and teaching the child to cope with the anxious feelings are the two primary principles that underlie this approach. Contingency management techniques entail using differential reinforcement to shape the phobic child's behavior. Desired behaviors (e.g., approaching phobic stimuli) are rewarded, and maladaptive behaviors (e.g., avoidance behaviors) are not. Self-control strategies use the cognitive tools of self-evaluation and self-reward to accomplish the same ends. Excellent reviews of the behavioral treatments of phobias are available elsewhere (Drobes and Strauss 1993; Marks 1987).

Although pharmacological treatments have not been shown to be effective for specific phobias, many children with specific phobias also have generalized anxiety or other anxiety disorders and may benefit from pharmacotherapy. Please refer to Fyer (1987) for a review of the pharmacological treatment of phobic disorders and to Riddle et al. (1999) and Velosa and Riddle (2000) for excellent comprehensive reviews of pharmacological treatment of pediatric anxiety disorders.

■ Panic Disorder

Adult studies have reported the efficacy of tricyclic antidepressants, monoamine oxidase inhibitors, selective serotonin reuptake inhibitors (SSRIs), and benzodiazepines for panic disorder (Schneier et al. 1990; Sheehan et al. 1981a; Spier et al. 1986). Although no controlled studies of the psychopharmacological treatment of panic disorder have been done in children, case reports suggest that childhood-onset panic disorder may be similar in its pharmacological response to that seen in adults (Biederman 1987; Black and Robbins 1990; Kutcher and MacKenzie 1988). Although no systematic treatment trials of SSRIs in children have been conducted, SSRIs are emerging in clinical practice as the first-line medication treatment of choice. Preliminary evidence in support of the use of paroxetine is provided by the 83% response rate reported in a recent open-label study of 18 children and adolescents with panic disorder (Masi et al. 2001). More systematic studies are necessary. Likewise, cognitive and behavioral treatments have proved effective in the treatment of adults with panic disorder (Barlow and Cerney 1988), and preliminary evidence suggests that they are also effective in children and adolescents (Drobes and Strauss 1993; Hoffman and Mattis 2000; Ollendick 1995).

■ Social Phobia

Results of a large-scale systematic study of fluvoxamine in children and adolescents with social phobia, separation anxiety disorder, or generalized anxiety disorder provide the first solid evidence of effective pharmacotherapy for social phobia in children and adolescents (Research Unit on Pediatric Psychopharmacology Anxiety Study Group 2001). In this study 128 children and adolescents (ages 6–17) were assigned to either fluvoxamine or placebo for 8 weeks. Seventy-six percent of the children in the fluvoxamine group showed significant improvement on the Clinical Global Impression Scale, as opposed to only 29% of children in the placebo group. Similarly, Birmaher et al. (1994) reported that the open treatment with fluoxetine of a mixed group of 21 children and adolescents with anxiety disorders (social phobia, overanxious disorder, or separation anxiety disorder) had generally favorable outcomes. The SSRIs should be considered the pharmacological treatments of choice. Phenelzine may be effective in patients who do not respond to SSRI treatment, but this agent should be used with great caution in adolescents and never in preadolescent children. In general, pharmacotherapy should not be used as the sole intervention for children with social phobia, although it may play an important role in a multimodal treatment plan that includes intensive behavioral intervention (Freeman et al. 2002).

To date, there have been 12 published studies demonstrating the efficacy of cognitive-behavioral treatment approaches for children or adolescents with social phobia. The treatment approaches used in 8 of these 12 studies were designed to treat child anxiety disorders in general (Barrett et al. 1996; Flannery-Schroeder and Kendall 2000; Kendall 1994; Kendall et al. 1997; Lumpkin et al. 2002; Silverman et al. 1999a, 1999b; Manassis et al. 2002). Although these studies did not focus on social phobia, children with social phobia were included in the trials. However, the strength of the treatment effect for social phobia cannot be measured directly from results of these more generalized anxiety treatment studies. Three studies have reported positive results for group treatments designed specifically to target social phobia in children or adolescents (Albano et al. 1995; Beidel et al. 2000; Hayward et al. 2000). To date, one study (Spence et al. 2000) has reported positive effects of two cognitive-behavioral interventions (individual CBT and CBT plus parental involvement) that specifically targeted social phobia in children and adolescents. Although the formats have differed somewhat across studies (e.g., group versus individual versus family; specific focus on social phobia versus anxiety disorders in general), four treatment components were present in all of the interventions: psychoeducation, expo-

sure, skill building (e.g., relaxation training, cognitive restructuring, social skills, problem-solving skills), and homework assignments (Kashdan and Herbert 2001). Pilot studies investigating the school-based (Masia et al. 2001) and community-based (Baer and Garland 2005) provision of cognitive-behavioral treatment to affected adolescents are also promising. Clearly, combined treatment trials are needed to study the relative efficacy of medication, cognitive-behavioral treatment, and their combination.

■ Selective Mutism

The evidence-based treatment literature on pharmacotherapy for selective mutism is limited. To date, the majority of this work has been single case studies using monoamine oxidase inhibitors or SSRIs (Black and Uhde 1992; Carlson et al. 1999; Golwyn and Sevlie 1999; Golwyn and Weinstock 1990; Harvey and Milne 1998; Thomsen et al. 1999; Wright et al. 1995). There have also been two more systematic studies using fluoxetine, one an open treatment trial (Dummit et al. 1996) and one a small, double-blind, placebo-controlled trial (Black and Uhde 1994). In the double-blind, placebo-controlled study of 16 children, fluoxetine was shown to be superior to placebo (Black and Uhde 1994). Subjects treated with fluoxetine were significantly more improved on parents' ratings of mutism change and global change at 12 weeks. Parents rated 4 of 6 fluoxetine-treated subjects but only 1 of 9 placebo-treated subjects as significantly improved after 12 weeks. Interestingly, of the 4 fluoxetine responders at 12 weeks, none had responded after 4 weeks of treatment, and only 1 had responded after 8 weeks of treatment. Clinician and teacher ratings did not indicate significant differences between treatment groups. Although improvement occurred, most subjects in both treatment groups remained very symptomatic at the end of the study period.

A sizable body of literature exists on empirical but uncontrolled studies regarding the behavioral treatment of selective mutism. The details of these studies are provided in several comprehensive reviews of this literature (Anstendig 1998; Cline and Baldwin 1994; Kratchowill 1981). Contingency management, exposure-based techniques, and self-modeling are the techniques most frequently employed. Although these studies have some methodological limitations, taken together they suggest that behavioral treatment approaches are often effective in the treatment of selective mutism.

Individual psychodynamically oriented therapy, play therapy, and family therapy are all very commonly used for children with selective mutism. However, the evidence base for these types of treatment is limited, and many methodological issues impede drawing conclusions about their efficacy. In the largest published studies of psychodynamic psychotherapy for selective mutism, Browne et al. (1963) and Wergeland (1979) concluded that the treatment was lengthy and the outcome poor.

Prognosis

Little is known about the outcome of children with specific phobia later in life. In a 5-year follow-up study of an epidemiological sample, Agras et al. (1972) found that of 10 children with diagnoses of phobias, all had either improved or recovered. Hampe et al. (1973) saw phobic children at 2-year follow-up and found that 80% were symptom free but that 7% had "serious fear reactions." Because specific phobias are amenable to behavioral treatment, one might hypothesize that treated patients would have a better long-term outcome.

Because panic disorder, social phobia, and selective mutism diagnoses have only recently received attention in children, the long-term outcome of these children is unknown. However, longitudinal studies with adults indicate that panic disorder and social phobia are often chronic disorders, and clinical experience suggests that this also tends to be the case for those with onset in childhood or adolescence (Black 1995, 1996).

Selective mutism, diagnosed according to DSM-IV-TR criteria, almost always resolves during childhood, with or without treatment. However, if selective mutism is viewed instead as a symptom of social phobia, the prognosis is poorer, because most children with selective mutism probably continue to have social phobia even after the selective mutism resolves (Black 1996).

Research Issues

None of the disorders described in this chapter have yet been adequately characterized. Specific phobia is the best described of these disorders, but few studies distinguish between exaggerated fears and the clinical cases. Longitudinal and outcome studies, family studies, and studies assessing the interaction of environmental and genetic factors in determining the risk for the development of these disorders are needed. Although the treatment literature has grown in the last decade, there is still a need for controlled treatment studies to systematically assess the effectiveness of disorder-specific pharmacological and psychosocial treatments, particularly when applied in combination.

References

Abelson JL, Alessi NE: Discussion of child panic revisited. J Am Acad Child Adolesc Psychiatry 31:114–116, 1992

Agras WS, Chapin HN, Oliveau DC: The natural history of phobia. Arch Gen Psychiatry 26:315–317, 1972

Albano AM, Marten PA, Holt CS, et al: Cognitive-behavioral group treatment for social phobia in adolescents: a preliminary study. J Nerv Ment Dis 183:649–656, 1995

American Psychiatric Association: Diagnostic and Statistical Manual of Mental Disorders, 4th Edition, Text Revision. Washington, DC, American Psychiatric Association, 2000

Anderson JC, Williams S, McGee R, et al: DSM-III disorders in preadolescent children. Arch Gen Psychiatry 44:69–76, 1987

Anstendig K: Selective mutism: a review of the treatment literature by modality from 1980–1996. Psychotherapy 35:381–391, 1998

Baer S, Garland EJ: Pilot study of community-based cognitive behavioral group therapy for adolescents with social phobia. J Am Acad Child Adolesc Psychiatry 44:258–264, 2005

Barlow DH: Current models of panic disorder and a view from emotion theory, in American Psychiatric Press Review of Psychiatry, Vol 7. Edited by Frances AJ, Hales RE. Washington, DC, American Psychiatric Press, 1988, pp 10–28

Barlow DH, Cerney JA: Psychological Treatment of Panic. New York, Guilford, 1988

Barrett PB, Dadds MR, Rapee RM: Family treatment of childhood anxiety: a controlled trial. J Consult Clin Psychol 64:333–342, 1996

Battaglia M, Bertella S, Bajo S, et al: Anticipation of age at onset in panic disorder. Am J Psychiatry 155:590–595, 1998

Beidel DC: Social phobia and overanxious disorder in school-age children. J Am Acad Child Adolesc Psychiatry 30:545–552, 1991

Beidel DC, Morris TL: Social phobia, in Anxiety Disorders in Children and Adolescents. Edited by March JS. New York, Guilford, 1995, pp 181–211

Beidel DC, Turner SM, Morris TL: Psychopathology of childhood social phobia. J Am Acad Child Adolesc Psychiatry 38:643–650, 1999

Beidel DC, Turner SM, Morris TL: Behavioral treatment of childhood social phobia. J Consult Clin Psychol 68:1072–1080, 2000

Bergman RL, Piacentini J, McCracken JT: Prevalence and description of selective mutism in a school-based sample. J Am Acad Child Adolesc Psychiatry 41:938–946, 2002

Biederman J: Clonazepam in the treatment of prepubertal children with panic-like symptoms. J Clin Psychiatry 48:38–41, 1987

Biederman J, Rosenbaum JF, Bolduc-Murphy EA, et al: Behavioral inhibition as a temperamental risk factor for anxiety disorders. Child Adolesc Psychiatr Clin N Am 2:667–684, 1993a

Biederman J, Rosenbaum JF, Bolduc-Murphy EA, et al: A 3-year follow-up of children with and without behavioral inhibition. J Am Acad Child Adolesc Psychiatry 32:814–821, 1993b

Biederman J, Faraone SV, Marrs A, et al: Panic disorder and agoraphobia in consecutively referred children and adolescents. J Am Acad Child Adolesc Psychiatry 36:214–223, 1997

Bird HR, Gould MS, Yager T, et al: Risk factors for maladjustment in Puerto Rican children. J Am Acad Child Adolesc Psychiatry 28:847–850, 1989

Birmaher B, Waterman GS, Ryan N, et al: Fluoxetine for childhood anxiety disorders. J Am Acad Child Adolesc Psychiatry 33:993–999, 1994

Black B: Separation anxiety disorder and panic disorder, in Anxiety Disorders in Children and Adolescents. Edited by March JS. New York, Guilford, 1995, pp 212–234

Black B: Social anxiety and selective mutism, in American Psychiatric Press Review of Psychiatry, Vol 15. Edited by Dickstein LJ, Riba MB, Oldham JM. Washington, DC, American Psychiatric Press, 1996, pp 469–495

Black B, Robbins DR: Panic disorder in children and adolescents. J Am Acad Child Adolesc Psychiatry 29:36–44, 1990

Black B, Uhde TW: Elective mutism as a variant of social phobia. J Am Acad Child Adolesc Psychiatry 31:1090–1094, 1992

Black B, Uhde TW: Treatment of elective mutism with fluoxetine: a double-blind, placebo-controlled study. J Am Acad Child Adolesc Psychiatry 33:1000–1006, 1994

Black B, Uhde TW: Psychiatric characteristics of children with selective mutism: a pilot study. J Am Acad Child Adolesc Psychiatry 34:847–856, 1995

Black B, Uhde TW, Robbins DR: Reply to Klein DF, Klein RG: Does panic disorder exist in childhood? (letter). J Am Acad Child Adolesc Psychiatry 29:834–835, 1990

Bradley SJ, Hood J: Psychiatrically referred adolescents with panic attacks: presenting symptoms, stressors, and comorbidity. J Am Acad Child Adolesc Psychiatry 32:826–829, 1993

Brown JB, Lloyd H: A controlled study of children not speaking at school. Journal of the Association of Workers With Maladjusted Children 3:49–63, 1975

Browne E, Wilson V, Laybourne PC: Diagnosis and treatment of elective mutism in children. J Am Acad Child Adolesc Psychiatry 2:605–617, 1963

Carlson JS, Kratochwill TR, Johnson HF: Sertraline treatment of 5 children diagnosed with selective mutism: a single-case research trial. J Child Adolesc Psychopharmacol 9:293–306, 1999

Clark DB, Bukstein OG, Smith MG, et al: Identifying anxiety disorders in adolescents hospitalized for alcohol abuse or dependence. Psychiatr Serv 46:618–620, 1995

Cline T, Baldwin S: Selective Mutism in Children. San Diego, CA, Singular, 1994

Coplan JD, Moreau D, Chaput F, et al: Salivary cortisol concentrations before and after carbon dioxide inhalations in children. Biol Psychiatry 51:326–333, 2002

Coryell W, Fyer A, Pine D, et al: Aberrant respiratory sensitivity to CO(2) as a trait of familial panic disorder. Biol Psychiatry 49:582–587, 2001

Costello EJ: Child psychiatric disorders and their correlates: a primary care pediatric sample. J Am Acad Child Adolesc Psychiatry 28:851–855, 1989

Costello EJ, Angold A: Epidemiology, in Anxiety Disorders in Children and Adolescents. Edited by March JS. New York, Guilford, 1995, pp 109–124

Costello EJ, Costello AJ, Edelbrock C, et al: Psychiatric disorders in pediatric primary care: prevalence and risk factors. Arch Gen Psychiatry 45:1107–1116, 1988

Crestani F, Lorez M, Baer K, et al: Decreased GABA-receptor clustering results in enhanced anxiety and a bias for threat cues. Nat Neurosci 2:833–839, 1999

Curry JF, Murphy LB: Comorbidity of anxiety disorders, in Anxiety Disorders in Children and Adolescents. Edited by March JS. New York, Guilford, 1995, pp 301–320

DeWit DJ, MacDonald K, Offord DR: Childhood stress and symptoms of drug dependence in adolescents and early adulthood: social phobia as a mediator. Am J Orthopsychiatry 69:61–71, 1999

Diler RS, Birmaher B, Brent DA, et al: Phenomenology of panic disorder in youth. Depress Anxiety 20:39–43, 2004

Dow SP, Sonies BC, Scheib D, et al: Practical guidelines for the assessment and treatment of selective mutism. J Am Acad Child Adolesc Psychiatry 34:836–846, 1995

Drobes DJ, Strauss CC: Behavioral treatment of childhood anxiety disorders. Child Adolesc Psychiatr Clin N Am 2:779–794, 1993

Dummit ES 3rd, Klein RG, Tancer NK, et al: Fluoxetine treatment of children with selective mutism: an open trial. J Am Acad Child Adolesc Psychiatry 35:615–621, 1996

Dummit ES 3rd, Klein RG, Tancer NK, et al: Systematic assessment of 50 children with selective mutism. J Am Acad Child Adolesc Psychiatry 36:653–660, 1997

Evans DW, Leckman JF, Carter A, et al: Ritual, habit, and perfectionism: the prevalence and development of compulsive-like behavior in normal young children. Child Dev 68:58–68, 1997

Flannery-Schroeder E, Kendall PC: Group and individual cognitive-behavioral treatments for youth with anxiety disorders: a randomized clinical trial. Cognit Ther Res 24:251–278, 2000

Francis G, Last CG, Strauss CC: Avoidant disorder and social phobia in children and adolescents. J Am Acad Child Adolesc Psychiatry 31:1086–1089, 1992

Freeman JB, Garcia AM, Leonard HL: Anxiety disorders, in Child and Adolescent Psychiatry: A Comprehensive Textbook, 3rd Edition. Edited by Lewis M. Baltimore, MD, Williams & Wilkins, 2002, pp 821–834

Fundudis T, Kolvin I, Garside RF: Speech Retarded and Deaf Children: Their Psychological Development. London, Academic Press, 1979

Fyer AJ: Simple phobia. Mod Probl Pharmacopsychiatry 22:174–192, 1987

Fyer AJ, Mannuzza S, Gallops MS, et al: Familial transmission of simple phobia and fears: a preliminary report. Arch Gen Psychiatry 47:252–256, 1990

Fyer AJ, Mannuzza S, Chapman TF, et al: A direct interview family study of social phobia. Arch Gen Psychiatry 50:286–293, 1993

Gittelman R, Klein DF: Relationship between separation anxiety and panic and agoraphobic disorders. Psychopathology 17 (suppl 1): 56–65, 1984

Golwyn DH, Sevlie CP: Phenelzine treatment of selective mutism in four prepubertal children. J Child Adolesc Psychopharmacol 9:109–113, 1999

Golwyn DH, Weinstock RC: Phenelzine treatment of elective mutism. J Clin Psychiatry 51:384–385, 1990

Goodwin RD, Gotlib IH: Panic attacks and psychopathology among youth. Acta Psychiatr Scand 109:216–221, 2004

Gray JA: The Neuropsychology of Anxiety. New York, Oxford University Press, 1982

Graziano AM, DeGiovanni IS, Garcia K: Behavioral treatment of children's fears: a review. Psychol Bull 86:804–830, 1979

Grillon C, Ameli R, Woods SW, et al: Fear-potentiated startle in humans: effects of anticipatory anxiety on the acoustic blink reflex. Psychophysiology 28:588–595, 1991

Grillon C, Dierker L, Merikangas K: Startle modulation in children at risk for anxiety disorders and/or alcoholism. J Am Acad Child Adolesc Psychiatry 36:925–932, 1997a

Grillon C, Pellowski M, Merikangas K, et al: Darkness facilitates the acoustic startle reflex in humans. Biol Psychiatry 42:453–460, 1997b

Grillon C, Dierker L, Merikangas K: Fear-potentiated startle in adolescent offspring of parents with anxiety disorders. Biol Psychiatry 44:990–997, 1998a

Grillon C, Morgan CA, Davis M, et al: Effect of darkness on acoustic startle in Vietnam veterans with PTSD. Am J Psychiatry 155:812–817, 1998b

Gullone E: The development of normal fear: a century of research. Clin Psychol Rev 20:429–451, 2000

Hampe E, Noble H, Miller LC, et al: Phobic children one and two years posttreatment. J Abnorm Psychol 82:446–453, 1973

Harvey BH, Milne M: Pharmacotherapy of selective mutism: two case studies of severe entrenched mutism responsive to adjunctive treatment with fluoxetine. South African Journal of Child and Adolescent Mental Health 10:59–66, 1998

Hayden TL: Classification of elective mutism. J Am Acad Child Psychiatry 19:118–133, 1980

Hayward C, Killen JD, Hammer LD, et al: Pubertal stage and panic attack history in sixth- and seventh-grade girls. Am J Psychiatry 149:1239–1243, 1992

Hayward C, Varady S, Albano AM, et al: Cognitive-behavioral group therapy for social phobia in female adolescents: results of a pilot study. J Am Acad Child Adolesc Psychiatry 39:721–726, 2000

Heimberg RG, Stein MB, Hiripi E: Trends in the prevalence of social phobia in the United States: a cohort analysis of changes over four decades. Eur Psychiatry 15:29–37, 2000

Hoffman EC, Mattis SG: A developmental adaptation of panic control treatment for panic disorder in adolescence. Cognitive and Behavioral Practice 7:253–261, 2000

Kagan J, Reznick JS, Snidman N: The physiology and psychology of behavioral inhibition in young children. Child Dev 58:1459–1473, 1987

Kashani JH, Orvaschel H: Anxiety disorders in mid-adolescence: a community sample. Am J Psychiatry 145:960–964, 1988

Kashani JH, Orvaschel H: A community study of anxiety in children and adolescents. Am J Psychiatry 147:313–318, 1990

Kashdan TB, Herbert JD: Social anxiety disorder in childhood and adolescence: current status and future directions. Clin Child Fam Psychol Rev 4:37–61, 2001

Kearney CA, Albano AM, Eisen AR, et al: The phenomenology of panic disorder in youngsters: an empirical study of a clinical sample. J Anxiety Disord 11:49–62, 1997

Kendall PC: Treating anxiety disorders in youth: results of a randomized clinical trial. J Consult Clin Psychol 62:100–110, 1994

Kendall PC, Flannery-Schroeder E, Panichelli-Mindel SM, et al: Therapy for youths with anxiety disorders: a second randomized clinical trial. J Consult Clin Psychol 65:366–380, 1997

Kendler KS, Neale MC, Kessler RC, et al: The genetic epidemiology of phobias in women: the interrelationship of agoraphobia, social phobia, situational phobia, and simple phobia. Arch Gen Psychiatry 49:273–281, 1992

Kessler RC, McGonagle KA, Zhao S, et al: Lifetime and 12-month prevalence of DSM-III-R psychiatric disorders in the United States: results from the National Comorbidity Survey. Arch Gen Psychiatry 51:8–19, 1994

King NJ, Gullone E, Tonge BJ, et al: Self-reports of panic attacks and manifest anxiety in adolescents. Behav Res Ther 31:111–116, 1993

King NJ, Ollendick TH, Mattis SG, et al: New clinical panic attacks in adolescents: prevalence, symptomatology, and associated features. Behav Change 13:171–183, 1997

Klein DF: Delineation of two drug-responsive anxiety syndromes. Psychopharmacologia 5:397–408, 1964

Klein DF: Anxiety reconceptualized, in Anxiety: New Research and Changing Concepts. Edited by Klein DF, Rabkin J. New York, Raven, 1981, pp 235–263

Klein DF: Testing the suffocation false alarm theory of panic disorder. Anxiety 1:144–148, 1994

Kolvin I, Fundudis T: Elective mute children: psychological development and background factors. J Child Psychol Psychiatry 22:219–232, 1981

Kopp S, Gillberg C: Selective mutism: a population-based study: a research note. J Child Psychol Psychiatry 38:257–262, 1997

Kratchowill TR: Selective Mutism: Implications for Research and Treatment. Hillsdale, NJ, Lawrence Erlbaum, 1981

Kristensen H: Selective mutism and comorbidity with developmental disorder/delay, anxiety disorder, and elimination disorder. J Am Acad Child Adolesc Psychiatry 39:249–256, 2000

Kumpulainen K, Rasanen E, Raaska H, et al: Selective mutism among second-graders in elementary school. Eur Child Adolesc Psychiatry 7:24–29, 1998

Kutcher SP, MacKenzie S: Successful clonazepam treatment of adolescents with panic disorder. J Clin Psychopharmacol 8:299–300, 1988

Lapouse R, Monk MA: Fears and worries in a representative sample of children. Am J Orthopsychiatry 29:223–248, 1959

Last CG, Beidel DC: Anxiety, in Child and Adolescent Psychiatry: A Comprehensive Textbook. Edited by Lewis M. Baltimore, MD, Williams & Wilkins, 1991, pp 281–292

Last CG, Strauss CG, Francis G: Comorbidity among childhood anxiety disorders. J Nerv Ment Dis 175:726–730, 1987

Last CG, Perrin S, Hersen M, et al: DSM-III-R anxiety disorders in children: sociodemographic and clinical characteristics. J Am Acad Child Adolesc Psychiatry 31:1070–1076, 1992

Leckman JF, Weissman MM, Merikangas KR, et al: Major depression and panic disorder. Psychopharmacol Bull 21:543–545, 1985

Leonard HL, Topol DA: Elective mutism, in Anxiety Disorders, Vol 2. Philadelphia, PA, WB Saunders, 1993, pp 695–707

Lewinsohn PM, Hops H, Roberts RE, et al: Adolescent psychopathology, I: prevalence and incidence of depression and other DSM-III-R disorders in high school students. J Abnorm Psychol 102:133–144, 1993

Liebowitz MR, Heimberg RG, Fresco DM: Social phobia or social anxiety disorder: what's in a name? (letter). Arch Gen Psychiatry 57:191–192, 2000

Lumpkin PW, Silverman WK, Weems CF, et al: Treating a heterogeneous set of anxiety disorders in youths with group cognitive behavioral therapy: a partially nonconcurrent multiple-baseline evaluation. Behav Ther 33:163–177, 2002

Malizia AL, Cunningham VJ, Bell CJ, et al: Decreased brain GABA(A)–benzodiazepine receptor binding in panic disorder: preliminary results from a quantitative PET study. Arch Gen Psychiatry 55:715–720, 1998

Manassis K, Mendlowitz SL, Scapillato D, et al: Group and individual cognitive-behavioral therapy for childhood anxiety disorders: a randomized trial. J Am Acad Child Adolesc Psychiatry 41:1423–1430, 2002

Marks IM: Fears, Phobias, and Rituals. New York, Oxford University Press, 1987

Masi G, Toni C, Mucci M, et al: Paroxetine in child and adolescent outpatients with panic disorder. J Child Adolesc Psychopharmacol 11:151–157, 2001

Masia CL, Klein RG, Storch EA, et al: School-based behavioral treatment for social anxiety disorder in adolescents: results of a pilot study. J Am Acad Child Adolesc Psychiatry 40:780–786, 2001

Merikangas KR, Avenevoli S, Dierker L, et al: Vulnerability factors among children at risk for anxiety disorders. Biol Psychiatry 46:1523–1535, 1999

Moreau D, Weissman MM: Panic disorder in children and adolescents: a review. Am J Psychiatry 149:1306–1314, 1992

Morris RJ, Kratochwill TR: Childhood fears and phobias, in The Practice of Child Therapy, 3rd Edition. Edited by Kratochwill TR, Morris RJ. Needham Heights, MA, Allyn & Bacon, 1998, pp 91–131

Nelles WB, Barlow DH: Do children panic? Clin Psychol Rev 8:359–372, 1988

Ollendick TH: Reliability and validity of the Revised Fear Surgery Schedule for Children (FSSC-R). Behav Res Ther 21:685–692, 1983

Ollendick TH: Cognitive-behavioral treatment of panic disorder with agoraphobia in adolescents: a multiple baseline design analysis. Behav Ther 26:517–531, 1995

Papp LA, Goetz R, Cole R, et al: Hypersensitivity to carbon dioxide in panic disorder. Am J Psychiatry 146:779–781, 1989

Pine DS: Development of the symptom of anxiety, in Child and Adolescent Psychiatry, 3rd Edition. Edited by Lewis M. Philadelphia, PA, Lippincott Williams & Wilkins, 2002, pp 343–351

Pine DS, Grun J: Research on pediatric anxiety: integrating affective neuroscience and developmental psychopathology. J Child Adolesc Psychopharmacol 9:1–12, 1999

Pine DS, Coplan JD, Papp LA, et al: Ventilatory physiology of children and adolescents with anxiety disorders. Arch Gen Psychiatry 55:123–129, 1998

Pine DS, Klein RG, Coplan JD, et al: Differential carbon dioxide sensitivity in childhood anxiety disorders and nonill comparison group. Arch Gen Psychiatry 57:960–967, 2000

Pine DS, Klein RG, Roberson-Nay R, et al: Response to 5% carbon dioxide in children and adolescents: relationship to panic disorder in parents and anxiety disorders in subjects. Arch Gen Psychiatry 62:73–80, 2005

Regier DA, Boyd JH, Burke JD, et al: One month of mental disorders in the United States based on five Epidemiologic Catchment Area sites. Arch Gen Psychiatry 45:977–986, 1988

Research Unit on Pediatric Psychopharmacology Anxiety Study Group: Fluvoxamine for the treatment of anxiety disorders in children and adolescents. N Engl J Med 344:1279–1285, 2001

Riddle MA, Bernstein GA, Cook EH, et al: Anxiolytics, adrenergic agents, and naltrexone. J Am Acad Child Adolesc Psychiatry 38:546–556, 1999

Rosenbaum JF, Biederman J, Gersten M, et al: Behavioral inhibition in children of parents with panic disorder and agoraphobia. Arch Gen Psychiatry 45:463–470, 1988

Roy-Byrne P, Geraci M, Uhde TW: Life events and the onset of panic disorder. Am J Psychiatry 143:1424–1427, 1986

Roy-Byrne P, Wingerson DK, Radant A, et al: Reduced benzodiazepine sensitivity in patients with panic disorder: comparison with patients with obsessive-compulsive disorder and normal subjects. Am J Psychiatry 153:1444–1449, 1996

Schneier FR, Liebowitz MR, Davies SO, et al: Fluoxetine in panic disorder. J Clin Psychopharmacol 10:119–121, 1990

Schneier FR, Johnson J, Hornig CD, et al: Social phobia: comorbidity and morbidity in an epidemiological sample. Arch Gen Psychiatry 49:282–289, 1992

Schwartz CE, Snidman N, Kagan J: Adolescent social anxiety as an outcome of inhibited temperament in childhood. J Am Acad Child Adolesc Psychiatry 38:1008–1015, 1999

Sheehan DV, Ballenger J, Jacobson G: Relative efficacy of monoamine oxidase inhibitors and tricyclic antidepressants in the treatment of endogenous anxiety, in Anxiety: New Research and Changing Concepts. Edited by Klein DF, Rabkin J. New York, Raven, 1981a, pp 47–67

Sheehan DV, Sheehan KE, Minichiello WE: Age of onset of phobic disorders: a reevaluation. Compr Psychiatry 22:544–553, 1981b

Silverman WK, Kurtines WM, Ginsburg GS, et al: Contingency management, self-control, and education support in the treatment of childhood phobic disorders: a randomized clinical trial. J Consult Clin Psychol 67:675–687, 1999a

Silverman WK, Kurtines WM, Ginsburg GS, et al: Treating anxiety disorders in children with group cognitive-behavioral therapy: a randomized clinical trial. J Consult Clin Psychol 67:995–1003, 1999b

Sinha SS, Coplan JD, Gorman JM, et al: Panic induced by carbon dioxide inhalation and lack of hypothalamic-pituitary-adrenal axis activation. Psychiatry Res 86:93–98, 1999

Solyom L, Ledwidge B, Solyom C: Delineating social phobia. Br J Psychiatry 149:464–470, 1986

Spence SH, Donovan C, Brechman-Toussaint M: Social skills, social outcomes, and cognitive features of childhood social phobia. J Abnorm Psychol 108:211–221, 1999

Spence SH, Donovan C, Brechman-Toussaint M: The treatment of childhood social phobia: the effectiveness of a social skills training-based, cognitive-behavioural intervention, with and without parental involvement. J Child Psychol Psychiatry 41:713–726, 2000

Spier SA, Tesar GE, Rosenbaum JF, et al: Treatment of panic disorder and agoraphobia with clonazepam. J Clin Psychiatry 47:238–242, 1986

Stein MB, Walker JR, Forde DR: Setting diagnostic thresholds for social phobia: considerations from a community survey of social anxiety. Am J Psychiatry 151:408–412, 1994

Steinhausen HC, Juzi C: Elective mutism: an analysis of 100 cases. J Am Acad Child Adolesc Psychiatry 35:606–614, 1996

Strauss CC, Last CG: Social and simple phobias in children. J Anxiety Disord 7:141–152, 1993

Suomi SJ, Kraemer GW, Baysinger CM, et al: Inherited and experiential factors associated with individual differences in anxious behavior displayed by rhesus monkeys, in Anxiety: New Research and Changing Concepts. Edited by Klein DF, Rabkin J. New York, Raven, 1981, pp 179–199

Tancer NK: Elective mutism: a review of the literature, in Advances in Clinical Child Psychology, Vol 14. Edited by Lahey BB, Kazdin AE. New York, Plenum, 1992, pp 265–288

Thomsen PH, Rasmussen G, Anderson CB: Elective mutism: a 17-year-old girl treated successfully with citalopram. Nord J Psychiatry 53:427–429, 1999

Thyer BA, Parrish RT, Curtis GC, et al: Ages of onset of DSM-III anxiety disorders. Compr Psychiatry 26:113–122, 1985

Turner SM, Beidel DC, Townsley RM: Social phobia: a comparison of specific and generalized subtypes and avoidant personality disorder. J Abnorm Psychol 101:326–331, 1992

Uhde TW, Tancer ME, Black B, et al: Phenomenology and neurobiology of social phobia: comparison with panic disorder. J Clin Psychiatry 52 (11, suppl):31–40, 1991

Uhde TW, Tancer ME, Rubinow DR, et al: Evidence for hypothalamo-growth hormone dysfunction in panic disorder: profile of growth hormone responses to clonidine, yohimbine, caffeine, glucose, GRF, and TRH in panic disorder patients versus healthy volunteers. Neuropsychopharmacology 6:101–118, 1992

Velosa JF, Riddle MA: Pharmacological treatment of anxiety disorders in children and adolescents. Child Adolesc Psychiatr Clin N Am 9:119–133, 2000

Verburg C, Griez E, Meijer J: A 35% carbon dioxide challenge in simple phobias. Acta Psychiatr Scand 90:420–423, 1994

von Korff MR, Eaton WW, Keyl PM: The epidemiology of panic attacks and panic disorder. Am J Epidemiol 122:970–981, 1985

Weissman MM, Leckman JE, Merikangas KR, et al: Depression and anxiety disorders in parents and children. Arch Gen Psychiatry 41:845–852, 1984

Wergeland H: Elective mutism. Acta Psychiatr Scand 59:218–228, 1979

Whitaker A, Johnson J, Shaffer D, et al: Uncommon troubles in young people: prevalence estimates of selected psychiatric disorders in a nonreferred adolescent population. Arch Gen Psychiatry 47:487–496, 1990

Wittchen HU, Stein MB, Kessler RC: Social fears and social phobia in a community sample of adolescents and young adults: prevalence, risk factors, and co-morbidity. Psychol Med 29:309–323, 1999

Wright HH, Cuccaro ML, Leonhardt TV, et al: Case study: fluoxetine in the multimodal treatment of a preschool child with selective mutism. J Am Acad Child Adolesc Psychiatry 34:857–862, 1995

Zimbardo PG: Shyness: What It Is and What to Do About It. New York, Addison-Wesley, 1977

Self-Assessment Questions

Select the single best response for each question.

20.1 To which of the following disorders does the DSM-IV-TR (American Psychiatric Association 2000) definition "a marked and persistent fear that is excessive or unreasonable, cued by the presence or anticipation of a specific object or situation" apply?

    A. Social phobia.

    B. Selective mutism.

    C. Specific phobia.

    D. Panic disorder.

    E. Anxiety disorder not otherwise specified.

20.2 All of the following statements regarding panic disorder are correct *except*

    A. Panic attacks are the hallmark of panic disorder.

    B. Panic disorder may occur with or without agoraphobia.

    C. Children with early development of separation anxiety disorder are at increased risk of later developing panic disorder.

    D. Symptoms, course of illness, and associated complicating conditions in children with panic disorder are very different from those in adults with panic disorder.

    E. Panic disorder may develop at any age during childhood or later.

20.3 Individuals with social phobia commonly fear which of the following social situations?

    A. Public speaking or performing.

    B. Attending social gatherings.

    C. Dealing with authorities.

    D. Asking for directions.

    E. All of the above.

20.4 In regard to the prevalence of selective mutism in children, which of the following statements is *true?*

    A. Prevalence estimates in children range from 3% to 5%.

    B. Selective mutism symptoms that occur upon starting school are likely to be unremitting.

    C. Variability in prevalence estimates may be due to vagueness in the DSM regarding the level of impairment required to meet diagnostic criteria.

    D. Scandinavian prevalence studies have reported lower rates of selective mutism than have U.S. studies among school-age children.

    E. Variability in prevalence estimates is unlikely to be related to differences in the consistent application of diagnostic criteria in study populations.

20.5 Which of the following descriptions refers to a *top-down* family genetic study of anxiety disorders?

    A. The evaluation of the prevalence of anxiety disorders in the offspring of adult probands.

    B. The evaluation of the prevalence of anxiety disorders in adult relatives of child probands.

    C. The longitudinal evaluation of young offspring of adult probands with anxiety disorders.

    D. The comparison of rates of co-occurrence of anxiety disorders in monozygotic twins.

    E. The comparison of rates of co-occurrence of anxiety disorders in dizygotic twins.

Posttraumatic Stress Disorder

Craig L. Donnelly, M.D., M.A.

John S. March, M.D., M.P.H.

Lisa Amaya-Jackson, M.D., M.P.H.

Historical Overview

It has long been recognized that the experience of extreme stress can exert profound and lasting changes on human cognition, emotion, and behavior. In the late 1970s and 1980s, childhood stress and trauma began to receive systematic and detailed empirical examination. The sophistication of the childhood trauma field emerged with the simultaneous development of a specific diagnostic nomenclature for stress disorders in adults and the publication of studies of children who experienced horrendous single-incident traumas. In one such incident, 26 children in Chowchilla, California, were kidnapped in a school bus and held in an underground bunker for 17 hours before escaping. Terr's (1979, 1981a, 1983a, 1983b, 1988) pioneering studies of these children, who were observed prospectively and individually, established many of the key manifestations of childhood posttraumatic stress disorder (PTSD).

In this chapter we present a basic review of pediatric PTSD. Interested readers may pursue more in-depth treatments of developmental approaches to PTSD (Pynoos 1994; Pynoos et al. 1995), assessment (McNally 1991), diagnosis and comorbidity (Amaya-Jackson and March 1995a, 1995b; March and Amaya-Jackson 1994), pharmacological treatment (Donnelly et al. 1999), psychosocial interventions (Pynoos and Nader 1993; Saigh 1992; Yule and Canterbury 1994), neurobiology (De Bellis et al. 1999a, 1999b), current recommended practice parameters for assessment and treatment (Cohen 1998), and other reviews of PTSD in childhood and adolescence (Perrin et al. 2000; Pfefferbaum 1997; Seedat et al. 2000; Terr 1996; Yule 1994).

Diagnostic Criteria and Clinical Findings

The diagnostic criteria for PTSD in children are the same as those used in adults. Four criteria must be satisfied to establish a DSM-IV-TR (American Psychiatric Association 2000) diagnosis of PTSD (Table 21–1). First, the individual must have been

Table 21–1.   DSM-IV-TR diagnostic criteria for posttraumatic stress disorder

A.   The person has been exposed to a traumatic event in which both of the following were present:

  (1)   the person experienced, witnessed, or was confronted with an event or events that involved actual or threatened death or serious injury, or a threat to the physical integrity of self or others

  (2)   the person's response involved intense fear, helplessness, or horror.   **Note:** In children, this may be expressed instead by disorganized or agitated behavior.

B.   The traumatic event is persistently reexperienced in one (or more) of the following ways:

  (1)   recurrent and intrusive distressing recollections of the event, including images, thoughts, or perceptions.   **Note:** In young children, repetitive play may occur in which themes or aspects of the trauma are expressed.

  (2)   recurrent distressing dreams of the event.   **Note:** In children, there may be frightening dreams without recognizable content.

  (3)   acting or feeling as if the traumatic event were recurring (includes a sense of reliving the experience, illusions, hallucinations, and dissociative flashback episodes, including those that occur on awakening or when intoxicated).   **Note:** In young children, trauma-specific reenactment may occur.

  (4)   intense psychological distress at exposure to internal or external cues that symbolize or resemble an aspect of the traumatic event

  (5)   physiological reactivity on exposure to internal or external cues that symbolize or resemble an aspect of the traumatic event

C.   Persistent avoidance of stimuli associated with the trauma and numbing of general responsiveness (not present before the trauma), as indicated by three (or more) of the following:

  (1)   efforts to avoid thoughts, feelings, or conversations associated with the trauma

  (2)   efforts to avoid activities, places, or people that arouse recollections of the trauma

  (3)   inability to recall an important aspect of the trauma

  (4)   markedly diminished interest or participation in significant activities

  (5)   feeling of detachment or estrangement from others

  (6)   restricted range of affect (e.g., unable to have loving feelings)

  (7)   sense of a foreshortened future (e.g., does not expect to have a career, marriage, children, or a normal life span)

D.   Persistent symptoms of increased arousal (not present before the trauma), as indicated by two (or more) of the following:

  (1)   difficulty falling or staying asleep

  (2)   irritability or outbursts of anger

  (3)   difficulty concentrating

  (4)   hypervigilance

  (5)   exaggerated startle response

E.   Duration of the disturbance (symptoms in Criteria B, C, and D) is more than 1 month.

F.   The disturbance causes clinically significant distress or impairment in social, occupational, or other important areas of functioning.

  Specify if:

  Acute: if duration of symptoms is less than 3 months

  Chronic: if duration of symptoms is 3 months or more

Table 21–1. DSM-IV-TR diagnostic criteria for posttraumatic stress disorder

Specify if:

    With Delayed Onset: if onset of symptoms is at least 6 months after the stressor

Source. Reprinted from American Psychiatric Association: *Diagnostic and Statistical Manual of Mental Disorders*, 4th Edition, Text Revision. Washington, DC, American Psychiatric Association, 2000. Copyright 2000 American Psychiatric Association. Used with permission.

exposed to a stressor of significant magnitude. There must follow the development of a triad of symptom clusters: subsequent reexperiencing of the event, avoidance of stimuli or numbing of general responsiveness, and persistent increased arousal. The stressor criterion defines the primary risk factor for PTSD and the essential feature of the diagnosis, namely, establishing exposure to a life-threatening event. The time course of the disorder can be variable, and PTSD may develop months or even years after the index trauma exposure. Symptoms must be debilitating and must be present for more than 1 month to meet the diagnostic criteria. Children who meet the symptom criteria but who do not meet the time criteria of symptom expression lasting for 1 month or more are considered under the category of acute stress disorder (Table 21–2).

■ Exposure to a Stressor

Objectively, PTSD stressors are characterized by threat to life, potential for physical injury, and an element of grotesqueness or horror that demarcates these events from less traumatic experiences, such as the expected death of a loved one from a serious illness or a highly embarrassing or humiliating personal event. Children react acutely to traumatic events with surprise, terror, and a sense of helplessness; these characterize the subjective features of the DSM-IV-TR PTSD stressor criterion. Characteristic stressors associated with PTSD in the pediatric population include kidnapping; serious animal bites; or severe injury due to burns, accidental shootings, and hit-

and-run accidents. Children are at special risk for PTSD from witnessing violence to a family member (e.g., rape or murder, suicide behavior, and spousal or sibling abuse). Also, as Saigh (1991) and others have pointed out, PTSD can result either from direct, witnessed, or verbal exposure or from "contaminant" effects of trauma indirectly experienced from a distance (Green 1995; Pfefferbaum et al. 2000).

In making the diagnosis of PTSD it is imperative that clinicians establish what might at first appear to be self-evident: that the traumatic event truly occurred and that the child was in fact exposed to it. Vague, secondhand, or unsubstantiated reports have no place in making the diagnosis of PTSD. It is known that PTSD is far more likely to occur after direct trauma exposure than after indirect exposure; however, it can occur in persons indirectly affected, such as those who have witnessed a violent injury to another or who have learned that a loved one was involved in a trauma (Green 1995). Nevertheless, caution is advised when attempting to delineate the traumatic exposure. Children's self-reports of trauma cannot be taken uncritically and automatically at face value, because it is known that even children with bona fide trauma histories often retain false details of their recollections of these real exposures (Terr 1979, 1981a, 1981b; also see Bremner et al. 2000). Memory is fluid and malleable, and children's recollections can be influenced both inadvertently and purposefully. Therefore, a neutral questioning stance on the part of the clinician is imperative, using both internal and external con-

---

Table 21–2. DSM-IV-TR diagnostic criteria for acute stress disorder

---

A. The person has been exposed to a traumatic event in which both of the following were present:

  (1) the person experienced, witnessed, or was confronted with an event or events that involved actual or threatened death or serious injury, or a threat to the physical integrity of self or others

  (2) the person's response involved intense fear, helplessness, or horror

B. Either while experiencing or after experiencing the distressing event, the individual has three (or more) of the following dissociative symptoms:

  (1) a subjective sense of numbing, detachment, or absence of emotional responsiveness

  (2) a reduction in awareness of his or her surroundings (e.g., "being in a daze")

  (3) derealization

  (4) depersonalization

  (5) dissociative amnesia (i.e., inability to recall an important aspect of the trauma)

C. The traumatic event is persistently reexperienced in at least one of the following ways: recurrent images, thoughts, dreams, illusions, flashback episodes, or a sense of reliving the experience; or distress on exposure to reminders of the traumatic event.

D. Marked avoidance of stimuli that arouse recollections of the trauma (e.g., thoughts, feelings, conversations, activities, places, people).

E. Marked symptoms of anxiety or increased arousal (e.g., difficulty sleeping, irritability, poor concentration, hypervigilance, exaggerated startle response, motor restlessness).

F. The disturbance causes clinically significant distress or impairment in social, occupational, or other important areas of functioning or impairs the individual's ability to pursue some necessary task, such as obtaining necessary assistance or mobilizing personal resources by telling family members about the traumatic experience.

G. The disturbance lasts for a minimum of 2 days and a maximum of 4 weeks and occurs within 4 weeks of the traumatic event.

H. The disturbance is not due to the direct physiological effects of a substance (e.g., a drug of abuse, a medication) or a general medical condition, is not better accounted for by brief psychotic disorder, and is not merely an exacerbation of a preexisting Axis I or Axis II disorder.

Source.   Reprinted from American Psychiatric Association: *Diagnostic and Statistical Manual of Mental Disorders*, 4th Edition, Text Revision. Washington, DC, American Psychiatric Association, 2000. Copyright 2000 American Psychiatric Association. Used with permission.

---

firmations. Child self-reports as gleaned in the clinical interview must be supplemented by parental histories and potentially important collateral information taken from other sources, including eyewitnesses, child protective teams, hospital records, and police documents. Careful attention to the nature of the stressor is mandatory. For example, physically abused boys may be at greater risk for developing externalizing behavior and conduct disorder that may hide or mask the presence of

PTSD, and the diagnosis may be missed in the absence of a thorough assessment of trauma exposure (Pelcowitz et al. 1994). Also, even though many sexually abused children do not meet strict diagnostic criteria for PTSD (Kendall-Tackett et al. 1993), clinicians must not underestimate the level of psychological impairment in this population.

Large-scale disasters like the Oklahoma City bombing of the Murrah Federal Building and the September 11th attack on the

World Trade Center may constitute an amalgam of traumatic experiences—including interpersonal violence, technological disaster, injury, loss of life, and displacement—as well as secondary traumatic phenomena. In cases of natural or technological disasters (e.g., an earthquake or a building collapse), the effect of trauma varies, depending not only on the severity of the disaster but also on the location, context, evacuation and recovery methods, advanced communication, popular media coverage, and disaster relief efforts.

Secondary adversities commonly befall children after tragedies—including displacement, relocation, attendance at a new school, separation from siblings, involuntary unemployment of a parent, and increased financial difficulties (Goenjian et al. 1994)—as well as changes in lifestyle and daily routines, which may be disruptive in and of themselves. Globally, the public health consequences of adversity secondary to trauma are immense. Medical procedures and rehabilitation may be ongoing for physical injuries and disability, and reintegration into school may be difficult. Children exposed to war atrocities may also experience malnutrition, deprivation, family disruption, loss, immigration, and resettlement. When the violence or disaster results in the death of a family member or a friend, an important interplay occurs between trauma and grief reactions, including continued preoccupation with the circumstances of the death and psychological upheavals among family members with different degrees of exposure (Pynoos et al. 1987b). Grief reactions and secondary depression in particular may complicate the reaction to a traumatic event.

Recent literature confirms that the objective magnitude of the stressor is directly proportional to the risk of developing PTSD (March 1993; McNally 1993). For example, in studies of the aftermath of a schoolyard sniper attack, Pynoos and Nader (1989a) and Pynoos et al. (1987b) showed that degree of exposure (proximity) was linearly related to the risk for PTSD symptoms.

Events that involve interpersonal violence or threat appear to be more likely to cause PTSD than technological or natural disasters (Yehuda 2002). PTSD occurs more frequently in those who experience rape and physical or sexual molestation than in those who are involved in accidents or natural disasters or who hear about traumatic events happening to others (Breslau et al. 1998). Traumas that are unpredictable or uncontrollable or that are perceived as lethal are more likely to invoke an intense response (Holbrook et al. 2001; Schreiber and Galai-Gat 1993).

■ Reexperiencing

Recall of traumatic exposure involves intense perceptual experiences and internal appraisals of the threat (Eth and Pynoos 1985). Children and adolescents with PTSD typically reexperience traumatic events in distressing intrusive thoughts or memories, in dreams, and (less commonly) in flashbacks. Reexperiencing may occur spontaneously or in response to traumatic reminders, called trauma triggers, that are linked to traumatic moments within the event itself. In addition, children mentally return to their experience, searching for ways to offset traumatic helplessness or to alter the outcome in thought and fantasy. In young children whose trauma exposure may have occurred preverbally before a narrative account and clear memory could be established, reexperiencing may take the form of fear reactions; reenactment; violent, odd, or repetitive posttraumatic actions; or distressing dreams and night terrors.

Children's traumatic dreams depict direct personal threat, even death, or threat of harm to others, especially family members, and they renew emotions associated with the experience.

Traumatic play refers to the repetitive dramatization in play of elements or themes of the event (Terr 1990). Children may involve siblings or peers in their traumatic play (Terr 1988). As with traumatic images, this play may recur because the child alters the action—for instance, by compulsively catching the bullet before it strikes. With time, the incorporation of traumatic elements may impede the normative uses of play (Pynoos and Nader 1990). The qualities of a persistent noxious theme, intensity, and repetitiveness that characterize traumatic play are in contrast to the usual fluidity, flexibility, and spontaneity that characterizes normal childhood play.

Reenactment behavior refers to conscious or unconscious replication of some aspect of the traumatic experience (Saylor et al. 1992; Terr 1990). In younger children, the behavior may derive from an "action memory." For example, a preschool child who was trapped in a well began to squeeze herself into small spaces. Adolescents especially may seek out opportunities to engage in reenactment behavior or thrill seeking and thus attempt to master or take command of the situation. Traumatic reminders may elicit acting out or dysfunctional behavior. For example, when one adolescent boy felt helpless in meeting a personal demand or confrontation, he would lie down on the floor in the way he had during a hostage taking.

Traumatic reminders—which may be technically defined as conditioned stimuli that provoke conditioned responses directly or indirectly related to the traumatic event itself—include the external circumstances of the event and the internal emotional and physical reactions of the child. The role of these reminders is in triggering physiological and psychological reactions and accounts for much of the phasic nature of the disorder. Common reminders include the following:

- Circumstances (e.g., location, time, preceding activity, clothes worn)
- Precipitating conditions (e.g., noises, high winds after experiencing a tornado, arguing)
- Other signs of danger (e.g., staring eyes, blaring horns, flashing lights)
- Endangering objects (e.g., trees, broken glass, weapons, belts)
- Situations presenting a sense of helplessness (e.g., cries for help, crying, fast heartbeat, a sinking feeling, ineffectualness, or moments of aloneness)

■ Avoidance of Stimuli or Numbing of General Responsiveness

Children with PTSD make conscious attempts to avoid traumatic reminders—namely, the thoughts, feelings, or activities that precipitate distressing recollections of the event. Cognitive suppression, distraction, and behavioral avoidance are particularly common, as is a frank refusal to talk about or discuss the trauma. However, children pay a high price for these survival strategies, because they inevitably affect other areas of functioning. The loss of previously acquired skills may cause a child to be less verbal or to regress to behaviors such as thumb sucking or enuresis. Rather than reporting feeling "numb," younger children report not wanting to know how they feel, tell of feeling alone with their subjective experience, or make efforts to keep an emotion from emerging (e.g., by going to sit alone). Children who are engaged in avoidance may appear deconcentrated and aloof. Other features of avoidance or numbing include periods of blank stares or looking dazed, withdrawal from social contact, and the appearance of being shut down. It is worth pointing out that a child's refusal to acknowledge or to talk about a potential traumatic experience does not, de facto, imply that the child is demonstrating the avoidance criterion of PTSD. The absence of evidence is not necessarily, in this case, evidence for diagnosis. When attempting to validate the diagnosis of PTSD, clinicians need to exert caution in this regard. Children will often refuse to directly discuss traumatic events whether or not they meet criteria for a diagnosis of PTSD.

Children may avoid specific thoughts, locations, objects, themes in their play, and behaviors that remind them of the incident. They may discontinue pleasurable activities to avoid excitement or fear. Diminished activity may represent a preoccupation with intrusive phenomena, a depressive reaction, an avoidance of affect-laden states or of traumatic reminders, or an effort to reduce the risk of further trauma.

Although earlier observations suggested a relative absence of major amnesia in children, more recent studies have reported a variety of memory disturbances (Pynoos and Nader 1989a). These disturbances may be introduced during recall rather than during perception or storage. Children may omit moments of extreme threat to life (at times screened by detailed recounting of other fearful moments); may distort proximity, duration, or sequencing; may introduce premonitions; and may minimize their life threat in other ways. Dissociative memory disturbances may also occur, especially in response to physical coercion, molestation, or abuse (Putnam and Trickett 1993).

■ Increased States of Arousal

Sleep disturbances, irritability, difficulty concentrating, hypervigilance, exaggerated startle responses, and outbursts of aggression represent a state of increased physiological arousal (Perry 1985; Perry and Pate 1994). The child is seen as being "on alert," hypervigilant, scanning, and ready to respond to any environmental threat (Ornitz and Pynoos 1989). Especially in school-age children, physiological reactivity may include somatic symptoms as a form of hyperarousal. Sleep disturbance may be severe and persistent; changes seen in sleep architecture have been noted in adult studies (Pitman 1993). Difficulty falling asleep, sleepwalking, and night terrors are common.

Finally, temporary or chronic difficulty in modulating aggression can make children act more irritable and quick to anger, resulting in a reduced tolerance for the normal behaviors, demands, and slights of peers and family members and in unusual acts of aggression or social withdrawal (Yule and Canterbury 1994). Often the externalizing behaviors, hyperreactivity, and irritability can be the most manifest of the symptom triad in children and adolescents with PTSD and may further complicate the diagnosis by masking other less obvious symptoms.

PTSD Complexity: From Individual Diagnosis to Population Frequency

Childhood and adolescent PTSD is a complex disorder with a myriad of symptom presentations. Like adults, children often present with multiple comorbid conditions adding still further layers of symptom complexity. PTSD is commonly misdiagnosed due to the failure of adequate trauma history taking on the part of some clinicians and due to the ease with which other clinicians make the diagnosis based simply on a history of trauma exposure in the midst of psychiatric symptoms.

Existing data suggest variability in prevalence ranging from 10% (Breslau et al. 1991) to as much as 40% (Richters 1993; Richters and Martinez 1993) in children and youths from violence-ridden neighborhoods. However, rates of PTSD vary widely depending on the nature of the trauma and the population studied—perhaps so widely, in fact, as to render large-population measures of incidence and prevalence relatively uninformative. In Terr's (1981b) cohort, for example, 100% of children developed PTSD, whereas rates of PTSD development in natural disasters are in the range of 3%–5% (Kessler et al. 1995).

It appears that children are more sensitive to the effects of trauma than adults, given the same trauma exposure, and consequently may exhibit higher rates of PTSD development.

Once established, PTSD in children is often both chronic and debilitating (March and Amaya-Jackson 1994; Nader et al. 1990; Terr 1983a), although the clinical course of PTSD in a given child can be highly variable. Factors responsible for the variability in course of illness include circumstantial ones (the nature of the stressor); attributes intrinsic to the child such as preexisting psychopathology, quality of attachment, and coping and resiliency strengths; and extrinsic influences that govern the nature of the recovery environment such as poverty or family support. In general, the more severe the stressor—in terms of intensity, duration, suddenness, and personal impact—the more prolonged the course. For those with mild exposure and minimum interpersonal impact, the symptoms of the trauma usually diminish within days or weeks of the event. Multiple adversities in the child's environment significantly add to the risk of comorbidity, and therefore to the chronicity and seriousness of the clinical condition.

For a variety of reasons, stress reactions in young people are increasingly common presentations in clinical settings. The opportunities for trauma exposure in modern life are numerous. In studies of PTSD in a rural North Carolina community, the median number of PTSD-magnitude stressors in children with posttraumatic symptomatology was five (March et al. 1995a). Contemporary society thus sets the stage for children to be exposed to a great variety of technological and interpersonal traumas on a scale that is perhaps unprecedented (e.g., the extensive media coverage of the September 11th attack on the World Trade Center). Given the great diversity of possible types of traumatic exposure, Terr (1991) provided a useful distinction between different traumatic processes: type I traumas (sudden and unpredictable, with a single-incident stressor) and type II traumas (chronic, expected, with a repeated stressor, typical of childhood physical and sexual abuse).

Developmental Considerations

The developmental stage exerts important influence over children's registration of danger, appraisals of threat, attribution of meaning, emotional and cognitive means of coping, toleration of their reactions, expectations about recovery, and effectiveness in addressing life changes (Pynoos 1994; Pynoos et al. 1995). Particularly problematic is the assessment of PTSD in infants and toddlers, in whom the lack of language development makes diagnosis difficult. The criteria set as evolved in DSM-IV-TR is not particularly sensitive to PTSD symptoms in infants and toddlers. Alternative criteria have been proposed that are more behaviorally anchored and are more sensitive to the likely manifestations of trauma in this early age group (Scheeringa et al. 1995; Zero to Three 1994).

Loss of acquired skills or failure to acquire new skills may manifest differently according to age. For example, younger children may become less verbal or may even experience mutism, enuresis, or thumb sucking in response to trauma. School-age children may show more inconsistency in behavior and mood, report forgetting recently acquired knowledge, and perform household chores as they did when they were younger. Adolescents may report becoming confused, similar to a younger child, or may exhibit dependency behaviors, become clingy, or withdraw from usual sources of emotional support.

Younger or temperamentally anxious children may overgeneralize threat and danger or be more socially reticent. Depressed children may have undue guilt. Impulsive children may exhibit increased hyperreactivity, explosiveness, and other problematic behaviors. Children may experience a renewal of symptoms or concerns due to prior stressful events (trauma reactivation), and, in the case of prior trauma, these reactions may significantly prolong recovery from the current traumatic episode.

The presence of PTSD in childhood or adolescence has a ripple effect throughout development. At present it is unknown whether it is "incurable" and remains as a lasting scar, as some researchers view it (Terr 1991), or whether it introduces an altered yet recoverable developmental trajectory that can be compensated for with appropriate interventions.

Comorbidity and Differential Diagnosis

Traumatized children frequently have symptoms of disorders other than PTSD, and children with other disorders often have PTSD as a comorbid diagnosis (Famularo et al. 1992; Ford et al. 2000; Gold-man et al. 1992; Pynoos et al. 1987a; Wozniak et al. 1999). There is reason to believe that comorbidities become more complicated with time; epidemiological studies sampling adults with child trauma histories indicate that serious and multiple comorbid conditions aggregate with PTSD (Breslau et al. 1998; Kessler et al. 1995; Muller et al. 2000). In traumatized children a wide variety of social behaviors have been reported to be abnormal, with problematic social behaviors serving both as a risk factor for and an outcome of traumatic experiences (Conaway and Hansen 1989).

In addition to true comorbidity, spurious comorbidity with PTSD results from overlap between criteria sets (e.g., affective constriction in PTSD overlaps with anhedonia in depression; symptoms of hypervigilance may mimic symptoms of generalized anxiety) and confounding similar symptoms of other diagnoses with those of PTSD (e.g., the inattention, impulsivity, and reactive defiance of attention-deficit/hyperactivity disorder and oppositional defiant disorder appear like the hyperarousal symptoms of PTSD). To clarify the diagnostic picture, careful questioning of parents, teachers, and especially the child vis-à-vis his or her internal experiences is necessary.

Traumatic experiences have an inherent potential to induce a variety of anxiety symptoms (Lonigan et al. 1994; March et al. 1995a). Many children experience increased attachment behaviors such as clinging, seeking reassurance, and worrying about the safety of family members or friends. Some children may be genetically prone to separation anxiety; others may have separation anxiety because of prior threats to important attachment bonds. However, most children respond directly to a traumatic event by activating attachment behaviors. A diagnosis of separation anxiety disorder is warranted when symptoms of separation anxiety interfere with the child's daily life, but the clinician must remember the reasonableness of the originating threat. Thus, reconstituting a safe environment must always precede otherwise premature attempts to enforce or encourage separation. The establishment of safety and assurance that basic needs are met must take place for a thorough and accurate differential diagnosis to be made and should certainly take place before any treatment is undertaken (Scheeringa 1999). Children who do not meet full criteria for PTSD often manifest symptoms of generalized anxiety disorder. It is important to remember the traumatic origin of the child's anxiety when designing a treatment plan for such children, who may otherwise be at risk for delayed-onset PTSD.

Other children display somatic rather than cognitive anxiety symptoms as a form of traumatic reenactment. These symptoms can resemble limited-symptom panic attacks, and without adequate treatment they may progress to panic disorder or to PTSD. Children may exhibit diffuse physical complaints derived from anxiety that may be related to the trauma, such as headache, stomachache, genital pain, or pain on urination.

Trauma-specific phobias are relatively easy to distinguish from PTSD in that they are more isolated, lack tonic arousal, do not readily generalize to new situations, and result in less psychosocial dysfunction than does PTSD.

Intrusive thoughts, urges, and images—not all of them pathological (Terr 1983b)—are found in several childhood psychiatric disorders other than PTSD. Intrusive phenomena following a traumatic event can often be distinguished from nontraumatic intrusions by the presence of trauma-specific contents, a subjective link made by the child with the trauma, or by contextual features. Obsessive-compulsive disorder is distinguished from PTSD in that obsessive-compulsive disorder usually lacks a PTSD-magnitude precipitant and trauma-specific intrusions.

Depressive-spectrum conditions are among the most common secondary comorbidities in PTSD and often constitute an important treatment focus (Yule 1992; Yule and Canterbury 1994). A full depressive syndrome is frequently a normal reaction to the loss of a loved one (Pynoos et al. 1987b). However, the trauma response often significantly interferes with the normal grief process. For example, reminiscing, an essential part of the bereavement process, can be drastically inhibited because the intrusive recollections of the traumatic event interfere with the child's effort to recall pleasant memories of the deceased (Pynoos et al. 1987b).

Schizophrenia, the delusional disorders, and brief reactive psychoses are readily differentiated from PTSD based on dissimilarities between psychotic intrusive thoughts and PTSD reexperiencing and the presence of otherwise intact reality testing in PTSD. Flashbacks, dissociative and hyperarousal symptoms, and isolated quasi-psychotic symptoms (e.g., seeing the face of the perpetrator around sleep onset) may transiently be present in the PTSD symptom presentation.

Self-mutilation, sexual or highly aggressive play, and suicidal behaviors may represent traumatic reenactments in children who have experienced sexual or physical abuse or who have been tortured, and these behaviors should always prompt a search for traumatic antecedents (Albach and Everaerd 1992).

As noted above, trauma can exacerbate, and PTSD can mimic, disruptive behavior disorders. Indeed, there appears to be an associated risk in children who have attention-deficit/hyperactivity disorder (ADHD) and oppositional defiant disorder for developing PTSD (Ford et al. 2000). A study of children after the Hamlet, North Carolina, fire showed that the development of PTSD exacerbated or led to disruptive behavior disorders (March et al. 1995a). However, before diagnosing oppositional defiant disorder, conduct disorder, or ADHD in a child who has experienced abuse or a life-threatening event, the clinician must rule out PTSD as the cause of the child's deteriorating school performance, inattention, irritability, or aggression. Substance abuse can complicate clinical presentations in adolescence, especially in teenagers who have trauma or abuse histories. Diagnoses such as conduct disorder and substance abuse should be addressed in their own right, even if the primary clinical focus is on PTSD.

Finally, it is important to recognize that not all reactions to traumatic events are necessarily pathological. This is especially true during the initial days and weeks following a traumatic event (Famularo et al. 1990; March 1991). If full syndrome criteria are present for less than 1 month, the diagnosis of acute stress disorder should be given.

Etiology and Pathogenesis

The interplay between an environmental event (i.e., the stressor) and a complex neurobiological system characterizes the pathogenesis of PTSD. With this cardinal fact in mind, the current conceptual framework for understanding psychological trauma has evolved primarily from three theoretical perspectives: psychoanalytic theory, social learning theory, and more recently, neurobiology.

■ Psychoanalytic Theory

In 1920, Freud noted that psychic trauma results when a traumatic stimulus overwhelms the ego and renders it helpless (S. Freud 1920/1955). Freud believed that the essential element in the pathogenesis of the traumatic response was the energy the trauma victim needed to utilize in warding off unbearable traumatic affects.

Freud also described the patient's "repetition compulsion" as an attempt to achieve mastery over the event by repeating themes of the trauma in actions of everyday life, leading to fixation on the trauma. Other psychodynamically defined defense mechanisms that are important in trauma work are suppression, repression, denial, dissociation, projection, doing-undoing, and identification with the aggressor.

■ Social Learning Theory

In contrast to psychoanalytic theory, a two-factor conditioning model derived from social learning theory frames PTSD as a stimulus-driven anxiety disorder in which both classical (factor 1) and instrumental or operant (factor 2) conditioning play important roles (Foa and Riggs 1995; Jones and Barlow 1990). In classical conditioning, the stressor or traumatic event acts as an unconditioned stimulus that elicits an unconditioned (reflexive) response characterized by physiological activation (fight-flight-freeze), extreme fear, and the cognitive perception of helplessness in the child. Cognitive, affective, physiological, and environmental cues accompanying the traumatic event then constitute conditioned stimuli, which, as mentioned earlier, are often called *traumatic reminders* or *trauma triggers*. Traumatic reminders, via stimulus generalization, become capable of eliciting a conditioned response in the form of PTSD symptoms. In instrumental conditioning, children quickly learn by trial and error how to reduce PTSD symptoms through cognitive and behavioral avoidance and sometimes anxiety-damping rituals.

Foa et al. (1989) summarized the literature on cognitive information processing in PTSD, hypothesizing that persons who have PTSD develop "fear structures" that are conditioned by both the event and the PTSD symptom picture. Fear structures are exceptionally sensitive to activation by internal and external cues reminiscent of the initiating trauma, including thoughts and affects incorporated during and after the event. Moreover, they contain automatic stimulus-response elements and verbal, somatic, and behavioral cues that attach to the meaning of the event. Symptoms may be maintained through the altered and inaccurate threat assessment that children with PTSD have established, whereby neutral stimuli are continuously being misappraised and perceived as threatening.

■ Neurobiology

Although neurobiology is conceptually separate from social learning theory, it is not difficult to imagine that fear structures are also represented at the neurobiological level (Perry 1985; Perry and Pate 1994). The literature on the neurobiology of PTSD in children and adolescents has begun to develop only in the past decade (De Bellis et al. 1994a, 1994b; Perry 1985; Perry and Pate 1994). Little is known about the specific neurobiological effects of early trauma on human growth and development. De Bellis et al. (1999a, 1999b) have extensively reviewed the psychobiology of pediatric PTSD.

It appears that early life trauma has an effect, not surprisingly, on a variety of central nervous system functions and anatomy as well as on neuroendocrine and immunological regulation (De Bellis et al. 1999a, 1999b; Heim et al. 2001; Heit et al. 1999; Wilson et al. 1999; Yehuda et al. 2001). Theoretical models, largely

based on dysregulation in the neurophysiological and neuroanatomical systems regulating the stress response, are gradually becoming more sophisticated (Ornitz and Pynoos 1989; Putnam and Trickett 1993) although the child and adolescent literature remains quite unsystematic and lags considerably behind adult research. Neurotransmitters implicated in traumatic stress include norepinephrine, serotonin, dopamine, γ-aminobutyric acid (GABA), excitatory amino acids, corticosteroids and their modulators, and endogenous opioids (De Bellis et al. 1994a, 1994b). De Bellis et al. (1999a, 1999b, 2001) showed that, compared with control children, maltreated children had smaller intracranial and cerebral volumes (but not hippocampal volumes) tracked over 2 years of development. Maltreated children were also shown to exhibit more suicidal ideation and behavior, greater depression, overall rates of psychopathology, and increased frequency of dissociation. Dysregulation in the hypothalamic-pituitary-adrenal axis and in secretion of cortisol (a "stress" hormone) is known to be present in both adults and children with PTSD (Cicchetti and Rogosch 2001; Yehuda 1998; Yehuda et al. 2001), although the specific abnormality tends to be variable. King et al. (2001) demonstrated that girls ages 5–7 years exposed to recent sexual abuse exhibited significantly lower salivary cortisol levels than age-matched control subjects. Although these findings are intriguing, the precise developmental implications for early-life dysregulation in hypothalamic-pituitary axis function have yet to be worked out.

Assessment

As in all psychiatric disorders, the first step in establishing a treatment program is a careful, thorough assessment that, in the case of PTSD, is stressor focused (Nader et al. 1991). Although semistructured interviews are useful for assessing psychiatric problems in children and adolescents, reliability and validity data for PTSD instruments have been slow to emerge (March and Albano 1996), and no structured instrument can replace a well-conducted series of clinical interviews in this most complex disorder. The most commonly used instrument—the Pynoos-Nader version of the Stress-Reaction Index—shows modest empirical support as a semistructured interview; it has been used as a self-report measure (Lonigan et al. 1991; March et al. 1995a) but does not adequately capture the DSM-IV criteria (American Psychiatric Association 1994), nor does it yield a DSM-IV diagnosis. With the support of the National Center for PTSD, Nader et al. (1994) developed the Clinician-Administered PTSD Scale—Child and Adolescent Version (CAPS-C). The CAPS-C allows for current and lifetime diagnoses and dimensional assessment of DSM-IV PTSD symptoms and collateral psychopathology. It is time consuming and demanding on the clinician to conduct and is probably best reserved for clinical-research settings.

A multimethod, multimodal evaluation is the preferred technique, including information from multiple sources (Amaya-Jackson and March 1993). In children younger than 48 months the most important trauma-variable predictor appears to be whether a caregiver was threatened, and therefore caregiver reports are crucial sources of clinical information (Scheeringa 1999). Parent–teacher measures, such as the Conners Parent and Teacher Rating Scales (Conners et al. 1995) and the SNAP IV (Swanson 1992) are efficient adjuncts for assessing collateral externalizing symptoms. Self-report measures, such as the Children's Depression Inventory (Kovacs 1985) and the Multidimensional Anxiety Scale for Children (March et al. 1995b), can be used to assess internalizing comorbidities.

Finally, the assessment of PTSD in children and adolescents must be embedded within developmental and social contexts. To some extent, because the DSM-IV-TR nosology is less sensitive to evaluation of early-life trauma and because it underemphasizes both developmental differences and social contextual factors, it is less than adequate for evaluating childhood-onset PTSD.

Treatment

■ Psychotherapy and Psychosocial Management

Other than case reports, few published treatment studies specifically focus on PTSD in children. However, researchers and clinicians have reported a variety of techniques that have proved valuable in clinical trauma work (Yule and Canterbury 1994). The adult PTSD literature points to tactics that may prove beneficial to children as well. In general, a "prevention-intervention" model—which incorporates triage for children exposed to stressors, support and strengthening of coping skills for anticipated grief and trauma responses, treatment of other disorders that may develop or become exacerbated in the context of PTSD, and treatment of acute PTSD symptoms—is recommended (Amaya-Jackson and March 1995a, 1995b; Pynoos and Nader 1993). The horrific effects of trauma may never be fully undone, and therefore "cure" may not be the appropriate treatment goal, but trauma victims can become well-functioning survivors if appropriate treatment is given and facilitation of healing takes place.

Solomon et al. (1992) reviewed empirical studies of psychotherapeutic, cognitive-behavioral, and drug treatments for PTSD. They correctly noted that the literature provides greater support for cognitive-behavioral treatment than for other treatments. Despite the lack of randomized controlled trials, the majority of child psychiatric clinicians questioned about their treatment strategies for PTSD utilized pharmacotherapy as a primary treatment element (Cohen et al. 2001). Treatment providers to children and adolescents are inevitably forced to operate from clinical consensus, uncontrolled trials, and downward extrapolation from adult studies.

The mainstay of treatment is usually an admixture of cognitive-behavioral, family-supportive, and psychodynamically informed psychotherapy, spread over several phases: brief preventive or initial therapy, long-term therapy, and pulsed intervention. Additional interventions include formal group and family therapy. Early preventive and initial therapy interventions are especially important in the setting of acute trauma, catching a window of opportunity when the youngster's symptoms are most prominent and the sealing over of affect has not had a chance to occur. Central to almost all treatment strategies is an emphasis on reexposing the individual to traumatic cues under safe conditions, incorporating reparative and mastery elements in a structured, supportive manner. An important point concerning psychotherapy for children with PTSD is that poorly conducted therapy at best can be a waste of precious time in the life of a child and at worst can be harmful and can inadvertently lead to retraumatization. Long-term therapy, especially in young children, can easily devolve into unfocused, repetitive sessions of "fiddling around." Therapists need to be diligent about continually rethinking the symptom picture, keeping focused on current dysfunction, and directing the therapy to specifically facilitate higher levels of adaptation and coping.

■ Initial Interventions

Critical incident stress debriefing and psychological first aid are techniques that are particularly applicable in crisis centers and in classrooms, although these techniques have no strong empirical support (Pynoos and Nader 1988, 1989b). Applications of these techniques typically involve groups of children gathering together in a specific setting. School settings in particular serve as an optimum site for immediate crisis intervention, ventilation, information processing, and screening of children who may need further evaluation (Motta 1994; Pynoos and Nader 1989b). Debriefing interviews with teachers and parents can help to identify, clarify, and normalize adults' and children's reactions to a traumatic event. During classroom discussions, children describe the traumatic event on a moment-to-moment basis, allowing clarification of traumatic and grief reactions as they affect current functioning.

In both individual therapy and group settings, free-form or semistructured projective play techniques such as spontaneous drawing, Winnicott's (1971) squiggle game, or Levy's (1939) preset play can be used as a means to express feelings, clarify confusion, and identify needs. Although it is often underestimated, simply allowing the time and a format for the basic human need to put experience into words and thus share traumatic events with others can be a potent early-phase intervention. Amaya-Jackson et al. (2003) described a protocol-based cognitive-behavioral treatment for PTSD designed to be used in groups of children as a school-based treatment intervention. This may be especially useful in situations where there are high rates of shared trauma exposure among populations of children in definable geographic regions such as neighborhoods or school districts.

The initial evaluation of children can incorporate many other interview techniques and goals that lead naturally into therapeutic intervention. Through the use of play, drawings, puppets, and role-playing, the child's experience as well as subjective meaning and attributions can be strategically explored. Clinicians must pay close attention to their own countertransference and rescue fantasies, the tendency to shy away from particularly upsetting aspects of the child's experiences, and well-intended but misguided attempts to spare the child distress when asking precise questions about the trauma. Children's reactions can at times be normalized, intervention fantasies can be acknowledged, traumatic reminders can be identified, and confusion and distortions can be clarified. The psychotherapeutic evaluation period should not be rushed, because it may take several sessions, especially in younger children, to develop a working therapeutic alliance and to detect emergent trauma themes in play assessment encounters.

An important but often neglected element of all types of therapy for pediatric PTSD is the initial didactic explanation to parents and children of the components of PTSD and the specific rationale for therapy, collectively referred to as psychoeducation. Children as well as adolescents need to understand the nature of their disorder and how their therapy relates to the bad things that have happened to them. Parents especially need to understand the rationale and basic behavioral principles of CBT, because by its very nature it requires some amount of discomfort during the course of treatment.

■ Brief Therapy

Trauma work frequently involves brief psychotherapy. Because controlled reex-posure to traumatic cues is an essential aspect of treatment, traumatic memories and associated specific reminders must be worked through in their entirety, both in therapy and in real-life activities. A key treatment concept necessary for successful "working through" is to approach the trauma as a series of traumatic moments, that is, sequential vivid memories of distress linked by less distressing narrative content (Pynoos and Nader 1988). Systematically strategizing recall in a moment-by-moment fashion minimizes cognitive and behavioral avoidance and thus promotes exposure and habituation of anxiety. Brief therapies may be most appropriate in situations where a child is seen soon after a traumatic exposure, in situations of single-incident trauma and when the target symptoms and goals of treatment are clearly defined and of a limited scope.

■ Cognitive-Behavioral Therapy

PTSD is the quintessential threat-induced anxiety disorder (March 1991; March and Amaya-Jackson 1994). As with other anxiety disorders, some clinicians believe that cognitive-behavioral therapy (CBT) optimized for the PTSD symptom picture may be the treatment of choice for PTSD symptoms per se and may be delivered both to individual children and in group-based therapeutic formats. Saigh (1992) made a persuasive case for the efficacy of CBT as a treatment of single-incident trauma in young persons. Deblinger et al. (1990, 1999) showed that CBT benefits children with PTSD caused by sexual abuse and that the benefits of therapy are durable until the 2-year follow-up. In a recently published randomized trial of more than 200 children, the majority of whom had sexual abuse-related PTSD, Cohen et al. (2004) demonstrated the superiority of manualized trauma-focused cognitive-behavior therapy (TF-CBT). Children in the TF-CBT group exhibited significant improvement in core PTSD symptoms as well as in depressive behavior, and parents exhibited improvement in depressive symptoms and effective parenting. This study lends further support to the effectiveness of trauma-focused therapy in the treatment of children with PTSD.

Theoretical Model Underlying PTSD and Its Treatment With CBT

Cognitive, affective, physiological, and environmental cues accompanying the traumatic event constitute conditioned stimuli, which, as noted earlier, are often called *traumatic reminders*. In turn, traumatic reminders become capable of eliciting fear (the conditioned response), which should decrease with prolonged, repeated exposure (habituation), assuming the absence of real threat. In the second (instrumental conditioning) stage, the individual learns to reduce trauma-related distress through cognitive and behavioral avoidance. These operant anxiety-reducing behaviors preclude the extinction of trauma-relevant anxiety and therefore are customarily targeted in exposure-based interventions.

Foa et al. (e.g., Foa and Riggs 1995; Foa and Rothbaum 1998) proposed that two sets of dysfunctional cognitions (i.e., schemas) underlie the development of this disorder: the world is indiscriminately dangerous and oneself (the victim) is extremely incompetent.

Typically, CBT for children with PTSD targets specific features of the PTSD symptom picture, using anxiety-management training, anger-coping, and exposure-based interventions. Numerous studies have shown that these interventions effectively reduce target symptoms in anxious children (Kendall 1991). By promoting ha-

bituation, exposure—encountering contact with the phobic stimulus until anxiety diminishes substantially—probably forms the core intervention in PTSD (Foa and Riggs 1995; Foa et al. 1989). When necessary, response prevention facilitates exposure by blocking rituals and avoidance behaviors, thereby undoing the reinforcing effects of avoidance. Anxiety-management training–which includes relaxation, breathing training, and cognitive restructuring—facilitates exposure, promotes provision of cognitive and behavioral corrective information, and enhances positive coping (Foa and Rothbaum 1992).

In all cases, CBT for other target symptoms must be integrated into the total treatment picture so that the trauma-relevant meaning of the symptoms to the child can be placed in an appropriate therapeutic context.

■ Group and Family-Based Therapy

Group and family therapy are additional interventions that can play an important role in treatment. Family therapy is particularly helpful in addressing the needs of children who are not receiving necessary emotional support within the family. Family members may have difficulty facing the child's distress or may lack necessary (but still teachable) skills to meet the child's needs adequately. Parents may be preoccupied with their own reactions and may not be aware of the child's symptoms. Families can be taught coping strategies, such as how to recognize and deal with traumatic reminders. In designing treatment interventions for young children, Scheeringa (1999) designed an eight-component package that places primary emphasis on parent-based interventions and on simply keeping the parent coming and engaged in therapy. Direct inclusion of parents in the treatment process may be especially important in situations involving intense interpersonal trauma such as in cases of intrafamilial physical or sexual abuse. Inclusion of parents and the use of group formats may also be useful in community shared trauma exposure such as Stubenbort et al. (2001) report in their use of CBT group therapy for children and adults after an air disaster.

Long-Term Treatment and Pulsed Intervention

A subgroup of children require long-term treatment. Exposure to massive violence, intrafamilial homicide or suicide, prolonged abuse, or repetitively distressing events suggests that brief trauma work may be insufficient. The presence of preexisting psychopathology in the child or a parent, a history of abuse, multiple foster placements, or ongoing exposure to a disruptive living situation also suggest a need for more intensive, longer-term intervention. "Pulsing" the treatment helps to prevent ongoing helplessness by minimizing dependence on the therapist as "the only one who really understands."

Medication Management

Although PTSD has an exogenous origin and requires psychological treatments, it is nevertheless, using Kardiner's (1941) term, a true *physioneurosis,* and psychotropic medication often proves helpful in allowing psychological treatment to progress. Unfortunately, few data exist to guide the use of medication in children and adolescents with PTSD (for review, see Donnelly et al. 1999). Yet, in a large sampling of treatment providers Cohen et al. (2001) found that 95% of medical practitioners who treat pediatric PTSD use pharmacotherapy, in combination with psychodynamic or cognitive-behavioral therapies. Medication use in children and adolescents with PTSD should be based on a stepwise approach in which broad-spectrum agents are considered first, followed by attention to comorbid diagnoses that are likely to be amenable to pharmacological intervention. Medication algorithms have been developed for such a stepwise approach in both adults and children (Donnelly and Amaya-Jackson 2002; Friedman et al. 2000).

Ideally, medications should decrease intrusions, avoidance, and anxious arousal; minimize impulsivity; improve sleep; treat secondary disorders; facilitate cognitive-behavioral psychotherapies; and improve functioning in daily life. It should be borne in mind that effective treatment of even one symptom in children with PTSD (e.g., improvement of sleep-onset disturbance) can have a positive ripple effect across multiple domains of functioning. Two selective serotonin reuptake inhibitors (SSRIs), paroxetine and sertraline, have recently received U.S. Food and Drug Administration (FDA) approval for the treatment of PTSD in adults (Beebe 2001; Brady et al. 2000; Marshall et al. 2001). Although much more limited than for adults, clinical experience is similar for children and adolescents.

The decision to use medication is based primarily on the types of target symptoms present that are likely to be responsive to medication (both core PTSD symptoms and comorbid condition symptoms), their severity, and the degree of disability that they cause. Although no medication currently has an FDA label indication for the treatment of PTSD in childhood, data from adult studies and clinical experience with other disorders in childhood provide guidance in selecting pharmacological agents. Pharmacotherapy may be an important component in the multimodal treatment of PTSD because it may offer relief from highly debilitating symptoms and buffer children against intense symptoms, allowing for easier confrontation of traumatic material in therapy and better functioning in life activities.

The SSRIs have received perhaps the most attention and are likely first-line choices in childhood owing to their broad-spectrum activity in anxiety, mood, and obsessive-compulsive spectrum disorders and the fact that they have demonstrated effectiveness in adult populations (Brady et al. 2000; Hidalgo and Davidson 2000; Marshall et al. 2001; van der Kolk et al. 1994) and are being actively investigated in childhood. Seedat et al. (2001) report the effectiveness of citalopram in a 12-week open-label trial in eight adolescents with moderate to severe PTSD. Subjects in their trial exhibited a 38% reduction in PTSD symptoms at the end of treatment (however, curiously, self-reported depressive symptoms failed to improve). The SSRIs can be effective in reducing trauma-associated re-experiencing, anxiety, and collateral mood symptoms, although they may be less effective in avoidance or numbing symptoms.

Adrenergic agents such as the α_2-adrenergic agonists clonidine and guanfacine and the β-adrenergic antagonist propranolol reduce sympathetic tone and may be effective in the symptoms of hyperarousal, impulsivity, activation, sleep problems, and nightmares seen in PTSD (De Bellis 1994b; Horrigan 1996; Marmar et al. 1993). Clonidine in particular has been shown to decrease startle responses and may target other symptoms of physiological lability, as measured by autonomic arousal (Ornitz and Pynoos 1989). Adrenergic agents deserve consideration in managing the hyperarousal, activation, motor hyperactivity, and sleep-onset problems often associated with PTSD in childhood.

The benzodiazepines have been used to treat anxiety disorders in children and adults, although there are few if any data to support their effectiveness in the core symptoms of PTSD (Friedman 1998). These agents (e.g., clonazepam, lorazepam) may have a minor role to play in reducing acute and intense symptoms of anxiety or agitation, or as a short-term adjunctive treatment to facilitate exposure tasks in psychotherapy. However, they should be used with caution in children and adolescents owing to their propensity to cause paradoxical disinhibition and their abuse potential. The benzodiazepines cannot be recommended as first- or second-line therapy at present.

The mood stabilizers may have a role to play in the treatment of childhood PTSD, especially in cases of severe affective instability. Lithium, valproate, and carbamazepine may reduce extreme mood lability and anger dyscontrol. Carbamazepine has received the most attention and has been shown to markedly reduce flashbacks, traumatic nightmares, intrusive recollections, and sleep disturbance in adults (Lipper et al. 1986). Looff et al. (1995) found carbamazepine to be highly effective in treating core PTSD symptoms in 22 of 28 patients with sexual abuse histories who had high rates of comorbidity with other disorders of children and adolescents.

Atypical neuroleptics such as risperidone, olanzapine, quetiapine, and ziprasidone may have a limited role to play in childhood PTSD but should be reserved for cases in which psychotic symptoms, severe aggression, or self-injurious behaviors are complicating management and first-line treatments are not containing these symptoms.

Cyproheptadine, a histaminergic agent with serotonin partial agonist/antagonist activity, is a safe agent that is commonly used in clinical practice for sleep-onset problems and traumatic nightmares. There is little in the way of controlled evidence for its efficacy; however, some investigators report benefits, and it carries few risks in the child and adolescent age group (Brophy 1991).

In summary, the state of knowledge regarding medication treatments for children and adolescents is in the earliest stages of development. There are no well-conducted randomized clinical trials to guide practitioners. Medication may have an important role in reducing debilitating symptoms of PTSD and providing a buffer for children while they confront difficult material in therapy and may also help to improve their general day-to-day functioning. A reasonable approach is to begin with a broad-spectrum agent such as an SSRI, which should target anxiety, mood, and re-experiencing symptoms. Adrenergic agents such as clonidine, either used alone or in combination with an SSRI, may be useful when symptoms of hyperarousal and impulsivity are problematic. Supplementing with a mood stabilizer may be necessary in severe affective dyscontrol. Similarly, introduction of an atypical neuroleptic may be necessary in cases of severe self-injurious behavior, dissociation, psychosis, or aggression. Comorbid conditions such as ADHD should of course be targeted with pharmacotherapy known to be effective, such as the psychostimulants.

Conclusion

PTSD is a common cause of psychiatric morbidity in children and adolescents. The disorder in youth is similar to that in adulthood, with differences primarily stemming from divergent stressors, the differential impact across stages of development, developmental themes, and family considerations. Children appear to be more sensitive to the effects of trauma, and early-life trauma exposure may set into play a complex sequence of events leading to development of multiple psychiatric disorders in adulthood. Treatment of PTSD in childhood involves debriefing and ventilation, psychoeducation of parent and child, brief psychotherapy, and pulsed long-term intervention using an admixture of psychodynamic, cognitive-behavioral, and pharmacological treatments.

References

Albach F, Everaerd W: Posttraumatic stress symptoms in victims of childhood incest. Psychother Psychosom 57:143–151, 1992

Amaya-Jackson L, March J: Post-traumatic stress disorder in children and adolescents, in Child Psychiatric Clinics of North America: Anxiety Disorders, Vol 2. Edited by Leonard HL. New York, WB Saunders, 1993, pp 639–654

Amaya-Jackson L, March J: Posttraumatic stress disorder, in Anxiety Disorders in Children and Adolescents. Edited by March J. New York, Guilford, 1995a, pp 276–300

Amaya-Jackson L, March J: Post-traumatic stress disorder in adolescents. Adolesc Med 6:251–270, 1995b

Amaya-Jackson L, Reynolds V, Murray MC, et al: Cognitive-behavioral treatment for pediatric posttraumatic stress disorder: protocol and application in school and community settings. Cognitive and Behavioral Practice 10(3), 2003

American Psychiatric Association: Diagnostic and Statistical Manual of Mental Disorders, 4th Edition. Washington, DC, American Psychiatric Association, 1994

American Psychiatric Association: Diagnostic and Statistical Manual of Mental Disorders, 4th Edition, Text Revision. Washington, DC, American Psychiatric Association, 2000

Beebe KL: Paroxetine in the treatment of PTSD: a 12-week, placebo-controlled, multicenter study. GlaxoSmithKline, 2001

Brady K, Pearlstein T, Asnis GM, et al: Efficacy and safety of sertraline treatment of post-traumatic stress disorder: a randomized controlled trial. JAMA 283:1837–1844, 2000

Bremner JD, Shobe KK, Kihlstrom JF: False memories in women with self-reported childhood sexual abuse: an empirical study. Psychol Sci 11:333–337, 2000

Breslau N, Davis GC, Andreski P, et al: Traumatic events and posttraumatic stress disorder in an urban population of young adults. Arch Gen Psychiatry 48:216–222, 1991

Breslau N, Kessler RC, Chilcoat-Schultz LR, et al: Trauma and posttraumatic stress disorder in the community: the 1996 Detroit Area Survey of Trauma. Arch Gen Psychiatry 55:626–632, 1998

Brophy MH: Cyproheptadine for combat nightmares in posttraumatic stress disorder and dream anxiety disorder. Mil Med 156:100–101, 1991

Cicchetti D, Rogosch FA: Diverse patterns of neuroendocrine activity in maltreated children. Dev Psychopathol 13:677–693, 2001

Cohen JA: Practice parameters for the assessment and treatment of children and adolescents with posttraumatic stress disorder. J Am Acad Child Adolesc Psychiatry 37 (10, suppl):4S–26S, 1998

Cohen JA, Mannarino AP, Rogal S: Treatment practices for childhood posttraumatic stress disorder. Child Abuse Negl 25:123–135, 2001

Cohen JA, Deblinger E, Mannarino AP, et al: A multisite, randomized controlled trial for children with sexual abuse-related PTSD symptoms. J Am Acad Child Adolesc Psychiatry 43:393–402, 2004

Conaway LP, Hansen DJ: Social behavior of physically abused and neglected children: a critical review. Clin Psychol Rev 9:627–652, 1989

Conners C, March J, Erhardt D, et al: Assessment of attention-deficit disorders. Journal of Psychoeducational Assessment 28:186–205, 1995

De Bellis MD, Chrousos GP, Dorn LD, et al: Hypothalamic-pituitary-adrenal axis dysregulation in sexually abused girls [see comments]. J Clin Endocrinol Metab 78:249–255, 1994a

De Bellis MD, Lefter L, Trickett PK, et al: Urinary catecholamine excretion in sexually abused girls. J Am Acad Child Adolesc Psychiatry 33:320–327, 1994b

De Bellis MD, Baum AS, Birmaher B, et al: A.E. Bennett Research Award. Developmental traumatology, I: biological stress systems. Biol Psychiatry 45:1259–1270, 1999a

De Bellis MD, Keshavan MS, Clark DB, et al: A.E. Bennett Research Award. Developmental traumatology, II: brain development. Biol Psychiatry 45:1271–1284, 1999b

De Bellis MD, Hall J, Boring AM, et al: A pilot longitudinal study of hippocampal volumes in pediatric maltreatment-related posttraumatic stress disorder. Biol Psychiatry 50:305–309, 2001

Deblinger E, McLeer SV, Henry D: Cognitive behavioral treatment for sexually abused children suffering post-traumatic stress: preliminary findings. J Am Acad Child Adolesc Psychiatry 29:747–752, 1990

Deblinger E, Steer RA, Lippmann J: Two-year follow-up study of cognitive behavioral therapy for sexually abused children suffering post-traumatic stress symptoms. Child Abuse Negl 23:1371–1378, 1999

Donnelly CL, Amaya-Jackson L: Post-traumatic stress disorder in children and adolescents: epidemiology, diagnosis, and treatment options. Paediatr Drugs 4:159–170, 2002

Donnelly CL, Amaya-Jackson L, March JS: Psychopharmacology of pediatric posttraumatic stress disorder. J Child Adolesc Psychopharmacol 9:203–220, 1999

Eth S, Pynoos RS: Post-Traumatic Stress Disorder in Children. Washington, DC, American Psychiatric Press, 1985

Famularo R, Kinscherff R, Fenton T: Symptom differences in acute and chronic presentation of childhood post-traumatic stress disorder. Child Abuse Negl 14:439–444, 1990

Famularo R, Kinscherff R, Fenton T: Psychiatric diagnoses of maltreated children: preliminary findings. J Am Acad Child Adolesc Psychiatry 31:863–867, 1992

Foa EB, Riggs DS: Posttraumatic stress disorder following assault: theoretical considerations and empirical findings. Current Directions in Psychological Science 4(2):61–65, 1995

Foa E, Rothbaum E: Cognitive-behavioral treatment of posttraumatic stress disorder, in Post-Traumatic Stress Disorder: A Behavioral Approach to Diagnosis and Treatment. Edited by Saigh P. Needham Heights, MA, Allyn & Bacon, 1992, pp 85–110

Foa EB, Rothbaum BO: Treating the Trauma of Rape. New York, Guilford, 1998

Foa E, Steketee G, Rothbaum B: Behavioral/cognitive conceptualizations of post-traumatic stress disorder. Behav Ther 20:155–176, 1989

Ford JD, Racusin R, Ellis CG, et al: Child maltreatment, other trauma exposure, and posttraumatic symptomatology among children with oppositional defiant and attention deficit hyperactivity disorders. Child Maltreat 5:205–217, 2000

Freud S: Beyond the pleasure principle (1920), in The Standard Edition of the Complete Psychological Works of Sigmund Freud, Vol 18. Translated and edited by Strachey J. London, Hogarth Press, 1955, pp 7–64

Friedman MJ: Current and future drug treatment for post-traumatic stress disorder patients. Psychiatr Ann 28:461–468, 1998

Friedman M, Davidson JR, Mellman TA, et al: Guidelines for pharmacotherapy and position paper on practice guidelines, in Effective Treatments for PTSD: Practice Guidelines From the International Society for Traumatic Stress Studies. Edited by Foa EB, Keane TM, Friedman MJ. New York, Guilford, 2000, pp 84–105

Goenjian AK, Najarian LM, Pynoos RS, et al: Posttraumatic stress disorder in elderly and younger adults after the 1988 earthquake in Armenia. Am J Psychiatry 151:895–901, 1994

Goldman SJ, D'Angelo EJ, DeMaso DR, et al: Physical and sexual abuse histories among children with borderline personality disorder. Am J Psychiatry 149:1723–1726, 1992

Green BL: Defining trauma: terminology and generic stressors dimensions. J Appl Soc Psychol 20:1632–1642, 1995

Heim C, Newport DJ, Bonsall R, et al: Altered pituitary-adrenal axis responses to provocative challenge tests in adult survivors of childhood abuse. Am J Psychiatry 158:575–581, 2001

Heit S, Graham Y, Nemeroff CB: Neurobiological effects of early trauma. Harv Ment Health Lett 16:4–6, 1999

Hidalgo RB, Davidson JR: Selective serotonin reuptake inhibitors in post-traumatic stress disorder. J Psychopharmacol 14:70–76, 2000

Holbrook TL, Hoyt DB, Stein MB, et al: Perceived threat to life predicts posttraumatic stress disorder after major trauma: risk factors and functional outcome. J Trauma 51:287–292, 2001

Horrigan JP: Guanfacine for posttraumatic stress disorder nightmares (letter). J Am Acad Child Adolesc Psychiatry 35:975–976, 1996

Jones JC, Barlow DH: The etiology of posttraumatic stress disorder. Clin Psychol Rev 10:299–328, 1990

Kardiner A: The Traumatic Neurosis of War. New York, Paul B Hoeber, 1941

Kendall P (ed): Child and Adolescent Therapy. New York, Guilford, 1991

Kendall-Tackett KA, Williams LM, Finkelhor D: Impact of sexual abuse on children: a review and synthesis of recent empirical studies. Psychol Bull 113:164–180, 1993

Kessler RC, Sonnega A, Bromet E, et al: Posttraumatic stress disorder in the National Comorbidity Survey. Arch Gen Psychiatry 52:1048–1060, 1995

King JA, Mandansky D, King S, et al: Early sexual abuse and low cortisol. Psychiatry Clin Neurosci 55:71–74, 2001

Kovacs M: The Children's Depression Inventory (CDI). Psychopharmacol Bull 21:995–998, 1985

Levy D: Release therapy. Am J Orthopsychiatry 9:713–736, 1939

Lipper S, Davidson JR, Grady TA, et al: Preliminary study of carbamazepine in posttraumatic stress disorder. Psychosomatics 27:849–854, 1986

Lonigan CJ, Shannon MP, Finch AJ, et al: Children's reactions to a natural disaster: symptom severity and degree of exposure. Advances in Behavior Research and Therapy 13(3):135–154, 1991

Lonigan CJ, Shannon MP, Taylor CM, et al: Children exposed to disaster, II: risk factors for the development of post-traumatic symptomatology. J Am Acad Child Adolesc Psychiatry 33:94–105, 1994

Looff D, Grimley P, Kuller F, et al: Carbamazepine for PTSD. J Am Acad Child Adolesc Psychiatry 34:703–704, 1995

March J: Post-traumatic stress in the emergency setting. Emergency Care Quarterly 7(1):74–81, 1991

March JS: What constitutes a stressor? The "Criterion A" issue, in Posttraumatic Stress Disorder: DSM-IV and Beyond. Edited by Davidson JRT, Foa EB. Washington, DC, American Psychiatric Press, 1993, pp 37–54

March JS, Albano AM: Assessment of anxiety in children and adolescents, in American Psychiatric Press Annual Review of Psychiatry, Vol 15. Edited by Dickstein LJ, Riba MB, Oldham JM. Washington, DC, American Psychiatric Press, 1996, pp 405–427

March JS, Amaya-Jackson L: Post-traumatic stress disorder in children and adolescents. PTSD Research Quarterly 4(4):1–7, 1994

March JS, Amaya-Jackson L, Costanzo P, et al: Post-traumatic stress in children and adolescents after an industrial fire. Paper presented at the annual meeting of the Anxiety Disorders Association of America, Pittsburgh, PA, April 1995a

March JS, Stallings P, Parker J, et al: The Multidimensional Anxiety Scale for Children (MASC): development and factor structure. Paper presented at the annual meeting of the Anxiety Disorders Association of America, Pittsburgh, PA, April 1995b

Marmar CR, Foy D, Kagan B, et al: An integrated approach for treating post-traumatic stress, in Post-Traumatic Stress Disorder: A Clinical Review. Edited by Pynoos RS. Lutherville, MD, Sidran Press, 1993

Marshall RD, Beebe KL, Oldham M, et al: Efficacy and safety of paroxetine treatment for chronic PTSD: a fixed-dose, placebo-controlled study. Am J Psychiatry 158:1982–1988, 2001

McNally RJ: Assessment of posttraumatic stress disorder in children. Psychol Assess 3:531–537, 1991

McNally RJ: Stressors that produce posttraumatic stress disorder in children, in Posttraumatic Stress Disorder: DSM-IV and Beyond. Edited by Davidson JRT, Foa EB. Washington, DC, American Psychiatric Press, 1993, pp 57–74

Motta RW: Identification of characteristics and causes of childhood posttraumatic stress disorder. Psychol Sch 31:49–56, 1994

Muller RT, Sicoli LA, Lemieux KE: Relationship between attachment style and posttraumatic stress symptomatology among adults who report the experience of childhood abuse. J Trauma Stress 13:321–332, 2000

Nader K, Pynoos RS, Fairbanks L, et al: Childhood PTSD reactions one year after a sniper attack. Am J Psychiatry 147:1526–1530, 1990

Nader K, Stuber M, Pynoos RS: Posttraumatic stress reactions in preschool children with catastrophic illness: assessment needs. Comprehensive Mental Health Care 1:223–239, 1991

Nader K, Blake D, Kriegler J, et al: Clinician Administered PTSD Scale for Children (CAPS-C), Current and Lifetime Diagnosis Version, and Instruction Manual. Los Angeles, CA, UCLA Neuropsychiatric Institute and National Center for PTSD, 1994

Ornitz E, Pynoos R: Startle modulation in children with post-traumatic stress disorder. Am J Psychiatry 146:866–870, 1989

Pelcowitz D, Kaplan S, Goldenberg B, et al: Posttraumatic stress disorder in physically abused adolescents. J Am Acad Child Adolesc Psychiatry 33:305–312, 1994

Perrin S, Smith P, Yule W: Practitioner review: the assessment and treatment of post-traumatic stress disorder in children and adolescents. J Child Psychol Psychiatry 41:277–289, 2000

Perry BD: Neurobiological sequelae of childhood trauma: posttraumatic stress disorders in children, in Catecholamine Function in Posttraumatic Stress Disorder: Emerging Concepts. Edited by Murburg M. Washington, DC, American Psychiatric Press, 1985, pp 233–255

Perry BD, Pate JE: Neurodevelopment and the Psychobiological Roots of Post-Traumatic Stress Disorder. Springfield, IL, Charles C Thomas, 1994

Pfefferbaum B: Posttraumatic stress disorder in children: a review of the past 10 years. J Am Acad Child Adolesc Psychiatry 36:1503–1511, 1997

Pfefferbaum B, Seale TW, McDonald NB, et al: Posttraumatic stress two years after the Oklahoma City bombing in youths geographically distant from the explosion. Psychiatry 63:358–370, 2000

Pitman RK: Biological findings in posttraumatic stress disorder: implications for DSM-IV classification, in Posttraumatic Stress Disorder: DSM-IV and Beyond. Edited by Davidson JRT, Foa EB. Washington, DC, American Psychiatric Press, 1993, pp 173–189

Putnam FW, Trickett PK: Child sexual abuse: a model of chronic trauma. Psychiatry 56:82–95, 1993

Pynoos RS: Traumatic Stress and Developmental Psychopathology in Children and Adolescents. Lutherville, MD, Sidran Press, 1994

Pynoos RS, Nader K: Psychological first aid and treatment approach to children exposed to community violence: research implications. J Trauma Stress 1:445–473, 1988

Pynoos RS, Nader K: Children's memory and proximity to violence. J Am Acad Child Adolesc Psychiatry 28:236–241, 1989a

Pynoos RS, Nader K: Prevention of Psychiatric Morbidity in Children After Disaster. Washington, DC, U.S. Government Printing Office, 1989b

Pynoos RS, Nader K: Children's exposure to violence and traumatic death. Psychiatr Ann 20:334–344, 1990

Pynoos RS, Nader K: Issues in the treatment of posttraumatic stress in children and adolescents, in International Handbook of Traumatic Stress Syndromes. Edited by Wilson JP, Raphael B. New York, Plenum, 1993, pp 535–549

Pynoos RS, Frederick CJ, Nader K, et al: Life threat and posttraumatic stress in school-age children. Arch Gen Psychiatry 44:1057–1063, 1987a

Pynoos RS, Nader K, Frederick CJ, et al: Grief reactions in school age children following a sniper attack at school. Isr J Psychiatry Relat Sci 24:53–63, 1987b

Pynoos RS, Steinberg AM, Wraith R: A Developmental Model of Childhood Traumatic Stress. New York, Wiley, 1995, pp 72–95

Richters J: Community violence and children's development: toward a research agenda for the 1990s. Psychiatry 56:3–6, 1993

Richters J, Martinez P: The NIMH Community Violence Project, I: children as victims and witnesses to violence. Psychiatry 56:7–21, 1993

Saigh PA: The development of posttraumatic stress disorder following four different types of traumatization. Behav Res Ther 29:213–216, 1991

Saigh PA: The behavioral treatment of child and adolescent posttraumatic stress disorder. Advances in Behaviour Research and Therapy 14:247–275, 1992

Saylor CF, Swenson CC, Powell P: Hurricane Hugo blows down the broccoli: preschoolers' post-disaster play and adjustment. Child Psychiatry Hum Dev 22:139–149, 1992

Scheeringa MS: Treatment for posttraumatic stress disorder in infants and toddlers. Journal of Systemic Therapies 18:21–31, 1999

Scheeringa MS, Zeanah CH, Drell MJ, et al: Two approaches to the diagnosis of posttraumatic stress disorder in infancy and early childhood. J Am Acad Child Adolesc Psychiatry 34:191–200, 1995

Schreiber S, Galai-Gat T: Uncontrolled pain following physical injury as the core-trauma in post-traumatic stress disorder. Pain 54:107–110, 1993

Seedat S, Kaminer D, Lockhat R, et al: An overview of post-traumatic stress disorder in children and adolescents. Primary Care Psychiatry 6:43–48, 2000

Seedat S, Lockhat R, Kaminer D, et al: An open trial of citalopram in adolescents with post-traumatic stress disorder. Int Clin Psychopharmacol 16:21–25, 2001

Solomon SD, Gerrity ET, Muff AM: Efficacy of treatments for posttraumatic stress disorder: an empirical review. JAMA 268:633–638, 1992

Stubenbort K, Donnelly GA, Cohen JA: Cognitive-behavioral group therapy for bereaved adults and children following an air disaster. Group Dyn 5:261–276, 2001

Swanson JM: School-Based Assessments and Interventions for ADD Students. Irvine, CA, KC Publications, 1992

Terr LC: Children of Chowchilla. Psychoanal Study Child 34:547–623, 1979

Terr LC: "Forbidden games": post-traumatic child's play. J Am Acad Child Adolesc Psychiatry 20:740–759, 1981a

Terr LC: Psychic trauma in children: observations following the Chowchilla school-bus kidnapping. Am J Psychiatry 138:14–19, 1981b

Terr LC: Chowchilla revisited: the effects of psychic trauma four years after a school-bus kidnapping. Am J Psychiatry 140:1543–1550, 1983a

Terr LC: Life attitudes, dreams, and psychic trauma in a group of "normal" children. J Am Acad Child Psychiatry 22:221–230, 1983b

Terr L: What happens to early memories of trauma? A study of twenty children under age five at the time of documented traumatic events. J Am Acad Child Adolesc Psychiatry 27:96–104, 1988

Terr LC: Too Scared to Cry: Psychic Trauma in Childhood. New York, Harper & Row, 1990

Terr LC: Childhood traumas: an outline and overview. Am J Psychiatry 148:10–20, 1991

Terr LC: Acute responses to external events and posttraumatic stress disorder, in Child and Adolescent Psychiatry: A Comprehensive Textbook, 2nd Edition. Edited by Lewis M. Baltimore, MD, Williams & Wilkins, 1996, pp 753–763

van der Kolk BA, Dreyfuss D, Michaels M, et al: Fluoxetine in posttraumatic stress disorder. J Clin Psychiatry 55:517–522, 1994

Wilson SN, van der Kolk B, Burbridge J, et al: Phenotype of blood lymphocytes in PTSD suggest chronic immune activation. Psychosomatics 40:222–225, 1999

Winnicott DW: Therapeutic Consultation in Child Psychiatry. New York, Basic Books, 1971

Wozniak J, Crawford MH, Biederman J, et al: Antecedents and complications of trauma in boys with ADHD: findings from a longitudinal study. J Am Acad Child Adolesc Psychiatry 38:48–56, 1999

Yehuda R: Recent developments in the neuroendocrinology of posttraumatic stress disorder. CNS Spectr 2 (suppl):22–29, 1998

Yehuda R: Post-traumatic stress disorder. N Engl J Med 346:108–114, 2002

Yehuda R, Hallig SL, Grossman R: Childhood trauma and risk for PTSD: relationship to intergenerational effects of trauma, parental PTSD and cortisol excretion. Dev Psychopathol 13:733–753, 2001

Yule W: Post-traumatic stress disorder in child survivors of shipping disasters: the sinking of the 'Jupiter.' Psychother Psychosom 57:200–205, 1992

Yule W: Posttraumatic stress disorders, in Child and Adolescent Psychiatry: Modern Approaches, 3rd Edition. Edited by Rutter M, Taylor E, Hersov L. Cambridge, MA, Blackwell Science, 1994, pp 392–406

Yule W, Canterbury R: The treatment of post traumatic stress disorder in children and adolescents. Int Rev Psychiatry 6:141–151, 1994

Zero to Three: Diagnostic classification: 0–3: Diagnostic Classification of Mental Health and Developmental Disorders of Infancy and Early Childhood. Arlington, VA, Zero to Three, 1994

Self-Assessment Questions

Select the single best response for each question.

21.1 In assessing a child for posttraumatic stress disorder (PTSD), clinicians should do all of the following *except*

A. Establish that the incident actually occurred.

B. Take children's self-reports of trauma at face value.

C. Supplement children's self-reports with histories from parents and others.

D. Remember that children's recollections may be influenced by others.

E. Use a neutral questioning stance.

21.2 Stimuli directly or indirectly related to a traumatic event that provoke conditioned responses are known as

A. Traumatic dreams.

B. Reenactment behavior.

C. Traumatic play.

D. Traumatic reminders.

E. None of the above.

21.3 Traumatized children frequently have symptoms of disorders other than PTSD. In addition to true comorbidity, spurious comorbidity with PTSD can result from 1) overlap between criteria sets and 2) confounding similar symptoms of other diagnoses with those of PTSD. Which of the following disorders overlaps with or has symptoms similar to those of PTSD?

A. Attention-deficit/hyperactivity disorder (ADHD).

B. Oppositional defiant disorder.

C. Major depressive disorder.

D. Generalized anxiety disorder.

E. All of the above.

21.4 Important principles in the psychotherapeutic treatment of children with PTSD include all of the following *except*

A. Reexposing the individual to traumatic cues under safe conditions.

B. Allowing the sessions to be unfocused so that unconscious material may be uncovered.

C. Keeping focused on the child's current dysfunction.

D. Being diligent about continually rethinking the symptom picture.

E. Directing the therapy to facilitate higher levels of adaptation and coping.

21.5 Which of the following antidepressants has been approved by the U.S. Food and Drug Administration (FDA) for the treatment of PTSD in adults and is often used to treat PTSD in children and adolescents?

A. Bupropion.

B. Nefazodone.

C. Imipramine.

D. Duloxetine.

E. Paroxetine.

Adjustment and Reactive Disorders

Gloria Reeves, M.D.

David Pruitt, M.D.

The diagnosis of adjustment disorder does not align easily with other categories of psychiatric illness. Although clinical practice teaches us to link stressors with presenting symptoms, most psychiatric diagnoses do not require a specific stressor to be identified or characterized. Diagnostic criteria tend to emphasize observable behaviors and internalized experiences, independent of environmental factors and external events. In contrast, the diagnostic criteria for adjustment disorder focus on the connection between stressors and psychological distress. This unique perspective offers an important option for clinicians who treat children and adolescents. Pediatric patients are often exposed to stressors beyond their control (e.g., parental divorce, financial stressors, relocation to a new home). The diagnosis of adjustment disorder elevates the importance of involving families and outside systems in treatment because it focuses on the impact of psychosocial stressors. This shift in focus may serve to destigmatize the individual patient and offer support to the child's family and community network.

The usefulness of the adjustment disorder diagnosis is challenged by the low volume of research available to characterize this disorder. The extensive review by Despland et al. (1995) of the adult literature on adjustment disorder between 1974 and November 1992 identified only 16 articles, with only 9 articles described as actual studies. Further research is warranted to help characterize the natural course of adjustment disorder as well as the unique features of this disorder during childhood.

Definition

DSM-IV-TR (American Psychiatric Association 2000) diagnostic criteria (Table 22–1) define adjustment disorder as the development of emotional or behavioral symptoms in response to a recent stressor and further define the disorder as occur-

---

Table 22–1.   DSM-IV-TR diagnostic criteria for adjustment disorders

---

A.   The development of emotional or behavioral symptoms in response to an identifiable stressor(s) occurring within 3 months of the onset of the stressor(s).

B.   These symptoms or behaviors are clinically significant as evidenced by either of the following:

(1)   marked distress that is in excess of what would be expected from exposure to the stressor

(2)   significant impairment in social or occupational (academic) functioning

C.   The stress-related disturbance does not meet the criteria for another specific Axis I disorder and is not merely an exacerbation of a preexisting Axis I or Axis II disorder.

D.   The symptoms do not represent bereavement.

E.   Once the stressor (or its consequences) has terminated, the symptoms do not persist for more than an additional 6 months.

Specify if:

  Acute: if the disturbance lasts less than 6 months
  Chronic: if the disturbance lasts for 6 months or longer

Adjustment disorders are coded based on the subtype, which is selected according to the predominant symptoms. The specific stressor(s) can be specified on Axis IV.

309.0	**With depressed mood**
309.24	**With anxiety**
309.28	**With mixed anxiety and depressed mood**
309.3	**With disturbance of conduct**
309.4	**With mixed disturbance of emotions and conduct**
309.9	**Unspecified**

Source.   Reprinted from American Psychiatric Association: *Diagnostic and Statistical Manual of Mental Disorders,* 4th Edition, Text Revision. Washington, DC, American Psychiatric Association, 2000. Copyright 2000 American Psychiatric Association. Used with permission.

---

ring within 3 months of the onset of the stressor. Symptoms must be beyond what would be expected for the given stressor and must result in significant impairment in social or academic functioning. Other Axis I conditions and bereavement must be excluded as a cause of the clinical presentation, and symptoms should resolve within 6 months of the termination of the stressor or its consequences. The course can be specified as either acute or chronic, depending on whether the duration of symptoms is less than or greater than 6 months. The diagnostic subtypes include adjustment disorder with either depressed mood, anxiety, mixed anxiety and depressed mood, disturbance of con-

duct, or mixed disturbance of emotions and conduct.

Differential Diagnosis

Stress-related diagnostic categories include posttraumatic stress disorder (PTSD) and bereavement. In PTSD, the stressor is specified as a traumatic event in which there is a serious threat to the safety of self or others and there is a well-defined profile of hyperarousal, avoidance, and reexperiencing symptoms. Bereavement is a diagnostic category used when the focus of stress is the loss of a loved one, particularly if "normal" grief reactions occur within the first few months after the death.

Depression and anxiety disorders should also be considered in the differential diagnosis. The distinction of these disorders from adjustment disorder may not be readily apparent. Both disorders may cause prominent shifts in mood or behavior, and both may be associated with psychosocial stressors. However, the diagnoses of anxiety or depressive disorders require more specific behavior and emotional symptom profiles, and symptoms are not necessarily linked to a specific stressor. With depressive and anxiety disorders, the symptoms do not have to occur within a specific time frame after onset of the stressor.

Cultural syndromes should also be considered in the differential diagnosis, although they are not considered to be pathological disorders. For example, "brain fag" is a West African cultural syndrome that describes energy, memory, and concentration difficulties that students experience in response to academic pressures. Changes in functioning that do not exceed the bounds of culturally sanctioned phenomena are considered "normal" and would not be expected to have negative long-term sequelae. Collateral information from family members or other members of the individual's culture of origin may be necessary to distinguish pathological symptoms from cultural phenomena.

Etiology

Although the diagnostic criteria clearly state that symptoms are associated with an identifiable stressor, there are important intrinsic factors that modulate the impact of a distressing event. Woolston (1988) discusses how an individual's level of cognitive development influences the interpretation of stressful events. For example, he points out that children are more likely than adults to link unrelated events as a cause-and-effect phenomenon. This may generate greater feelings of guilt or distress if the child feels involved in causing an uncontrollable event. Sanger et al. (1993) surveyed a group of 50 children with idiopathic epilepsy, ages 5–16 years, to determine what they thought was the cause of their seizures. Only 41% of the respondents identified their seizure disorder as a dysfunction of the brain. One child assumed that her seizures were related to overeating.

A child's level of psychological development also will modulate the response to stressors. An external stressor may have greater impact in causing distress if it amplifies preexisting issues, such as poor self-esteem (Woolston 1988). The capacity to engage adaptive defense mechanisms will also modulate the impact of a stressor. A child using more primitive defense mechanisms may be less effective in managing distress and thus more vulnerable to developing symptoms.

In a prospective study, bias in self-perception of competence, either positive or negative, was demonstrated to be associated with adjustment problems during adolescence (DuBois and Silverthorn 2004). An inflated sense of competence may impair social skills (i.e., reduce social support), whereas negative perception of competence may be associated with a negative cognitive style (i.e., increased depression and anxiety).

At a physiological level, individual neurohormonal responses to stressors may alter the subjective sense of distress after an event. If the stressor is adjustment to a chronic illness, the physiological changes related to the illness may mimic psychiatric symptoms (e.g., anemia causing fatigue or hypoglycemia causing anxiety or poor concentration). Side effects of treatment can also be mislabeled as psychiatric symptoms (e.g., increased sleep from a sedating medication).

Relationships play an important and complex role in how children respond to stressful events. For example, maternal depression is associated with adjustment problems in youth. This finding may be related to increased genetic vulnerability of mood symptoms, disrupted parenting/attachment issues, as well as increased stress of the parent in managing a difficult child. Thus, causal relationships are bidirectional between parent and child (Elgar et al. 2004). Chronic difficulties with peers are also associated with maladjustment (Ladd and Troop-Gordon 2003).

Prevalence

Initial studies of adjustment disorder in clinical populations have generally shown its prevalence to be high (Newcorn and Strain 1992). A retrospective study of all psychiatric patients admitted in 1989 through a suburban hospital emergency department revealed that 7.1% of adults and 34.4% of adolescents had an adjustment disorder admission diagnosis. The most common subtype of adjustment disorder in adults and adolescents was adjustment disorder with depressed mood (Greenberg et al. 1995). In a sample of more than 11,000 patients at a university-based clinic, 10% of all patients and 16% of patients under the age of 18 years were diagnosed with adjustment disorder. There was no significant difference in prevalence between male and female patients (Mezzich et al. 1989).

Clinical Presentation and Course of Illness

Kovacs et al. (1994) conducted a prospective study of 30 child psychiatric patients, ages 8–13 years, with a research-defined diagnosis of adjustment disorder. To meet criteria, subjects needed to have at least three clinically significant symptoms in the relevant symptom domain. These patients were compared with 26 control subjects, who were also matched for comorbidity rates. For patients diagnosed with adjustment disorder with depressed mood, the most common symptoms were sadness, decreased pleasure, self-deprecation, and irritability. More than half (58%) of these patients indicated a history of suicidal ideation at some point after onset of the stressor. The identified stressors included new school year (30%), change in family situation (23%), peer rejection (13%), parental illness (10%), death of parent or grandparent (7%), move (7%), or other (10%). Median time to recovery after onset of symptoms was 7 months, and close to 100% of the study population had resolution of symptoms within 2 years. Compared with the control group, there was no evidence of long-term sequelae over an 8-year follow-up assessment.

Andreasen and Hoenk (1982) examined the predictive value of the adjustment disorder diagnosis by conducting a 5-year follow-up of a cohort of adolescents (n=52) and adults (n=48) who were diagnosed with adjustment disorder. The adults fared better than the adolescents; 71% of adults and 44% of the adolescents were assessed to be free from psychiatric illness at follow-up (an additional 13% of adolescents were well but had intervening problems during the 5-year period). In regard to diagnostic subtypes, patients with disturbance of conduct tended to have poorer outcomes than did patients with depressed mood. Whether the initial adjustment disorder diagnosis was made in an inpatient or an outpatient setting was not significant in predicting good outcome. The most common follow-up diagnoses in the adolescent group were major depressive disorder (19%), antisocial personality disorder (19%), alcoholism (17%), and substance abuse (12%).

Fabrega et al. (1987) addressed the specificity of the adjustment disorder diagnosis by examining symptomatology in more than 5,000 patients who were assessed in a walk-in psychiatric clinic (15% of the patients were younger than 19 years of age). Diagnostic evaluations were completed using a semistructured interview format. Patients were divided into three groups: those with no psychiatric diagnosis (1.6%), those with the sole diagnosis of adjustment disorder (2.3%), and those with specific Axis I or Axis II diagnoses (96.1%). The third group included patients with adjustment disorder diagnoses and a comorbid psychiatric diagnosis. Patients with the sole diagnosis of adjustment disorder rated higher on measures of psychosocial stressors than did patients with a specific diagnosis (i.e., other than adjustment disorder), but the adjustment disorder patients rated lower on all indicators of psychopathology. Patients with diagnoses of adjustment disorder also scored higher on psychopathology measures than did patients with no diagnosable mental illness. Fabrega et al. (1987) concluded that adjustment disorder serves a useful purpose as a transitional illness category because it describes a population with psychopathology intermediate between people with psychosocial stressors but no diagnosable disorder and people with stressors who meet criteria for a disorder other than adjustment disorder.

In one study, readmission rates for patients with a diagnosis of adjustment disorder with depressed or anxious mood were found to be lower than rates for patients with an anxiety or depressive disorder diagnosis (Jones et al. 2002). However, diagnoses were based solely on clinical interview and did not include structured assessments.

Specific Stressors and Resilience Factors

Because adjustment disorder is related specifically to stressors, investigation of children's reactions to different types of stressors may help to determine prevention and treatment interventions. One major stressor experienced by many children is adjustment to illness.

Chronic illness is a risk factor for behavioral and emotional problems in children (Kovacs et al. 1995; Newcorn and Strain 1992; Perrin et al. 1993). Kovacs et al. (1995) investigated childhood adjustment to the onset of juvenile diabetes. The study assessed a cohort of 92 children hospitalized for acute-onset diabetes. Within 6 months of the hospitalization, the most common psychiatric diagnosis was adjustment disorder. The first month after the diagnosis was the period of greatest vulnerability; 73% of the adjustment disorder diagnoses were made during that time frame. This increased vulnerability may be related to physiological factors, because a patient's glucose levels often have not stabilized during this early phase of treatment. This period is also the time when patients and families need the greatest support and when prevention efforts are the most critical. The short-term psychiatric outcomes for the children in this study were good. All children eventually recovered from the adjustment disorder, and the average time to recovery was 3 months. However, the presence of adjustment disorder was a risk factor for other psychiatric illnesses during the next 5 years.

Perrin et al. (1993) investigated perceptions of adjustment in children with chronic health conditions, including grand mal and petit mal seizure disorders, cerebral palsy, and visible orthopedic conditions (e.g., rheumatoid arthritis, scoliosis). The investigators attempted to recruit subjects who were not in an acute health crisis, so they excluded children who had been diagnosed with a chronic illness less than 6 months before, or had been hospitalized less than 6 months previously, or did not attend school regularly. Measures of psychosocial adjustment were completed by the children, their parents, and their teachers. Children with chronic illness were compared with a community control group.

All three observers (child, parent, and teacher) rated children with chronic orthopedic conditions (including rheumatoid arthritis and scoliosis) as equally or better adjusted than same-age peers. The overall assessment of child adjustment in this group was higher than for other health conditions The authors suggested that a visible condition may elicit more support from others to alleviate stress. All of the teachers were aware of the health problems in this group, whereas only half the teachers knew about the health condition in the epileptic group. However, children with cerebral palsy received higher ratings of adjustment from self- and teacher reports than from parental reports. Perrin et al. (1993) hypothesized that patients with cerebral palsy have had their conditions most of their lives, so they probably do not think of themselves as being ill, whereas the parents are acutely aware of how many services and how much care the children needed throughout their development.

Perrin et al. (1993) also surveyed mothers about their beliefs regarding control of their children's epilepsy. Mothers who felt they had control over the prevention of their children's seizures tended to rate their epileptic children as better adjusted than did mothers who felt they had little impact on the prevention of their children's seizures. Thus, parental perceptions involved a complex interaction between the parents' experience of observing and interacting with their child and their individual beliefs about their capacity to control the child's health condition.

Treatment

Few research data are available on treatment options for adjustment disorder. However, it can be ascertained from the review described in the previous section that treatment should be strongly influenced by the child's situation. Because family members may be involved in the identified stressor and they have considerable influence on a child's perception and experience of stressors, they are an important part of the treatment equation. Family interventions can help eliminate labeling of the child in the "sick role" and may provide relief to others affected by the stress. Elgar et al. (2004) identified the need for future research to determine 1) whether combining parent training with treatment for parental psychopathology (e.g., maternal depression) is more effective than treatment with either intervention alone and 2) the optimal order/timing of these interventions to improve child and family functioning. Unlike stressors identified in PTSD, which may be more extreme and less common, stressors identified in adjustment disorder may occur quite frequently in a given population. This allows for easier identification of patients for group interventions and prevention efforts. Pharmacological treatment of adjustment disorder may be considered to target the child's reactive symptoms and alleviate immediate distress around the onset of a stressor. However, adjustment disorder is usually short-lived, and little is known about any long-term benefit in pharmacological treatment to prevent later onset of other psychiatric illnesses. Longer-term follow-up of children with adjustment disorder may be helpful in clarifying the merits of various interventions.

Conclusion

The diagnostic category of adjustment disorder appears to describe a unique reaction to stress, distinct from those experienced by children with other psychiatric illnesses. The adjustment disorder diagnosis offers clinicians the option of conceptualizing a child's difficulties in the framework of a stress reaction, which may be helpful in destigmatizing the child's problems and enlisting the participation of families and other systems in treatment.

However, it is not always clear how to operationally define the diagnosis. Researchers developed more stringent diagnostic criteria (e.g., presence of four or more active symptoms) to help distinguish these patients more clearly from children who experience stress but who function reasonably well. The time frame defined for symptomatology is also problematic. The judgment of when a stressor began and when it has resolved is often subjective and is therefore susceptible to poor interrater reliability. Longitudinal research is needed to clarify the usefulness of this diagnosis in predicting future risk of maladjustment and psychiatric illness. This information could be applied in developing prevention efforts and in planning treatment interventions.

References

American Psychiatric Association: Diagnostic and Statistical Manual of Mental Disorders, 4th Edition, Text Revision. Washington, DC, American Psychiatric Association, 2000

American Psychiatric Association: Diagnostic and Statistical Manual of Mental Disorders, 4th Edition, Text Revision. Washington, DC, American Psychiatric Association, 2000

Andreasen NC, Hoenk PR: The predictive value of adjustment disorders: a follow-up study. Am J Psychiatry 139:584–590, 1982

Despland JN, Monod L, Ferrero F: Clinical relevance of adjustment disorder in DSM-III-R and DSM-IV. Compr Psychiatry 36:454–460, 1995

DuBois DL, Silverthorn N: Bias in self-perceptions and internalizing and externalizing problems in adjustment during early adolescence: a prospective investigation. J Clin Child Adolesc Psychol 33:373–381, 2004

Elgar FJ, McGrath PJ, Waschbusch DA, et al: Mutual influences on maternal depression and child adjustment problems. Clin Psychol Rev 24:441–459, 2004

Fabrega H, Mezzich JE, Mezzich AC: Adjustment disorder as a marginal or transitional illness category in DSM-III. Arch Gen Psychiatry 44:567–572, 1987

Greenberg WM, Rosenfeld DN, Ortega EA: Adjustment disorder as an admission diagnosis. Am J Psychiatry 152:459–461, 1995

Jones R, Yates WR, Zhou MH: Readmission rates for adjustment disorders: comparison with other mood disorders. J Affect Disord 71:199–203, 2002

Kovacs M, Gatsonis C, Pollock M, et al: A controlled prospective study of DSM-III adjustment disorder in childhood. Arch Gen Psychiatry 51:535–541, 1994

Kovacs M, Ho V, Pollock MH: Criterion and predictive validity of the diagnosis of adjustment disorder: a prospective study of youths with new-onset insulin-dependent diabetes mellitus. Am J Psychiatry 152:523–528, 1995

Ladd GW, Troop-Gordon W: The role of chronic peer difficulties in the development of children's psychological adjustment problems. Child Dev 74:1344–1367, 2003

Mezzich JE, Fabrega H Jr, Coffman GA, et al: DSM-III disorders in a large sample of psychiatric patients: frequency and specificity of diagnoses. Am J Psychiatry 146:212–219, 1989

Newcorn JH, Strain J: Adjustment disorder in children and adolescents. J Am Acad Child Adolesc Psychiatry 31:318–326, 1992

Perrin EC, Ayoub CC, Willett JB: In the eyes of the beholder: family and maternal influences on perceptions of adjustment of children with a chronic illness. J Dev Behav Pediatr 14:94–105, 1993

Sanger MS, Perrin EC, Sandler HA: Development in children's causal theories of their seizure disorders. J Dev Behav Pediatr 14:88–93, 1993

Woolston JL: Theoretical considerations of the adjustment disorders. J Am Acad Child Adolesc Psychiatry 27:280–287, 1988

Self-Assessment Questions

Select the single best response for each question.

22.1 The diagnosis of adjustment disorder in children and adolescents

　A. Has a focus similar to that in other psychiatric disorders, emphasizing observable symptoms and internalized experiences as primary components of the condition.

　B. Elevates the importance of families and outside systems because of its emphasis on psychosocial stressors.

　C. Requires that symptoms develop within 6 months of the onset of the stressors.

　D. Requires that the presenting symptoms be similar to what would be expected for any child exposed to the stressor in question.

　E. Is warranted when symptoms continue for years after the termination of the stressor.

22.2 All of the following factors can likely amplify the impact of an identifiable stressor on a child *except*

　A. Cognitive immaturity.

　B. Preexisting low self-esteem.

　C. More primitive defense mechanisms.

　D. More accurate understanding of cause-and-effect relationships.

　E. Treatment side effects.

22.3 In Kovacs et al.'s (1994) controlled prospective study of children with adjustment disorder, which of the following findings was reported?

　A. More than half of the study group children reported a history of suicidal ideation after the onset of the stressor.

　B. More than half of the study population had suffered the death of a parent.

　C. The median time to recovery after symptom onset was 3 months.

　D. Close to 100% recovery was reported in the study population within 12 months.

　E. The study group evidenced significantly more long-term sequelae compared with the control group.

22.4 In Kovacs et al.'s (1995) study of children hospitalized for acute-onset diabetes, all of the following findings were reported *except*

　A. Seventy-three percent of adjustment disorder diagnoses were made during the first month after the diabetes diagnosis.

　B. The first month posthospitalization was the period of greatest psychological vulnerability.

　C. Greater vulnerability during the first month postdiagnosis may be related to physiological factors.

　D. Short-term psychiatric outcomes for the study population were poor.

　E. The presence of adjustment disorder was a risk factor for developing other psychiatric illnesses within the next 5 years.

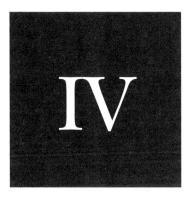

Disorders
Affecting
Somatic
Function

Infant and Childhood Obesity

Joseph L. Woolston, M.D.

David Szydlo, M.D., Ph.D.

Natural History of Infantile and Childhood-Onset Obesity

The study of the natural history of obesity in infancy and early childhood is in its preliminary stages. Data about the typical course of this disorder are contradictory. Some investigators suggest that early-onset obesity is a chronic and steadily progressive disorder with very few remissions (Charney et al. 1976; Eid (1970). Other investigators (Poskitt 1980; Shapiro et al. 1984) report that obesity in infancy is a poorer predictor of later-childhood obesity than was believed previously.

The incidence and prevalence of obesity in early childhood are not nearly as well studied as those of obesity in adulthood. The few studies that have been conducted indicate that the prevalence of obesity in preschool-age children is 5%–10% (Maloney and Klykylo 1983). Obesity tends to follow throughout life, and according to Whitaker et al. (1997) its presence at any age will increase the risk of persistence at subsequent ages. This means that although most obese infants will not remain so, they have a

higher risk of becoming obese children. These children are in turn more likely to be obese adolescents, who could very likely become obese adults. Power et al. (1997) concluded that overweight in children younger than age 3 years is not a predictor of future obesity, unless at least one parent is also obese. After that age, the likelihood that obesity will persist into adulthood increases with age and is higher in children with severe obesity. For example, after age 6 years, the probability that obesity will persist exceeds 50%, and 70%–80% of adolescents who are obese will remain so as adults.

Currently, the population of the United States appears to be experiencing an epidemic of childhood obesity. The prevalence of the most severe cases—defined as a body mass index (BMI, expressed as weight/height^2 or kg/m^2) for age over the ninety-fifth percentile—has virtually doubled since 1980, reaching 25%–30%, whereas the prevalence of standard cases (BMI for age over the eighty-fifth percentile) has increased about 50% (Gortmaker et al. 1987; Moran 1999). Furthermore, on the basis of the National Health Examination Survey and the National Health and Nutrition Examination Surveys, the prevalence of obesity was shown to increase by 54% in children ages 6–11 years and by 39% in adolescents ages 12–17 years. The prevalence of severe obesity jumped 98% and 64% within these groups, respectively. Hispanic, Native American, and black patients tend to be more affected than other populations (Kumanyika 1993). Overweight alone has almost tripled in children (ages 6–19 years) between 1970 and 1999, according to a report by the Centers for Disease Control and Prevention (2002), putting the proportion of overweight children ages 6–11 years at 13%, and of adolescents ages 12–19 years at 14%. This epidemics appear to be the result of cultural factors that promote excessive caloric intake and inadequate caloric expenditure.

Classification Schema for Infantile Obesity

One of the most obvious explanations for the contradictory results of various studies of infantile obesity is that it is an etiologically heterogeneous syndrome. Many authors (e.g., Maloney and Klykylo 1983; Stunkard 1975, 1980) have identified multiple factors, including emotional, socioeconomic, genetic, developmental, energetic, and neurological factors, that contribute to the development of obesity.

However, virtually no attempts have been made to subdivide forms of juvenile-onset obesity into phenomenologically homogeneous groupings. Although such an attempt might be seen as reductionistic, it is warranted by the evidence of heterogeneity in this syndrome. In this subtyping schema, endogenous and exogenous obesity should be differentiated. Endogenous obesity should be classified according to specific organic etiology.

Causes of exogenous obesity should be subdivided into simple excessive caloric intake and genetic/familial, psychogenic, and mixed factors.

■ Endogenous Obesity

A primary focus of clinicians who are studying the etiology of infantile obesity is determining specific organic dysfunctions that produce endogenous obesity. This *endogenous* form of obesity is in contradistinction to *exogenous* obesity, in which no physical dysfunction is present other than an excess caloric intake. Endogenous obesity is caused by discrete genetic, endocrinological, or neurological syndromes. Hormonal causes include hypothyroidism, hypercortisolism, primary hyperinsulinism, pseudohypoparathyroidism, acquired hypothalamic problems (e.g., tumors, infections, traumatic syndromes, vascular lesions). Genetic syndromes include Alström, Bardet-Biedl, Beckwith-Wiedemann, Börjeson-Forssman-Lehmann, Cohen, familial lipodystrophy, Fröhlich's, Kleine-Levin, Klinefelter's, Laurence-Moon, Mauriac, Prader-Willi, and Turner's. Of special research interest is the fact that Prader-Willi syndrome appears to be associated with a microdeletion of the proximal long arm of chromosome 15, band q11.2 (Donlon 1988). This is the first specifically defined gene alteration associated with a syndrome involving obesity, insatiable appetite, mental retardation, hypogonadism, and strabismus. Other genetic associations have also been made to leptin and β_3-adrenergic receptor.

Although clinicians often suspect that these organic syndromes have an etiological role in obesity in early childhood, they occur quite rarely, probably in less than 1% of obese patients. In addition, exogenous and endogenous obesity can be easily distinguished: Children with endogenous obesity usually are below the twenty-fifth percentile in height and have delayed bone age; a family history of obesity is uncommon, and there tend to be associated findings on physical examination. Children with exogenous obesity usually are above the fiftieth percentile in height and have an advanced bone age.

■ Exogenous Obesity: Obesity of Simple Excessive Caloric Intake

Obesity of simple excessive caloric intake results when a primary caretaker overfeeds the infant because of misinformation or cultural practice. The infant and the caretaker do not have any psychiatric disorders, and the family history for obesity is negative. This form of infantile obesity is relatively responsive to dietary intervention, assuming that the cultural attitudes that influence feeding can be modified. The age at onset can range from the neonatal period to early childhood, and the course may be rapid or gradual. The vast majority of infants and young children in the United States today are part of the current epidemic related to simple excessive caloric intake.

■ Genetic/Familial Obesity

In genetic/familial obesity, an underlying genetic or familial vulnerability to obesity is presumed. No evidence of psychopathology or nutritional misinformation is seen, but the family history for obesity is positive. In addition, the child may have characteristics associated with a so-called difficult temperament (low rhythm/predictability and low persistence/attention). Although both the age at onset and course are variable, usually the obesity is gradual and progressive, starting by age 5 or 6 years. Intervention has rather poor results, especially if it is introduced after the obesity has been present for several years.

A family line analysis of obesity indicated that a strong correlation exists between body weight of parents and that of their children. For example, by age 17 years, the children of obese parents are three times more likely to be obese than are the children of lean parents. If one sibling is overweight, the possibility that a second sibling will be overweight is 40% (Garn and Clark 1976). If two siblings are overweight, the possibility that the third sibling will be overweight is 80% (Garn and Clark 1976). According to the American Academy of Child and Adolescent Psychiatry (1997), if one parent is obese, there is a 50% chance that the children will also be obese, and when both parents are obese, the children have an 80% chance of being obese. These data seem to support a genetic basis for obesity, but one must keep other nongenetic but family-related factors in mind. Garn and Clark (1976) also found that if one spouse is overweight, the likelihood that the other spouse will be overweight is 30%. This finding obviously cannot be explained by genetic factors.

The familial factors related to infantile obesity are less clear. Poskitt (1980) reported no significant difference between the number of overweight and normal-weight infants who had one or two overweight parents. But by age 5 years, 78% of the overweight and only 35% of the normal-weight children had at least one overweight parent. This difference was significant and showed that the relative risk of a child being overweight with at least one overweight parent was more than five times that for a child with two normal-weight parents.

Well-designed genetic studies involving monozygotic and dizygotic concordance (Stunkard et al. 1986a) and adoption samples (Price and Gottesman 1991; Stunkard et al. 1986b, Van Itallie 1988) support a strong genetic contribution to all forms of body habitus, ranging from fatness to thinness. In a more recent study, Proietto and Thorburn (1994) suggested that abnormalities at the fat-cell level could be acquired but could also be genetic. Hirsch and Leibel (1998) described five different genes that are capable of causing obesity in mice (each with a human homologue).

■ **Psychogenic Obesity**

In psychogenic obesity, the family history for obesity may be negative and no evidence of nutritional misinformation may be found, but the infant and/or primary caretaker has strong evidence of psychopathology. Current data indicate two specific types of psychogenic obesity—one related to a traumatic separation from the primary caretaker and the other related to severe, chronic familial disorganization. The first type of psychogenic obesity has a sudden onset (usually before age 3 years) and can progress rapidly. Intervention must address the psychological and nutritional needs of the child and primary caretaker. Because the etiology is related to psychology more than to genetics, the results of intervention will be more variable than the rather poor prognosis for familial obesity. The second type of psychogenic obesity is associated with severely disorganized families in which the child's developmental needs are either ignored or misperceived. In these families, infants and toddlers are fed at the slightest sign of distress.

Studies of psychiatric disorders in obese adults have been as contradictory as studies of other aspects of obesity. Although many authors have reported no objective data indicating an increased incidence of psychopathology in obese adolescents and adults (McCance 1961; Shipman and Plesset 1963), other authors such as Bruch (1973) and Stunkard (1975) have reported the opposite. Silverstone (1969) attempted to reconcile these

discrepant reports by proposing a new categorization that differentiates between late-onset obesity secondary to a gradual accumulation of fat and early-onset obesity characterized by a sudden increase in weight caused by anxiety-driven overeating. Some authors have attempted to relate obesity to personality disorders (Sansone et al. 2000) or psychiatric pathology (Delvin et al. 2000), but the results are far from conclusive.

Very little is known about psychopathology in infantile obesity. In one report, Kahn (1973) described a sample of 73 obese children younger than 3 years. He found that 32% of these children had a sudden weight gain after a major, traumatic separation from their primary caretakers. This report alludes to a discrete syndrome related to traumatic separation that results in a sudden onset of obesity.

Another type of psychogenic obesity of infancy and early childhood occurs in the context of a disorganized family in which the child's needs are poorly perceived and even more poorly differentiated (Christoffel and Forsyth 1985). Typically, any sign of distress in the infant or toddler is responded to by feeding and/or neglect. Szydlo (1999) described the three most common psychogenic findings in a group of obese children ages 4–14 years as being 1) early separation from their mothers (before 24 months of age), 2) family dysfunctionality, and 3) exposure to traumatic and/or violent events.

The observed psychosocial characteristics of obesity parallel features of failure to thrive of psychosocial origin (Barbero and Shaheen 1967; Leonard et al. 1966). Children with this form of psychogenic obesity have severely disrupted and disorganized families. Factors that contribute to and are an expression of family dysfunction include separation of the parents, parental abuse of alcohol or drugs, and failure to maintain a stable living environment. The severe family disorganization not only is related to the etiology of obesity but also is a major obstacle to treatment because it frequently results in poor medical care, failure to follow through with management plans, and, sometimes, hostility toward health care professionals. The family members often deny the severity—or even the existence—of the problem.

In one study, the parents of all patients were unable to set limits, which also was evident in other parent–child interactions (Kahn 1973). Some mothers were depressed. Case reports (Boxer and Miller 1987; Woolston and Forsyth 1989) described a high level of parental noncompliance, direct undermining, and lack of parents' participation in the treatment of their child.

Some authors have attributed obesity in adolescence to defensive processes that are related to growing up, sexuality, and intimacy. This hypothesis has been described only in individual accounts from mental health professionals working with this age group. A study based on the defensive element of obesity concluded that for some sexually abused women, obesity may have an adaptive function (Wiederman et al. 1999).

■ Iatrogenic Obesity

Although many pharmacological agents produce weight gain, some of the atypical antipsychotics are particularly prone to cause this side effect (Martin et al. 2003). Unfortunately, these same agents also cause insulin resistance, leading to a greater risk of type 2 diabetes mellitus. This form of obesity may occur in conjunction with obesity caused by other factors.

■ Obesity of Mixed Etiology

In obesity of mixed etiology, more than one of the previously listed etiologies is found. It is obvious that infants who are overfed, who have a positive family history for obesity, and who have significant psychological disturbances will have a very resistant form of obesity. Each factor acts synergistically to maintain the obesity despite vigorous intervention. A clustering of these three etiological factors is not uncommon.

Complications

Children and adolescents are exposed to a great number of health risks related to being overweight and/or obese. Many of these are preventable, but unfortunately, most studies indicate that there is a rising number of children with unhealthy body composition, which in turn has immediate and long-term negative effects on them. Pediatricians and child psychiatrists are finding that diseases typically seen in adults are now increasingly seen in children and adolescents; such diseases include asthma, sleep apnea and other sleep disorders, pickwickian syndrome, hypertension, high cholesterol and dyslipidemia, syndrome X, type 2 diabetes, insulin resistance, hyperandrogenemia, menstrual abnormalities, gallbladder disease, liver steatosis, liver fibrosis and/or cirrhosis, and orthopedic complications such as degenerative arthritis and slipped femoral epiphysis (Bao et al. 1994; Dietz 1998; Freedman et al. 1999; Pinhas-Hamiel et al. 1996).

The negative psychological effects and cognitive complications of these diseases can last a lifetime: neurocognitive deficits; depression and other emotional problems; social difficulties and rejection; stigma; struggles with self-image, self-esteem, and insecurity; and body image distortion. At times, especially under the effects of media, family, and peer pressure, unplanned and unmanaged radical dieting and heavy exercising take the nutritional dysregulation process to the opposite side of the continuum, resulting in other eating disorders such as anorexia nervosa, bulimia nervosa, and binge eating disorder.

Treatment Approaches

No obesity treatment can claim long-term efficacy, despite the many algorithms that exist to define effective intervention modalities, such as self-help, pharmacological treatment, psychological therapies of all sorts, education, and surgery. A plethora of treatment options based on unproven explanatory models (e.g., the food addiction model) have been proposed in the popular media in an attempt to respond both to the need of patients who buy into the "look slim" mentality and the despair of obese patients who have impaired health and psychosocial dysfunction.

Unfortunately, a model of linear causality is still frequently employed to evaluate and treat infantile and childhood obesity. Typically, the clinician searches for a specific cause, especially organic or endogenous. However, this search usually is futile, because endogenous obesity is quite rare and virtually never occurs in children who are ranked above the twenty-fifth percentile in height. The clinician then often focuses on a very narrow nutritional approach. This focus is closer to the biological underpinnings of the problem—a positive balance between caloric intake and expenditure—but it frequently ignores the powerful biopsychosocial influences that permit or encourage the child to overeat and underexercise. As would be expected, a multidisciplinary team approach is necessary to assess and treat such a multifactorial, chronic disorder (Boxer and Miller 1987; Woolston and Forsyth 1989). An ideal multidisciplinary team consists of a pediatrician, develop-

mental psychologist, child psychiatrist, social worker, nurse, and nutritionist. The team assesses the child's physical, developmental, psychiatric, familial, adaptive, functional, and maturational status. Because childhood obesity is so complex and severe, an inpatient evaluation may be required. The family's involvement is the most important variable in successful treatment. Pharmacological and nonpharmacological management combinations have been tried, with sufficient short-term success (Greenberg et al. 1999).

The clinician must perform a full medical assessment of the child to determine concomitant disorders, sequelae, and possible causes of obesity. Disorders such as slipped femoral epiphysis, diabetes mellitus, hypoxia, papilledema, sleep apnea, hypertension, cardiomegaly, pneumonia, polycythemia, and pickwickian syndrome may result from obesity and must be treated vigorously. This is critical in pickwickian syndrome because the respiratory hypoventilation and daytime hypersomnolence associated with severe obesity have a reported mortality of 40% in children (Boxer and Miller 1987). Prader-Willi syndrome should be aggressively approached because of the behavioral problems in this group, although current therapies do not seem to help in the behavioral manifestations of the disorder (Akefeldt and Gillberg 1999). Because of the apparent correlation between severe familial disorganization and some cases of infantile obesity, the child should be examined for other medical problems associated with neglect, such as inadequate immunization, lead poisoning, iron deficiency, and tuberculosis.

The therapist must carefully assess developmental, cognitive, and emotional status to define various psychological and developmental strengths and weaknesses. If the child is older than 30 months of age, he or she should be enrolled in an early intervention school program. The child should be examined for specific psychiatric disorders, such as attention-deficit/hyperactivity disorder, anxiety disorders, mood disorders, and oppositional defiant disorder.

In addition to evaluating all aspects of family functioning, the therapist must assess potential mental health and social resources for the family. The overall nutritional state of the child, the caloric intake for weight maintenance, and perhaps the nutritional status of other family members should be determined. The daily functioning of the child and family, including feeding and other mealtime behavior, should be ascertained, and specific behaviors that must be eliminated or strengthened should be identified. In this manner, the team evaluates the overall strengths and weaknesses of the child and family to discover the multiple factors behind the child's excessive caloric intake and inadequate caloric expenditure. As with other severe growth and eating disorders, the child may need to be removed from the home. This most restrictive alternative must be seen as a relatively undesirable intervention because the problem frequently reemerges when the child returns to the home.

The proposed subtyping schema for exogenous obesity helps to guide specific treatment approaches. Infants with simple excessive caloric intake respond well to parental nutritional counseling and the implementation of a more appropriate, balanced diet. Preliminary data contradict conventional wisdom by indicating that children with genetic/familial obesity also may have a relatively good response to brief, family-based behavioral intervention. A study by Epstein et al. (1990) using a prospective, randomized, controlled experimental design reported that an 8-week behavioral intervention program for both the obese child and his or her parents significantly reduced the obesity in the child at the end of the 10-year follow-up period. Unfortunately, this study's results have not been replicated. Levine et al. (2001) showed that a short-term family behavioral program was successful in containing weight gain for most children in their trial, as well as in improving the children's mood and eating disorder symptomatology.

Although pharmacotherapy has not been studied in the treatment of childhood obesity, several medications have been tested extensively for the treatment of adult obesity. Unfortunately, the most promising medications proved to be either ineffective (fluoxetine [Levine et al. 1989]) or unsafe (fenfluramine plus phentermine [Fishman 1999]). Sibutramine has been researched for use both in combination with diet and exercise (Berube-Parent et al. 2001) and on its own, as continuously or intermittently administered (Wirth and Krause 2001). Weight loss in all trials was achieved, but contradictory information exists as to the side effects and risks of using this new drug (Taflinski and Chojnacka 2000). Research on safety and efficacy in children is needed for all of these agents and newer ones. New pharmacological treatments developed from the results of the *ob* gene discoveries may become powerful treatments for obesity.

References

Akefeldt A, Gillberg C: Behavior and personality characteristics of children and young adults with Prader-Willi syndrome: a controlled study. J Am Acad Child Adolesc Psychiatry 38:761–769, 1999

American Academy of Child and Adolescent Psychiatry: Obesity in children and teens. Facts for Families Series (79). Washington, DC, American Academy of Child and Adolescent Psychiatry, 1997. Available at: http://www.aacap.org/publications/factsfam/79.htm. Accessed May 4, 2003.

Bao W, Srinvasan SR, Wattigney WA, et al: Persistence of multiple cardiovascular risk clustering related to syndrome X from childhood to young adulthood. Arch Intern Med 154:1842–1847, 1994

Barbero G, Shaheen E: Environmental failure to thrive: a clinical interview. J Pediatr 73:690–698, 1967

Berube-Parent S, Prud'homme D, St-Pierre S, et al: Obesity treatment with a progressive clinical tri-therapy combining sibutramine and supervised diet-exercise intervention. Int J Obes Relat Metab Disord 25:1144–1153, 2001

Boxer GH, Miller BD: Treatment of a 7-year-old boy with obesity-hypoventilation (Pickwickian syndrome) on a psychosomatic inpatient unit. J Am Acad Child Adolesc Psychiatry 5:798–805, 1987

Bruch H: Eating Disorders: Obesity, Anorexia Nervosa, and the Person Within. New York, Basic Books, 1973

Centers for Disease Control and Prevention: Prevalence of overweight among children and adolescents: United States, 1999. Hyattsville, MD, National Center for Health Statistics, 2002

Charney E, Chamblee H, McBride M, et al: The childhood antecedents of adult obesity: do chubby infants become obese adults? N Engl J Med 195:6–9, 1976

Christoffel KK, Forsyth BWC: The ineffective parent, childhood obesity syndrome (abstract). Paper presented at the 25th annual meeting of the Ambulatory Pediatric Association, New York, September 1985

Delvin MJ, Yanovski SZ, Wilson GT: Obesity: what mental health professionals need to know. Am J Psychiatry 157:854–866, 2000

Dietz W: Health consequences of obesity in youth: childhood predictors of adult disease. Am J Dis Child Pediatr 101:518–525, 1998

Donlon TA: Similar molecular deletions on chromosome 15q11.2 are encountered in both the Prader-Willi and Angelman syndromes. Hum Genet 80:322–328, 1988

Eid EE: Follow-up study of physical growth of children who had excessive weight gain in the first six months of life. BMJ 2:72–76, 1970

Epstein LH, Valoski A, Wing RR, et al: Ten-year follow-up of behavioral, family-based treatment for obese children. JAMA 264:2519–2523, 1990

Fishman AP: Aminorex to fen/phen: an epidemic foretold. Circulation 99:156–161, 1999

Freedman DS, Dietz WH, Srinivasan SR, et al: The relation of overweight to cardiovascular risk factors among children and adolescents: the Bogulusa Heart Study. Pediatrics 103:1175–1182, 1999

Garn SM, Clark DC: Trends in fatness and the origins of obesity: Ad Hoc Committee to Review the Ten-State Nutrition Survey. Pediatrics 57:443–456, 1976

Gortmaker SL, Dietz WH Jr, Sobol AM, et al: Increasing pediatric obesity in the United States. Am J Dis Child 141:535–540, 1987

Greenberg I, Chan S, Blackburn GL: Nonpharmacological and pharmacological management of weight gain. J Clin Psychiatry 60:31–36, 1999

Hirsch J, Leibel RL: The genetics of obesity. Hosp Pract 33:55–59, 62–65, 69–70, 1998

Kahn EJ: Obesity in children, in The Psychology of Obesity: Dynamics and Treatment. Edited by Kiell N. Springfield, IL, Charles C Thomas, 1973, pp 121–146

Kumanyika S: Ethnicity and obesity development in children. Ann N Y Acad Sci 699:81–92, 1993

Leonard M, Rhymes J, Solnit AJ: Failure to thrive in infants. Am J Dis Child 111:600–612, 1966

Levine LR, Enas GG, Thompson WL, et al: Use of fluoxetine, a selective serotonin uptake inhibitor, in the treatment of obesity: a dose-response study (with a commentary by Weintraub M). Int J Obes Relat Metab Disord 13:635–645, 1989

Levine MD, Ringham RM, Kalarchian MA, et al: Is family-based behavioral weight control appropriate for severe pediatric obesity? Int J Eat Disord 30:318–328, 2001

Maloney MJ, Klykylo WM: An overview of anorexia nervosa, bulimia, and obesity in children and adolescents. J Am Acad Child Psychiatry 22:99–107, 1983

Martin A, Scahill L, Charney DS, et al: Antipsychotic agents: traditional and atypical, in Pediatric Psychopharmacology: Principles and Practice. Edited by Martin A, Scahill L, Charney DS, et al. New York, Oxford University Press, 2003, pp 328–340

McCance C: Psychiatric factors in obesity. Dissertation for diploma in psychological medicine, University of London, London, England, 1961

Moran R: The evaluation and treatment of childhood obesity. Am Fam Physician 59:859–873, 1999

Pinhas-Hamiel O, Dolan LM, Daniels SR, et al: Increased incidence of non-insulin-dependant diabetes mellitus among adolescents. J Pediatr 128:608–615, 1996

Poskitt EME: Obese from infancy: a re-evaluation. Topics in Pediatrics 2:81–89, 1980

Power C, Lake JK, Cole TJ: Measurement and long-term health risks of child and adolescent fatness. Int J Obes Relat Metab Disord 21:507–526, 1997

Price RA, Gottesman II: Body fat in identical twins reared apart: roles for genes and environment. Behav Genet 21:1–7, 1991

Proietto J, Thorburn AW: Animal models of obesity—theories of aetiology. Baillieres Clin Endocrinol Metab 8:509–525, 1994

Sansone RA, Wiederman MW, Sansone LA: The prevalence of borderline personality disorder among individuals with obesity: a critical review of the literature. Eating Behaviors 1:94–104, 2000

Shapiro LR, Crawford PB, Clark MJ: Obesity prognosis: a longitudinal study of children from age six months to nine years. Am J Public Health 74:968–972, 1984

Shipman MG, Plesset M: Anxiety and depression in obese dieters. Arch Gen Psychiatry 8:530–535, 1963

Silverstone JT: Psychological factors in obesity, in Obesity: Medical and Scientific Aspects. Edited by Baird IM, Howard AN. London, E & S Livingstone, 1969, pp 45–55

Stunkard AJ: Obesity, in American Handbook of Psychiatry. Edited by Reiser MF. New York, Basic Books, 1975, pp 325–333

Stunkard AJ: Obesity, in Comprehensive Textbook of Psychiatry, 3rd Edition. Edited by Kaplan HI, Freedman AM, Sadock BJ. Baltimore, MD, Williams & Wilkins, 1980, pp 1872–1881

Stunkard AJ, Foch TT, Hrubec A: A twin study of human obesity. JAMA 256:51–54, 1986a

Stunkard AJ, Sørensen TIA, Hanis C, et al: An adoption study of human obesity. N Engl J Med 314:193–198, 1986b

Szydlo D: Psychological and familial determinants of eating disorders: causes and effects. Keynote lecture. National Conference on Psychiatric Disorders. American British Cawdray Hospital, Mexico, October 1999

Taflinski T, Chojnacka J: Sibutramine-associated psychotic episode. Am J Psychiatry 157:2057–2058, 2000

Van Itallie TB: Obesity, Genetics and ponderal set point. Clinical Neuropharmacology 11 (suppl 1):1–7, 1988

Whitaker RC, Wright JA, Pepe MS, et al: Predicting obesity in young adulthood from childhood and parental obesity. N Engl J Med 337:869–873, 1997

Wiederman MW, Sansone RA, Sansone LA: Obesity among sexually abused women: an adaptive function for some? Women Health 29:89–100, 1999

Wirth A, Krause J: Long-term weight loss with sibutramine: a randomized controlled trial. JAMA 286:1331–1339, 2001

Woolston JL, Forsyth B: Obesity of infancy and early childhood: a diagnostic schema, in Advances in Clinical Child Psychology, Vol 12. Edited by Lahey BB, Kazdin AE. New York, Plenum, 1989, pp 179–192

Self-Assessment Questions

Select the single best response for each question.

23.1 The prevalence of obesity in early childhood is not nearly as well studied as the prevalence of obesity in adulthood. However, the few studies that have been conducted indicate the prevalence of obesity in preschool children to be in the range of

    A. 0–5%.
    B. 5%–10%.
    C. 10%–15%.
    D. 15%–20%.
    E. 20%–25%.

23.2 According to a report by the Centers for Disease Control and Prevention (2002), the prevalence of obesity in children between the ages of 6 and 19 years is in the range of

    A. 2%–5%.
    B. 6%–8%.
    C. 13%–14%.
    D. 21%–23%.
    E. 30%–33%.

23.3 According to the American Academy of Child and Adolescent Psychiatry (1997), if one parent is obese, children have what percentage chance of being obese?

    A. 10%.
    B. 30%.
    C. 40%.
    D. 50%.
    E. 70%.

23.4 Which of the following statements concerning the genetic/familial form of obesity is *true?*

    A. There is evidence of psychopathology in the child or parent.
    B. Evidence of nutritional misinformation is seen.
    C. The family history for obesity is negative.
    D. The obesity has a sudden onset, usually around ages 12–13 years.
    E. The child may have characteristics associated with "difficult temperament."

23.5 Which of the following statements regarding psychogenic obesity is *true?*

    A. There is evidence of psychopathology in the child or parent.
    B. There is no evidence of nutritional misinformation.
    C. The family history for obesity is negative.
    D. In one type, associated with traumatic separation from the primary caregiver, there is a sudden onset, usually before age 3 years.
    E. All of the above.

Anorexia Nervosa and Bulimia Nervosa

David B. Herzog, M.D.

Kamryn T. Eddy, M.A.

Eugene V. Beresin, M.D.

Eating disorders are prevalent problems most commonly observed in late adolescent and young adult women and often associated with psychiatric comorbidity and medical complications. Among the eating disorders, anorexia nervosa and bulimia nervosa have received the most clinical research attention over the past several decades. While both are characterized by an overwhelming desire for thinness, anorexia nervosa is marked by extreme weight loss, body image disturbance, and an intense fear of weight gain, and bulimia nervosa is marked by binge eating, compensatory behaviors, and an overvaluation of weight and shape. Preoccupation with food, weight, and shape are common features to patients with eating disorders.

The medical community has recognized anorexia nervosa as a diagnosis since the turn of the nineteenth century. In contrast, bulimia nervosa was not formally recognized as a clinical diagnosis until 1979 by Gerald Russell.

In this chapter, we describe the diagnostic criteria, clinical findings, differential diagnoses, epidemiology, etiology, treatment, and prognosis of anorexia nervosa and bulimia nervosa.

Anorexia Nervosa

■ Diagnostic Criteria

Anorexia nervosa typically has its onset in an adolescent female who perceives herself to be overweight. Patients with anorexia nervosa commonly lose weight by restricting their food intake, excessively exercising, inducing vomiting after meals, and abusing laxatives, diuretics, or diet pills. DSM-IV-TR (American Psychiatric Association 2000) criteria for the disorder are shown in Table 24–1.

Within anorexia nervosa, DSM-IV-TR

Table 24–1.   DSM-IV-TR diagnostic criteria for anorexia nervosa

---

A.   Refusal to maintain body weight at or above a minimally normal weight for age and height (e.g., weight loss leading to maintenance of body weight less than 85% of that expected; or failure to make expected weight gain during period of growth, leading to body weight less than 85% of that expected).

B.   Intense fear of gaining weight or becoming fat, even though underweight.

C.   Disturbance in the way in which one's body weight or shape is experienced, undue influence of body weight or shape on self-evaluation, or denial of the seriousness of the current low body weight.

D.   In postmenarcheal females, amenorrhea, i.e., the absence of at least three consecutive menstrual cycles. (A woman is considered to have amenorrhea if her periods occur only following hormone [e.g., estrogen] administration.)

Specify type:

    Restricting type: during the current episode of anorexia nervosa, the person has not regularly engaged in binge-eating or purging behavior (i.e., self-induced vomiting or the misuse of laxatives, diuretics, or enemas)

    Binge-eating/purging type: during the current episode of anorexia nervosa, the person has regularly engaged in binge-eating or purging behavior (i.e., self-induced vomiting or the misuse of laxatives, diuretics, or enemas)

Source.   Reprinted from American Psychiatric Association: *Diagnostic and Statistical Manual of Mental Disorders*, 4th Edition, Text Revision. Washington, DC, American Psychiatric Association, 2000. Copyright 2000 American Psychiatric Association. Used with permission.

---

distinguishes between two subtypes—restricting and binge-eating/purging—based on presence or absence of bulimic symptoms. When compared with patients with restricting anorexia, those with the binge-eating/purging type may be more likely to have comorbid impulsivity, including substance use disorders, personality disorders, mood lability, and suicidality (American Psychiatric Association 2000). Additionally, they may have more severe medical complications as their low weight is compounded by binge/purge behaviors. Notably, however, the majority of patients with restricting anorexia develop bulimic symptoms during the course of the disorder (Bulik et al. 1997; Eddy et al. 2002).

■ Clinical Features

Physical Symptoms

Common physical complaints include cold intolerance, dizziness, constipation, abdominal discomfort, and bloating. Despite malnutrition, the patient is often hyperactive; lethargy may indicate fluid and electrolyte imbalance, cardiovascular compromise or severe depression.

Physical Examination

Patients with anorexia may wear multiple layers of bulky clothing. Adolescent anorexic patients tend to appear younger than their chronological age, whereas those with chronic anorexia may look considerably older than their age. Cachexia and breast atrophy are noticeable. The skin is often dry and may be yellow-tinged due to carotenemia. Bradycardia, hypotension, hypokalemia, lanugo, alopecia, and edema are common (Becker et al. 1999). Dental erosion and dorsal surface hand lesions (Russell's sign; Russell 1985) are noted in anorexic patients who self-induce vomiting.

Medical Complications

Anorexia nervosa is associated with multiple medical complications secondary to starvation (Rome and Ammerman 2003; Rome et al. 2003). Additionally, in patients with the binge-eating/purging type, these complications may also be secondary to bulimic symptoms (described more fully below; see Bulimia Nervosa, Medical Complications).

Cardiac complications. Electrocardiographic abnormalities are common among anorexic patients and typically normalize with refeeding (Panagiotopoulos et al. 2000). Low voltage, bradycardia, T-wave inversions, and ST segment depression may be found separately or in conjunction with arrhythmias (Kreipe and Harris 1992). Prolonged QT intervals and emetine-induced myocardial damage may be life threatening (Gottdiener et al. 1978). Those who vomit or abuse diuretics are at greatest risk for fatal cardiovascular complications (arrhythmias) because of resulting electrolyte imbalances.

Hematological changes. Mild anemia, leukopenia, and thrombocytopenia are often observed but usually reverse with refeeding.

Gastrointestinal complications. Decreased gastric motility, delayed gastric emptying, and constipation are often found in patients with restricting anorexia (1983). The use of metoclopramide or edrophonium as well as weight restoration may result in dissipation of these symptoms (Buchman et al. 1994). Pancreatitis has also been reported. Liver enzyme and amylase levels may be elevated but will reverse with refeeding. Acute gastric dilation and rupture and acute vascular compression of the duodenum leading to intestinal obstruction are rare but have a high mortality.

Renal abnormalities. Dehydration may result in increased levels of blood urea nitrogen. Polyuria often develops and may be traced to the decrease in renal concentrating capacity and an abnormality in vaso-

pressin secretion, which may produce partial diabetes insipidus. Peripheral edema is present in 20% of patients, usually during refeeding and rehydration. Weight restoration reverses these symptoms, although vasopressin abnormalities may persist for some time.

Neurological abnormalities. Neurological abnormalities are rarely found on physical examination and extensive neurological assessment is usually unwarranted, except in atypical presentations (e.g., prepubertal females, males, and treatment nonresponders). Magnetic resonance imaging studies have revealed enlarged ventricles and cortical sulci in adolescent patients associated with degree of weight loss (Katzman et al. 1996). Yet even in weight-restored patients, magnetic resonance images reveal smaller gray-matter volumes and larger sulcal cerebrospinal fluid volumes compared with those of control subjects, suggesting that anorexia nervosa may have long-lasting effects on the brain (Katzman et al. 1997; Lambe et al. 1997).

Endocrine complications. A hallmark of anorexia nervosa is amenorrhea, most often resulting from starvation-induced hypogonadism. However, in 20%–30% of patients, amenorrhea precedes weight loss and often persists despite weight recovery (Becker et al. 1999). In one community-based study, Misra et al. (2004) found that adolescents with anorexia nervosa were significantly less likely than healthy control subjects to be premenarchal despite comparable bone maturity. Clinical signs of hypothyroidism may be present due to decreased levels of triiodothyronine; primary hypothyroidism is rare because serum thyroxine and thyroid-stimulating hormone levels are usually in the low-normal to normal range. Reduced levels of growth hormone binding protein, insulin-like growth factor, and insulin-like growth factor binding protein-3 may explain growth retardation in anorexic patients (Golden et al. 1994; Misra et al. 2004); these levels revert to normal after nutritional rehabilitation. Decreased serum leptin levels in anorexia correlate highly with weight, body fat percentage, and insulin-like growth factor I (IGF-I) (Grinspoon et al. 1996; Misra et al. 2004).

Skeletal complications. Bone mineral density is reduced at several skeletal sites in most women with anorexia nervosa. In a community sample (N=130), Grinspoon et al. (2000) found that bone mineral density was reduced by at least 1 standard deviation in 92% of patients and by at least 2.5 standard deviations in 38% of patients. Diagnosis of anorexia for at least 1 year, adolescent onset, at least 6 months of amenorrhea, lower body mass index, low calcium intake (<600 mg/day), and fewer than 3 weekly hours of physical activity, were all predictive of adolescent osteopenia (Biller et al. 1989; Castro et al. 2000; Misra et al. 2004; Turner et al. 2001). Although bone density increases with weight gain, the persistence of osteopenia despite recovery may indicate bone mineral loss during adolescence is not completely reversible. Premenarchal anorexic patients whose disorder remits during adolescence may have better bone mineral density repletion (Jagielska et al. 2001).

Recent studies have focused on the association between low bone formation and low levels of IGF-I in the development of osteopenia (Grinspoon et al. 1996; Misra et al. 2004; Soyka et al. 1999). To date, no studies have shown estrogen administration to be effective in preventing bone loss, and no other effective drug treatment has been found.

Psychological Assessment

Patients with anorexia nervosa constitute a heterogeneous population. The prototypic patient manifests severe body-image distortion, interoceptive disturbance, and a pervasive sense of ineffectiveness (Bruch 1973). Personality characteristics include obsessionality, interpersonal insecurity, minimization of emotional expression, intolerance of anger, perfectionism, identity confusion, rigid control over impulses, low self-esteem, competitiveness, envy, and increased sense of responsibility and guilt (Strober 2004; Westen and Harnden-Fischer 2001). Ambivalence about sexual and emotional maturation, separation anxiety, and fears of being controlled are often areas of conflict. Axis I comorbidity most often includes major depression, reported in 50%–70% of patients (Herzog et al. 1999; Ivarsson et al. 2000) and anxiety disorders (e.g., obsessive-compulsive disorder), reported in 50% of patients (Braun et al. 1994; Bulik et al. 1997). Substance abuse and personality disorders are also prevalent (Herzog et al. 1999).

The affective range of expression for patients with anorexia is highly variable. Most often, the patient's affect is restricted and depressive features may be inferred from the patient's behavior; suicidal ideation may be present. The patient often has a limited capacity for self-observation or personal insight. Cognitive impairments, such as diminished attention and short-term memory, or obsessive thinking about food, may be starvation-induced.

■ Differential Diagnosis

Initial medical assessment must address the possibility that organic illness may mimic signs and symptoms of anorexia nervosa. Physical disorders with clinical symptoms common to those of anorexia include diabetes mellitus, colitis, thyroid disease, inflammatory bowel disease, acid peptic diseases, Addison's disease, intestinal motility disorders such as achalasia, and brain tumors. Psychiatric disorders that may manifest weight loss and bingeing or purging include conversion disorders, schizophrenia, and mood disorders (American Psychiatric Association 2004).

Epidemiology

According to large-scale population and archival surveys, lifetime prevalence of anorexia nervosa is estimated at 0.5% (American Psychiatric Association 2004). However, concerns about weight and shape among young girls are widespread (Field et al. 1999, 2003; Maloney et al. 1989) and meta-analytic review indicates these more prevalent dieting behaviors and body dissatisfaction represent risk factors for the development of eating disorders (Stice 2002).

Approximately 90%–95% of patients with anorexia are female (Hoek 2002). Age at onset ranges from preteen to adulthood with bimodal peaks at ages 13–14 and 17–18 years (Hoek and van Hoeken 2003). Recent studies indicate anorexia is prevalent across ethnicity and socioeconomic status. Younger, higher-weight, well-educated minority females who are more closely aligned with "white, middle-class values" may be at increased risk compared with other minorities (Crago et al. 1996). Notably, one large self-report health survey indicated that although socioeconomic status was associated with unhealthy dieting behaviors in adolescent females, it was not correlated with clinically significant eating-disorder behaviors (Rogers et al. 1997).

Etiology

High-Risk Populations

Involvement in activities that require highly focused attention on weight and appearance, including ballet, long-distance running, gymnastics, ice skating, and modeling, may increase risk for anorexia nervosa (e.g., O'Connor et al. 1996; Sundgot-Borgen and Torstveit 2004). Other suscep-

tible groups include chronically ill women with diseases like cystic fibrosis, diabetes, and spina bifida (e.g., Neumark-Sztainer et al. 1995; Rodin and Daneman 1992; Silber et al. 1999), and mood disorders, particularly depression (Garfinkel et al. 1987), and women with professions that require high standards of achievement (Herzog et al. 1987a). Although men constitute a smaller statistical group of anorexic patients, particular subgroups including athletes (e.g., runners, wrestlers) and male homosexuals may be at increased risk (e.g., Carlat et al. 1997).

Pathogenesis

Multiple perspectives on the pathogenesis of anorexia exist. The most comprehensive picture emerging suggests that a combination of psychodevelopmental, sociocultural, genetic, and neurochemical factors are implicated in the onset of the disorder (Becker et al. 1999; Fairburn et al. 1999; Garner 1993; Patton et al. 1999).

Individual development. From a psychodynamic perspective, anorexia nervosa results in a patient's attempts to solve intrapsychic conflicts. Eating symptoms are conceptualized as a behavioral manifestation of emotional conflict where purging behaviors help the patient to achieve affective homeostasis by ridding herself of painful affect and retaining a sense of accomplishment by furthering weight loss (Herzog et al. 1987b).

Developmental theory hypothesized that the infant's primary sense of trust in others, self-confidence, gratification of needs, and accurate affective and interoceptive awareness depend on the ability of the caretaker, typically the mother, to respond appropriately to the child. When a mother imposes her own needs on the child, serious consequences may result. For example, when feeding takes place because of the mother's need to quiet the child rather than when the child is hungry, the child develops uncertainty about her inner states and his or her ability to evoke care from the mother. The child feels drawn to comply with the needs of her mother to maintain this fragile connection on which the child's survival depends (Bruch 1982). This compliance and primacy of the mother's needs over the child's can occur outside of the feeding situation as well, leaving the child feeling increasingly controlled and devalued.

Further, mothers of anorexic patients can be self-sacrificing in their care of others while in denial of their own impulses and appetites. Like their children, they are exquisitely sensitive to perceived rejection, hostility, and conflict. This mother–child relationship makes it difficult for the child to take responsibility for her own feelings and to express aggression toward the mother, as wielding it could result in loss of the mother either by her destruction or abandonment. Hostility is projected to the external world, which is then viewed as dangerous and untrustworthy. The typical profile of fathers poses additional conflicts for the child. The mother's deferentiality is matched by a complementary entitlement to this behavior in the father. Underneath the father's professional success and mastery frequently lie serious problems in self-esteem and basic trust that are similar to their wives' issues—a needy, dependent side that is often denied. Such men usually distrust women and perceive them as powerful in their ability to betray and abandon them. They frequently manage this distrust by attempting to dominate women.

Thus, while family relationships may appear fine on the surface, the parents are often emotionally isolated; each has grave difficulties in intimacy and trust, yet they remain bound together in a self-sustaining cycle. The parents' relationship, although not consciously understood by the anor-exic child, is perceived as somehow troubled, dangerous, and, at times, terrifying. It certainly does not represent an attainable model of male–female relationships; it is one that the anorexic child consciously and unconsciously avoids, largely through symptoms. The female child is terrified of becoming the woman her mother is and simultaneously is distrustful of relationships with men.

Approval and affection are seen as unreliable states that can quickly become negative and disapproving. Ambivalence is poorly tolerated. Anorexic patients protect themselves from the hostile elements by using ritualistic algorithms of good and bad (Gordon et al. 1989; Kernberg 1975). Although the anorexic patient fiercely defends against aggression, largely by denial and projection, such defenses are rarely capable of keeping angry impulses unconscious. An inadequate defensive structure further contributes to low self-esteem and profound guilt. Aggression is acted out through self-directed punitive attacks (e.g., self-starvation, -deprivation, and -deprecation), combined with a passive-aggressive assault on the family (starvation in the face of others' frantic attempts to rescue the patient). Concomitantly, the inner experience is not of aggression but rather of a noble, ascetic, powerful activity that makes the child feel special and misunderstood by the world.

From a personality perspective, individuals are considered to be vulnerable to the development of anorexia nervosa on the basis of certain temperamental characteristics, including emotional constraint, perfectionism, and rigidity (Karwautz et al. 2002; Klump et al. 2000; Strober 1980, 2004; Vitousek and Manke 1994; Westen and Harnden-Fischer 2001). Adolescence may be an unsettling and frightening period marked by physical changes inherent in pubertal development, and increasing social and psychosexual demands. For individuals with the aforementioned character-istics in particular, who are temperamen-tally averse to sudden changes and much of what the transition from childhood to ado-lescence and adulthood entails, retreat into structure and rigidity (across all do-mains, including eating) can provide a fa-miliar sense of security. While providing a relief from the physical and emotional changes and demands associated with ado-lescence, anorexia nervosa simultaneously causes physical and emotional debilitation; this dilemma renders the disease all the more difficult for the patient to extract her-self from (Strober 2004).

Family perspectives. Family theorists at-tempt to understand anorexia nervosa in the context of family interaction in which the family is the unit of dysfunction and treatment, with the identified patient as the symptom bearer. Anorexic families often present a conflict-free exterior that masks lack of intimacy, enmeshment, overprotection, rigidity, and lack of con-flict resolution (Minuchin et al. 1978). The role of the anorexic is to divert atten-tion from impending family conflict; the symptoms serve as a stabilizing force for the family. As the patient becomes increas-ingly thin, she becomes increasingly de-pendent on and inseparable from the family (Minuchin 1984). In these families, excessive nurturance seemed to under-mine the daughter's efforts at separation; her attempts at genuine self-expression were neglected (Humphrey 1989).

Sociocultural factors. Notably, anorexia nervosa tends to affect females almost 10 times as frequently as males and tends to arise at times of sexual maturation includ-ing menarche and puberty. The reason that anorexia afflicts mostly females may be associated with femininity and the fe-male role in society, but the nature of this pattern is speculative. Researchers have attributed this distribution to the greater

cultural pressures on women toward thin-ness, which is commonly portrayed in Western culture (e.g., via values, media) as a prerequisite to success and beauty.

An additionally powerful social force is the difference in socialization between girls and boys. Gilligan (1982) demonstrated that girls are brought up to espouse "fem-inine" values, including service to others, attention to relationships, and interdepen-dence, while boys are trained to be autono-mous, self-directed, and rule-oriented in their relationships. As modern culture is transforming traditional models of female role definition by encouraging girls to be more autonomous, self-directed, and rule-oriented, girls are left in a double bind. For some, anorexia may be a response to these pressures of socialization.

Biological factors. Genetic factors in the transmission of anorexia nervosa among family members are at the forefront of re-search on the disorder. Results of popula-tion-based twin studies as well as clinical samples suggest significant genetic and nonshared environmental influences on anorexic symptomatology (Klump et al. 2001; Wade et al. 2000). In a review of six family studies on eating disorders, Strober (1995) found that anorexia is several times more common in biological rela-tives of index patients than in the general population. Strong indications of a ge-netic component contributing to the ex-pression of anorexia nervosa prompted a recent multisite genetic study, which pro-vided initial evidence for the presence of a susceptibility locus on chromosome 1p (Grice et al. 2002).

Neurochemically, starvation itself pro-duces extensive changes in hypothalamic and metabolic functioning and anorexia nervosa is further associated with changes in the noradrenergic, serotonergic, dopa-minergic, and opioid neurotransmitter sys-tems and with alterations in neuromodulators such as corticotropin-releasing hormone (Fava et al. 1989). Research indicates that under certain circumstances, hypothalamic epinephrine and serotonin induce loss of appetite, whereas norepinephrine increases food intake (Stoving et al. 1999). Dysregulated serotonin levels in women with anorexia that persist postrecovery suggest that this neurotransmitter may contribute to the development of the disorder (Frank et al. 2001; Kaye 1997; Stoving et al. 1999). This finding is supported by controlled family studies of patients with anorexia that find elevated familial risk of mood disorders among first- and second-degree relatives of index patients (Strober et al. 1990).

Biological research on mechanisms of perception and taste in anorexia nervosa has indicated an abnormal sensory response to high-calorie foods may be responsible for bingeing behaviors (Sunday et al. 1992). An alternative view, the set-point hypothesis, expects emaciated anorexic patients to show initially elevated taste preferences for calorie-dense foods, followed by decreased levels after nutritional therapy. Drewnowski et al. (1987) found that optimal sugar-to-fat ratios were elevated among patients with anorexia, even following weight gain. Abnormal taste profiles may be an enduring characteristic in patients with eating disorders.

Early Warning Signs

Early warning signs of anorexia nervosa that may be observed by family members or primary care physicians are changes in eating behaviors and weight-related concerns (e.g., not eating with the family, nighttime eating, increased body concerns in normal or underweight females), physical changes (e.g., weight loss, amenorrhea), changes in social behaviors (e.g., avoidance of activities, isolation), and mood-related changes (e.g., loss of self-esteem, depressed mood, irritability).

■ Treatment

Treatment of anorexia nervosa presents unique difficulties (Strober 2004). Anorexia nervosa is largely an ego-syntonic disorder and patients are typically resistant to initiating treatment focused on weight gain. Often, patients do not come to medical attention until they have lost a considerable amount of weight (Maloney and Klykylo 1983). The patient may be difficult to engage and the clinician may forge an initial alliance drawing on some area of acknowledged symptomatic difficulty. In the absence of an identified problem, the clinician may develop an alliance by empathically understanding the patient's perspective. Her condition forces others to pay attention and take control when, paradoxically, this is precisely what she fears. This pattern of a literal starvation for attention and caretaking, coupled with isolation and resistance, is played out in dyadic control struggles, both in the family and with the clinician. Hence, sensitivity and empathy for the patient, along with steadfast adherence to basic physical safety guidelines, is necessary for assessment or treatment to proceed. Although many anorexic patients will view limits on safety as evidence of further imposed "control," often there is a sense of relief (usually unconscious) that someone is taking over a situation gone out of control (Beresin et al. 1989; Lock 2002).

To date, randomized controlled clinical trials for anorexia nervosa are limited. The majority of research in this area has involved the study of family therapy for adolescent anorexia nervosa (described further below).

Evaluation of the anorexic patient should incorporate a team approach and include medical, psychiatric, family, and nutritional assessments. The first determination in the evaluation of the anorexic patient is often whether inpatient treatment is indicated (see Table 24–2).

Table 24–2. Level of care criteria for patients with eating disorders

	Level of care				
Characteristic	Level 1: outpatient	Level 2: intensive outpatient	Level 3: partial hospitalization (full-day outpatient care)	Level 4: residential treatment center	Level 5: inpatient hospitalization
Medical complications	Medically stable to the extent that more extensive medical monitoring, as defined in levels 4 and 5, is not required			Medically stable to the extent that intravenous fluids, nasogastric tube feedings, or multiple daily laboratory tests are not needed	For adults: heart rate <40 bpm; blood pressure <90/60 mm Hg; glucose <60 mg/dL; potassium <3 mEq/L; electrolyte imbalance; temperature <97.0 °F; dehydration; or hepatic, renal, or cardiovascular organ compromise requiring acute treatment For children and adolescents: heart rate in the 40s; orthostatic blood pressure changes (>20-bpm increase in heart rate or >10- to 20-mm Hg drop); blood pressure below 80/50 mm Hg; hypokalemia or hypophosphatemia
Suicidality	No intent or plan			Possible plan but no intent	Intent and plan

Table 24–2. Level of care criteria for patients with eating disorders (*continued*)

Characteristic	Level of care				
	Level 1: outpatient	Level 2: intensive outpatient	Level 3: partial hospitalization (full-day outpatient care)	Level 4: residential treatment center	Level 5: inpatient hospitalization
Weight as percentage of healthy body weight (for children, determining factor is rate of weight loss)	>85%	>80%	>75%	<85%	<75% (for children and adolescents: acute weight decline with food refusal even if not <75% below healthy body weight)
Motivation to recover, including cooperativeness, insight, and ability to control obsessive thoughts	Fair to good	Fair	Partial; preoccupied with ego-syntonic thoughts more than 3 hours a day; cooperative	Poor to fair; preoccupied with ego-syntonic thoughts 4–6 hours a day; cooperative with highly structured treatment	Very poor to poor; preoccupied with ego-syntonic thoughts; uncooperative with treatment or cooperative only in highly structured environment
Comorbid disorders (substance abuse, depression, anxiety)	Presence of comorbid condition may influence choice of level of care				Any existing psychiatric disorder that would require hospitalization
Structure needed for eating/gaining weight	Self-sufficient		Needs some structure to gain weight	Needs supervision at all meals or will restrict	Needs supervision during and after all meals or nasogastric/special feeding

Table 24–2.   Level of care criteria for patients with eating disorders *(continued)*

Characteristic	Level of care				
	Level 1: outpatient	Level 2: intensive outpatient	Level 3: partial hospitalization (full-day outpatient care)	Level 4: residential treatment center	Level 5: inpatient hospitalization
Impairment and ability to care for self; ability to control exercise	Able to exercise for fitness, but able to control compulsive exercising		Structure required to prevent patient from compulsive exercising	Complete role impairment, cannot eat and gain weight by self; structure required to prevent patient from compulsive exercising	
Purging behavior (laxatives and diuretics)	Can greatly reduce purging in nonstructured settings; no significant medical complications such as electrocardiogram abnormalities or others suggesting the need for hospitalization			Can ask for and use support or use skills if desires to purge	Needs supervision during and after all meals and in bathrooms
Environmental stress	Others able to provide adequate emotional and practical support and structure		Others able to provide at least limited support and structure	Severe family conflict, problems, or absence so as unable to provide structured treatment in home, or lives alone without adequate support system	
Treatment availability/ living situation	Lives near treatment setting			Too distant to live at home	

Inpatient Treatment

Inpatient treatment of anorexia nervosa is mandated by the severity of the patient's physical and psychological status. If indicated, hospitalization must be viewed as one phase in long-term treatment that will also include outpatient care.

Criteria are suggested by the American Academy of Child and Adolescent Psychiatry for hospitalization of children and adolescents with anorexia nervosa. Body mass index (BMI; kg/m^2) is used to indicate the degree of severity of anorexia nervosa in an individual. A BMI of $17.5 \ kg/m^2$ correlates with a body weight of less than 85% of the expected, indicating underweight. Inpatient treatment should incorporate a comprehensive psychiatric evaluation, a medical examination, appropriate laboratory studies, and close observation (Andersen et al. 1985). During the course of hospitalization, a team approach must be used and may include a psychiatrist, pediatrician, nutritionist, family therapist, recreational therapist, educator, and nursing staff.

The patient may be hospitalized either on a pediatric or a psychiatric ward based on the needs of the patient and the expertise of the staff. Patients with severe depression in the midst of a family crisis or in severe denial can receive more effective treatment on a psychiatric ward; those who primarily need nutritional repletion can often be treated adequately on a medical ward. One innovative treatment design is the pediatric day unit (Danziger et al. 1988), where parents are incorporated into the day-to-day interventions of patient care. This approach seeks to eliminate the punitive aspects of patient separation from parents. Parental supervision of patient behavior and meals aids in the restoration of positive patient and parental interaction.

The inpatient treatment program must have a nutritional rehabilitation protocol to which all treating clinicians can agree, and the treatment regimen must be explained to the patient prior to hospitalization. The staff, patient, and family must be aware that the administration of a feeding regimen is a life-saving act rather than a punishment. At the time of admission, a target weight for discharge should be established. The American Psychiatric Association suggests a healthy target weight "at which normal menstruation and ovulation are restored" or, for premenarchal girls, a weight at which "normal physical and sexual development resumes" (American Psychiatric Association Work Group on Eating Disorders 2000). However, some patients may continue to menstruate at low weights and others may not regain menses with weight gain; therefore, the minimum target weight is often estimated at 90% of ideal weight for height according to standard tables (American Psychiatric Association Work Group on Eating Disorders 2000). The target weight must be sufficiently high to protect the patient from bordering on a medically precarious state, and should be maintained for a period prior to discharge. Once the patient has reached the target weight, a reasonable range should be established to allow for day-to-day fluctuations. Once weight is increased to a medically stable level, the patient will be more psychologically amenable to other treatment modalities.

Limitations in health care coverage have reduced lengths of hospital stays. Currently, national data show that the average number of days of inpatient and outpatient treatment for an eating disorder is less than the minimum recommended by standards of care (Striegel-Moore et al. 2000). As a result, many anorexic patients who are still underweight are being discharged prematurely, which has been associated with increased risk of rehospitalization (Baran et al. 1995). For some patients, day treatment programs can ease the transition from inpatient to outpatient therapy.

Outpatient Treatment

In most cases, a multimodal approach incorporating several therapeutic techniques is necessary. The core outpatient treatment for anorexic patients should include a biopsychosocial approach involving ongoing medical management as well as family and individual psychotherapy. Additional treatment options group therapy, pharmacotherapy, and nutritional counseling. Currently, although many treatment techniques seem to be effective for anorexia, only five randomized, controlled clinical trials of treatment for adolescent anorexia nervosa have been published. These five studies generally support the use of the Maudsley method of family therapy to treat adolescent anorexia.

Family therapy.   Family therapy may be initially introduced to the family as a means of support for coping with the adolescent's anorexia nervosa. It is often not clear that family problems have led to the onset or maintenance of the eating disorder, yet families are uniformly affected by the anorexia and family therapies use a variety of techniques with anorexic families.

In the 1980s, Russell and colleagues at the Maudsley Hospital developed a new family treatment for use with anorexia nervosa. This therapy approach has become known as the Maudsley method and has been tested with adolescents with anorexia nervosa in five published clinical trials (Eisler et al. 1997, 2000; Geist et al. 2000; Le Grange et al. 1992; Robin et al. 1994, 1999; Russell et al. 1987). This treatment suggests that the family, instead of being viewed as problematic or "pathological," should be used by the therapist as an important resource to help patients recover (Lock and Le Grange 2001; Lock et al. 2001). The treatment involves three stages, including refeeding the patient, helping the patient and her family to negotiate new patterns of relationships, and

addressing adolescent identity issues relating to individuation; these are described fully in the family therapy treatment manual (Lock et al. 2001).

While the Maudsley method builds on early family therapy approaches described by Selvini-Palazzoli (1978) and Minuchin et al. (1978), it offers a novel approach by enlisting the parents as resources, which has demonstrated efficacy in randomized controlled clinical trials. The earlier approaches involved conceptualizing and reformulating the child's "disease" to the "symptoms" of a family in distress. In this context the problem became viewed as a larger familial process in which all members play a part rather than as the individual's illness (Selvini-Palazzoli 1978). As such, the communication and affective patterns of all of the family members would be addressed and restructured to provide support and tolerable independence to the patient (Minuchin 1984; Minuchin et al. 1978).

Currently, family therapy using the Maudsley method is regarded as the treatment of choice for adolescent anorexia nervosa. Long-term benefits from this form of family therapy have been shown to be stronger in patients with early-onset anorexia nervosa who are treated at an early stage in the disorder (Eisler et al. 1997).

Individual psychotherapy.   Although family therapy for adolescent patients has received the most research attention and empirical support, individual psychotherapy is the most widely used outpatient treatment of anorexia in the community. The goal of psychotherapy is to help the patient achieve a more adaptive capacity for self-regulation than current eating behaviors. The therapist establishes trust by acknowledging the patient's ongoing pain and recognizing the multiple determinants of the disorder (social, psychopathological, genetic, biological, behavioral, and familial).

The patient is often reassured by the therapist's knowledge about eating disorders and relieved to discover that the therapist neither minimizes nor is repulsed by the patient's symptoms. Given the patient's precarious medical status, clinicians should create a "therapeutic envelope" designed to provide a safety net for the patient if weight or vital signs fall below agreed-on minimums (Hamburg et al. 1989). Clear guidelines regarding weight, vital signs, and hospitalization should be established early in treatment and can be formalized as a contract.

A wide range of psychotherapeutic theoretical orientations and techniques have been advocated including cognitive behavioral, supportive, psychoeducational, and insight-oriented therapies. While the treatment rationale and specific therapeutic techniques employed may differ by theoretical approach, many common elements exist and the goals of treatment are similar. Because a fundamental problem for the anorexic patient often lies in the earliest dyadic relationships, the therapist must be aware of the patient's distrust of relationships. The therapist should be empathic and accurately "mirror" the perceived wants, needs, and feelings of the patient. It is important that the therapist be tolerant, undemanding, consistent, flexible, and able to empathize with the patient, sharing and tolerating affect without denial, resistance, or criticism. An effective therapeutic alliance demonstrates that relationships can sustain anger, conflict, and misunderstanding (Beresin et al. 1989).

Psychotherapy with the anorexic patient is a slow, difficult, process. Transferential anger and devaluation, suspension of therapy, boundary difficulties, critical illness, and hospitalization may occur throughout the course of therapy. Erroneous assumptions are discussed, and conflicts that may be embodied in the eating symptoms may be addressed. Over time,

the experience of the therapists' consistency in care and boundary maintenance may also facilitate the patient's ability to make effective use of additional forms of treatment. A multimodal approach to care is optimal because clinical experience suggests that psychotherapy alone is not adequate to treat patients with anorexia nervosa (American Psychiatric Association Work Group on Eating Disorders 2000).

Group therapy. Anorexic patients often express little interest in group treatments because they are socially avoidant and mistrustful. Moreover, their competitiveness can result in substantial weight loss for group members unless at least a few members are well on their way toward recovery. Yet, in the group setting, patients find it helpful to learn that others experience the same feelings and symptoms. The goal of group therapy is to decrease the patient's feelings of isolation by creating a nonthreatening environment in which patients may share thoughts and feelings (Piazza et al. 1983; Rollins and Piazza 1981).

A recent development that practitioners should be aware of is the increasingly common use of online Web sites that offer eating disorder information or host chat rooms and group discussions (American Psychiatric Association Work Group on Eating Disorders 2000). In fact, some of these sites provide explicit instructions on how to lose weight or purge more effectively. Thus lack of professional supervision on these sites may have detrimental effects; patient and family use of the Internet for information and support should be monitored.

Pharmacotherapy

Medication should not constitute the sole treatment for anorexia nervosa but can be helpful when used adjunctively to support weight restoration, prevent relapse, and treat psychiatric comorbidity. Several of the selective serotonin reuptake inhibitors have been evaluated in patients with anorexia and while none seems to aid specifically in weight restoration (Attia et al. 1998; Strober et al. 1999), fluoxetine has conferred some advantage in reducing risk of relapse in patients who are weight restored (Gwirtsman et al. 1990; Hsu 1995; Kaye et al. 1991, 2001). Additionally, a number of uncontrolled studies and case reports have examined the use of neuroleptics in patients with anorexia (Powers and Santana 2004). This research suggests that some neuroleptics (e.g., olanzapine) may be used to facilitate weight gain in anorexic patients, perhaps in part through a reduction of anxiety and depressive symptoms (e.g., Barbarich et al. 2004). However, potentially serious side effects associated with neuroleptic administration (e.g., increased glucose, lipids, QTc, risk of tardive dyskinesia) need to be considered prior to prescription. Research examining a range of other medications, including clomipramine, lithium, thiothixene, pimozide, sulpiride, and naloxone, has yielded negative or equivocal results.

It is noteworthy, however, that clinical psychopharmacological trials in patients with anorexia nervosa have typically included adult samples. To date, only one randomized controlled clinical psychopharmacological trial of adolescents with anorexia nervosa exists (Biederman et al. 1985), in which investigators found that the tricyclic antidepressant amitriptyline showed no benefit and conferred no advantage over placebo or individual supportive therapy in the treatment of adolescent anorexia.

Further, it is important to emphasize that psychotropic medication should be prescribed only in the context of psychotherapy. Given the medical severity of the illness, medication should be closely monitored and low dosages are necessary initially to reduce side effects in this low-weight population. The following principles are essential in prescribing psychotropics to malnourished, dehydrated, and physically compromised patients who are often resistant to such treatment: 1) educate the patient and family about the use and effects of medication; 2) select the specific target symptoms (e.g., obsessions, depression), or comorbid conditions (e.g., depression); 3) start at a low dose and increase slowly; and 4) monitor serum levels of the medication, vital signs, and electrocardiograms.

Prognosis

The course of anorexia nervosa is variable but can often be chronic and marked by relapse. A comprehensive meta-analysis of 119 studies including 5,590 patients with anorexia indicated that over long-term follow-up (up to 29 years; mode of 5–10 years), less than one-half of surviving patients will achieve full recovery, one-third will improve, and 20% will remain chronically ill (Steinhausen 2002). In one 7.5-year prospective follow-up study, predictors of full recovery included higher body weight at intake and shorter duration of intake episode. Early treatment for adolescents with anorexia predicts a better outcome. Further, the majority of anorexic patients engage in bingeing and purging behaviors during the course of the disorder (Casper et al. 1980; Eckert et al. 1995; Eddy et al. 2002).

The mortality rate for anorexia nervosa, 0.56% per year, is more than 12 times as high as that for young women in the general population (Becker et al. 1999). An 11-year follow-up study of women with eating disorders had a mortality rate of 5.1% for the subjects with anorexia nervosa, where three of the seven deaths were due to suicide (Franko et al. 2004; Herzog et al. 2000). In a survey of 14 outcome studies, Herzog et al. (1988) found that 24% of the deaths reported were due to suicide. Factors found to predict death in women with anorexia nervosa include abnormally low serum albumin levels and low weight at intake (Herzog et al. 1997), poor social functioning (Lowe et al. 2001), longer duration of illness, bingeing and purging, comorbid substance abuse, and comorbid affective disorders (Herzog et al. 2000). Although death is commonly due to suicide, it is also frequently ascribed to inanition. However, the exact cause of death is often unclear.

Bulimia Nervosa

■ Diagnostic Criteria

Bulimia nervosa typically has its onset in a late adolescence or early adulthood in individuals who are of normal weight or slight overweight, and may onset following a period of dieting. The disorder is currently defined in DSM-IV-TR (American Psychiatric Association 2000) on the basis of recurrent binge eating and compensatory behaviors and related cognitions. Binge eating is defined as the consumption of an objectively large amount of food within a short period of time, accompanied by the subjective experience of loss of control over eating. During a binge, people with bulimia tend to eat rapidly and consume a large amount of food (ranging from several hundred to thousands of calories) (Rossiter and Agras 1990). The experience of loss of control over eating can involve difficulty resisting the urge to eat, eating more rapidly than usual, and eating calorie-dense foods that are typically avoided outside of binge episodes. Compensatory behaviors are used to counteract the effects of a binge and include self-induced vomiting; misuse of laxatives, diuretics, and enemas; fasting; or excessive exercise. DSM-IV-TR criteria for bulimia are shown in Table 24–3.

Within bulimia nervosa, DSM-IV-TR distinguishes between two subtypes—purging and nonpurging—based on the type of compensatory behaviors employed; the majority of patients with bulimia present with the purging type (i.e., compensatory behaviors including vomiting, laxatives, diuretics). While individuals with bulimia often use more than one type of compensatory behaviors, 80%–90% engage in self-induced vomiting (American Psychiatric Association 2000). Patients with purging type bulimia tend to have more psychiatric and medical comorbidity than those with nonpurging type. As noted previously, up to 50% of patients with anorexia nervosa will develop bulimic symptomatology; crossover from bulimia nervosa to anorexia nervosa is less likely (Kassett et al. 1988).

■ Clinical Features

Physical Symptoms

Patients with bulimia nervosa often complain of peripheral edema, bloating, weakness, fatigue, dental problems, and finger calluses (Rome and Ammerman 2003; Rome et al. 2003).

Physical Examination

Patients with bulimia nervosa are typically within the healthy weight range, although a subset is overweight or obese. The few physical findings associated with bulimia are highly specific and secondary to self-induced vomiting (Lasater and Mehler 2001). These include transient facial swelling and peliosis (purpura), and calluses or abrasions on the dorsal area of the hand (Russell's sign; Russell 1985).

Medical Complications

Medical complications associated with bulimia nervosa are most often secondary to purging, but may also be associated with malnutrition and binge eating.

Laboratory findings.   Purging through vomiting and misuse of laxatives or diuret-

Table 24–3. DSM-IV-TR diagnostic criteria for bulimia nervosa

A. Recurrent episodes of binge eating. An episode of binge eating is characterized by both of the following:

  (1) eating, in a discrete period of time (e.g., within any 2-hour period), an amount of food that is definitely larger than most people would eat during a similar period of time and under similar circumstances

  (2) a sense of lack of control over eating during the episode (e.g., a feeling that one cannot stop eating or control what or how much one is eating)

B. Recurrent inappropriate compensatory behavior in order to prevent weight gain, such as self-induced vomiting; misuse of laxatives, diuretics, enemas, or other medications; fasting; or excessive exercise.

C. The binge eating and inappropriate compensatory behaviors both occur, on average, at least twice a week for 3 months.

D. Self-evaluation is unduly influenced by body shape and weight.

E. The disturbance does not occur exclusively during episodes of anorexia nervosa.

Specify type:

  Purging type: during the current episode of bulimia nervosa, the person has regularly engaged in self-induced vomiting or the misuse of laxatives, diuretics, or enemas

  Nonpurging type: during the current episode of bulimia nervosa, the person has used other inappropriate compensatory behaviors, such as fasting or excessive exercise, but has not regularly engaged in self-induced vomiting or the misuse of laxatives, diuretics, or enemas

Source. Reprinted from American Psychiatric Association: *Diagnostic and Statistical Manual of Mental Disorders*, 4th Edition, Text Revision. Washington, DC, American Psychiatric Association, 2000. Copyright 2000 American Psychiatric Association. Used with permission.

ics can result in serious electrolyte and acid-based complications (Lasater and Mehler 2001). Hypokalemia secondary to purging is less common but can lead to significant cardiac problems including arrhythmias, muscle weakness, and tetany (Mitchell et al. 1991). Metabolic alkalosis is more common secondary to purging. Pseudo-Bartter's syndrome may also develop if fluid levels are not increased (Mehler and Andersen 1999). Lower-extremity edema is also present when purging is stopped; due to high levels of aldosterone (leading to salt retention and edema) and typically resolves when purging is stopped.

Oral problems. Chronic regurgitation of acidic gastric contents can lead to a range of oral complications. Enamel erosion (perimolysis) and gum recession, typically on the lingual surface of front teeth, is

irreversible and quite common in patients with purging bulimia (Altshuler 1990). Swelling of the parotid glands (and occasionally the submandibular glands) due to salivary gland hypertrophy (sialadenosis) can occur in up to half of patients with bulimia and is related to frequency of self-induced vomiting (Mandel and Kaynar 1992). This problem as well as associated elevation of serum amylase levels are transient and should remit when purging is discontinued. Additionally, dry mouth, oral mucosal erythema, and cheilitis may be present (Spigset 1991); vitamin B_{12} deficiency should be assessed.

Gastrointestinal problems. Gastrointestinal difficulties are common in patients with bulimia and are often related to purging. Vomiting can lead to esophageal disorders including esophagitis, chest pain, dyspepsia, gastroesophageal reflux disease, esophageal rupture, hiatal hernias, and Barrett's esophagus. Difficulties associated with laxative abuse include irritable bowel syndrome, melancosis coli, and an atonic or cathartic colon. Additionally, constipation can result when laxatives are first discontinued and should remit within approximately 3 weeks (Colton et al. 1999). For these patients, exercise, fluid intake, and fiber increase can be helpful.

Cardiovascular problems. Excessive purging can result in volume depletion related to dizziness, hypotension, and syncope; as noted above, purging-related hypokalemia can also relate to arrhythmias. Use of ipecac to induce vomiting can result in skeletal muscle myopathy or even fatal cardiomyopathy. Rates of mitral valve prolapse are also elevated in patients with bulimia nervosa (Johnson et al. 1986).

Psychological Assessment

Patients with bulimia nervosa are preoccupied with eating, weight and shape, and tend to have marked body dissatisfaction and low mood. Associated Axis I comorbidity often includes mood, anxiety, and substance use disorders. Approximately half of patients with bulimia nervosa report a lifetime history of a mood or anxiety disorder, with depression, social phobia, and obsessive-compulsive disorder being particularly common (Braun et al. 1994; Bulik et al. 1997; Herzog et al. 1999; Ivarsson et al. 2000). While depression may precede the onset, have simultaneous onset, or follow the eating disorder onset, anxiety disorders most often precede the onset of the eating disorder. A substantial minority of patients with bulimia nervosa also reports a lifetime history of substance use disorders, with alcohol abuse being the most common.

The diagnostic group of patients with bulimia nervosa seems to be heterogeneous with regard to personality (Westen and Harnden-Fischer 2001) but may include patients with perfectionism, identity confusion, impulse dysregulation, low self-esteem, guilt, and shame. Research indicates that a subset of patients with bulimia can be characterized as multi-impulsive or dysregulated across multiple domains including eating, affect, interpersonal functioning, and sexuality, for example. Bulimic patients with dysregulated personality styles are more likely to present with comorbid substance use disorders, Cluster B Axis II disorders, self-destructive and self-injurious behaviors, and kleptomania (Herzog et al. 1999).

While the affective range of patients with bulimia is variable, patients tend to be depressive but less constricted than patients with anorexia and more aware of their feelings. Preoccupation with eating, weight, and shape are present but patients are often able to articulate feelings and triggers associated with the binge/purge cycle.

■ Differential Diagnosis

In the initial medical and psychiatric assessments it is important to address the possibility that a range of conditions may produce features similar to symptoms of bulimia nervosa (American Psychiatric Association 2000). Neurological disorders that impact appetite regulation and eating behaviors including brain tumors (e.g., pituitary or hypothalamic), and syndromes such as Klein-Levin or Kluver-Bucy need to be ruled out. Gastrointestinal disorders (e.g., malabsorption, ulcers, enteritis) should be considered. Additionally hormonal disorders relating to malnutrition and hypometabolism (e.g., adrenal disease, diabetes mellitus, pituitary dysfunction, hyperparathyroidism) should be ruled out. Psychiatric conditions including major depressive disorder and borderline personality disorder may be characterized by appetite dysregulation and binge eating or may be comorbid with bulimia nervosa. When binge eating and/or purging exist only in the context of anorexia nervosa, a bulimia diagnosis is not assigned.

■ Epidemiology

Population surveys indicate a 1%–4% lifetime prevalence rate of bulimia nervosa (American Psychiatric Association 2000), although estimates are higher within population subsets including college women (Pyle and Mitchell 1986). As noted above, dieting behaviors, weight and shape concerns, as well as binge eating, are prevalent in school-age children and adolescents, all of which may be precursors to threshold eating disorders (Stice 2002).

As with anorexia, approximately 90%–95% of patients with bulimia are female (Hoek 2002). Age at onset tends to be somewhat later than in anorexia, occurring in late adolescence and early adulthood, and may coincide with a time of transition (e.g., high school to college) or psychosocial stress (American Psychiatric Association 2000). Research indicates that bulimic attitudes and behaviors are widespread across ethnic and racial groups while findings regarding bulimia nervosa are unclear, with some investigators suggesting African American women are less likely than Caucasian women to meet criteria for bulimia nervosa (Striegel-Moore et al. 2003). Notably, however, eating disorders are more commonly seen in industrialized nations in which a thin female appearance is valued.

■ Etiology

High-Risk Populations

As with patients with anorexia nervosa, involvement in activities where weight and appearance are central (e.g., ballet, long-distance running) may increase risk for bulimia (O'Connor et al. 1996; Sundgot-Borgen and Torstveit 2004). Furthermore, patients with certain physical conditions including insulin-dependent diabetes mellitus may be particularly vulnerable to the development of bulimia nervosa (Rodin 2002). Similarly, particular subgroups of males including athletes (e.g., wrestlers) and male homosexuals may be at increased risk (Russell and Keel 2002).

Pathogenesis

As in anorexia nervosa, a multifactorial conceptualization of the etiology of bulimia nervosa exists, implicating psychological, biological, and social factors.

Individual development. Psychodynamically, individuals with bulimia nervosa share a number of traits with anorexic patients, such as perfectionism, difficulty with affect regulation, pervasive low self-esteem, and conflict aversion. They are also sensitive to rejection and fear abandonment. However, patients with bulimia nervosa tend to be more impulsive and overtly self-destructive, manifested by purging, shoplifting, promiscuous sex, and abuse of drugs and alcohol, particularly when compared with patients with restricting anorexia. Another major difference lies in the ego-dystonic experience of their eating disorder. Bingeing and purging typically produces intolerable feelings of shame and self-loathing. Thus bulimic patients have far more difficulty denying their illness, and live in torment. While some of these personality traits have biological roots, many are derivative of the deeply ingrained family problems. Bulimic families differ from anorexic families in a high degree of overt conflict, hostility and criticism. Parents tend to be less involved, unsupportive, and more distressed than in families with restrictive anorexia nervosa. Family volatility, coupled with impaired empathic parent–child relationships tends to produce children who are troubled with fears of abandonment, betrayal, and retaliation.

These hostile interactions may produce children who develop borderline personality traits as a function of traumatic and disruptive attachments. Bulimic patients thus tend to display a greater degree of suicidal ideation, feelings of victimization and chaotic interpersonal relationships.

Personality theory suggests that these characteristics of perfectionism, affect dysregulation, low self-esteem or negative affect, and conflict aversion are vulnerability factors predictive of the bulimic symptoms that emerge. Perfectionism is often characterized by dichotomous thinking, in which something or someone is either all good or all bad. This type of thinking may relate to the bulimic patient's alternation between strict dieting and binge eating; the patient who is engaging in strict dieting may have difficulty maintaining her limited intake, and, believing she has already failed, may engage in overeating (Fairburn et al. 1993; Polivy and Herman 1993). At the same time, her failure to adhere to her diet and her fall into binge eating leaves the patient feeling out of control and lowers her self-esteem and -efficacy. To regain a sense of control and to improve her self-esteem, she begins the cycle of dieting again. Additionally, the binge eating and purging have been hypothesized to serve as regulation strategies for coping with negative affect (Polivy and Herman 1993). Likewise, both overeating and purging are acts of self-destruction, which may reflect the patient's internalized emotionality (e.g., anger) that she is averse to expressing outwardly. As in anorexia nervosa, the symptoms of bulimia are at once coping strategies consonant with the patient's personality style, and resultant in physical deterioration.

Family perspectives. Clinical writings and research have indicated the existence of disturbances in mother–child dyadic relationships, as well as familial relationships, in patients with bulimia nervosa. Bulimic patients, as noted above, often have attachment difficulties, and families tend to be high in conflict, low in cohesion, less independent, and more achievement oriented (e.g., Crowther et al. 2002; Latzer et al. 2002). Further, the findings from one large community-based study indicated that parental problems, including low child–parent contact and high parental expectations, as well as parent difficulties with alcohol, may be risk factors for bulimia nervosa (Fairburn et al. 1997). Yet the nature of the relationship between family dysfunction variables and bulimic symptoms is often unclear with regard to directionality.

Sociocultural factors. The role of sociocultural factors in the pathogenesis of bulimia nervosa is supported by the increased prevalence of the disorder in industrialized nations. Media images of ideal beauty are inundating in Western society and yet they are unrealistically thin for most women; women with a childhood history of overweight and obesity may be at particular risk (Fairburn et al. 1997). Over time, the presentation of these unrealistic images leads to internalization of a thin body ideal and associated body dissatisfaction, both of which predict dieting and bulimic symptoms (for a review, see Stice 2002). Further, cross-cultural research indicates that exposure to Western beauty ideals influences the development of eating disorder pathology (Becker et al. 2002). It is likely that the confluence of multiple psychological, biological, and sociocultural factors predicts the development of bulimia nervosa.

Biological factors. The role of biology and genetic factors in the development of bulimia nervosa have received considerable attention in the last decade. The biological model is supported by the higher concordance of monozygotic than dizygotic twins, which implicates genetic factors. On the basis of twin studies heritability estimates for bulimia nervosa range from 31%–83% (Bulik et al. 1998; Kendler et al. 1991; Wade et al. 2000). Genetic studies are currently underway and although it is unlikely that a single gene will be identified as predictive of bulimia nervosa, preliminary findings suggest there are significant links between presence of bulimia nervosa and chromosome 10p (Bulik et al. 2003).

Further support for biological factors include the dietary restraint model of bulimia nervosa, which suggests that patient-induced dietary restraint leads to binge eating. Neurotransmitters, including serotonin, play a role in appetite, satiation, food selection, and eating pattern, all of which may be disrupted for patients with bulimia nervosa (Mitchell and deZwaan 1993). Additionally, the appetite-inducing neuropeptide Y and peptide YY have been found to be elevated in patients with bulimia nervosa (Kaye et al. 1990). Cholecystokinin, which is a hormone associated with the experience of satiety and discontinuation of eating behavior, has been found to be low in some patients with bulimia nervosa (Bailer and Kaye 2003). The disruption of these neuronal systems may be implicated in bulimia nervosa.

Early Warning Signs

Early warning signs in the detection of bulimia nervosa are similar to those of anorexia nervosa. Family members and physicians may note changes in eating behaviors and weight-related concerns (e.g., an increase in secrecy associated with eating), physical changes (e.g., signs of malnutrition including thinning hair), as well as interpersonal- and mood-related changes.

■ Treatment

As in the treatment of anorexia nervosa, treatment for bulimia nervosa often involves multiple components, the most common of which are psychosocial and pharmacological. Patients with bulimia nervosa often manifest shame and embarrassment with regard to their binge/purge symptoms. They tend to experience their symptoms as ego dystonic, unlike patients with anorexia nervosa. There is often considerable ambivalence in these patients who on the one hand describe feeling out of control with their eating behaviors and may have a wish for immediate relief and therefore be interested in beginning a treatment that will help them regain stability over their eating. Yet simultaneously, they may be hesitant to implement recommendations, demonstrating significant fears that discontinuing the binge/purge cycle will result in weight gain, which they believe would be unbearable. Determining motivation and readiness to change is important early on in treatment.

The primary aims of treatment for bulimia nervosa are to reduce and eliminate binge/purge behaviors, to modify unhealthy attitudes towards weight and shape, and to encourage healthier coping styles. Comprehensive initial assessment is warranted to determine an appropriate and individualized treatment course. For a subset of patients, bulimia nervosa may be complicated by a concomitant medical condition; in these cases prioritizing the severity of various medical problems is necessary in treatment planning (see Table 24–2).

Inpatient Treatment

Inpatient treatment of bulimia nervosa is not frequently indicated but may be necessary when mandated by the severity of the patient's physical health secondary to binge/purge behaviors, due to medical instability associated with medical morbidity (e.g., diabetes), or due to safety concerns related to severe depression or suicidality. Additionally, for the patient who is unable to manage her binge/purge behaviors on an outpatient basis, the structure of an inpatient setting may be helpful in disrupting the binge/purge cycle.

Outpatient Treatment

Psychotherapy. Although bulimia nervosa often onsets during adolescence and is a prevalent problem among adolescent females, to date there have been no published randomized controlled clinical trials of treatment for adolescent bulimia nervosa. Among adults, several psychosocial interventions have received empirical support for the treatment of bulimia nervosa, and currently, psychotherapy is regarded as the first-line of treatment for the disorder. Results from the adult literature suggest that these therapies may be effective in adolescent patients. The examination of the efficacy of these therapies in adolescents is warranted.

Cognitive-behavioral therapy (CBT) has received the strongest empirical support for the treatment of bulimia nervosa, achieving 80% reductions in bingeing and purging behavior in patients and leading to full recovery in approximately half of patients (Agras et al. 2000; Wilson et al. 2002). Further, CBT is particularly effective in improving distorted cognitions related to eating, weight, and shape, which may protect against relapse. The treatment is typically short-term and focused, comprising 15–20 sessions held over a 4- to 5-month period. CBT for bulimia nervosa operates along the dietary restraint model of bulimia nervosa. Within this model, dietary restraint leads to binge eating and subsequent compensatory behaviors, both of which reinforce concern about eating, weight, and shape, and in turn drive the bulimic cycle (Fairburn et al. 1993, 2003). CBT intervenes in this cycle by targeting dietary restraint and in turn reducing and eliminating binge eating and purging, and simultaneously addressing dysfunctional eating, weight, and shape cognitions. The

key components of treatment include psychoeducation around healthy eating and the implications of disordered eating behaviors, the prescription of "regular" eating, self-monitoring (in the form of daily food logs), and restructuring of distorted cognitions around eating, weight, and shape. While CBT can be delivered in an individual, group, or self-help manualized format, meta-analytic review indicates that individual treatment confers an advantage over group treatment (Thompson-Brenner et al. 2003). CBT-focused self-help and guided self-help approaches have demonstrated efficacy and although response rates with self-help are not as high as with individual CBT, advantages include the wide availability and low cost.

Interpersonal psychotherapy (IPT) has demonstrated comparable rates of improvement and recovery to CBT in the treatment of bulimia nervosa, although it appears to work somewhat less quickly. First developed by Klerman et al. (1984) for the treatment of depression, IPT has been modified for use with bulimia nervosa (Fairburn 1997). In contrast to CBT, IPT targets interpersonal functioning rather than maladaptive eating behaviors and cognitions. The IPT model of bulimia nervosa suggests that interpersonal difficulties lead to low self-esteem and dysphoria, and that bingeing and purging are used as coping mechanisms to regulate affect. Thus, through a short-term focused treatment, IPT aims to address interpersonal difficulties, which leads to improvements in bulimic symptoms that often accrue even posttreatment.

Yet in spite of the efficacy of CBT and IPT in addressing bulimic symptoms, approximately 50% of patients remain symptomatic posttreatment (Thompson-Brenner et al. 2003). Presently treatment trials are designed to deconstruct CBT and IPT approaches to identify mechanisms of change in order to determine what is working and why treatment is not effective for all patients. Integrated therapies, which incorporate elements of different treatment modalities, are more representative of treatment used in the community and attempts to study them in controlled treatment trials are under way. One example of this is an enhanced version of CBT (CBT-E), which incorporates cognitive behavioral principles, interpersonal aspects, affect regulation strategies taken from dialectical behavior therapy, and other techniques all in an individualized approach as they apply to the patient. Preliminary findings suggest high rates of improvement and recovery for difficult-to-treat patients. These more integrative therapy approaches may also be effective in addressing comorbidity and maladaptive personality styles involved in the etiology and maintenance of bulimic symptoms.

A significant limitation of these clinical trials for bulimia nervosa is that patient samples are most often adult; the generalizability of these findings to adolescents with the disorder is unclear. These empirically supported treatments are described in detail in treatment manuals available for use by treating clinicians. Notably, however, these manuals are not routinely used outside of research and academic institutions (Haas and Clopton 2003). In a naturalistic study of community-based clinicians treating adult patients with bulimia nervosa, Thompson-Brenner and Westen (2005a, 2005b) found that treatment in the community was longer in duration and more theoretically integrative than the treatments tested in randomized controlled clinical trials. The investigators found that community-based clinicians tended to employ many techniques similar to those described in the treatment manuals but were flexible with their use of cognitive behavioral and psychody-

namic principles based on the individual needs of the patient (e.g., considering the patient's personality style, comorbidity). The clinician's ability to be flexible (e.g., employing more cognitive behavioral techniques, employing more dynamic principles) predicted a more positive patient posttreatment outcome.

Family therapy. Although there is less research to support the use of family therapy to treat bulimia nervosa, a series of case reports and noncontrolled studies have indicated its utility with bulimia (Le Grange et al. 2003). There is some evidence to suggest that a family therapy approach to the treatment of bulimia nervosa (using the Maudsley model) may be helpful, particularly for younger patients who are living with their parents, and for older patients who have ongoing conflicts with their parents (e.g., Woodside et al. 1996a, 1996b). Multisite controlled treatment trials of family therapy for adolescent bulimia nervosa are currently in progress.

Group therapy. Both cognitive behavioral and interpersonal therapies have been modified for use in group format. While these modified therapies do appear useful for treatment of bulimia nervosa, the magnitude of treatment effects are less than those of individual therapy (Thompson-Brenner et al. 2003). Additionally, supportive group treatment may be a helpful adjunctive to individual therapy. Patients may benefit from meeting with others who are experiencing the same difficulties by alleviating shame associated with the eating disorder, supporting one another, and in building social skills. There is some evidence to support the inclusion of dietary counseling in group treatments for bulimia (Laessle et al. 1987).

As with patients with anorexia, the use of online Web sites offering eating disorder information or group discussion should be monitored for patients with bulimia and family members, as with patients with anorexia (American Psychiatric Association Work Group on Eating Disorders 2000).

Pharmacotherapy

Pharmacotherapy has also demonstrated utility in the treatment of bulimia nervosa, specifically in the reduction of bingeing and purging symptoms. In particular, antidepressant therapy has been widely studied in adults with bulimia nervosa, demonstrating mean reductions in bulimic symptoms of approximately 70% and posttreatment abstinence rates of approximately 30% (for a review, see Agras 1997). Currently, the selective serotonin reuptake inhibitor (SSRI) fluoxetine is the only medication approved by the FDA for the treatment of bulimia nervosa (recommended dosage: 60 mg qd). While preliminary research has indicated other SSRIs may be equally helpful in the reduction of binge/purge symptoms, randomized controlled trials involving long-term follow-up are not yet available. Further, earlier studies indicated the utility of tricyclic antidepressants, particularly desipramine, in the treatment of bulimic symptoms; however, SSRIs tend to be better tolerated (Zhu and Walsh 2002). Generally, monoamine oxidase inhibitors are avoided in patients with bulimia nervosa due to nutritional instability associated with binge/purge behaviors. Similarly, the antidepressant bupropion is contraindicated due to an increased risk of seizures in patients with bulimia nervosa.

Antidepressant medication is useful for the treatment of bulimic symptoms independent of whether the patient suffers from comorbid depression (Walsh et al. 1991). This finding argues against an antidepressant effect and leaves the mechanism of action of the utility of antidepressants in addressing bulimic symptoms unclear. Given the role of serotonin in appetite regulation, it is possible that antidepressants act on serotonin to reduce binge eating.

Other medications that have been tested include the opiate agonist naltrexone, the anticonvulsant topiramate, and sibutramine, which have all demonstrated preliminary efficacy with patients with bulimia nervosa (Appolinario et al. 2003; McElroy et al. 2003).

Yet in spite of the utility of psychotropic medications, particularly antidepressants, in the treatment of bulimic symptoms, they appear to be generally less effective than psychotherapy alone. There is some evidence that medication in conjunction with psychotherapy confers and advantage over either modality alone but this advantage appears to be minimal (Nakash-Eisikovits et al. 2002).

Similar to the psychotherapy literature, however, clinical trials including adolescent patients are limited and the applicability of these findings to younger patients is not clear. Although there have been no published randomized controlled psychopharmacological clinical trials for adolescents with bulimia nervosa, one recent open trial suggests fluoxetine may be helpful in treating adolescent patients (Kotler et al. 2003). However, given the lack of controlled clinical trials of these medications among child and adolescent patients—those with eating disorders, as well as those with other psychiatric disorders—prescription of psychotropic medications among younger patients should be made cautiously and their use should be monitored closely by the prescribing clinician. Education about the use and effects of medication with patients and family members is critical.

Adjunctive Treatments

A medical assessment is indicated in patients with bulimia nervosa and ongoing medical management may be useful particularly to treat patients with complications, those discontinuing laxative and/or diuretic abuse, as well as those taking psychotropic medications. Nutritional counseling, which is often a component of psychotherapy (e.g., CBT), may also be helpful to provide additional structure, support, and education for patients who have difficulty meal planning and regulating their eating (Laessle et al. 1987).

■ Prognosis

The longitudinal course of bulimia nervosa is variable but as with anorexia nervosa, it may be chronic and relapsing. Longitudinal research suggest that 50%–75% of patients with bulimia nervosa will achieve full recovery from their eating disorder (Fairburn et al. 2000; Fichter and Quadflieg 1997; Herzog et al. 1999), although approximately one-third of these will go on to relapse (Herzog et al. 1999; Keel and Mitchell 1997). A small minority of patients seem to present with chronic bulimia nervosa. It appears that a longer duration of illness, history of unsuccessful treatment attempts, comorbid substance abuse, and Cluster B personality disorders, are predictive of a worse outcome for patients with bulimia nervosa.

■ Research Issues

Eating disorders research is advancing, and within this area issues of nosology and classification, etiology, risk, and maintenance, and treatment development and outcome, are central.

First, investigating valid and reliable diagnostic criteria is a priority. Additional research is necessary to address the eating disorder categories and their associated subdivisions (i.e., subtypes). Given the considerable overlap in symptomatology among diagnostic groups as well as the likelihood of diagnostic migration, some have argued that an alternative system of eating disorder description/categorization be considered (Fairburn et al. 2003).

Second, in regard to etiology, risk, and maintenance of anorexia and bulimia nervosa, biological research is currently underway. It is likely that ongoing large-scale family studies of anorexia nervosa and bulimia nervosa will increase our understanding of the etiological role of genetics in these disorders. Prospective longitudinal studies on the naturalistic course of anorexia and bulimia nervosa will establish base rates of short-interval and long-term recovery, chronicity, and mortality. Further, current research in the areas of cognitive functioning and neuroimaging are helping to elucidate patterns of cognitive impairment as well as identifying neural systems implicated in anorexia and bulimia nervosa. Additional research on the neurochemistry (neurotransmitter systems and neuromodulators) of anorexia and bulimia nervosa and on changes in the central nervous system that precede onset is necessary to increase our understanding of the pathophysiology and to develop more effective pharmacological and cognitive-behavioral treatments (Fava et al. 1989). Similarly, research on the pattern of sensory responsiveness to sweets and fat during childhood or early adolescence may determine early psychobiological markers for eating disorders (Grill 1985). Investigations of osteoporosis, a frequent and severe complication of anorexia nervosa, will elucidate mediating mechanisms and appropriate treatment.

Third, with regard to treatment, ongoing research is aimed at elucidating mechanisms of action for effective treatments, isolating components of treatment in order to establish their relation to outcome, and developing and testing new and integrative therapies in order to continue to improve outcomes. However, a significant gap in the literature exists with regard to the use of psychotherapy and pharmacotherapy interventions with child and adolescent patients with eating disorders, particularly those with bulimia nervosa. Research in this area is critical to determine whether downward extensions of treatments that have demonstrated efficacy with adults is appropriate, or whether novel interventions are warranted. Further, bridging the gap between research and clinical practice is a priority.

Conclusion

Both anorexia nervosa and bulimia nervosa are life-threatening conditions that have come to the forefront of public attention in the last several decades. The successful collaboration of clinical researchers from all disciplines is necessary to further the understanding of the pathogenesis and treatment of these disorders.

References

Agras WS: Pharmacotherapy of bulimia nervosa and binge eating disorder: longer-term outcomes. Psychopharmacol Bull 33:433–436, 1997

Agras WS, Crow SJ, Halmi KA, et al: Outcome predictors for the cognitive behavior treatment of bulimia nervosa: data from a multisite study. Am J Psychiatry 157:1302–1308, 2000

Altshuler BD: Eating disorder patients. Recognition and intervention. J Dent Hyg 64:119–125, 1990

American Psychiatric Association: Diagnostic and Statistical Manual of Mental Disorders, 4th Edition, Text Revision. Washington, DC, American Psychiatric Association, 2000

American Psychiatric Association Work Group on Eating Disorders: Practice guideline for the treatment of patients with eating disorders (revision). Am J Psychiatry 157 (suppl 1): 1–39, 2000

Andersen AE, Morse CL, Santmyer KS: Inpatient treatment for anorexia nervosa, in Handbook of Psychotherapy for Anorexia Nervosa and Bulimia. Edited by Garner DM, Garfinkel PE. New York, Guilford, 1985, pp 311–343

Appolinario JC, Bacaltchuk J, Sichieri R, et al: A randomized, double-blind, placebo-controlled study of sibutramine in the treatment of binge-eating disorder. Arch Gen Psychiatry 60:1109–1116, 2003

Attia E, Haiman C, Walsh BT, et al: Does fluoxetine augment the inpatient treatment of anorexia nervosa? Am J Psychiatry 155:548–551, 1998

Bailer UF, Kaye WH: A review of neuropeptide and neuroendocrine dysregulation in anorexia and bulimia nervosa. Curr Drug Targets CNS Neurol Disord 2:53–59, 2003

Baran SA, Weltzin TE, Kaye WH: Low discharge weight and outcome in anorexia nervosa. Am J Psychiatry 152:1070–1072, 1995

Barbarich NC, McConaha CW, Gaskill J, et al: An open trial of olanzapine in anorexia nervosa. J Clin Psychiatry 65:1480–1482, 2004

Becker AE, Grinspoon SK, Klibanski AK, et al: Eating disorders. N Engl J Med 340:1092–1098, 1999

Becker AE, Burwell RA, Gilman SE, et al: Eating behaviours and attitudes following prolonged exposure to television among ethnic Fijian adolescent girls. Br J Psychiatry 180:509–514, 2002

Beresin EV, Gordon C, Herzog DB: The process of recovering from anorexia nervosa, in Psychoanalysis and Eating Disorders. Edited by Bemporad JR, Herzog DB. New York, Guilford, 1989, pp 103–130

Biederman J, Herzog DB, Rivinus TM, et al: Amitriptyline in the treatment of anorexia nervosa: a double-blind, placebo-controlled study. J Clin Psychopharmacol 5:10–16, 1985

Biller BMK, Saxe V, Herzog DB, et al: Mechanisms of osteoporosis in adult and adolescent women with anorexia nervosa. J Clin Endocrinol Metab 68:548–554, 1989

Braun DL, Sunday SR, Halmi KA: Psychiatric comorbidity in patients with eating disorders. Psychol Med 24:859–867, 1994

Bruch H: Eating Disorders. New York, Basic Books, 1973

Bruch H: Anorexia nervosa: therapy and theory. Am J Psychiatry 139:1531–1538, 1982

Buchman AL, Ament ME, Weiner M, et al: Reversal of megaduodenum and duodenal dysmotility associated with improvement in nutritional status in primary anorexia nervosa. Dig Dis Sci 39:433–440, 1994

Bulik C, Sullivan PF, Fear J, et al: Predictors of the development of bulimia nervosa in women with anorexia nervosa. J Nerv Ment Dis 185:704–707, 1997

Bulik CM, Sullivan PF, Kendler KS: Heritability of binge-eating and broadly defined bulimia nervosa. Biol Psychiatry 44:1210–1218, 1998

Bulik CM, Sullivan PF, Wade TD, et al: Twin studies of eating disorders: a review. Int J Eat Disord 27:1–20, 2003

Carlat DJ, Camargo CA Jr, Herzog DB: Eating disorders in males: a report on 135 patients. Am J Psychiatry 154:1127–1132, 1997

Casper RC, Eckert ED, Halmi KA, et al: Bulimia: its incidence and clinical importance in patients with anorexia nervosa. Arch Gen Psychiatry 37:1030–1035, 1980

Castro J, Lazaro L, Pons F, et al: Predictors of bone mineral density reduction in adolescents with anorexia nervosa. J Am Acad Child Adolesc Psychiatry 39:1365–1370, 2000

Colton P, Woodside DB, Kaplan AS: Laxative withdrawal in eating disorders: treatment protocol and 3 to 20-month follow-up. Int J Eat Disord 25:311–317, 1999

Crago M, Shisslak CM, Estes LS: Eating disturbances among American minority groups: a review. Int J Eat Disord 19:239–248, 1996

Crowther JH, Kichler JC, Sherwood NE: The role of familial factors in bulimia nervosa. Eat Disord: J Tx Prevent 10:141–151, 2002

Danziger Y, Carol CA, Varsano I, et al: Parental involvement in treatment of patients with anorexia nervosa in a pediatric day-care unit. Pediatrics 81:159–162, 1988

Drewnowski A, Halmi KA, Pierce B, et al: Taste and eating disorders. Am J Clin Nutr 46:442–450, 1987

Eckert ED, Halmi KA, Marchi P, et al: Ten-year follow-up of anorexia nervosa: clinical course and outcome. Psychol Med 25:143–156, 1995

Eddy KT, Keel, PK, Dorer DJ, et al: A longitudinal comparison of anorexia nervosa subtypes. Int J Eat Disord 31:191–201, 2002

Eisler I, Dare C, Russell GFM, et al: Family and individual therapy in anorexia nervosa: a 5-year follow-up. Arch Gen Psychiatry 54:1025–1030, 1997

Eisler I, Dare C, Hodes M, et al: Family therapy for adolescent anorexia nervosa: the results of a controlled comparison of two family interventions. J Child Psychol Psychiatry 41:727–736, 2000

Fairburn CG: Interpersonal psychotherapy for bulimia nervosa, in Handbook of Treatment for Eating Disorders. Edited by Garner DM, Garfinkel PE. New York, Guilford, 1997, pp 278–294

Fairburn CG, Marcus MD, Wilson GT: Cognitive-behavioral therapy for binge eating and bulimia nervosa: a comprehensive treatment manual, in Binge Eating: Nature, Assessment, and Treatment. Edited by Fairburn CG, Wilson GT. New York, Guilford, 1993, pp 361–404

Fairburn CG, Welch SL, Doll HA, et al: Risk factors for bulimia nervosa. A community-based case-control study. Arch Gen Psychiatry 54:509–517, 1997

Fairburn CG, Cooper Z, Doll HA, et al: Risk factors for anorexia nervosa: three integrated case-control comparisons. Arch Gen Psychiatry 56:468–476, 1999

Fairburn CG, Cooper Z, Doll HA, et al: The natural course of bulimia nervosa and binge eating disorder in young women. Arch Gen Psychiatry 57:659–665, 2000

Fairburn CG, Cooper Z, Shafran R: Cognitive behaviour therapy for eating disorders: a "transdiagnostic" theory and treatment. Behav Res Ther 41:509–528, 2003

Fava M, Copeland PM, Schweiger U, et al: Neurochemical abnormalities of anorexia nervosa and bulimia nervosa. Am J Psychiatry 146:963–971, 1989

Fichter M, Quadflieg N: Six-year course of bulimia nervosa. Int J Eat Disord 22:361–384, 1997

Field AE, Carmago CA Jr, Taylor CB, et al: Overweight, weight concerns, and bulimic behaviors among girls and boys. J Am Acad Child Adolesc Psychiatry 38:754–760, 1999

Field AE, Austin SB, Taylor CB, et al: Relation between dieting and weight change among preadolescents and adolescents. Pediatrics 112:900–906, 2003

Frank GK, Kaye WH, Weltzin TE, et al: Altered response to meta-chlorophenylpiperazine in anorexia nervosa: support for a persistent alteration of serotonin activity after short-term weight restoration. Int J Eat Disord 30:57–68, 2001

Franko DL, Keel PK, Dorer DJ, et al: What predicts suicide attempts in women with eating disorders? Psychol Med 34:843–853, 2004

Garfinkel PE, Garner DM, Goldbloom DS: Eating disorders: implications for the 1990s. Can J Psychiatry 32:624–630, 1987

Garner DM: Pathogenesis of anorexia nervosa. Lancet 341:1631–1635, 1993

Geist R, Heinmaa M, Stephens D, et al: Comparison of family therapy and family group psychoeducation in adolescents with anorexia nervosa. Can J Psychiatry 45:173–178, 2000

Gilligan C: In a Different Voice: Psychological Theory and Women's Development. Cambridge, MA, Harvard University Press, 1982

Golden NH, Kreitzer P, Jacobson MS, et al: Disturbances in growth hormone secretion and action in adolescents with anorexia nervosa. J Pediatr 125:655–660, 1994

Gordon C, Beresin E, Herzog DB: The parent's relationship and the child's illness in anorexia nervosa. J Am Acad Psychoanal 17:29–42, 1989

Gottdiener JS, Gross HA, Henry WL, et al: Effects of self-induced starvation on cardiac size and function in anorexia nervosa. Circulation 58:426–433, 1978

Grice DE, Halmi KA, Fichter MM, et al: Evidence for a susceptibility gene for anorexia nervosa on chromosome 1. Am J Hum Genet 70:787–792, 2002

Grill HJ: Introduction: physiological mechanisms in conditioned taste aversions. Ann N Y Acad Sci 443:67–88, 1985

Grinspoon S, Baum H, Lee K, et al: Effects of short-term recombinant human insulin-like growth factor 1 administration on bone turnover in osteopenic women with anorexia nervosa. J Clin Endocrinol Metab 81:3864–3870, 1996

Grinspoon S, Thomas E, Pitts S, et al: Prevalence and predictive factors for regional osteopenia in women with anorexia nervosa. Ann Intern Med 133:790–794, 2000

Gwirtsman HE, Guze BH, Yager J, et al: Fluoxetine treatment of anorexia nervosa: an open clinical trial. J Clin Psychiatry 51:378–382, 1990

Haas HL, Clopton JR: Comparing clinical and research treatments for eating disorders. Int J Eat Disord 33:412–420, 2003

Hamburg P, Herzog DB, Brotman AW, et al: The treatment resistant eating disordered patient. Psychiatr Ann 19:494–499, 1989

Herzog DB, Borus JF, Hamburg P, et al: Substance abuse, eating behaviors, and social impairment of medical students. J Med Educ 62:651–657, 1987a

Herzog DB, Hamburg P, Brotman AW: Psychotherapy and eating disorders: an affirmative view. Int J Eat Disord 6:545–550, 1987b

Herzog DB, Keller MB, Lavori PW: Outcome in anorexia nervosa and bulimia nervosa: a review of the literature. J Nerv Ment Dis 176:131–143, 1988

Herzog W, Deter HC, Fiehn W, et al: Medical findings and predictors of long-term physical outcome in anorexia nervosa: a prospective 12-year follow-up study. Psychol Med 27:269–279, 1997

Herzog DB, Dorer DJ, Keel PK, et al: Recovery and relapse in anorexia and bulimia nervosa: a 7.5-year follow-up study. J Am Acad Child Adolesc Psychiatry 38:829–837, 1999

Herzog DB, Greenwood DN, Dorer DJ, et al: Mortality in eating disorders: a descriptive study. Int J Eat Disord 28:20–26, 2000

Hoek HW: Distribution of eating disorders, in Eating Disorders and Obesity: A Comprehensive Handbook. Edited by Fairburn CG, Brownell KD. New York, Guilford, 2002, pp 233–237

Hoek HW, van Hoeken D: Review of the prevalence and incidence of eating disorders. Int J Eat Disord 34:383-396, 2003

Hsu LK: Psychopharmacology in anorexia nervosa. Symposium presented at the annual meeting of the American Psychiatric Association, Miami, FL, May 1995

Humphrey LL: Observed family interactions among subtypes of eating disorders using structural analysis of social behavior. J Consult Clin Psychol 57:206–214, 1989

Ivarsson T, Rastam M, Wentz E, et al: Depressive disorders in teenage-onset anorexia nervosa: a controlled longitudinal partly community-based study. Compr Psychiatry 41:398–403, 2000

Jagielska G, Wolanczyk T, Komender J, et al: Bone mineral content and bone mineral density in adolescent girls with anorexia nervosa: a longitudinal study. Acta Psychiatr Scand 104:131–137, 2001

Johnson GL, Humphries LL, Shirley PB, et al: Mitral valve prolapse in patients with anorexia nervosa and bulimia. Arch Intern Med 146:1525–1529, 1986

Karwautz A, Rabe-Hesketh S, Collier DA: Premorbid psychiatric morbidity, comorbidity, and personality in patients with anorexia nervosa compared to their healthy sisters. Eur Eat Disord Rev 10:255–270, 2002

Kassett JA, Gwirtsman HE, Kaye WH, et al: Pattern of onset of bulimic symptoms in anorexia nervosa. Am J Psychiatry 145:1287–1288, 1988

Katzman DK, Lambe EK, Mikulis DJ, et al: Cerebral gray matter and white matter volume deficits in adolescent girls with anorexia nervosa. J Pediatr 129:794–803, 1996

Katzman DK, Zipursky RB, Lambe EK, et al: A longitudinal magnetic resonance imaging study of brain changes in adolescents with anorexia nervosa. Arch Pediatr Adolesc Med 151:793–797, 1997

Kaye WH: Anorexia nervosa, obsessional behavior, and serotonin. Psychopharmacol Bull 33:335–344, 1997

Kaye WH, Berrettini W, Gwirtzman H, et al: Altered cerebrospinal neuropeptide Y and peptide YY immunoreactivity in anorexia and bulimia nervosa. Arch Gen Psychiatry 47:548–556, 1990

Kaye WH, Weltzin TE, Hsu LK, et al: An open trial of fluoxetine in patients with anorexia nervosa. J Clin Psychiatry 52:464–471, 1991

Kaye WH, Nagata T, Weltzin TE, et al: Double-blind placebo-controlled administration of fluoxetine in restricting- and restricting-purging-type anorexia nervosa. Biol Psychiatry 49:644–652, 2001

Keel PK, Mitchell JE: Outcome in bulimia nervosa. Am J Psychiatry 154:313–321, 1997

Kendler KS, MacLean C, Neale M, et al: The genetic epidemiology of bulimia nervosa. Am J Psychiatry 148:1627–1637, 1991

Kernberg O: Borderline Conditions and Pathological Narcissism. Northvale, NJ, Jason Aronson, 1975

Klerman GL, Weissman MM, Rounsaville BJ, et al: Interpersonal Psychotherapy of Depression. New York, Basic Books, 1984

Klump KL, Bulik CM, Pollice C, et al: Temperament and character in women with anorexia nervosa. J Nerv Ment Dis 188:559–567, 2000

Klump KL, Miller KB, Keel PK, et al: Genetic and environmental influences on anorexia nervosa syndromes in a population-based twin sample. Psychol Med 31:737–740, 2001

Kotler LA, Devlin MJ, Davies M, et al: An open trial of fluoxetine for adolescents with bulimia nervosa. J Child Adolesc Psychopharmacol 13:329–335, 2003

Kreipe RE, Harris JP: Myocardial impairment resulting from eating disorders. Pediatric Annals 21:760–768, 1992

Laessle RG, Waadt S, Pirke KM: A structured behaviorally oriented group treatment for bulimia nervosa. Psychother Psychosom 48:141–145, 1987

Lambe EK, Katzman DK, Mikulis DJ, et al: Cerebral gray matter volume deficits after weight recovery from anorexia nervosa. Arch Gen Psychiatry 54:537–542, 1997

Lasater LM, Mehler PS: Medical complications of bulimia nervosa. Eat Behav 2:279–292, 2001

Latzer Y, Hochdorf Z, Bachar E: Attachment style and family functioning as discriminating factors in eating disorders. Contemporary Family Therapy: An International Journal 24:581–599, 2002

Le Grange D, Eisler I, Dare C, et al: Evaluation of family treatments in adolescent anorexia nervosa—a pilot study. Int J Eat Disord 12:347–357, 1992

Le Grange D, Lock J, Dymek M: Family-based therapy for adolescents with bulimia nervosa. Am J Psychother 57:237–251, 2003

Lock J: Treating adolescents with eating disorders in the family context. Empirical and theoretical considerations. Child Adolesc Psychiatr Clin North Am 11:331–342, 2002

Lock J, Le Grange D: Can family-based treatment of anorexia nervosa be manualized? J Psychother Pract Res 10:253–261, 2001

Lock J, Le Grange D, Agras WS, et al: Treatment Manual for Anorexia Nervosa: A Family-Based Approach. New York, Guilford, 2001

Lowe B, Zipfel S, Buchholz C, et al: Long-term outcome of anorexia nervosa in a prospective 21-year follow-up study. Psychol Med 31:881–890, 2001

Maloney M, Klykylo WM: An overview of anorexia nervosa, bulimia, and obesity in children and adolescents. J Am Acad Child Psychiatry 22:99–107, 1983

Maloney M, McGuire J, Daniels SR, et al: Dieting behavior and eating attitudes in children. Pediatrics 84:482–489, 1989

Mandel L, Kaynar A: Bulimia and parotid swelling: a review and case report. J Oral Maxillofac Surg 50:1122–1125, 1992

McElroy SL, Hudson JI, Malhotra S, et al: Citalopram in the treatment of binge-eating disorder: a placebo-controlled trial. J Clin Psychiatry 64:807–813, 2003

Mehler PS, Andersen AE: Eating Disorders: A Guide to Medical Care and Complications. Baltimore, MD, Johns Hopkins University Press, 1999

Minuchin S: Family Kaleidoscope. Cambridge, MA, Harvard University Press, 1984

Minuchin S, Rosman BL, Baker L: Psychosomatic Families: Anorexia Nervosa in Context. Cambridge, MA, Harvard University Press, 1978

Misra M, Aggarwal A, Miller KK, et al: Effects of anorexia nervosa on clinical, hematologic, biochemical, and bone density parameters in community-dwelling adolescent girls. Pediatrics 114:1574–1583, 2004

Mitchell JE, deZwaan M: Pharmacological treatments of binge eating, in Binge Eating: Nature, Assessment, and Treatment. Edited by Fairburn CG, Wilson CT. New York, Guilford, 1993, pp 250–269

Mitchell JE, Specker SM, de Zwaan M: Comorbidity and medical complications of bulimia nervosa. J Clin Psychiatry 52 (suppl):13–20, 1991

Nakash-Eisikovits O, Dierberger A, Westen D: A multidimensional meta-analysis of pharmacotherapy for bulimia nervosa: summarizing the range of outcomes in controlled clinical trials. Harv Rev Psychiatry 10:193–211, 2002

Neumark-Sztainer D, Story M, Resnick MD, et al: Body dissatisfaction and unhealthy weight-control practices among adolescents with and without chronic illness: a population-based study. Arch Pediatr Adolesc Med 149:1330–1335, 1995

O'Connor P, Lewis R, Kirchner E, et al: Eating disorder symptoms in former female college gymnasts: Relations with body compositions. Am J Clin Nutr 64:840–843, 1996

Panagiotopoulos C, McCrindle BW, Hick K, et al: Electrocardiographic findings in adolescents with eating disorders. Pediatrics 105:1100–1105, 2000

Patton GC, Selzer R, Coffey C, et al: Onset of eating disorders: population based cohort over 3 years. BMJ 318:765–768, 1999

Piazza E, Carni JD, Kelly J, et al: Group psychotherapy for anorexia nervosa. J Am Acad Child Psychiatry 22:276–278, 1983

Polivy J, Herman CP: Etiology of binge eating: psychological mechanisms, in Binge Eating: Nature, Assessment, and Treatment. Edited by Fairburn CG, Wilson GT. New York, Guilford, 1993, pp 173–205

Powers PS, Santana C: Available pharmacological treatments for anorexia nervosa. Expert Opin Pharmacother 5:2287–2292, 2004

Pyle RL, Mitchell JE: The prevalence of bulimia in selected samples. Adolesc Psychiatry 13:241–252, 1986

Robin AL, Siegel PT, Koepke T, et al: Family therapy versus individual therapy for adolescent females with anorexia nervosa. J Dev Behav Ped 15:111–116, 1994

Robin AL, Siegel PT, Moye AW, et al: A controlled comparison of family versus individual therapy for adolescents with anorexia nervosa. J Am Acad Child Adolesc Psychiatry 38:1482–1489, 1999

Rodin G: Eating disorders in diabetes mellitus, in Eating Disorders and Obesity: A Comprehensive Handbook, 2nd Edition. Edited by Brownell KD, Fairburn CG. New York, Guilford, 2002, pp 286–292

Rodin G, Daneman D: Eating disorders and IDDM: a problematic association. Diabetes Care 15:1402–1412, 1992

Rogers L, Resnick MD, Mitchell JE, et al: The relationship between socioeconomic status and eating-disordered behaviors in a community sample of adolescent girls. Int J Eat Disord 22:15–23, 1997

Rollins N, Piazza E: Anorexia nervosa: a quantitative approach to follow-up. J Am Acad Child Adolesc Psychiatry 20:167–183, 1981

Rome ES, Ammerman S: Medical complications of eating disorders: an update. J Adolesc Health 33:418–426, 2003

Rome ES, Ammerman S, Rosen DS, et al: Children and adolescents with eating disorders: the state of the art. Pediatrics 111:98–108, 2003

Rossiter EM, Agras WS: An empirical test of DSM-III-R definition of a binge. Int J Eat Disord 9:513–518, 1990

Russell CJ, Keel PK: Homosexuality as a specific risk factor for eating disorders in men. Int J Eat Disord 31:300–306, 2002

Russell GFM, Szmukler GI, Dare C, et al: An evaluation of family therapy in anorexia nervosa and bulimia nervosa. Arch Gen Psychiatry 44:1047–1056, 1987

Russell GFM: Anorexia and bulimia nervosa, in Child and Adolescent Psychiatry: Modern Approaches. Edited by Rutter M, Hersor L. Oxford, UK, Blackwell Scientific, 1985, pp 625–637

Russell GFM: Bulimia nervosa: an ominous variant of anorexia nervosa. Psychol Med 9:429–448, 1979

Selvini-Palazzoli M: Self-Starvation: From Individual to Family Therapy in the Treatment of Anorexia Nervosa. Northvale, NJ, Jason Aronson, 1978

Silber TJ, Shaer C, Atkins D: Eating disorders in adolescents and young women with spina bifida. Int J Eat Disord 25:457–461, 1999

Soyka LA, Grinspoon S, Levitsky LL, et al: The effects of anorexia nervosa on bone metabolism in female adolescents. J Clin Endocrinol Metab 84:4489–4496, 1999

Spigset O: Oral symptoms in bulimia nervosa. A survey of 34 cases. Acta Odontol Scand 49:335–339, 1991

Steinhausen HC: The outcome of anorexia nervosa in the 20th century. Am J Psychiatry 159:1284–1293, 2002

Stice E: Risk and maintenance factors for eating pathology: a meta-analytic review. Psychological Bulletin 128:825–848, 2002

Stoving RK, Hangaard J, Hansen-Nord M, et al: A review of endocrine changes in anorexia nervosa. J Psychiatr Res 33:139–152, 1999

Striegel-Moore RH, Leslie D, Petrill SA, et al: One-year use and cost of inpatient and outpatient services among female and male patients with an eating disorder: evidence from a national database of health insurance claims. Int J Eat Disord 27:381–389, 2000

Striegel-Moore RH, Dohm FA, Kraemer HC, et al: Eating disorders in white and black women. Am J Psychiatry 160:1326–1331, 2003

Strober M: Personality and symptomatological features in young, nonchronic anorexia nervosa patients. J Psychosom Res 24:353–359, 1980

Strober M: Family genetic perspectives on anorexia nervosa and bulimia nervosa, in Eating Disorders and Obesity: A Comprehensive Handbook. Edited by Brownell KD, Fairburn CG. New York, Guilford, 1995, pp 212–218

Strober M: Managing the chronic, treatment-resistant patient with anorexia nervosa. Int J Eat Disord 36:245–255, 2004

Strober M, Lampert C, Morrell W, et al: A controlled family study of anorexia nervosa: evidence of familial aggregation and lack of shared transmission with affective disorders. Int J Eat Disord 9:239–253, 1990

Strober M, Pataki C, Freeman R, et al: No effect if adjunctive fluoxetine on eating behavior or weight phobia during the inpatient treatment of anorexia nervosa: an historical case-control study. J Child Adolesc Psychopharmacol 9:195–201, 1999

Sunday SR, Einhorn A, Halmi KA: Relationship of perceived macronutrient and caloric content to affective conditions about food in eating-disordered, restrained, and unrestrained subjects. Am J Clin Nutr 55:362–371, 1992

Sundgot-Borgen J, Torstveit MK: Prevalence of eating disorders in elite athletes is higher than in the general population. Clin J Sport Med 14:25–32, 2004

Thompson-Brenner H, Glass S, Westen D: A multidimensional meta-analysis of psychotherapy for bulimia nervosa. Clinical Psychology: Science & Practice 10: 269–287, 2003

Thompson-Brenner H, Westen D: A naturalistic study of psychotherapy for bulimia nervosa, part 1: comorbidity and therapeutic outcome. J Nerv Ment Dis 193:573–584, 2005a

Thompson-Brenner H, Westen D: A naturalistic study of psychotherapy for bulimia nervosa, part 2: therapeutic interventions in the community. J Nerv Ment Dis 193:585–595, 2005b

Turner JM, Bulsara MK, McDermott BM, et al: Predictors of low bone density in young adolescent females with anorexia nervosa and other dieting disorders. Int J Eating Disord 30:245–251, 2001

Vitousek K, Manke F: Personality variables and disorders in anorexia nervosa and bulimia nervosa. J Abnorm Psychol 103:137–147, 1994

Wade TD, Bulik CM, Neale M, et al: Anorexia nervosa and major depression: an examination of shared genetic and environmental risk factors. Am J Psychiatry 157:469–471, 2000

Walsh BT, Hadigan CM, Devlin MJ, et al: Long-term outcome of antidepressant treatment for bulimia nervosa. Am J Psychiatry 148: 1206–1212, 1991

Westen D, Harnden-Fischer J: Personality profiles in eating disorders: rethinking the distinction between Axis I and Axis II. Am J Psychiatry 158:547–562, 2001

Wilson GT, Fairburn CC, Agras WS, et al: Cognitive-behavioral therapy for bulimia nervosa: time course and mechanisms of change. J Consult Clin Psychol 70:267274, 2002

Woodside DB, Shekter-Wolfson LF, Garfinkel PE, et al: Family functioning in anxiety and eating disorders—a comparative study. Compr Psychiatry 37:139–143, 1996a

Woodside DB, Swinson RP, Kuch K, et al: Long-term follow-up of patient-reported family functioning in eating disorders after intensive day hospital treatment. J Psychosom Res 41:269–277, 1996b

Zhu AJ, Walsh BT: Pharmacological treatment of eating disorders. Can J Psychiatry 47:227–234, 2002

Self-Assessment Questions

Select the single best response for each question.

24.1 The DSM-IV-TR (American Psychiatric Association 2000) diagnostic criteria for anorexia nervosa include which of the following?

A. Body weight less than 50% of that expected.
B. Body height less than 85% of that expected.
C. Apathy to weight change.
D. Amenorrhea in postmenarcheal females.
E. Loss of interest in body habitus.

24.2 Common signs and symptoms associated with anorexia nervosa include which of the following?

A. Heat intolerance.
B. Tachycardia.
C. Diarrhea.
D. Breast engorgement.
E. Growth of lanugo hair.

24.3 Which of the following medical complications is *not* routinely associated with anorexia nervosa?

A. Arrhythmias.
B. Leukopenia.
C. Neurological abnormalities.
D. Decreased gastric motility.
E. Decreased bone mineral density.

24.4 Which of the following statements regarding the use of pharmacotherapy in the treatment of anorexia nervosa is *true*?

A. Medication has no adjunctive role.
B. Multiple psychotropic medications have been shown to effectively reverse the disorder.
C. Clomipramine and lithium have shown positive effects in clinical studies.
D. Fluoxetine may have a role in maintaining weight in weight-recovered anorexia patients.
E. Pharmacotherapy has been shown to be superior to combined medication–psychotherapy treatment in several studies.

24.5 DSM-IV-TR (American Psychiatric Association 2000) diagnostic criteria for bulimia nervosa include all of the following *except*

   A. The individual engages in recurrent episodes of binge eating.
   B. The individual engages in recurrent inappropriate compensatory behavior to prevent weight gain.
   C. Binge eating and inappropriate compensatory behaviors both occur, on average, at least weekly for 6 months.
   D. Self-evaluation is unduly influenced by body shape and weight.
   E. The disturbance does not occur exclusively during episodes of anorexia nervosa.

24.6 Compared with normal-weight individuals, persons with bulimia nervosa demonstrate elevations of which of the following neuropeptides and hormones?

   A. Neuropeptide Y.
   B. Cholecystokinin.
   C. Leptin.
   D. Cortisol.
   E. None of the above.

24.7 Which of the following antidepressants has been studied most extensively in bulimia nervosa and has been shown to be effective in its treatment?

   A. Venlafaxine.
   B. Mirtazapine.
   C. Fluvoxamine.
   D. Bupropion.
   E. Fluoxetine.

Tic Disorders

Robert A. King, M.D.

James F. Leckman, M.D.

Definition

Tics are abrupt, purposeless, recurrent, stereotyped movements or sounds. They are frequently experienced as being involuntary or as occurring in response to an irresistible impulse (Leckman et al. 1999a). Tics can sometimes, with effort, be briefly suppressed or deferred. The frequency of tics can vary over the day in response to changing environmental circumstances. Over the course of weeks to months, a pattern of waxing and waning of tic symptoms is common. Tics may exactly mimic voluntary movements or speech, or they may have an exaggerated or more forceful character.

Simple tics are sudden, brief, meaningless tics occurring singly; in contrast, complex tics involve movements or vocalizations orchestrated into longer or more purposeful-appearing constellations. Common simple motor tics include grimaces, rapid head or limb jerks, shrugs, and abdominal tensing. Among the most common simple vocal tics are sniffs, barks, coughs, guttural throat clearing, and other expiratory vocalizations. Examples of complex motor tics are biting, throwing, hitting, skipping, touching objects or self, dystonic postures, and gestures, which may be obscene (copropraxia) or compulsive imitations (echopraxia). Complex vocal tics range from dysfluencies and aberrations in prosody through formed syllables, words, or phrases; such phrases often take the form of stereotyped ejaculations (e.g., "shut up!," "you bet!"), obscenities (coprolalia), or echoing others (echolalia) or oneself (palilalia).

The intensity, frequency, and diversity of tics cover a wide gamut of severity, ranging from transient simple tics that occur fleetingly in many school-age children to the persistent, variegated multiple vocal and motor tics of Tourette's disorder. In some individuals, tics appear as apparently isolated phenomena. In others, they may be associated with learning difficulties, impulsivity, inattentiveness, emotional lability, or obsessive-compulsive phenomena (King and Scahill 2001).

DSM-IV-TR (American Psychiatric Association 2000) lists three specific disorders—transient tic disorder, chronic motor or vocal tic disorder, and Tourette's disorder, which are distinguished on the basis of frequency, persistence, and variety of tics.

Despite the apparent precision of the DSM-IV-TR frequency and duration criteria, however, it is unclear to what extent they truly demarcate distinctive syndromes with differing etiologies, symptomatic concomitants, or clinical courses rather than points on a spectrum of symptomatic severity in the expression of a common underlying genetic vulnerability.

Clinical Findings

■ Transient Tic Disorder

Transient tics are very common in prepubertal children, with boys being more often affected than girls. The most common transient tics involve the face, head, neck, or arms. Transient vocal tics are much more rare. Transient tics run a waxing and waning course, which is often exacerbated by stress, excitement, or fatigue. Children are often unaware of their tics or may try to rationalize them away (e.g., "I just sniffed because I had a cold"). Indeed, forceful, repetitive blinking, sniffing, or throat clearing often results in visits to the optometrist, allergist, or pediatrician. Transient tics in childhood are by definition time-limited and in most cases are nonimpairing. In the absence of a positive family tic history, however, there are no clear clinical guidelines to predict which mild motor tics of recent onset are likely to remit and which are likely to persist or effloresce. Family studies suggest that in some individuals transient tic disorder represents a mild phenotypical expression of the Tourette's syndrome gene and a marker of genetic risk for that individual's offspring (Kurlan et al. 1988). Whether other forms of transient tics exist that have alternative genetic determinants remains to be determined.

■ Chronic Motor or Vocal Tic Disorder

The most common chronic tics are motor tics, especially those of the face, head, neck, and arms. In evaluating adults with chronic tics, a careful history often reveals that the tics have been present since childhood; in retrospect, some such individuals may have met the criteria for Tourette's disorder as children, but now manifest only either chronic motor or vocal tics as a residual condition.

■ Tourette's Syndrome (Chronic Motor and Phonic Tic Disorder)

Chronic motor and phonic tic disorder was first described in 1885 by Georges Gilles de la Tourette, who described what he considered its cardinal features: convulsive muscular jerks, inarticulate shouts, and coprolalia. He also noted that individual symptoms waxed and waned and that, although some patients' tic symptoms worsened over time, there was no general mental deterioration.

The initial symptoms of Tourette's syndrome most frequently appear between ages 5 and 8 years. Initially, they may resemble the transient motor tics of childhood in that they are often mild and transient and involve the face, head, or upper extremities. With time, however, the tics become persistent and increase in diversity and distribution, often progressing from the upper parts of the body to involve the trunk and legs (rostral-caudal progression). Initially most motor tics are simple ones (e.g., blinks, arm or head jerks, grimaces), but with time more complex motor tics such as biting, clapping, touching, or orchestrated simultaneous multiple movements may appear as well.

The onset of motor tics usually precedes that of vocal tics. However, in some cases simple vocal tics such as sniffing or compulsive throat clearing may be the first symptoms. Initial vocal tics are most often simple and include sniffing, chirps, throat clearing, grunts, coughs, or squeaks. Later, vocal tics may increase in complexity, with inappropriate blurting out of formed syllables, words, and phrases or compulsive repetition of either the patient's own utterances (palilalia) or those of others (echolalia). Speech fluency and prosody may be paroxysmally altered. Despite its traditional association with Tourette's syndrome, coprolalia does not usually appear until around puberty and occurs in fewer than one-third of cases.

The variety and temporal patterning of tics is virtually limitless (Leckman et al. 1999a). Individual tics may wax and wane over weeks or months; they may even disappear, only to be replaced in time by others. Tics may occur singly or as part of complex combinations of motor and vocal tics involving many parts of the body. Frequency may range from isolated occurrences a few times a week to bouts that last for hours and leave the patient frightened and exhausted. The intensity of tics may vary from those so minimal that only the patient is aware of them to explosive outbursts that resound throughout the house or result in physical damage to the self or to surroundings.

Children may be unaware of or may deny or minimize their symptoms. Efforts may be made to camouflage the tic-like nature of a gesture or to substitute a less objectionable exclamation for an offensive one. Patients may be able to suppress tics more or less successfully for a period of time (e.g., in church or while performing) but then experience a paroxysm of tics once they relax their guard. As a result, teachers and parents may have divergent impressions of tic severity or be misled into thinking that the tics are voluntary and could be eliminated if only the child would exert more willpower. Tics markedly decrease or disappear during sleep and are exacerbated by stress, excitement, fatigue, and illness (Silva et al. 1995; Surwillo et al. 1978).

Although the course of tics in any individual case is unpredictable, early adolescence is usually the period of greatest severity, with most individuals experiencing a diminution or even disappearance of tics by early adulthood (Leckman et al. 1998). (Comorbid difficulties, however—such as obsessions, compulsions, anxiety, and attention-deficit disorder–like symptoms—may persist unabated.) Most adolescent or adult patients with Tourette's syndrome report that their tics are often preceded by a premonitory sensation or urge to perform the tic (Bliss 1980; Leckman et al. 1993). These bodily urges—often described as an intense urge, pressure, or itch—and the effort necessary to suppress them are often more debilitating and distracting than the tics themselves. Performing the tic, which is experienced as being at least partially voluntary, produces transient relief. Some patients report the need to repeat a complex tic "one more time" or until they have gotten the action "just right" (e.g., complete or symmetrical) (Leckman et al. 1994).

When tic symptoms are prominent, they frequently take a serious toll on children's self-esteem and social confidence. Beyond exposing the child to gibes and reproaches, the tics leave the child feeling out of control of his or her own body and mental processes. The very boundaries of the self and the distinction between what is actively willed versus what is involuntarily experienced are called into question (Cohen 1991).

■ Associated Conditions

Not all of the psychological difficulties of individuals with Tourette's syndrome result from stigma or shame. Impulsivity, distractibility, anxiety proneness, mood lability or depression, and learning difficulties are often associated with the syndrome and may even antedate the onset of tics (King and Scahill 2001). Indeed, for many children these associated symptoms, especially symptoms of attention-deficit/hyperactivity disorder (ADHD), are potentially greater sources of social and functional impairment than are the tics themselves (Stokes et al. 1991).

The increased rates of anxiety seen in individuals with Tourette's syndrome may be a reflection of their increased autonomic reactivity (Chappell et al. 1994). Individuals with Tourette's syndrome also frequently have neuropsychological impairments in fine motor coordination, visuomotor integration, and executive functioning, often manifested in poor handwriting, disorganized papers, and difficulty copying figures and designs (Schultz et al. 1999).

By adulthood, as many as 40% of patients with Tourette's syndrome also meet the criteria for an associated diagnosis of obsessive-compulsive disorder (OCD). Some compulsions—such as tapping, kissing, biting, and sexual touching—may be impossible to distinguish from complex motor tics. Other obsessions and compulsions may range from ordering behaviors (e.g., "evening up") or needing to get an action "just right" through full-blown ego-dystonic obsessions and compulsions (e.g., washing, checking). Careful inquiry often reveals recurrent, intrusive, and unwanted thoughts or images (frequently concerning aggression, sex, or other emotionally charged issues), as well as a relentless preoccupation with resisting compulsive urges. Tic-related OCD appears to differ from cases of OCD without a history of tics in terms of phenomenology, neurobiological features, and treatment response (King et al. 2005; Leckman et al. 1995; Miguel et al. 2001). Compared with non-tic-related OCD, tic-related OCD appears to have a greater male preponderance, earlier onset, and a greater predominance of 1) obsessions and compulsions concerning religion, sex, and aggression; and 2) compulsions involving repeating, counting, ordering, arranging, and symmetry; in addition, tic-related compulsions are more likely to feel driven by "just right" phenomena and urges rather than by anxiety.

Differential Diagnosis

In its fully developed form, with both simple and complex motor and phonic tics present, Tourette's syndrome is easily distinguished from other neurological conditions. However, when motor tics occur in isolation, the differential diagnosis must include other dyskinesias: myoclonus, choreoathetosis, dystonia, akathisia, paroxysmal and tardive dyskinesias, and excessive startle syndromes (Jankovic 2001). The presentation and natural history of the tic disorders are usually sufficiently distinctive to permit diagnosis on clinical grounds without extensive diagnostic tests. Few other conditions show the combination of childhood onset and abrupt but intermittent movements that are temporarily suppressible. The distribution, timing, and kinesthetics of tics usually distinguish them from the unilateral pattern of ballismus; the twisting, frequently sustained movements of dystonia; and the inability to sustain contractions that characterizes chorea.

Clinical context is also a helpful guide. For example, acute and tardive akathisia and dyskinesias are usually associated with starting or stopping neuroleptic medication. Chorea often occurs in the context of a genetic or metabolic disorder (e.g., Wilson's disease or Huntington's chorea) or, in the case of Sydenham's chorea, a poststreptococcal autoimmune reaction.

Children with OCD may sometimes have to touch, tap, blink, or look in certain compulsive patterns, but these movements are usually deliberate and associated with specific ideation or situations and with an absence of sporadic, random tics. Psychogenic tics (conversion disorder) usually lack the characteristic pattern of early simple tics that wax and wane over time. Stereotypies are repetitive behaviors most often found in children with pervasive developmental disorders or other poorly relating children (Rapin 2001) (although they may also occur occasionally in children with good social relating); in contrast to the multiplicity of waxing and waning tics seen in Tourette's syndrome, stereotypies typically remain unchanged over years or months and appear to be soothing or pleasurable, rather than intrusive or distressing. Children with frequent cursing sometimes raise the question of coprolalia; it is rare, however, to see tic-related coprolalia without a plethora of simple motor or vocal tics. Although coprolalia may occur in the context of anger or upset, it is most distinctive in contexts where there is no apparent motivation to curse.

Epidemiology

Tics are common among school-age children, with as many as 18% of boys and 11% of girls found to have "tics" (Scahill et al. 2001b; Snider et al. 2002).

At one time, Tourette's syndrome was considered extremely rare. Whereas with greater awareness, many more cases now come to clinical attention, it has also become clear that there exist many mild, undiagnosed cases. Most population-based surveys yield prevalence estimates of Tourette's syndrome in the range of 5–10 per 10,000, with children being more likely to be identified than adults and males more commonly affected than females (Scahill et al. 2001b); a few studies have found substantially higher rates when school-based observational techniques are used (Mason et al. 1998).

One longitudinal study (Peterson et al. 2001a) assessed the presence of tics, OCD, ADHD, and other comorbid disorders in an epidemiological sample of children at four time points beginning in childhood and continuing into early adulthood. When the subjects were seen at age 1–10 years, the prevalence of tics was 17.7%; in adolescence the rate of tics in the same children was 2%–3%, suggesting that most childhood tics remit by adolescence. Childhood tics were associated with increased rates in adolescence of OCD and other anxiety symptoms. Adolescents with tics were more likely to have or develop OCD, depressive symptoms, and conduct disorder. In young adolescents with tics, the presence of comorbid ADHD predicted the persistence of tics into later adolescence; the presence of comorbid OCD and phobias predicted persistence of tics into early adulthood. However, tics were not significantly associated with ADHD either cross-sectionally or prospectively.

Etiology

Tourette's syndrome provides a paradigm for other childhood-onset neuropsychiatric disorders: an apparent genetically determined vulnerability, age-dependent expression of symptoms reflecting maturational factors, sexual dimorphism, stress-dependent fluctuations in symptom severity, and apparent environmental influences on the phenotypical expression of the underlying genotype (Leckman and Cohen 1999).

■ Genetic Factors

Monozygotic twin pairs show a markedly higher concordance rate for Tourette's syndrome (53%) than do dizygotic twins (only 8%); if concordance is measured by the broader criteria of the presence of any tics in the co-twin, the monozygotic concordance rate increases to 77% versus 23% for dizygotic twin pairs (Price et al. 1985). These figures suggest a strong genetic factor in Tourette's syndrome as well as a common genetic determinant for both Tourette's syndrome and milder tic symptoms. The existence of monozygotic pairs discordant for the presence of tics or tic severity, however, also suggests that nongenetic factors play a role in determining the phenotypical expression of the presumed genetic vulnerability to Tourette's syndrome.

Family studies indicate that at least 60% of cases of Tourette's syndrome are familial. However, these same studies suggest that what is transmitted in the families of probands with Tourette's syndrome is not simply vulnerability to Tourette's syndrome per se but rather vulnerability to a broad range of tic or obsessive-compulsive symptoms. Thus, the phenotypical expression of the presumed Tourette's syndrome genotype is highly variable, with the inherited diathesis manifesting itself in the form of either tics or obsessive-compulsive symptoms of varying severity. Gender-related, stress-related, and other as yet poorly understood factors appear to modify the form and severity of phenotypical expression.

Although some family data are consistent with a single autosomal locus, other polygenic models may need to be considered. For example, whereas a single locus may confer vulnerability to tic-spectrum disorders, other loci may help determine the severity or phenotypical presentation (Pauls et al. 1999).

The family data also point to common genetic factors at work in both tic disorders and some cases of OCD (Pauls et al. 1995, 1999). As previously noted, OCD is a common associated diagnosis in patients with Tourette's syndrome. Furthermore, first-degree relatives of patients with Tourette's syndrome have an increased prevalence of OCD that may occur unaccompanied by any tic symptoms. This increased risk of OCD among first-degree relatives is unaffected by whether the probands have both Tourette's syndrome and obsessive-compulsive disorder or Tourette's syndrome alone. This suggests that the OCD seen in such families represents an alternative phenotypical expression of the Tourette's syndrome gene.

The Tourette Syndrome International Consortium for Genetics' (1999) genomewide scans of affected sibling pairs and high-density families have yielded maps of genomic regions of interest; among these are two areas on chromosomes 4q and 8p. A complementary approach of examining rare cases of cytogenetic abnormalities co-segregating with Tourette's syndrome and related disorders has pointed to regions on chromosomes 3p, 7q, 8q, 9p, and 18q (State et al. 2003). Other investigators have identified a promising site located at 11q23.

■ Neuroanatomical Correlates

The basal ganglia and their connections provide the most likely neuroanatomical substrate of Tourette's syndrome (and related obsessive-compulsive phenomena) (Leckman and Riddle 2000; Peterson et al. 1999). With extensive connections to the sensorimotor and associational cortex, the basal ganglia play a crucial role in integrating sensorimotor information and motor control. These structures are functionally organized into multiple parallel cortico-striato-thalamo-cortical circuits that process information associated with the planning and performance of motor routines. It is these neural loops that permit the adaptive formation of habits—acquired semiautomatic routines linking sensory cues and motor actions (Leckman and Riddle 2000). Failure of inhibition in specific subcircuits may produce the premonitory sensations and urges, compulsions, and movements associated with Tourette's syndrome and related forms of OCD (as well as the inattention and impulsivity found in patients with comorbid ADHD).

Leckman and Riddle (2000) proposed that "tics or stereotypies may be best seen as those prewired bits of behavior that are available to be assembled into habits" (p. 350). The relative functional balance between the striosomal and matrix compartments of the striatum may determine the vulnerability to tic-like dopamine-mediated stereotypies; these two compartments receive their respective inputs from limbic structures and from motor and sensorimotor areas. Dysregulation in the activity of the neurons at the striosomal-matrix boundary could potentially result in the too-ready release of (or failure to inhibit) preformed motor routines in response to external or internal stimuli.

The basal ganglia are rich in dopamine and other neurotransmitters implicated in the pathogenesis of Tourette's syndrome by neuropharmacological evidence. For example, a single photon emission computed tomographic (SPECT) study of monozygotic twins with Tourette's syndrome revealed increased dopamine receptor availability in the caudate nuclei of the more severely affected co-twins (Wolf et al. 1996). (Postmortem studies of Tourette's syndrome patients also suggest altered neurotransmitter levels in the basal ganglia [Anderson et al. 1999].)

Both adults and children with Tourette's syndrome have smaller mean caudate and lenticular volumes (Peterson et al. 2003), with decreased lenticular volume associated with the presence of comorbid OCD and the persistence of tic symptoms into adulthood (Bloch et al. 2005). In addition to basal ganglia abnormalities, subjects with Tourette's syndrome also have altered regional cortical volumes, some of which are associated with greater worst-ever tic severity, suggesting decreased inhibitory reserves available to help suppress tic impulses (Peterson et al. 2001b). Functional magnetic resonance imaging studies of Tourette's syndrome subjects during voluntary tic suppression reveal activation of the ventral prefrontal cortex and caudate nucleus associated with bilateral deactivation of the putamen and globus pallidus, which are likely substrates for the generation of tic activity (Peterson et al. 1998).

Deficits in intracortical inhibition are seen in the decreased duration in adults with Tourette's syndrome (relative to control subjects with no tic disorder) of the usual silencing of spontaneous cortical discharge produced by transcranial magnetic stimulation over the motor cortex (Ziemann et al. 1997).

■ Neurochemical Correlates

One line of research into the pathogenesis of tic disorders concerns possible defects in neurotransmitter or neuromodulator regulation, especially in systems located in the basal ganglia and related brain structures (Anderson et al. 1999).

Support for the role of altered dopaminergic functioning in Tourette's syndrome comes from the clinical observation that neuroleptics, which preferentially block central dopaminergic receptors, are clinically useful in partially suppressing tics. In contrast, dopaminergic agonists such as dextroamphetamine, methylphenidate, and cocaine frequently exacerbate tics.

A preliminary SPECT study of unmedicated adults with Tourette's syndrome found a significantly increased density of striatal presynaptic dopamine uptake sites in the basal ganglia (Malison et al. 1995).

A possible modulating role for the

noradrenergic system in the course of Tourette's syndrome is suggested by the observations that stress exacerbates many tics (Silva et al. 1995; Surwillo et al. 1978) and that alpha-adrenergic receptor blockers, such as clonidine and guanfacine, may ameliorate some tics, as well as the impulsivity seen in some patients with ADHD (Tourette's Syndrome Study Group 2002). Individuals with Tourette's syndrome show a heightened reactivity of the adrenergic sympathetic system and of the hypothalamic-pituitary-adrenal axis in response to stress (Chappell et al. 1994). This apparent increase in noradrenergic response to stress may help account for the exacerbation of tics in response to stress.

■ Perinatal Factors

The lack of complete concordance for tics among monozygotic twins indicates nongenetic influences on the phenotypical expression of the Tourette's syndrome gene. Among monozygotic twin pairs discordant for Tourette's syndrome, the twin who subsequently develops tics appears to be usually the twin with the lower birth weight (Leckman et al. 1990). Furthermore, SPECT studies show that monozygotic co-twins with more severe tics have greater numbers of dopamine receptor sites in the caudate nucleus (Wolf et al. 1996). Stressful maternal life circumstances during pregnancy and the severity of first-trimester nausea and vomiting appear to be risk factors for the later development of tic disorder (Leckman et al. 1990). Such perinatal stressors have been shown to produce enduring heightened neurobiological responsivity to stress.

Gender-specific prenatal hormonal factors may also account for some of the sexually dimorphic aspects of the phenotypical expression of the putative Tou-

rette's syndrome gene, such as its apparently greater penetrance in males. Prenatal androgen levels are known to have dramatic and permanent effects on the functional organization of the developing nervous system, and it is therefore possible that androgens or other gender-related factors favoring symptomatic expression of the Tourette's syndrome gene exert their effects prenatally on the developing male nervous system (Peterson et al. 1995).

■ Autoimmune Factors

A potentially important biological subtype of tic disorder has been proposed by Swedo et al. (1998), who have suggested that aberrant autoimmune mechanisms triggered by group A beta-hemolytic streptococcal infection may produce a spectrum of disorders including tics and OCD; they have termed this putative group of disorders *pediatric autoimmune neuropsychiatric disorders associated with streptococcal infection* (PANDAS) (see also Chapter 18, "Obsessive-Compulsive Disorder," in this volume). Sydenham's chorea (St. Vitus' dance), now recognized as a late sequela of rheumatic fever, is often accompanied by the appearance of tics, mood changes, OCD, ADHD, and anxiety (Mercadante et al. 2001; Swedo et al. 1993). Swedo et al. described a series of children in whom exacerbations of OCD or tics were accompanied by positive streptococcal throat cultures and increased antistreptococcal and antineuronal antibodies without any evidence of rheumatic fever. This clinical syndrome appears to be characterized by sudden onset of symptoms, episodic course, and abrupt symptom exacerbations, which may also be accompanied by adventitious movements.

After the observations of Kiessling et al. (1993) and Swedo et al. (1994), other studies noted the presence of antineuronal or antinuclear antibodies in patients with Tourette's syndrome or OCD (see Singer and Loiselle 2003). Given the existence of genetic vulnerability factors for rheumatic fever and other autoimmune disorders, it will be important to determine whether genetic factors also play a role in possible autoimmune or streptococcal-related forms of tics.

The existence of autoimmune or streptococcal-related forms of tic disorder may have important clinical and preventive implications. In a systematic treatment trial in a series of children meeting the criteria for PANDAS, plasmapheresis or intravenous immunoglobulin infusion produced a dramatic improvement, sustained for up to a year, that was significantly superior to placebo infusion (Perlmutter et al. 1999). Because promiscuous use of antibiotics carries its own individual and public health risks, antibiotic prophylaxis should be reserved only for cases with well-documented recurrent streptococcal-linked exacerbations (Garvey et al. 1999). At present, it seems prudent to maintain a readiness to culture children with Tourette's syndrome or OCD who complain of sore throat or who have been exposed to streptococcus.

Because streptococcal infections, tics, and obsessive-compulsive symptoms are all common in the school-age population, further research is needed to refine the identification of cases where there is a true causal link and to clarify the pathophysiological mechanisms involved (Kurlan and Kaplan 2004; Mercadante et al. 2001; Singer and Loiselle 2003).

Treatment

Treatment must begin with a careful, comprehensive evaluation of the patient's psychological, social, and educational or vocational adjustment. The diagnosis of an identifiable tic disorder does not obviate the need for a thorough medical, developmental, family, and psychosocial history and assessment. The impact of the symptoms on the patient's self-concept, family and peer relations, and classroom participation must be assessed in the context of the patient's and family's overall strengths and weaknesses (Leckman et al. 1999b).

Structured instruments, such as the Yale Global Tic Severity Scale, are helpful in collecting standardized symptom data and provide useful baseline information for any therapeutic intervention (Scahill et al. 1999). The challenges facing patients with tic disorders (and their families) vary with the changing manifestations of the disorder and the vicissitudes of normal development. Because chronic tic disorder and Tourette's syndrome are chronic conditions, the ongoing availability of a supportive clinician is an invaluable asset for both patient and family in anticipating and dealing with difficulties (King et al. 1999; Leckman et al. 1999b).

■ Supportive, Educational, and Psychotherapeutic Interventions

Education about the nature and course of tic disorders can help relieve some of the worries and mistaken impressions families have concerning Tourette's syndrome. It is essential, however, to learn what meanings the symptoms and diagnosis carry for the patient and family. Helping the child, parents, and school understand the child's symptoms as manifestations of a neuropsychiatric disorder can help "decriminalize" symptoms previously regarded as willful, provocative, or crazy. Parents are usually relieved to learn that, in contrast to the extreme picture often presented in the lay press, most cases are not relentlessly progressive and improve by adulthood.

Collaboration with the school is important in obtaining appropriate special educational services and gaining teachers' support in dealing with peer ostracism or teasing.

Chronic tic disorders are not *caused* by psychological factors. However, symptoms are often exacerbated by stress or emotional arousal, and in turn, the tic disorders are themselves the source of considerable psychosocial difficulty. Thus, although psychotherapy will not eliminate chronic tics, it may nonetheless play an important role in reducing stress, addressing low self-esteem, and ameliorating family or internal conflicts that relate to the tics.

Cognitive-behavioral interventions such as exposure and response prevention may be useful for obsessive-compulsive symptoms associated with Tourette's syndrome, although tic-related compulsions that are driven by "just right" phenomena and premonitory urges, rather than by anxiety, may benefit more from a habit-reversal approach (King et al. 1999). Habit-reversal techniques have also been successfully employed with tics (Piacentini and Chang 2001).

The Tourette Syndrome Association can provide educational materials, advocacy resources, and supportive contact with other families with Tourette's syndrome.

■ Pharmacological Treatment

Medication is indicated in tic disorder only when potential benefits appear to outweigh potential side effects. For a detailed review of the pharmacotherapy of tic disorders, see King et al. (2003). The indications and choice of medication will differ depending on whether the target symptoms are the tics themselves or the associated symptoms of inattention, impulsivity, or obsessive-compulsive disor-

der. There is no evidence that medication affects the prognosis or underlying course of the illness.

Physical discomfort, social stigmatization, and interference with classroom participation are all indications for a trial of medication for tics.

Although the most potent tic-suppressing medications are neuroleptics and related dopamine blocking agents (see below), their frequent side effects warrant limiting their use to more severe cases of Tourette's syndrome or to those unresponsive to other medication. A more benign first-choice medication for tics, especially in mild cases, is one of the alpha-adrenergic agents, such as clonidine or guanfacine; although these agents are less potent and less consistently effective than the neuroleptics, they have fewer serious side effects (Leckman et al. 1991; Scahill et al. 2001a; Tourette's Syndrome Study Group 2002). Unlike the neuroleptics, which are usually given in a single bedtime dose to reduce sedation, clonidine or guanfacine must be given in divided doses (usually 3–4 times a day for clonidine, 2–3 times a day for guanfacine) to maintain tic control. Clonidine is best started with a single 0.05-mg dose (0.025 mg for younger children) each morning. If this is tolerated well, additional doses of 0.025–0.05 mg are added at weekly intervals, first at lunch or early afternoon and then after school. If tics are troublesome in the evening, an additional suppertime dose may be added. If necessary, the strength of each dose may be gradually increased in small increments up to a daily total of about 0.3 mg; beyond this level, side effects usually become problematic. (The corresponding starting dose for guanfacine is 0.5 mg, with increases in 0.25-mg increments up to a total of 3 mg, if necessary, in three divided doses.) The response to clonidine or guanfacine is usually gradual, sometimes requiring several weeks to become apparent. Beyond reducing tics, clonidine and guanfacine also frequently have a beneficial effect on the inattentiveness, distractibility, and emotional lability seen in many children with Tourette's syndrome (Leckman et al. 1991; Tourette's Syndrome Study Group 2002); guanfacine appears superior to clonidine in this regard, with less sedation and a longer duration of action (Scahill et al. 2001a).

The principal side effect of clonidine is dose-related sedation, which occurs in about 10%–20% of patients. Other side effects of guanfacine and clonidine include irritability, dry mouth, orthostatic hypotension, and, rarely, cardiac arrhythmias.

The most potent medications for tics are the various neuroleptic drugs. Of these, the typical neuroleptics—haloperidol, fluphenazine, and pimozide, which are relatively specific dopamine type 2 receptor (D_2) antagonists—have been most widely studied and used the longest. About 60%–90% of patients with Tourette's syndrome respond to these medications.

Despite the potency of the neuroleptic drugs, the side effects frequently associated with these agents limit their usefulness. Acute dystonias, akathisia, drowsiness, cognitive blunting, medication-induced dysphoria, or separation anxiety often necessitate reducing or discontinuing these medications or lead to patient noncompliance. The possibility of tardive dyskinesias, especially with the older typical neuroleptics, also makes their long-term use potentially worrisome.

The availability of the newer atypical neuroleptics has provided more acceptable alternatives to the typical neuroleptics. Of these, systematic data support the usefulness of risperidone (Bruggeman et al. 2001; Scahill et al. 2003), olanzapine (Onofrj et al. 2000), and ziprasidone (Sallee et al. 2000) for suppressing tics. The demonstrated lack of efficacy of clozapine is a reminder that not all atypical neuroleptics are effective for tics. Although these agents promise to carry a lower long-term risk of tardive dyskinesias than do the typical neuroleptics, acute dyskinesias, sedation, and dysphoria can occur with the atypical agents as well. Excessive weight gain is especially a problem with risperidone and olanzapine. As with pimozide, ziprasidone may cause cardiac conduction abnormalities (such as prolonged QTc interval); hence, electrocardiographic monitoring before and after initiating medication is desirable, as is caution regarding coadministration of medications (such as macrolide antibiotics) that may interfere with cytochrome metabolism, resulting in potentially fatal drug interactions.

Neuroleptic medication is best initiated at a low dose (e.g., 0.25 mg of haloperidol, 0.5 mg of risperidone, or 1 mg of pimozide), with gradual increments of the same amount every 1–2 weeks if the tic symptoms remain bothersome. Increases and decreases in dosage should be made slowly, because the therapeutic response to medication is often gradual, and rebounds in tic severity after abrupt withdrawal of medication can obscure the underlying course of the symptoms.

Many patients with Tourette's syndrome continue to suffer troublesome tics even on optimal doses of neuroleptic or alpha-adrenergic drugs. Because of the side effects associated with polypharmacy, these individuals pose a difficult therapeutic challenge.

Pergolide is a mixed D_2/D_1 agonist that in lower doses is believed to reduce dopaminergic transmission through its effect on presynaptic D_2 autoreceptors. In a 6-week placebo-controlled crossover study in children, Gilbert and colleagues (2000) found that pergolide (mean dose: 200 micrograms; range: 150–300 micrograms) produced a significant decrease in total tic severity scores relative to placebo. Because of limitations in the study design, however, further studies are needed.

Nicotinergic agents, such as nicotine or mecamylamine, may augment the tic-suppressing effectiveness of neuroleptics, perhaps by prolonged inactivation of ace-tylcholinergic nicotinic receptor subtypes. For example, in several open trials and one placebo-controlled trial (Silver et al. 2001a), application of a transdermal nicotine patch (7 mg/day) for one to several days produced a substantial reduction of tics in patients whose tics were inadequately controlled with an optimal maintenance dose of neuroleptic. (Longer periods of application are undesirable because they may produce nicotine addiction.) Improvement may be maintained for up to a month after a single period of nicotine patch application, but it appears to dissipate over longer periods. Some individuals may experience nausea or vomiting from the nicotine transdermal patch, in some cases severe enough to require its removal.

Studies of mecamylamine (a nicotinergic agent) for the treatment of tics have been difficult to interpret. However, a recent double-blind, placebo-controlled study of mecamylamine, up to 7.5 mg/day, found it to be ineffective as a monotherapy for subjects with Tourette's syndrome (Silver et al. 2001b).

Baclofen, a muscle relaxant that influences gamma-aminobutyric acid neurotransmission, has been studied for the treatment of tics, with equivocal results (Singer et al. 2001).

Injections of diluted botulinum toxin have been studied in patients with Tourette's syndrome (Marras et al. 2001). In most cases, benefit was limited to the anatomical areas injected. The most common side effects were soreness, often bothersome muscle weakness, ptosis, and mild transient dysphagia. Injection appeared to be most effective for eyelid and vocal tics. Direct injection of the vocal cords was reported to be effective in several cases of severe vocal tics, but it also produced the adverse effect of hypophonia (Kwak et al. 2000). These studies thus suggest that botulinum toxin injection may be useful for ameliorating specific severe or impairing tics but do not produce overall improvement of tics at untreated sites. Botulinum toxin treatment also has the disadvantage that injections usually have to be repeated every few weeks.

Apart from the tics themselves, the inattention, distractibility, or obsessions and compulsions that accompany Tourette's syndrome may require pharmacological intervention.

Treatment of ADHD in Individuals With Tourette's Syndrome

The ADHD symptoms that accompany Tourette's syndrome are often more impairing for children than the tics themselves (Stokes et al. 1991). Because stimulants may increase tics (or precipitate de novo tics) in a small number of children, the approach to treating comorbid tics and ADHD has been controversial. Some studies (e.g., Gadow et al. 1995) have found no increase in tics in children with ADHD and tics who were treated with methylphenidate; other trials have found little or no increase in *average* tic scores, but clinically significant increases in a handful of subjects (Gadow et al. 1999; Law and Schachar 1999; Varley et al. 2001).

Alternatives to stimulant medication that have proved useful in controlled trials for the treatment of comorbid ADHD and tics include clonidine (Leckman et al. 1991; Tourette's Syndrome Study Group 2002); guanfacine (Scahill et al. 2001a); and deprenyl (Feigin et al. 1996). Tricyclic antidepressant drugs such as desipramine (Singer et al. 1995) and nortriptyline (Spencer et al. 1993) also appear to be useful, although careful electrocardio-graphic monitoring appears warranted in light of concerns regarding possible arrhythmias and cardiac conduction effects (Riddle et al. 1993). Although in one series of 100 children with tics and comorbid ADHD, atomoxetine did not increase tics (McCracken et al. 2003), cases of atomoxetine-linked tic exacerbation have been reported (Lee et al. 2004).

Our personal preference for the treatment of children with ADHD and moderately severe tics is to first try an alpha-adrenergic agent, preferably guanfacine, because this may be helpful both for tics and for ADHD symptoms. If ADHD symptoms remain impairing, however, a low dose of a stimulant or atomoxetine might be tried next, after appropriate discussion of the potential risks and benefits. A recent randomized study (Tourette's Syndrome Study Group 2002) compared methylphenidate alone, clonidine alone, methylphenidate and clonidine combined, and placebo alone in children with ADHD and tics. Clonidine alone and methylphenidate alone were more effective than placebo in reducing ADHD symptoms, with combined clonidine and methylphenidate producing the greatest benefit; clonidine appeared to be most helpful for impulsivity and hyperactivity, whereas methylphenidate appeared most useful for inattention. The authors concluded that methylphenidate, alone or in combination, did not increase tics over the short-term period of the trial. Although the lack of adverse cardiac effects in this study was reassuring, further studies are warranted in light of the controversy over the safety of such drug combinations (Swanson et al. 1999; Wilens and Spencer 1999).

Treatment of OCD in Individuals With Chronic Tic Disorder

Obsessive-compulsive symptoms plague many patients with Tourette's syndrome, even when their tics have diminished spontaneously or in response to medication treatment. Depending on the type of OCD symptoms experienced, exposure and response-prevention or habit-reversal techniques may be an important component in the treatment of these patients (King et al. 1999, 2005; Piacentini and Chang 2001).

The various selective serotonin reuptake inhibitor (SSRI) medications have been used successfully in children with combined tic disorder and OCD (Riddle et al. 1990; Scahill et al. 1997; Wehr and Namerow 2001). As is true for SSRIs in other children, the SSRIs are generally well tolerated in children with combined tics and OCD, with behavioral activation (Riddle et al. 1991) the most common troublesome side effect. Although tic exacerbations or de novo tics have been reported with SSRI administration (Fennig et al. 1994), this is relatively uncommon (Scahill et al. 1997).

As noted above, however, tic-related forms of OCD appear to differ from non-tic-related OCD in terms of phenomenology and treatment response (King et al. 2005; Leckman et al. 1995; Miguel et al. 2001). For example, compared with non-tic-related OCD, tic-related OCD is less responsive to SSRI monotherapy (McDougle et al. 1994). Addition of a neuroleptic—such as haloperidol (McDougle et al. 1994), risperidone (McDougle et al. 2000), or olanzapine (Bogetto et al. 2000)—appears to improve treatment response to an SSRI.

Patients with tic disorders and their families should be cautioned about all drug use, both licit and illicit. Sympathomimetic agents ranging from decongestants through speed and cocaine markedly exacerbate tics. Older patients may experiment with alcohol, nicotine, or cannabinoids in an attempt to self-medicate their tics.

References

American Psychiatric Association: Diagnostic and Statistical Manual of Mental Disorders, 4th Edition, Text Revision. Washington, DC, American Psychiatric Association, 2000

Anderson GM, Leckman JF, Cohen DJ: Neurochemical and neuropeptide systems, in Tourette's Syndrome—Tics, Obsessions, Compulsions: Developmental Psychopathology and Clinical Care. Edited by Leckman JF, Cohen DJ. New York, Wiley, 1999, pp 261–281

Bliss J: Sensory experiences of Gilles de la Tourette syndrome. Arch Gen Psychiatry 37:1343–1347, 1980

Bloch MH, Leckman JF, Zhu H, et al: Caudate volumes in childhood predict symptom severity in adults with Tourette syndrome. Neurology 65:1253–1258, 2005

Bogetto F, Bellino S, Vaschetto P, et al: Olanzapine augmentation of fluvoxamine-refractory obsessive-compulsive disorder (OCD): a 12-week open trial. Psychiatry Res 96:91–98, 2000

Bruggeman R, van der Linden C, Buitelaar JK, et al: Risperidone versus pimozide in Tourette's disorder: a comparative double-blind parallel-group study. J Clin Psychiatry 62:50–56, 2001

Chappell PB, Riddle M, Anderson G, et al: Enhanced stress responsivity of Tourette syndrome patients undergoing lumbar puncture. Biol Psychiatry 36:35–43, 1994

Cohen DJ: Tourette's syndrome: a model disorder for integrating psychoanalytic and biological perspectives. Int Rev Psychoanal 18:195–209, 1991

Feigin A, Kurlan R, McDermott MP, et al: A controlled trial of deprenyl in children with Tourette's syndrome and attention deficit hyperactivity disorder. Neurology 46:965–968, 1996

Fennig S, Naisberg Fennig S, Pato M, et al: Emergence of symptoms of Tourette's syndrome during fluvoxamine treatment of obsessive-compulsive disorder. Br J Psychiatry 164:839–841, 1994

Gadow KD, Sverd J, Sprafkin J, et al: Efficacy of methylphenidate for attention-deficit hyperactivity disorder in children with tic disorder. Arch Gen Psychiatry 52:444–455, 1995

Gadow KD, Sverd J, Sprafkin J, et al: Long-term methylphenidate therapy in children with comorbid attention-deficit hyperactivity disorder and chronic multiple tic disorder. Arch Gen Psychiatry 56:330–336, 1999

Garvey MA, Perlmutter SJ, Allen AJ, et al: A pilot study of penicillin prophylaxis for neuropsychiatric exacerbations triggered by streptococcal infection. Biol Psychiatry 45:1564–1571, 1999

Gilbert DL, Sethuraman G, Sine L, et al: Tourette's syndrome improvement with pergolide in a randomized, double-blind, crossover trial. Neurology 54:1310–1315, 2000

Gilles de la Tourette G: Etude sur une affection nerveuse caractérisée par de l'incoordination motrice accompagnée d'echolalie et de coprolalie. Arch Neurol (Paris) 9:19–42, 158–200, 1885

Jankovic J: Differential diagnosis and etiology of tics, in Tourette Syndrome and Associated Disorders. (Advances in Neurology Series, Vol 85). Edited by Cohen DJ, Jankovic J, Goetz C. Philadelphia, PA, Lippincott Williams & Wilkins, 2001, pp 15–29

Kiessling LS, Marcotte AC, Culpepper L: Antineuronal antibodies: tics and obsessive compulsive symptoms. J Dev Behav Pediatr 14:281–282, 1993

King RA, Scahill L: Emotional and behavioral difficulties associated with Tourette's syndrome, in Tourette Syndrome and Associated Disorders (Advances in Neurology Series, Vol 85). Edited by Cohen DJ, Jankovic J, Goetz C. Philadelphia, PA, Lippincott Williams & Wilkins, 2001, pp 79–88

King RA, Scahill L, Findley D: Psychosocial and behavioral treatments in Tourette's syndrome, in Tourette's Syndrome—Tics, Obsessions, Compulsions: Developmental Psychopathology and Clinical Care. Edited by Leckman JF, Cohen DJ. New York, Wiley, 1999, pp 338–359

King RA, Scahill L, Lombroso PJ, et al: Tourette's syndrome and other tic disorders, in Pediatric Psychopharmacology: Principles and Practice. Edited by Martin A, Scahill L, Charney DS, Leckman JF. New York, Oxford University Press, 2003, pp 526–542

King RA, Findley D, Scahill L, et al: Obsessive-compulsive disorder in Tourette's syndrome, in Handbook of Tourette's Syndrome and Related Tic and Behavioral Disorders, 2nd Edition. Edited by Kurlan R. New York, Marcel Dekker, 2005, pp 427–453

Kurlan R, Kaplan EL: The pediatric autoimmune neuropsychiatric disorders associated with streptococcal infection (PANDAS) etiology for tics and obsessive-compulsive symptoms: hypothesis or entity? Practical considerations for the clinician. Pediatrics 113:883–886, 2004

Kurlan R, Behr J, Medved L, et al: Transient tic disorder and the spectrum of Tourette's syndrome. Arch Neurol 45:1200–1201, 1988

Kwak CH, Hanna PA, Jankovic J: Botulinum toxin in the treatment of tics. Arch Neurol 57:1190–1193, 2000

Law SF, Schachar RJ: Do typical clinical doses of methylphenidate cause tics in children treated for attention-deficit hyperactivity disorder? J Am Acad Child Adolesc Psychiatry 38:944–951, 1999

Leckman JF, Cohen DJ: Evolving models of pathogenesis, in Tourette's Syndrome—Tics, Obsessions, Compulsions: Developmental Psychopathology and Clinical Care. Edited by Leckman JF, Cohen DJ. New York, Wiley, 1999, pp 155–176

Leckman JF, Riddle M: Tourette's syndrome: when habit forming systems form habits of their own? Neuron 28:349–354, 2000

Leckman JF, Dolnansky ES, Hardin MT, et al: Perinatal factors in the expression of Tourette's syndrome: an exploratory study. J Am Acad Child Adolesc Psychiatry 29:220–226, 1990

Leckman JF, Hardin MT, Riddle MA, et al: Clonidine treatment of Gilles de la Tourette's syndrome. Arch Gen Psychiatry 48:324–328, 1991

Leckman JF, Walker DE, Cohen DJ: Premonitory urges in Tourette's syndrome. Am J Psychiatry 150:98–102, 1993

Leckman JF, Walker DE, Goodman WK, et al: "Just right" perceptions associated with compulsive behaviors in Tourette's syndrome. Am J Psychiatry 151, 675–680, 1994

Leckman JF, Grice DE, Barr LC, et al: Tic-related vs. non-tic related obsessive compulsive disorder. Anxiety 1:208–215, 1995

Leckman JF, Zhang H, Vitale A, et al: Course of tic severity in Tourette syndrome: the first two decades. Pediatrics 102:14–19, 1998

Leckman JF, King RA, Cohen DJ: Tics and tic disorders, in Tourette's Syndrome—Tics, Obsessions, Compulsions: Developmental Psychopathology and Clinical Care. Edited by Leckman JF, Cohen DJ. New York, Wiley, 1999a, pp 23–42

Leckman JF, King RA, Scahill L, et al: Yale approach to assessment and treatment, in Tourette's Syndrome—Tics, Obsessions, Compulsions: Developmental Psychopathology and Clinical Care. Edited by Leckman JF, Cohen DJ. New York, Wiley, 1999b, pp 285–308

Lee TS, Lee TD, Lombroso PJ, et al: Atomoxetine and tics in ADHD. J Am Acad Child Adolesc Psychiatry 43:1068–1069, 2004

Malison RT, McDougle CJ, van Dyck CH, et al: [123I]Beta-CIT SPECT imaging demonstrates increased striatal dopamine transporter binding in Tourette's syndrome. Am J Psychiatry 152:1359–1361, 1995

Marras C, Andrews D, Sime E, et al: Botulinum toxin for simple motor tics: a randomized, double-blind, controlled clinical trial. Neurology 56:605–610, 2001

Mason A, Banerjee S, Eapen V, et al: The prevalence of Tourette syndrome in a mainstream school population. Dev Med Child Neurol 40:292–296, 1998

McCracken JT, Sallee FR, Leonard HL, et al: Improvement of ADHD by atomoxetine in children with tic disorders. Paper presented at the annual meeting of the American Academy of Child and Adolescent Psychiatry, Miami, FL, October 14–19, 2003

McDougle CJ, Goodman WK, Leckman JF, et al: Haloperidol addition in fluvoxamine-refractory obsessive compulsive disorder: a double blind placebo-controlled study in patients with and without tics. Arch Gen Psychiatry 51:302–308, 1994

McDougle CJ, Epperson CN, Pelton GH, et al: A double-blind, placebo-controlled study of risperidone addition in serotonin reuptake inhibitor-refractory obsessive-compulsive disorder. Arch Gen Psychiatry 57:794–801, 2000

Mercadante MT, Hounie AG, Diniz JB, et al: The basal ganglia and immune-based neuropsychiatric disorders. Psychiatr Ann 31:534–540, 2001

Miguel EC, do Rosario-Campos MC, Shavitt RG, et al: The tic-related obsessive-compulsive disorder: phenotype and treatment implications, in Tourette Syndrome and Associated Disorders (Advances in Neurology Series, Vol 85). Edited by Cohen DJ, Jankovic J, Goetz C. Philadelphia, PA, Lippincott Williams & Wilkins, 2001, pp 43–56

Onofrj M, Paci C, D'Andreamatteo G, et al: Olanzapine in severe Gilles de la Tourette syndrome: a 52-week double-blind crossover study vs low-dose pimozide. J Neurol 247:443–446, 2000

Pauls DL, Alsobrook J, Goodman W, et al: A family study of obsessive-compulsive disorder. Am J Psychiatry 152:76–84, 1995

Pauls DL, Alsobrook JP II, Gelernter J, et al: Genetic vulnerability, in Tourette's Syndrome—Tics, Obsessions, Compulsions: Developmental Psychopathology and Clinical Care. Edited by Leckman JF, Cohen DJ. New York, Wiley, 1999, pp 194–212

Perlmutter SJ, Leitman SF, Garvey MA, et al: Therapeutic plasma exchange and intravenous immunoglobulin for obsessive-compulsive disorder and tic disorders in childhood. Lancet 354:1153–1158, 1999

Peterson BS, Leckman JF, Cohen DJ: Tourette's syndrome: a genetically predisposed and an environmentally specified developmental psychopathology, in Developmental Psychopathology, Vol 2: Risk, Disorder, and Adaptation. Edited by Cicchetti D, Cohen DJ. New York, Wiley, 1995, pp 213–242

Peterson BS, Skudlarski P, Anderson AW, et al: A functional magnetic resonance imaging study of tic suppression in Tourette syndrome. Arch Gen Psychiatry 55:326–333, 1998

Peterson BS, Leckman JF, Arnsten A, et al: Neuroanatomical circuitry, in Tourette's Syndrome—Tics, Obsessions, Compulsions: Developmental Psychopathology and Clinical Care. Edited by Leckman JF, Cohen DJ. New York, Wiley, 1999, pp 230–260

Peterson BS, Pine DS, Cohen P, et al: Prospective, longitudinal study of tic, obsessive-compulsive, and attention-deficit/hyperactivity disorders in an epidemiological sample. J Am Acad Child Adolesc Psychiatry 40:685–695, 2001a

Peterson BS, Staib L, Scahill L, et al: Regional brain and ventricular volumes in Tourette syndrome. Arch Gen Psychiatry 58:427–440, 2001b

Peterson BS, Thomas P, Kane M, et al: Basal ganglia volumes in patients with Gilles de la Tourette's syndrome. Arch Gen Psychiatry 60:415–424, 2003

Piacentini J, Chang S: Behavioral treatments for Tourette syndrome and tic disorders: state of the art, in Tourette Syndrome and Associated Disorders (Advances in Neurology Series, Vol 85). Edited by Cohen DJ, Jankovic J, Goetz C. Philadelphia, PA, Lippincott Williams & Wilkins, 2001, pp 319–331

Price RA, Kidd KK, Cohen DJ, et al: A twin study of Tourette syndrome. Arch Gen Psychiatry 42:815–820, 1985

Rapin I: Autism spectrum disorders: relevance to Tourette syndrome, in Tourette Syndrome and Associated Disorders (Advances in Neurology Series, Vol 85). Edited by Cohen DJ, Jankovic J, Goetz C. Philadelphia, PA, Lippincott Williams & Wilkins, 2001, pp 89–101

Riddle MA, Hardin MT, King R, et al: Fluoxetine treatment of children and adolescents with Tourette's and obsessive-compulsive disorders: preliminary clinical experience. J Am Acad Child Adolesc Psychiatry 29:45–48, 1990

Riddle MA, King RA, Hardin MT, et al: Behavioral side effects of fluoxetine in children and adolescents. J Child Adolesc Psychopharmacol 3:193–198, 1991

Riddle MA, Geller B, Ryan N: Another sudden death in a child treated with desipramine. J Am Acad Child Adolesc Psychiatry 32:792–797, 1993

Sallee FR, Kurlan R, Goetz CG, et al: Ziprasidone treatment of children and adolescents with Tourette's syndrome: a pilot study. J Am Acad Child Adolesc Psychiatry 39:292–299, 2000

Scahill L, Riddle MA, King RA, et al: Fluoxetine has no marked effect on tic symptoms in patients with Tourette's syndrome: a double-blind placebo-controlled study. J Child Adolesc Psychopharmacol 7:75–85, 1997

Scahill L, King RA, Schultz RT, et al: Selection and use of diagnostic and clinical rating instruments, in Tourette's Syndrome—Tics, Obsessions, Compulsions: Developmental Psychopathology and Clinical Care. Edited by Leckman JF, Cohen DJ. New York, Wiley, 1999, pp 310–324

Scahill L, Chappell PB, Kim YS, et al: A placebo-controlled study of guanfacine in the treatment of children with tic disorders and attention deficit hyperactivity disorder. Am J Psychiatry 158:1067–1074, 2001a

Scahill L, Tanner C, Dure L: The epidemiology of tics and Tourette syndrome in children and adolescents, in Tourette Syndrome and Associated Disorders (Advances in Neurology Series, Vol 85). Edited by Cohen DJ, Jankovic J, Goetz C. Philadelphia, PA, Lippincott Williams & Wilkins, 2001b, pp 261–271

Scahill L, Leckman JF, Schultz RT, et al: A placebo-controlled trial of risperidone in Tourette syndrome. Neurology 60:1130–1135, 2003

Schultz RT, Carter AS, Scahill L, et al: Neuropsychological findings, in Tourette's Syndrome—Tics, Obsessions, Compulsions: Developmental Psychopathology and Clinical Care. Edited by Leckman JF, Cohen DJ. New York, Wiley, 1999, pp 80–103

Silva RR, Munoz DM, Barickman J, et al: Environmental factors and related fluctuation of symptoms in children and adolescents with Tourette's disorder. J Child Psychol Psychiatry 36:305–312, 1995

Silver AA, Shytle RD, Philipp MK, et al: Transdermal nicotine and haloperidol in Tourette's disorder: a double-blind placebo-controlled study. J Clin Psychiatry 62:707–714, 2001a

Silver AA, Shytle RD, Sheehan KH, et al: Multicenter, double-blind, placebo-controlled study of mecamylamine monotherapy for Tourette's disorder. J Am Acad Child Adolesc Psychiatry 40:1103–1110, 2001b

Singer HS, Loiselle C: PANDAS: a commentary. J Psychosom Res 55:31–39, 2003

Singer H, Brown J, Quaskey S, et al: The treatment of attention-deficit hyperactivity disorder in Tourette's syndrome: a double-blind placebo-controlled study with clonidine and desipramine. Pediatrics 95:74–81, 1995

Singer HS, Wendlandt J, Krieger M, et al: Baclofen treatment in Tourette syndrome: a double-blind, placebo-controlled, crossover trial. Neurology 56:599–604, 2001

Snider LA, Seligman LD, Ketchen BR, et al: Tics and problem behaviors in schoolchildren: prevalence, characterization, and associations. Pediatrics 110(2 pt 1):331–336, 2002

Spencer T, Biederman J, Wilens T, et al: Nortriptyline treatment of children with attention-deficit hyperactivity disorder and tic disorder or Tourette's syndrome. J Am Acad Child Adolesc Psychiatry 32:205–210, 1993

State M, Greally JM, Cuker A, et al: Epigenetic abnormalities associated with a chromosome 18(q21-q22) inversion and a Gilles de la Tourette syndrome phenotype. Proc Natl Acad Sci USA 100:4684–4689, 2003

Stokes A, Bawden HN, Camfield PR, et al: Peer problems in Tourette's disorder. Pediatrics 87:936–942, 1991

Surwillo WW, Shafii M, Barrett CL: Gilles de la Tourette syndrome: a 20-month study of the effects of stressful life events and haloperidol on symptom frequency. J Nerv Ment Dis 166:812–816, 1978

Swanson JM, Connor DF, Cantwell D: Combining methylphenidate and clonidine: ill-advised. J Am Acad Child Adolesc Psychiatry 38:617–619, 1999

Swedo SE, Leonard HL, Schapiro MB, et al: Sydenham's chorea: physical and psychological symptoms of St Vitus Dance. Pediatrics 91:706–713, 1993

Swedo SE, Leonard HL, Kiessling LS: Speculations on anti-neuronal antibody-mediated neuropsychiatric disorders of childhood. Pediatrics 93:323–326, 1994

Swedo SE, Leonard HL, Garvey M, et al: Pediatric autoimmune neuropsychiatric disorders associated with streptococcal infections: clinical description of the first 50 cases. Am J Psychiatry 155:264–271, 1998

Tourette Syndrome International Consortium for Genetics: A complete genome screen in sib pairs affected by Gilles de la Tourette syndrome. Am J Hum Genet 65:1428–1436, 1999

Tourette's Syndrome Study Group: Treatment of ADHD in children with Tourette's syndrome: a randomized controlled trial. Neurology 58:527–536, 2002

Varley CK, Vincent J, Varley P, et al: Emergence of tics in children with attention deficit hyperactivity disorder treated with stimulant medications. Compr Psychiatry 42:228–233, 2001

Wehr AM, Namerow LB: Citalopram for OCD and Tourette's syndrome. J Am Acad Child Adolesc Psychiatry 40:740–741, 2001

Wilens TE, Spencer TJ, Swanson JM, et al: Combining methylphenidate and clonidine: a clinically sound medication option. J Am Acad Child Adolesc Psychiatry 38:614–616; discussion 619–622, 1999

Wolf SS, Jones DW, Knable MB, et al: Tourette syndrome: prediction of phenotypic variation in monozygotic twins by caudate nucleus D_2 receptor binding. Science 273:1225–1227, 1996

Ziemann U, Paulus W, Rothenberger A: Decreased motor inhibition in Tourette's disorder: evidence from transcranial magnetic stimulation. Am J Psychiatry 154:277–284, 1997

Self-Assessment Questions

Select the single best response for each question.

25.1 Which of the following statements regarding transient tic disorder is *true*?

    A. Transient tics are very rare among prepubertal children.

    B. Girls are more often affected than boys.

    C. Transient tics run a waxing and waning course.

    D. Transient tics most commonly involve the trunk and lower extremities.

    E. Transient vocal tics are common.

25.2 All of the following statements regarding Tourette's syndrome are correct *except*

    A. Chronic motor and phonic tic disorder was first described in 1885 by Georges Gilles de la Tourette.

    B. Initial symptoms of Tourette's syndrome most frequently appear between the ages of 5 and 8 years.

    C. Tic symptoms may wax and wane over time.

    D. Vocal tics usually precede motor tics.

    E. Children may be able to suppress tics for periods of time.

25.3 The most likely neuroanatomical substrate of Tourette's syndrome is

    A. The thalamus.

    B. The pituitary.

    C. The prefrontal cortex.

    D. The basal ganglia.

    E. The amygdala.

25.4 Which of the following psychotropic agents is least likely to exacerbate tics?

    A. Haloperidol.

    B. L-dopa.

    C. Dextroamphetamine.

    D. Methylphenidate.

    E. Cocaine.

25.5 Side effects of clonidine in the treatment of tic disorders include all of the following *except*

    A. Sedation.

    B. Irritability.

    C. Dry mouth.

    D. Cardiac arrhythmias.

    E. Hypertension.

Disorders of Elimination

Thomas Walsh, M.D.

Edgardo Menvielle, M.D.

Deepa Khushlani, M.D.

The disorders of elimination—enuresis and encopresis—represent an inability to achieve or maintain control of bodily functions. These disorders are not uncommon and can cause significant distress for both the child and the family. The presenting symptoms of elimination disorders are seen by a variety of health professionals, occasionally as symptoms of other disorders. In this chapter we review the causes, sequelae, and treatment of each of these disorders.

Enuresis

Enuresis is the repeated involuntary or intentional discharge of urine beyond the expected age for controlling urination (in the absence of a definable physical disorder). According to DSM-IV-TR (American Psychiatric Association 2000), the disorder is present when voiding of urine occurs at least twice a week for at least 3 months or causes clinically significant distress or im-

pairment in functioning (Table 26–1). Primary enuresis occurs in children who have never controlled their wetting for an extended period; secondary enuresis is the reemergence of wetting after a continuous period of control of 6 months or longer. Enuresis may be characterized as *nocturnal* (the most common), *diurnal* (more frequent in children younger than 5 years), and *mixed*.

■ Clinical Features

About 80% of patients with enuresis have primary enuresis. Left untreated, the remission rate is 10%–20% per year, which gradually increases with age. Primary enuresis therefore can be viewed as a self-limiting disorder, with enuresis continuing into adulthood in 1% of patients (Forsythe and Redmond 1974).

Although most children with enuresis do not have a coexisting psychiatric disorder, the prevalence of emotional–behav-

Table 26–1. DSM-IV-TR diagnostic criteria for enuresis

A. Repeated voiding of urine into bed or clothes (whether involuntary or intentional).

B. The behavior is clinically significant as manifested by either a frequency of twice a week for at least 3 consecutive months or the presence of clinically significant distress or impairment in social, academic (occupational), or other important areas of functioning.

C. Chronological age is at least 5 years (or equivalent developmental level).

D. The behavior is not due exclusively to the direct physiological effect of a substance (e.g., a diuretic) or a general medical condition (e.g., diabetes, spina bifida, a seizure disorder).

Specify type:

Nocturnal only
Diurnal only
Nocturnal and diurnal

Source. Reprinted from American Psychiatric Association: *Diagnostic and Statistical Manual of Mental Disorders,* 4th Edition, Text Revision. Washington, DC, American Psychiatric Association, 2000. Copyright 2000, American Psychiatric Association. Used with permission.

ioral disorders is greater than in the general population (Friman et al. 1998; Rutter 1989). Associations have been demonstrated with attention-deficit/hyperactivity disorder (Biederman et al. 1995) and with anxiety disorders, specifically selective mutism (Kristensen 2000). Coexisting disorders include encopresis and developmental delays. No association has been demonstrated between enuresis and tics, nail biting, temper tantrums, fire setting, or cruelty to animals (Felthous and Bernhard 1978; Oppel et al. 1968).

Psychosocial impairment in children with enuresis can result from the effect of enuresis on the child's self-esteem, the degree to which the disorder causes so-cial isolation and ostracism by peers, and the negative response of caregivers (e.g., anger, punishment, and rejection). Impairment also may be a result of coexisting disorders. Although the number of enuretic children with coexisting emotional–behavioral problems is small, children for whom help is sought may have more behavioral symptoms (Couchells et al. 1981).

■ **Differential Diagnosis**

A diagnosis of enuresis assumes the absence of identifiable physical causes. Any condition causing increased urine output can cause enuresis; therefore, diabetes mellitus and diabetes insipidus must be considered, as well as increased fluid intake with psychogenic causes. Urinary tract infection, especially in girls, must be ruled out, as must seizure disorders, renal insufficiency, neurological disorders that affect bladder innervation, neuroleptic-induced enuresis, and urinary tract anatomical dysfunctions. All of these can be readily ruled out by careful clinical assessment based on history, physical examination, urinalysis, and urine culture when necessary, with further assessment only as clinically indicated.

■ **Epidemiology**

Enuresis is as common in girls as in boys between ages 4 and 6 years. Beyond that age range the difference in prevalence increases steadily; by age 11 boys are twice as likely as girls to be symptomatic. Nocturnal enuresis occurs in 15% of 5-year-olds, with a decrease of about 15% per year thereafter. At age 7, 15% of boys have involuntary wetting less often than once a week, and 7% have involuntary wetting at least once a week. Commonly, boys from the latter group are those referred for treatment (Shaffer 1985).

Approximately 75% of enuretic children have a first-degree relative with a history of enuresis. When both parents have a positive history, 77% of the children are enuretic; when one parent is affected, 44% of the children are enuretic (Bakwin 1973). The relationship of enuresis to a range of psychosocial factors—including family, social, and economic background—once was thought to be significant but has since been questioned (Fergusson et al. 1986).

■ Etiology

No single cause of enuresis has been identified. Primary enuresis has been viewed as representing a maturational delay, with multiple factors contributing to this theory. Genetic studies have demonstrated a high incidence of enuresis in parents and siblings of bed wetters, with the suggestion of subtypes based on a variety of modes of genetic transmission (von Gontard et al. 1999). Investigation of the endogenous production of the antidiuretic hormone arginine vasopressin initially indicated that enuresis might be a result of a failure to achieve the expected diurnal variation of antidiuretic hormone (Medel et al. 1998; Norgaard et al. 1989). Although this has led to better understanding of the physiology of the disorder, the findings have been inconclusive. Physiological research has been extended to the role of urine osmolality and renal tubular function (Mikkelsen 2001).

Investigations of enuresis as a disorder of sleep have determined that no association exists between enuresis and any particular stage of sleep (Mikkelsen et al. 1980). A better understanding of the role of sleep may lead to the identification of subtypes of the disorder (Neveus et al. 1999). Enuresis has been related to abnormalities in bladder size, function, or anatomy, but these anatomical factors appear to account for only a minority of patients.

Secondary enuresis can be a manifesta-tion of stress in children, especially those between ages 4 and 6 years. Environmental stressors, such as a move to a new home, birth of a sibling, hospitalization, or child abuse, may cause a transient regression in bladder control. Although there is no evidence to support the notion that enuresis has a symbolic meaning, a relationship can be found between psychiatric disorders and enuresis, with cause and effect being different in individual cases (Rutter 1989). In some children with daytime wetting, a lack of awareness of internal cues may be an etiological factor.

■ Treatment

Multiple treatment modalities exist for functional enuresis. However, one point is central to applying all modalities: enuresis is mostly a self-limited, benign disorder. It is necessary to provide reassurance and support to prevent secondary emotional effects on self-esteem and family relationships and to prevent shame and guilt from developing from the symptoms. Excessive investigation and overaggressive treatment of all types should be avoided.

Treatment should be preceded by a period of observation during which there is open discussion of the problem, tracking of symptoms by using a chart, and positive reinforcement of dry periods. Simple interventions such as late fluid restrictions and encouragement of night-time urination may be tried. This pretreatment period sometimes produces significant and lasting remission of symptoms.

The most effective treatment for primary enuresis is the enuresis alarm, a conditioning device with an alarm triggered by the child's voiding. Various designs of this apparatus are available, ranging from the conventional bell and pad to more compact and sensitive systems.

Explanations for the success of this treatment are based on behavioral theories—including classical conditioning, avoidance learning, and social learning—but these are not adequate explanations of its efficacy. The success rate for the enuresis alarm is good: 60%–80% of patients initially respond to the alarm, with some relapse. Because of the relapse rate, a second course of treatment is often necessary (Forsythe and Butler 1989). Dry bed training (including positive reinforcement for inhibiting urination, retention-control training, positive-practice nighttime awakening, cleanliness training, and aversive consequences) has been used but does not appear to be effective when used without the enuresis alarm (Butler 1998). For maximum effect, compliance in using the enuresis alarm must be addressed. When a family fails to continue using the alarm, the clinician must be sensitive to the family's difficulties in sustaining treatment and must offer guidance and support.

A number of pharmacological agents have been used with some success to treat enuresis. Tricyclic antidepressants and desmopressin (deamino-8-D-arginine vasopressin [DDAVP]) have proved beneficial (Monda and Husmann 1995); stimulants, sedatives, and anticholinergic agents have not.

Tricyclic antidepressants, especially imipramine, have been widely studied and used in the treatment of enuresis (Bindelglas and Dee 1978; Fritz et al. 1994). The mechanism of action of imipramine is uncertain. Effective doses are in the 25- to 75-mg range, with a decrease in frequent wetting in most cases, but total remission in only about 30%; significant relapse occurs after discontinuing imipramine. Potential cardiac conduction abnormalities and other unwanted side effects and risk of fatal toxicity on overdose, intentional or otherwise, must be considered when using imipramine.

DDAVP, an analog of the antidiuretic hormone vasopressin, has been found to be effective in the treatment of enuresis and has replaced imipramine as the most-used pharmacological agent (Mikkelsen 2001; Thompson and Rey 1995). The postulated mechanism is decreased nighttime urine output to a point that does not exceed bladder capacity, thus eliminating nighttime wetting. DDAVP is administered in doses of 200–400 µg orally (20–40 µg intranasally) and produces a remission of symptoms comparable to that of imipramine with a similarly significant relapse rate (Hjalmas et al. 1998). The relatively rare occurrence of hyponatremia and possible seizures is a consideration in its use (Muller et al. 2004).

In general, pharmacological interventions are useful when rapid, short-term relief from symptoms must be achieved, when symptoms become the source of conflict in relationships within a family, or when symptoms create or exacerbate maladaptive behavior in the child and other methods have failed.

The clinician's decision to treat is an important one for each child; the benefits need to justify a sometimes prolonged and complex treatment process. Because it appears that children have improved self-concept following successful treatment and that treatment failure does not have adverse emotional effects, treatment of this condition should be considered (Moffatt 1989).

■ Prognosis

Because enuresis is mostly self-limiting and effective treatment is available, prognosis is good. In children with coexisting disorders or significant secondary emotional complications, appropriate intervention is necessary for successful outcome.

Encopresis

According to DSM-IV-TR, encopresis is the repeated involuntary or intentional passage of feces into inappropriate places by children older than 4 years or with a mental equivalent to age 4 years. Encopresis is not exclusively due to the effect of a substance, such as a laxative, or to a medical condition, except when medical conditions result in constipation. The frequency required to meet DSM-IV-TR criteria is at least one event per month for at least 3 months (Table 26–2).

■ Clinical Features

In primary encopresis, the disturbance is not preceded by a period of fecal continence; secondary encopresis is preceded by a period of fecal continence lasting at least 1 year. The secondary type may account for as many as 50%–60% of all cases (Walker et al. 1988). Different types of encopresis can be described based on the outcome of bowel training, awareness of defecation, presence of chronic constipation, and psychological precipitants of soiling episodes. In children who achieve adequate bowel control but who deposit feces in inappropriate places in response to family stress or as a purposeful act, the soiling episode may represent episodic behavioral disorganization or regression under stress or an act of defiance or reprisal toward caregivers. Children who have never achieved appropriate bowel control and who may have a history of inadequate, unsuccessful toilet training may be unaware of the soiling or may be aware but unable to control it.

Encopresis with constipation and overflow incontinence is the most common type (85%–95%). Children with this disorder either have never achieved bowel control or have achieved control but proper functioning is not maintained because of constipation leading to fecal impaction

Table 26–2. DSM-IV-TR diagnostic criteria for encopresis

A. Repeated passage of feces into inappropriate places (e.g., clothing or floor) whether involuntary or intentional.

B. At least one such event a month for at least 3 months.

C. Chronological age is at least 4 years (or equivalent developmental level).

D. The behavior is not due exclusively to the direct physiological effects of a substance (e.g., laxatives) or a general medical condition except through a mechanism involving constipation.

Code as follows:

787.6 With constipation and overflow incontinence
307.7 Without constipation and overflow incontinence

Source. Reprinted from American Psychiatric Association: *Diagnostic and Statistical Manual of Mental Disorders,* 4th Edition, Text Revision. Washington, DC, American Psychiatric Association, 2000. Copyright 2000, American Psychiatric Association. Used with permission.

and overflow. This group has infrequent bowel movements and frequent accidents (often more than two a day) in the form of small stains of liquid stool (Doleys 1983; Levine 1982).

Cases not involving constipation and feces overflow are characterized by intentional depositing or smearing of feces in a prominent location. This type of encopresis is associated with defiant behaviors, that is, as a covert expression of anger. Smearing may occur accidentally in the child's attempt to clean or hide feces passed involuntarily.

Some children want to avoid embarrassing situations, and they may hide soiled clothes and deny the soiling, appearing mortified when the problem is discussed. Others appear either unconcerned, unaware, or indifferent to the offensive odor.

Most children with functional encopresis do not appear to have significant behavioral problems (Gabel et al. 1986). However, the social ostracism that many children with encopresis experience may lead to low self-esteem and poor peer relationships. Because primary care providers may manage many cases of encopresis associated with underlying constipation, children who are referred to psychiatrists may represent either a more severely affected group or those who have comorbid behavior disorders (Friman et al. 1988).

■ Differential Diagnosis

Functional encopresis must be distinguished from structural organic causes of encopresis, such as aganglionic megacolon (Hirschsprung's disease). Although severe cases of aganglionic megacolon are detected soon after birth, mild cases may go undetected until later in life. Functional encopresis also should be distinguished from chronic or intermittent diarrhea due to organic disorders such as Crohn's disease or irritable bowel syndrome or the use of laxatives. A medical condition that causes constipation allows for a concurrent diagnosis of encopresis; however, the diagnosis is not warranted when fecal incontinence is related to nonconstipating conditions such as chronic diarrhea. A plain abdominal roentgenogram can aid diagnosis and management of encopresis (Rockney et al. 1995).

■ Epidemiology

Functional encopresis is estimated to affect between 1.5% and 7.5% of children of elementary school age (Walker et al. 1988). This range of reported incidence results from the various diagnostic criteria used in these studies. In children, secondary encopresis rarely starts after age 8 years. Primary encopresis apparently is more common in lower socioeconomic classes and is three to four times more common in boys than in girls. It is generally believed that encopresis is underreported (Doleys 1983; Hersov 1985).

■ Etiology

No single pathophysiological or psychodynamic explanation accounts for all cases of encopresis. Combinations of maturational and psychosocial factors may be involved, including precipitating psychosocial stressors such as parental divorce, sibling rivalry, or starting school. In one case series of 63 children, boys with primary encopresis were more likely to have developmental delays and enuresis, whereas boys with secondary encopresis were more likely to have conduct disorders (Foreman and Thambirajah 1996).

Anismus, the lack of relaxation of the external anal sphincter during defecation, is observed in 75% of cases of encopresis (Sentovich et al. 1998). However, it remains unclear whether this neuromuscular dysfunction precedes or follows constipation. Chronic constipation may result from a combination of factors. The retention of feces may result from painful defecation because of an anal fissure, a struggle between the parent and the child over bowel training, or a phobic avoidance of the toilet based on a real or imaginary negative experience. Constipation leads to fecal impaction, and liquid feces tend to leak around the impaction. The child's attempts to prevent involuntary passage of feces by anal contraction may increase the amount of retained feces. With rectal distention, the internal anal sphincter becomes weak and underresponsive, and the sensation of passage of feces through the rectum decreases. The child may lose awareness of the passage of stools, and his or her sense of smell becomes habituated to the foul odor (this may be most relevant for older children who appear to lack an age-appropriate social concern). In primary encopresis, constipation is often established before the child has mastered bowel control skills.

Psychodynamic factors generally focus on the mother-child relationship or on a fixation on anal self-stimulation as a source of pleasure (Clarck et al. 1990). Proposed causes include rigid, perfectionist parents; coercive training; and the mother's ambivalence toward the child's need for autonomy (Anthony 1957; Easson 1960; Pinkerton 1958). Family-constellation factors—such as an uninvolved, passive father and a domineering, overinvolved, or depressed mother—have been implicated as well (Bemporad et al. 1971). Posttraumatic encopresis associated with anal sexual assault has been observed (Boon 1991), and an association with behavior problems, learning difficulties, and emotional disorders has been made (Cox et al. 2002)

■ Treatment

The goal of treatment is the child's regular independent use of the toilet and the resolution of coexisting problems. The therapeutic approach should be based on the type of encopresis, and medical, behavioral, and psychotherapeutic interventions should be used as indicated. Careful evaluation, including both medical and psychosocial assessment, and a period of observation to record soiling, accompanied by open discussion of the symptoms, should precede any intervention. Medical and behavioral interventions vary according to the characteristics of each child's soiling. The treatment principles for children who retain feces include educating the child and parents about the problem, disimpacting the bowel, and training the child in bowel control (Brooks et al. 2000). Education about the symptom, the mechanism of retention, and the rationale for the intervention is used as the initial strategy to recruit both parent and child as active participants collaborating to solve the problem

(Landman and Rappaport 1985).

A necessary medical intervention is to remove the blockage of feces in the bowel, which is usually done with laxatives or enemas. It is best to avoid enemas in children with a history of abuse. After the bowel is clean, several management measures are used to prevent reimpaction and to gain continence control (Seth and Heyman 1994). Diet modification with an increase in the child's intake of dietary fiber and water helps to facilitate bowel function and to prevent impaction. Behavioral intervention using toilet training (10-minute sittings 20 minutes after meals) is instituted to increase the chance of bowel movements in the toilet utilizing the gastroileal reflex. Appropriate bowel movements and accident-free days are reinforced through praise or tangible rewards. Aversive consequences for soiling accidents, such as showering and washing the soiled clothes, also reinforce the child's self-monitoring (Doleys 1983; Gerber and Meyer 1965; Houts and Peterson 1986; Young 1973). The initial promise of biofeedback therapy was not supported by subsequent studies that failed to demonstrate superiority to the conventional approach of catharsis, diet modification, educational intervention, and behavioral training (Loening-Baucke 1990, 1995; Nolan et al. 1998). Biofeedback may still have a use as an adjunctive treatment. Because of the chronic nature of constipation, ongoing medical management of recurring constipation may be required for months or years.

Pharmacological agents may have some role in the treatment of nonretentive encopresis. Some studies have reported symptomatic improvement with imipramine and amitriptyline (Dossetor et al. 1998; Mikkelsen 1996). Tricyclic antidepressants exacerbate constipation and therefore are contraindicated in retentive encopresis.

When significant comorbid psychopathology is present in the individual and family, appropriate psychotherapeutic intervention is indicated. Associated psychopathology may be a factor in the etiology of encopresis, especially in children who have shown adequate bowel control. In other cases, psychopathology may result from the encopresis and may impede the effectiveness of bowel control training. Although psychiatric intervention may be needed to treat coexisting primary psychiatric disorders, psychotherapy may also be needed to treat secondary maladaptive patterns, even though self-esteem may improve with simple relief of the symptoms. Family therapy is useful when the child and family must disengage from interactions that perpetuate the problem (Margolies and Gilstein 1983–1984).

■ Prognosis

The prevalence of functional encopresis gradually declines from a peak at age 6 years in boys and 8 years in girls to almost complete disappearance by age 16 years in both boys and girls (Rex et al. 1992). Soiling at night is associated with a poorer prognosis than is soiling during the day. Other indicators of poor prognosis are nonchalant attitude, associated conduct problems, and soiling as an expression of aggression (Landman and Rappaport 1985; Levine 1982).

Research Issues

Compared with enuresis, there is a paucity of research on encopresis, possibly reflecting the relative rarity of encopresis (Mikkelsen 2001). Because maturational factors are so important in diagnosing both enuresis and encopresis, further research is needed to explore the relationship between the two, to define the pathophysiology of each, and to explore common links to other developmental disorders. In addition, the relationship between maturational and emotional factors needs further investigation. Because these disorders are treated by primary-care physicians, urologists, gastroenterologists, and psychiatrists, issues related to developing common definitions and integrated treatment approaches must be explored. More data need to be collected to understand whether the types of disorders treated differ among various practitioners and whether the various treatment approaches are efficacious.

References

American Psychiatric Association: Diagnostic and Statistical Manual of Mental Disorders, 4th Edition, Text Revision. Washington, DC, American Psychiatric Association, 2000

Anthony EJ: An experimental approach to the psychology of childhood: encopresis. Br J Med Psychol 30:146–175, 1957

Bakwin H: The genetics of enuresis, in Bladder Control and Enuresis. Edited by Kolvin L, MacKeith RC, Meadow SR. London, Heinemann Medical, 1973, pp 73–77

Bemporad JR, Pfeifer CM, Gibbs L, et al: Characteristics of encopretic patients and their families. J Am Acad Child Psychiatry 10:272–292, 1971

Biederman J, Santangelo SL, Faraone SV: Clinical correlates of enuresis in ADHD and non-ADHD children. J Child Psychol Psychiatry 36:865–877, 1995

Bindelglas PM, Dee G: Enuresis treatment with imipramine hydrochloride: a 10-year follow-up study. Am J Psychiatry 135:1549–1552, 1978

Boon F: Encopresis and sexual assault (letter). J Am Acad Child Adolesc Psychiatry 30:509–510, 1991

Brooks RC, Copen RM, Cox DJ, et al: Review of the treatment literature for encopresis, functional constipation, and stool-toileting refusal. Ann Behav Med 22:260–267, 2000

Butler RJ: Annotation: night wetting in children: psychological aspects. J Child Psychol Psychiatry 39:453–463, 1998

Clarck AF, Tayler PJ, Bhate SR: Nocturnal fecal soiling and anal masturbation. Arch Dis Child 65:1367–1368, 1990

Couchells SM, Johnson SB, Carter R, et al: Behavioral and environmental characteristics of treated and untreated enuretic children and matched nonenuretic controls. J Pediatr 99:812–816, 1981

Cox DJ, Morris JB Jr, Borowitz SM, et al: Psychological differences between children with and without chronic encopresis. J Pediatr Psychol 27:585–591, 2002

Doleys DM: Enuresis and encopresis, in Handbook of Child Psychopathology. Edited by Ollendick TH, Hersen M. New York, Plenum, 1983, pp 201–226

Dossetor D, Stiefel I, Gomes L: A case of predominantly nocturnal soiling treated with amitriptyline. Eur Child Adolesc Psychiatry 7:114–118, 1998

Easson RL: Encopresis-psychogenic soiling. Can Med Assoc J 82:624–628, 1960

Felthous AR, Bernhard H: Enuresis, firesetting, and cruelty to animals: the significance of two-thirds of this triad. J Forensic Sci 45:240–246, 1978

Fergusson DM, Horwood LJ, Shannon FT: Factors related to the age of attainment of nocturnal bladder control: an 8-year longitudinal study. Pediatrics 78:884–890, 1986

Foreman DM, Thambirajah MS: Conduct disorder, enuresis and specific developmental delays in two types of encopresis: a casenote study of 63 boys. Eur Child Adolesc Psychiatry 5:33–37, 1996

Forsythe WL, Butler RJ: Fifty years of enuretic alarms. Arch Dis Child 64:879–885, 1989

Forsythe WL, Redmond A: Enuresis and spontaneous cure rate of 1,129 enuretics. Arch Dis Child 49:259–265, 1974

Friman PC, Mathews JR, Finney JW, et al: Do encopretic children have clinically significant behavioral problems? Pediatrics 82(3 pt 2):407–409, 1988

Friman PC, Handwerk ML, Swerer SM, et al: Do children with primary nocturnal enuresis have clinically significant behavior problems? Arch Pediatr Adolesc Med 152:537–539, 1998

Fritz GK, Rockney RM, Yeung AS: Plasma levels and efficacy of imipramine treatment for enuresis. J Am Acad Child Adolesc Psychiatry 33:60–64, 1994

Gabel S, Hegeders AM, Wald A, et al: Prevalence of behavior problems and mental health utilization among encopretic children: implications for behavioral pediatrics. J Dev Behav Pediatr 7:293–297, 1986

Gerber H, Meyer V: Behavior therapy and encopresis: the complexities involved in treatment. Behav Res Ther 2:227–231, 1965

Hersov L: Faecal soiling, in Child and Adolescent Psychiatry: Modern Approaches, 2nd Edition. Edited by Rutter M, Hersov L. St. Louis, MO, CV Mosby, 1985, pp 482–489

Hjalmas K, Hanson E, Hellstrom AL, et al: Long-term treatment with desmopressin in children with primary monosymptomatic nocturnal enuresis: an open multicentre study. Swedish Enuresis Trial (SWEET) Group. Br J Urol 82:704–709, 1998

Houts AC, Peterson JK: Treatment of a retentive encopretic child using contingency management and diet modification with stimulus control. J Pediatr Psychol 11:375–383, 1986

Kristensen H: Selective mutism and comorbidity with developmental disorder/delay, anxiety disorder, and elimination disorder. J Am Acad Child Adolesc Psychiatry 39:249–256, 2000

Landman GB, Rappaport L: Pediatric management of severe treatment-resistant encopresis. J Dev Behav Pediatr 6:349–351, 1985

Levine MD: Encopresis: its potentiation, evaluation and alleviation. Pediatr Clin North Am 29:315–330, 1982

Loening-Baucke V: Modulation of abnormal defecation by biofeedback treatment in chronically constipated children with encopresis. J Pediatr 116:214–222, 1990

Loening-Baucke V: Biofeedback treatment for chronic constipation and encopresis in childhood, I: long-term outcome. Pediatrics 96:105–110, 1995

Margolies R, Gilstein K: A systems approach to the treatment of chronic encopresis. Int J Psychiatry Med 13:141–151, 1983–1984

Medel R, Dieguez S, Brindo M, et al: Monosymptomatic primary enuresis: differences between patients responding or not responding to oral desmopressin. Br J Urol 81:46–49, 1998

Mikkelsen EJ: Modern approaches to enuresis and encopresis, sleep stage, and drug response, in Child and Adolescent Psychiatry, 2nd Edition. Edited by Lewis M. Baltimore, MD, Williams & Wilkins, 1996, pp 593–601

Mikkelsen EJ: Enuresis and encopresis: ten years of progress. J Am Acad Child Adolesc Psychiatry 40:1146–1158, 2001

Mikkelsen EJ, Rapoport JL, Nee L, et al: Childhood enuresis, I: sleep patterns and psychopathology. Arch Gen Psychiatry 37:1139–1145, 1980

Moffatt MEK: Nocturnal enuresis: psychological implications of treatment and nontreatment. J Pediatr 114(4 pt 2): 697–704, 1989

Monda JM, Husmann DA: Primary nocturnal enuresis: a comparison among observation, imipramine, desmopressin acetate and bed-wetting alarm systems. J Urol 154:745–748, 1995

Muller D, Roehr CC, Eggert P: Comparative tolerability of drug treatment for nocturnal enuresis in children. Drug Saf 27:717–727, 2004

Neveus T, Hetta J, Cnattingius S, et al: Depth of sleep and sleep habits among enuretic and incontinent children. Acta Paediatr 88:748–752, 1999

Nolan T, Castro-Smith T, Coffey C, et al: Randomized control trial of biofeedback training in persistent encopresis with anismus. Arch Dis Child 79:131–135, 1998

Norgaard JP, Rittig S, Djurhuus JC: Nocturnal enuresis: an approach to treatment based on pathogenesis. J Pediatr 114(4 pt 2):705–710, 1989

Oppel WC, Harper PA, Rider RV: Social, psychological and neurological factors associated with enuresis. Pediatrics 42:627–641, 1968

Pinkerton P: Psychogenic megacolon in children: the implications of bowel negativism. Arch Dis Child 33:371–398, 1958

Rex DK, Fitzgerald JF, Goulet RJ: Chronic constipation with encopresis persisting beyond 15 years of age. Dis Colon Rectum 35:242–244, 1992

Rockney RM, McQuade WH, Days AL: The plain abdominal roentgenogram in the management of encopresis. Arch Pediatr Adolesc Med 149:623–627, 1995

Rutter M: Isle of Wight revisited: twenty-five years of child psychiatric epidemiology. J Am Acad Child Adolesc Psychiatry 28:633–653, 1989

Sentovich SM, Kauffman SS, Cali RL: Pudendal nerve function in normal and encopretic children. J Pediatr Gastroenterol Nutr 26:70–72, 1998

Seth R, Heyman MB: Management of constipation and encopresis in infants and children. Gastroenterol Clin North Am 23:621–636, 1994

Shaffer D: Enuresis, in Child Psychiatry: Modern Approaches, 2nd Edition. Edited by Rutter M, Hersov L. Oxford, UK, Blackwell Scientific, 1985, pp 465–481

Thompson S, Rey JM: Functional enuresis: is desmopressin the answer? J Am Acad Child Adolesc Psychiatry 34:266–271, 1995

von Gontard A, Eiberg H, Hollmann E, et al: Molecular genetics of nocturnal enuresis: linkage to a locus on chromosome 22. Scand J Urol Nephrol Suppl 202:76–80, 1999

Walker CE, Milling L, Bonner B: Incontinence disorders: enuresis and encopresis, in Handbook of Pediatric Psychology. Edited by Routh D. New York, Guilford, 1988, pp 263–298

Young GC: The treatment of childhood encopresis by conditioned gastro-ileal reflex training. Behav Res Ther 11:499–503, 1973

Self-Assessment Questions

Select the single best response for each question.

26.1 Which of the following statements regarding the clinical presentation of enuresis is *true?*

  A. About 80% of patients with enuresis have primary enuresis.
  B. Without treatment, the remission rate is 30%–50% per year, which decreases with age.
  C. Enuresis continues into adulthood in approximately 8% of cases.
  D. There is no identified increase prevalence of emotional–behavioral disorders in the enuretic population, when compared to the general population.
  E. Clear association between enuresis and tic disorders has been demonstrated.

26.2 Which of the following circumstances would be consistent with a child meeting DSM-IV-TR (American Psychiatric Association 2000) diagnostic criteria for enuresis?

  A. The child must be at least 3 years of age and demonstrate repeated voiding of urine in his or her bed or clothes at least twice weekly for 3 consecutive months.
  B. The child must be at least 3 years of age and demonstrate repeated voiding of urine in his or her bed or clothes at least five times weekly for 6 consecutive months.
  C. The child must be at least 3 years of age and demonstrate repeated voiding of urine in his or her bed or clothes that is not due to a physiological condition.
  D. The child must be at least 5 years of age and demonstrate repeated voiding of urine in his or her bed or clothes at least twice weekly for 3 consecutive months.
  E. The child must be at least 5 years of age and demonstrate repeated voiding of urine in his or her bed or clothes at least five times weekly for 6 consecutive months.

26.3 All of the statements regarding treatment of enuresis are correct *except*

  A. Enuresis is largely a self-limited, benign disorder.
  B. It is important to provide reassurance support to prevent secondary emotional effects.
  C. Treatment should be preceded by a period of observation and tracking of symptoms.
  D. The most effective treatment for primary enuresis is the enuresis alarm.
  E. Pharmacological interventions include desmopressin (DDAVP), imipramine, and methylphenidate.

26.4 Which of the following statements regarding encopresis is *true?*

  A. Primary encopresis is not preceded by a period of fecal continence.
  B. Secondary encopresis may account for 10%–20% of all cases.
  C. Encopresis resulting from constipation and overflow incontinence is a rare form of the disorder.
  D. Children with encopresis characterized by intentional depositing or smearing of feces are less likely to demonstrate defiant behaviors than are children with encopresis with overflow incontinence.
  E. Most children with functional encopresis demonstrate severe behavioral problems.

26.5 Which of the following statements regarding the treatment of encopresis is *true?*

  A. Treatment typically includes medical interventions alone.
  B. Treatment requires little evaluation because of the ease with which encopresis is diagnosed.
  C. Treatment in children who retain feces should include education, disimpaction, and bowel training.
  D. Treatment should not include aversive consequences for soiling accidents.
  E. Biofeedback appears to be the most effective available treatment.

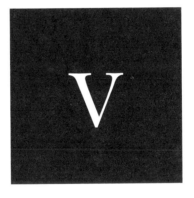

Special Issues

27

Physical and Sexual Abuse of Children

Paramjit T. Joshi, M.D.

Jay A. Salpekar, M.D.

Peter T. Daniolos, M.D.

Definitions

Child abuse continues to be a serious pediatric and social problem all over the world. In the Child Abuse Prevention, Adoption and Family Services Act of 1988, physical abuse was defined as "the physical injury of a child under 18 years of age by a person who is responsible for the child's welfare, under circumstances which indicate that the child's health or welfare is harmed or threatened" (Kaplan 1996, p. 1034). For the National Incidence Study, physical abuse was defined as being present when a child younger than age 18 experiences nonaccidental injury (harm standard) or risk of injury (endangerment standard) as a result of having been hit with a hand or other object or having been kicked, shaken, thrown, burned, stabbed, or choked by a parent or parent substitute (Sedlak and Broadhurst 1996). *Child neglect* is differentiated from child abuse and refers to the failure of the responsible caretaking adults to provide adequate physical care and supervision. This chapter focuses on physical abuse.

Sexual abuse most commonly refers to any activity within a spectrum ranging from inappropriate physical touching to sexual intercourse or rape. For decades child sexual abuse has continued to elude specific definition despite the efforts of researchers, therapists, and child advocates (Haugaard 2000). Important considerations include the wide range of normative sexual behavior and development among children and adolescents (Ryan 2000). Children may exhibit a wide range of sexual behaviors, even in circumstances where abuse may not be present (Friedrich et al. 1998). Children are very impressionable and model behavior that they see in adults. Eroticized behavior, increased sexual interest, and sexual play may result from numerous influences beyond potential abuse, including inadvertent observation of adults engaged in sexual activity, oedipal fantasies, manic or hypomanic states, or exposure to pornographic materials and television (Yates 1997). *Sexual play* generally involves mutually interested children at similar ages and developmental stages and does not involve coercion (American Academy of Pediatrics 1999). *Incest* refers to the sexual abuse of children within the context of the nuclear family, generally involving sexual activity between a parent and child or among siblings.

Legal definitions of abuse generally involve sexual contact between an adult and a minor child (Green 1993). If both the perpetrator and the victim are minors, abuse can be understood to have occurred, provided that there is a significant discrepancy in age or there is coercion involved. Some have defined age discrepancies of 4–5 years as being more definitive for an abuse scenario, but there is not a commonly accepted age difference defining abuse of a minor by another minor.

Epidemiology

The work of Kempe et al. (1962), who first described the battered child syndrome, led to the recognition of child abuse as a major pediatric, psychiatric, and social problem. By 1965 child protective services were established throughout the United States, and all 50 states passed laws requiring mandatory medical reporting of child abuse and neglect. During the 1970s, cases of incest and sexual abuse were increasingly reported (Green 1993). However, sexual abuse is still significantly underreported.

A report issued by the National Child Abuse and Neglect Data System of the U.S. Department of Health and Human Services in 2001 noted 826,000 victims of maltreatment nationwide, declining from over 900,000 children in 1998. The overall number of victimized children has continued to decline since 1993, when a

record high of 1,018,692 incidents was reported. Reasons for this decline are not well understood (Putnam 2003). Parents continued to be the main perpetrators. Almost 60% of all victims experienced neglect, while 21.3% experienced physical abuse and 11.3% were sexually abused. Data from the National Violence Against Women Survey revealed that whereas men were more likely to have experienced physical abuse as a child, the psychological and behavioral effects of abuse were more detrimental in female victims (M.P. Thompson et al. 2004). Fisher et al. (1997) studied a community probability sample of 665 youngsters, ages 9–17 years, and found that an alarming 25.9% had experienced abuse, as defined by behaviors such as severe punishment or infliction of physical injury.

The number of child fatalities caused by maltreatment remained unchanged at about 1,100. Younger children are at greatest risk for fatal maltreatment. In a 1998 report by the U.S. Department of Health and Human Services (Kaplan et al. 1999) it was documented that more than 75% of maltreatment fatalities in 1996 involved children younger than 3 years of age. Boys are at significantly increased risk. Other risk factors include having been born to a mother younger than 21 years, non–European American ethnicity, or products of multiple births (Keenan et al. 2003). Homicides occurring during the first week of life are almost exclusively perpetrated by mothers. Mothers and fathers were equally likely to fatally injure their children ages 1 week–13 years. However, fathers committed 63% of parent-perpetrated homicides among 13- to 15-year-olds and were responsible for 80% of those occurring in 16- to 19-year-olds (Kuntz and Bahr 1996).

Some studies report that 10%–25% of girls are sexually victimized in some manner before age 18 years (Fergusson et al.

1996). One study reports incidence as high as 34% (Wyatt et al. 1999). The most common age of initial sexual abuse is between 8 and 11 years of age (Kempe 1978; Muram 2001). A 1999 U.S. Department of Health and Human Services report also noted an overall downward trend in the incidence of child sexual abuse. Nationwide child protective services organizations reported 90,000 sexual abuse victims (U.S. Department of Health and Human Services 2001) down from 114,000 cases in 1994 (Finkelhor and Berliner 1995). Male parents or male parent figures continued to be the most common perpetrators of sexual abuse (U.S. Department of Health and Human Services 2001). Women are reported as abusers in a distinct minority of cases, and adolescents are reported to be the perpetrators in 20% of cases (American Academy of Pediatrics 1999).

Sexual abuse of boys has been less well studied and may be more significantly underreported and untreated (Moody 1999). Retrospective surveys have found that as many as 18% of males older than 18 years report having been victims of childhood sexual abuse (Finkelhor et al. 1990; Holmes and Slap 1998). Boys seem less likely to disclose abuse, generally for fear of disbelief, retribution, or social stigma and reluctance to admit vulnerability (Holmes and Slap 1998; Yates 1997). Perpetrators of abuse against boys are most likely to be male and unrelated to the victim (Holmes and Slap 1998). Studies have also shown that sexually abused boys are more likely to ultimately express a homosexual identity compared with boys without such a history (Fromuth and Burkhart 1989). However, if the perpetrator is female, boys may be even more disinclined to report abuse and less likely to be supported by caregivers when abuse is reported (Holmes and Slap 1998; Peluso and Putman 1996).

Etiology

The prevailing model of the etiology of abuse is an ecological one (Belsky 1980). Most experts believe that physical and sexual abuse results from a combination of factors both within parents and children, and in conjunction with their specific environment. Green (1993) believed that environmental stress, compounded by parental personality traits and characteristics of the child, created a climate leading to abuse. Child abuse tends to occur in multiproblem families—parental mental illness and substance abuse, lack of social supports, poverty, single parenthood, minority ethnicity, lack of acculturation, the presence of four or more children in a family, young parental age, stressful events, and exposure to family violence are all known risk factors (R.A. Thompson 1994). Sexual abuse tends to occur in families with significant instability and with characterological or personality disorder as opposed to major mental illness. Whereas sexual abuse is prevalent in all socioeconomic classes (Fergusson et al. 1996), physical abuse and neglect may be more common in lower socioeconomic classes (Wissow 1995). Abusers have racial, religious, and ethnic distributions similar to the general population (Ryan et al. 1996).

Risk factors that may predict recurrence of abuse include young age of the victim; number of previous referrals to child protective services; and caretaker characteristics such as emotional impairment, substance abuse, lack of social support, presence of domestic violence, and history of childhood abuse (English et al. 1999). Risk factors in the child, such as prematurity, mental retardation, and physical handicaps, could increase the likelihood of abuse (Cicchetti and Toth 1995). Children with cognitive deficits may have impaired judgment and decreased ability to tolerate and verbally communicate feelings, and as a result, react aggressively and become more vulnerable to maltreatment (Lewis 1992). Martin and Elmer (1992) found a history of low birth weight in 19% of an abused cohort compared with a 9.2% general prevalence at the time. These children may be more vulnerable to abuse because of excessive crying or behavior that is difficult to manage.

Themes of social isolation, enmeshment, and role confusion are common for families in which the father sexually abuses a daughter. Rigid patriarchal structure and a poor marital relationship are frequent. Such fathers may have an unstable job history, abuse alcohol, or be sexually and emotionally rejected by the spouse (Yates 1997). The incestuous father then seeks gratification from the daughter as an alternative to pursuing extramarital affairs (Mrazek and Mrazek 1981; Schetky and Green 1988). Some reports suggest that deep religiosity or social inhibition may lead to the selection of intrafamilial sexual abuse rather than adulterous affairs (Yates 1997).

Egeland et al. (1993) found that maltreated mothers who were able to break the intergenerational cycle of abuse reported receiving emotional support from a foster parent or relative when they were children, which in turn enhanced their self-worth and ability to be effective parents. These positive experiences challenged their negative caregiving models and helped them work through their own experiences of being abused. It is widely believed that abuse during childhood can lead to victims abusing their own offspring (Kaufman and Zigler 1987; Oliver 1993; Straus et al. 1980). However, methodological issues in many studies have limited research attempting to confirm this phenomenon (Ertem 2000). In only 4 of 10 English language published studies between 1965 and 2000, were the relative risks of maltreatment in the children of parent victims found to be significantly increased. However, one rigorously designed controlled study (Ertem 2000) did find that "primiparous mothers of low socioeconomic status who reported clearly defined severe physical abuse during childhood were 12.6 times more likely to abuse their children than mothers who had emotionally supportive parents." For sexual abuse, one study indicated that 35% of male perpetrators were themselves abused, and the likelihood of male victims becoming perpetrators was increased if the abuser was a female relative (Glasser et al. 2001). Mothers who were abused as children may unconsciously recreate scenarios of abuse by transferring parental roles to a daughter, who then becomes incestuously involved with an abusive father (Yates 1997).

Research has been more clear as to the important question of how intergenerational continuity of abuse can be interrupted (Egeland 1988). Studies of women who "broke the cycle of abuse" suggest that continuity of abuse is not the rule; many abused children grow up to be competent, nonabusive parents (Herman 1992). Maltreated mothers who were able to break the intergenerational cycle of abuse reported having received emotional support from a foster parent or relative when they were children, which in turn enhanced their self-worth and ability to be effective parents. These positive experiences challenged their negative caregiving models and helped them work through their own experiences of being abused (Egeland et al. 1993).

Profiles of Perpetrators

Perpetrators have a wide variety of character and personality pathology. However, a common theme among abusers is that they regard their victims not as independent but instead as narcissistic extensions of themselves, existing only for the purposes of their own gratification (Glasser et al. 2001). Green (1997) described characteristics of abusive parents, including a background of deprivation and abuse and a high prevalence of psychopathology and psychiatric impairment (especially antisocial personality disorder, alcoholism, and major depression). Abusive fathers were often characterized by extreme jealousy of their spouse's attention toward the targeted child, stemming from their own maternal deprivation in childhood and unresolved sibling rivalry. Furthermore, Smith et al. (1973) reported that half of their sample of abusive mothers were of borderline or subaverage intelligence. Several controlled studies of abusive mothers have reported significantly lower self-esteem in comparison with the control mothers (Anderson and Lauderdale 1982; Evans 1980; Rosen and Stein 1980). It is postulated that social isolation reduces exposure of the parent to other parents who could provide a normal and corrective parenting model.

Abusers select children on the basis of age, gender, and physical characteristics—all of which primarily reflect their emotional needs. Those who have been abused may select victims with characteristics that match their own appearance or age when they were first abused. Abusers have been described as passive and inadequate in most aspects of their lives; contact with children gives them feelings of power and control (Hilton and Mezey 1996). Sexual perpetrators may associate themselves with events or circumstances where they have access to children. Examples include youth group activities, schools, recreational facilities, or locations near playgrounds or other areas

that youths may frequently be found. Abusers may seek to "groom" victims, offering them gifts or money in order to gain their trust prior to engaging in any abusive behavior (Hilton and Mezey 1996). Perpetrators are usually gender specific regarding their victims; those who select both male and female victims may have more severe psychopathology (Hilton and Mezey 1996). Intrafamilial victimization or victimization by known perpetrators is generally more common than sexual abuse from an unknown or extrafamilial source (Faller 1994). Less is known about female perpetrators of abuse. Women are less likely to be reported as sexual abusers (Bell 1999). Up to half of female perpetrators reported were adolescent babysitters (Holmes and Slap 1998). Women were less likely to sexually abuse younger boys, and the boys were far less likely to report the abuse or to believe themselves to have been abused (Bell 1999).

Children and adolescents constitute a significant percentage of perpetrators of sexual abuse. Approximately 30%–50% of the instances of sexual abuse are perpetrated by those younger than 18 years, and most young perpetrators initially engage in abusive acts before age 15 years (American Academy of Child and Adolescent Psychiatry 1999). The Federal Bureau of Investigation indicates that 15% of those arrested for forcible rape were younger than 18 years (Ryan et al. 1996). The Uniform Data Collection System developed by the National Adolescent Perpetrator Network has extensively collected sociodemographic information on perpetrators (Ryan et al. 1996). In the study by Ryan and colleagues, nearly 40% of abusive youths reported having been sexually abused themselves. More than 60% were known to school systems as having truancy or behavior or learning problems at school. The majority of female adolescents who abuse have themselves been abused. These adolescents were generally abused at younger ages and were three times as likely to have been abused by a female (American Academy of Child and Adolescent Psychiatry 1999; Mathews et al. 1997). Sexually abusive youths most frequently have comorbid conduct disorder (CD), mood disorders, and anxiety disorders (American Academy of Child and Adolescent Psychiatry 1999). The number of psychiatric diagnoses increases as the age of first offense decreases (Shaw et al. 1996).

Clinical Presentation of Child Abuse

Children who are victims of abuse exhibit a variety of emotional and behavioral symptoms. Documentation of all injuries is crucial, with photographic documentation of cutaneous findings. One must consider the possibility of physical abuse in every child who presents with an injury. The age at onset of the sexual abuse plays an important role in subsequent presenting symptoms. The clinician should obtain a careful and thorough history and complete a comprehensive physical examination in every injured child, including radiological and laboratory studies. Indicators suggesting possible abuse include lack of a reasonable explanation for the injury; contradictory, changing, or vague history of the injury; observation of an inappropriate history for the injury; an excessive or inadequate level of concern; and delay in seeking medical attention (Cheung 1999). In addition, a parent who blames an injury on the child's sibling or claims that it was self-inflicted, or a parent with unrealistic and premature expectations of the child, could also be suggestive of abuse (Green 1997). The behavioral observations and findings on clinical examination of the

child described below should suggest an inflicted injury.

■ Behavioral Observations of Physical and Sexual Abuse

The clinician needs to be sensitive to and aware of certain frequently observed behaviors that have been associated with abuse in children.

- Unusually fearful and docile, distrustful, and/or guarded
- Wary of physical contact
- On the alert for danger
- Attempts to meet parents' needs by role reversal
- Afraid to go home
- Angry reactions and delinquent behaviors
- Hypersexual behavior, self-exposing
- Artwork or play with themes of sexual activity or aggression
- Substance abuse
- Suicidality
- Fire-setting behavior

■ Medical Findings of Physical Abuse

The physician should closely examine an injured child for suspicious physical findings suggesting abuse (Cheung 1999; DeAngelis 1992):

- Cutaneous injuries, such as bruises or lacerations in the shape of an object or multiple bruises in areas that are difficult to injure in play (e.g., upper arms, medial thighs)
- Stocking glove distribution burns suggesting immersion, burns on the perineum, burns in recognizable shapes (e.g., an iron), cigarette burns, and especially multiple burns in various stages of healing
- Head injuries, including complex skull fractures with intracranial hemorrhage, retinal hemorrhage, bilateral ocular in-

jury, dental injury, or traumatic hair loss with scalp hematomas

- Ear injuries, including twisting injuries of the lobe and ruptured tympanic membranes
- Skeletal injuries, including posterior rib fractures (especially when there are multiple fractures), multiple fractures in different stages of healing, metaphyseal fractures in long bones of infants, spiral fractures, and femur fractures in a nonambulatory child; also, radiological signs of subperiosteal hemorrhage, epiphyseal separation, periosteal shearing, and periosteal calcification
- Abdominal injuries, including hepatic hematoma, laceration, or hemorrhage and duodenal hematoma or perforation
- Anogenital injuries such as lacerations, scarring or bruising of genitalia, and anal dilatation or scarring
- Chest injuries such as pulmonary contusion, pneumothorax, or pleural effusion

Special attention needs to be paid when examining an infant or toddler for possible physical abuse. In 1972, pediatric radiologist John Caffey coined the term *whiplash shaken baby syndrome* to describe a constellation of clinical findings in infants and toddlers, including retinal hemorrhages, subdural or subarachnoid hemorrhages, and little or no evidence of external cranial trauma. It was postulated that whiplash forces caused subdural hematomas by tearing cortical bridging veins. Serious injuries in infants are rarely accidental unless there is a clear explanation. Head injuries are the leading cause of traumatic childhood death and of child abuse fatalities.

Radiological documentation of skeletal injuries may be the best and first source of evidence of alleged abuse. High-definition radiographs read by a pediatric radi-

ologist are optimal (Scherl et al. 2000). A skeletal survey to identify recent and old fractures is indicated in a child less than age 2 years with suspicious bruising or fractures. Such surveys are not as helpful in children over age 5 years (American Academy of Pediatrics 2001; Bulloch et al. 2000; Cadzow and Armstrong 2000). Bone scans should be performed to identify subtle fractures in children younger than 5 years of age. A magnetic resonance imaging (MRI) study can better identify epiphyseal separations if they are suspected from the plain films. Ultrasound may also be indicated to identify epiphyseal injury (Toomey and Bernstein 2001). Both MRI and computed tomography (CT) scans can assist in determining when the injuries occurred and can also substantiate repeated injuries by documenting changes in the chemical states of hemoglobin in affected areas (Sato et al. 1989). In the event of suspected brain or head injury, a CT scan is the first-line imaging investigation, with its sensitivity to intraparenchymal, subarachnoid, subdural, and epidural hemorrhage and also to mass effect. Due to its relative insensitivity to subarachnoid blood and fractures, an MRI study is considered complementary to a CT scan and should ideally be obtained 2–3 days later if possible. Because MRI may fail to detect acute bleeding, its use should be delayed for 5–7 days in acutely ill children (Cheung 1999). Thoracoabdominal trauma is best evaluated initially by CT scanning (Toomey and Bernstein 2001).

■ Medical Findings of Sexual Abuse

Frequently, the presenting complaints of victims of sexual abuse are vague and may take the form of abdominal pain, headaches, enuresis, encopresis, and sleep dysregulation. Children are often highly secretive or vague regarding such complaints for fear of reprisals coming from the perpetrator. Certain physical findings such as irritation of the vulva, repeated urinary tract infections, hematuria, blood in the stool, or anal fissures can be commonly identified in sexually abused children but are nevertheless nonspecific.

Pediatric consultation is of paramount importance to appropriately consider alternative diagnostic possibilities. Sometimes the presenting symptoms, such as rectal or genital bleeding or sexually transmitted diseases, are highly suggestive of sexual abuse. Specific findings, such as a dilated hymen or anus, bruising, scarring, or perianal tearing, are important findings to discern and to document appropriately (American Academy of Child and Adolescent Psychiatry 1999; Atabaki and Paradise 1999; Hobbs et al. 1995). The presence of sexually transmitted diseases may or may not confirm the occurrence of sexual activity or abuse. Generally, gonorrhea, genital herpes, or syphilis definitively diagnosed in a child outside of the perinatal period usually confirms the occurrence of sexual activity and possible sexual abuse. The presence of human immunodeficiency virus (HIV), chlamydia, or anogenital condylomata acuminata should raise suspicion for sexual abuse but may not represent diagnostic certainty (American Academy of Child and Adolescent Psychiatry 1997; Atabaki and Paradise 1999). Definitive findings confirming sexual activity include pregnancy or the presence of semen. Pregnancy in an adolescent should always prompt an inquiry as to the possibility of sexual abuse. A sexual abuse history is often present in adolescents who become sexually active early, and some reports indicate that up to two-thirds of pregnant adolescents have experienced sexual abuse (Elders and Albert 1998). Emergency room physicians are commonly called on to perform acute evaluations that include crisis management and evidence collection. Physical examination should be done promptly. However, if the abuse has occurred within the past 72 hours, physical examinations should be performed immediately with the goal of obtaining reliable physical evidence. It is recommended that a physician trained in conducting sexual abuse evaluations perform the examination. The examination should be done a minimum number of times by the smallest possible number of clinicians. The assessment should be done as part of a comprehensive physical examination to deemphasize the genital findings. Sexually abused children frequently do not have corroborating physical findings (American Academy of Child and Adolescent Psychiatry 1997). Obtaining evidence from a physical examination is exquisitely important; if physical evidence is present, perpetrators are 2.5 times as likely to receive legal consequences (Palusci et al. 1999).

The American Academy of Pediatrics (1999) has outlined comprehensive guidelines for the necessary physical examination after sexual abuse; among them are the following:

- The examination should not cause additional emotional trauma. Appropriate time must be allowed to account for the child's anxiety.
- Careful explanation of every step should precede the examination.
- Particular attention needs to be given to examination of the mouth, genitals, perineal region, anus, buttocks, and thighs.
- A supportive adult known to the child, as well as a nursing chaperone, should be present.
- The examination should be thorough, including developmental, growth, mental, and emotional factors as well as physical findings.

- History taking should be thorough and ideally should be obtained before the physical examination.
- Care should be taken not to suggest answers to questions.
- If collection of forensic samples is imperative and the child is unable to cooperate, use of sedation should be considered.
- Appropriate agency reporting and thorough documentation of findings as well as the child's statements and behavior are essential.
- The physician should offer reassurance, such as "Your body will heal and recover" (Elders and Albert 1998).

Diagnostic Considerations and Comorbidity

There is increasing evidence that children who are victims of abuse have varying symptoms and sequelae, stemming from the variability in timing, duration, frequency, and specific characteristics of the abuse as well as an individual child's resilience and vulnerability to particular major mental illness. In reviewing the psychological effects of abuse, Cicchetti and Toth (1995) noted a wide range of effects, such as affective dysregulation, disruptive and aggressive behaviors, insecure and atypical attachment patterns, impaired peer relationships with either increased aggression or social withdrawal, and academic underachievement. The same authors also found a high rate of other comorbid psychiatric disorders, including depression, CD, attention-deficit/ hyperactivity disorder (ADHD), oppositional defiant disorder (ODD), and posttraumatic stress disorder (PTSD). Others have reported abuse to be significantly associated with global impairment, poor social competence, major depression, CD, ODD, agoraphobia, overanxious disorder, ADHD, and substance abuse (Famularo et al. 1992; Fisher et al. 1997; Kaplan et al. 1998; Livingston et al. 1993).

Two categories of trauma have been described by Terr (1991). Type I trauma produces typical symptoms of PTSD after a one-time, sudden traumatic event. Type II trauma is the result of long-term repeated exposure to trauma, similar to what many physically or sexually abused youths experience. Type II trauma often results in an array of coping mechanisms such as denial and dissociation rather than symptoms characteristic of PTSD. Terr also noted that CD, ADHD, depression, and dissociative disorders were common conditions in children with histories of type II trauma. Pelcovitz et al. (1994) likewise found higher prevalences of depression, CD, and ODD in their sample of physically abused youths.

Four factors have been suggested to describe the extent to which a child is traumatized by sexual abuse. These include traumatic sexualization, powerlessness, stigmatization, and betrayal, rendering the youngster powerless, leading to feelings of fear, anxiety, and helplessness (Finkelhor and Browne 1986). Schetky and Green (1988) cite other factors that influence the sexually abused child's symptomatology and outcome. These are the age and developmental level of the child; the onset, duration, and frequency of the abuse; the degree of coercion and physical trauma; the relationship between the child and the perpetrator; the child's preexisting personality; and the interaction between acute and long-term variables.

■ Neurodevelopmental Impact of Abuse

Traumatic events are overwhelming, and lead to disrupted brain homeostasis and a maladaptive compensatory response (Perry and Pollard 1998). Sustained stress leads to overstimulation of the hypothalamic-pituitary-adrenal (HPA) axis and subsequently to elevated cortisol levels (Bremner et al. 2003). Theoretically, all parts of the brain may be affected: the cortex, limbic system, midbrain, and brain stem, with powerful traumatic memories created. Altered cortical homeostasis affects cognitive or narrative memory, altered limbic homeostasis affects emotional memory, altered midbrain homeostasis affects motor memory, and altered brain-stem homeostasis may affect physiological state memories (Castro-Alamancos and Connors 1996; LeDoux et al. 1989; Perry and Pollard 1998; Phillips and LeDoux 1992; Perez 1994).

Altered brain homeostasis affects natural stress responses of hyperarousal and dissociation. Hyperarousal, or "fight or flight," naturally involves activation of the sympathetic nervous system via the norepinephrine neurons in the locus coeruleus of the midbrain. Interaction between the locus coeruleus and the HPA axis results in increase in the release of adrenocorticotropin and cortisol to prepare the body for defense (Perry and Pollard 1998). Arousal, startle responses, vigilance, irritability, and sleep are all affected by this activation. Abused youths exhibit impaired sleep efficiency, prolonged sleep latency, and increased activity during sleep (Glod et al. 1997). Chronic activation of the HPA axis and resulting cortisol system alteration may damage the hippocampus (Sapolsky 1996). Adults with PTSD due to severe sexual or physical abuse exhibit decreased hippocampal size, as detected with MRI and positron emission tomography (PET) scans (Bremner et al. 1995, 1997, 2003). Such findings may explain the memory impairment often present in victims of abuse. Studies of abused children have revealed hippocampal and limbic abnormalities, which in turn predispose to memory deficits and emotional dysregulation. Following the acute fear response, the brain creates a set of memories that can be trig-gered by reminders of the trauma. Affected children thus remain in a persistent state of fear, with hypersensitivity and reactivity (Perry and Pollard 1998). The only response to the pain of the abuse may be to activate dissociative mechanisms involving disengagement from the external world by using primitive psychological defenses such as depersonalization, derealization, numbing, and—in extreme cases—catatonia (Perry and Pollard 1998). Dissociation is protective and allows the child to psychologically survive the abuse. Over time, however, it often becomes maladaptive, emerging at inappropriate times.

Cognitive and academic impairment in maltreated youths have been consistently documented in a number of studies (Cahill et al. 1999; Coster et al. 1989; Fox et al. 1988; McFadyen and Kitson 1996; Perry and Pollard 1998). In severely abused children, frontotemporal and anterior brain electroencephalographic abnormalities have been noted (Ito et al. 1993, 1998). Language delays have been reported in abused youths (Fox et al. 1988). Studies of preschool children report significantly decreased intelligence compared with control subjects (Vondra et al. 1990). Wodarski et al. (1990) studied a group of physically abused youths and found that 60% of the neglected youths and 55% of the abused youths had repeated at least one grade, compared with 24% of the comparison group. A 3-year follow-up study of this population found that the language and mathematics scores dropped in the abused group.

■ Attachment Dysregulation

A child's internal representation of his or her attachment figure depends on the availability and responsiveness of the caregiver (Main and Hesse 1990). Research has shown that the way a child thinks about his or her relationship with the primary caregivers is related to the child's self-esteem, social competence, peer relationships, arousal, distress, and psychopathology (Crowell 1995). Over time, the infant develops a set of expectations about future interactions based on previous experiences of interactions with the primary caregiver (Bowlby 1982). Ainsworth et al. (1978) proposed that an infant securely attaches to a mother who is sensitive to the infant's needs. Insensitive or unresponsive parenting leads to insecure attachments, subcategorized insecure attachments as anxious/avoidant, anxious/ambivalent and disorganized attachment. Abusive parenting is associated with insecure attachments, often of the disorganized type, which in turn often leads to later psychopathology in the infant. In a review of the impact of child maltreatment on subsequent attachment patterns (Morton and Browne 1998), 11 of 13 studies found that compared with control children, significantly more maltreated infants displayed insecure attachments. Children exposed to abusive parenting are excessively sensitized in their arousal level, emotional regulation, and behavioral reactivity and are at risk for later developing neuropsychiatric problems (Perry and Pollard 1998). Conversely, Gunnar (1998) suggested that the security of attachment between an infant and caregiver buffers stress by downregulating the HPA axis. Numerous studies have identified the key role of a responsive, predictable, and nurturing caregiver in the development of a healthy neurobiological stress response (Perry and Pollard 1998). During the first 2 years of life, there is a genetically programmed overproduction of axons, dendrites, and synapses in the brain, with subsequent pruning of those not used (Singer 1995). The environment thus influences which synaptic connections survive (Glaser 2000), possibly explaining the power of physical abuse in derailing secure attachments and healthy outcomes. The work of Lyons-Ruth et al. (1990) and of

Beardslee et al. (1997) has shown that healthy infant–parent attachment promotes optimal development and protects against adverse outcomes.

■ Aggression

The most frequent sequelae of abuse is aggression. Abused preschool children engage in aggressive behavior more frequently than their peers (Klimes-Dougan and Kistner 1990), and they more often attribute hostile intent to their peers (Dodge et al. 1990). Abused children have also been reported to be at risk for violent criminal behavior in adolescence (Herrenkohl et al. 1997) and in adulthood (Widom 1989). Adolescents with a history of abuse are also reported to engage in more aggression with their peers and within their dating relationships (Wolfe et al.1998). Pathological defense mechanisms may also play a role, including identification with the aggressor. It is known that the repeated infliction of pain can lead to aggression, well illustrated in the training of fighting dogs and bulls (Berkowitz 1984). Lewis (1996) wrote that abusive experiences provide a model for violence, teach aggression through reinforcement, inflict pain, and cause central nervous system injuries associated with impulsivity, emotional lability, and impaired judgment. Furthermore, this experience creates a sense of being endangered and thus increases paranoid feelings and diminishes the child's capacity to recognize feelings and put them into words, not actions.

■ Substance Abuse and Self-Injurious Behavior

Children may resort to behaviors that facilitate opioid mediated dissociation, such as rocking, head banging, and self-mutilation, with these painful stimuli activating the brain's endogenous opiates. Abused children are also more likely to develop substance abuse, likely in a self-medicating fashion. Alcohol serves to reduce anxiety, opiates trigger soothing dissociation, and stimulants activate meso-limbic dopaminergic reward areas in children with few true rewards in their lives (Perry and Pollard 1998).

■ Attention-Deficit/Hyperactivity Disorder

Studies of abused children have documented a higher prevalence of ADHD in abused children and adolescents. Several explanations have been postulated. It is possible that children who have ADHD are more likely to provoke abusive behaviors in adults. Impulsive parents could directly transmit ADHD genetically to their children. However, it is also plausible that the trauma of abuse itself plays a causal role in the development of ADHD symptoms (Famularo et al. 1992; Kaplan et al. 1994; Weinstein et al. 2000; Weiss et al. 1999).

■ Depression and Suicide

Abused infants are prone to affective withdrawal, diminished capacity for pleasure, and a tendency to exhibit negative affects such as sadness and distress (Green 1997). Major depression or dysthymia was reported in 27% of children of latency age who had been abused (Green 1997). Approximately 8% of children and adolescents with documented abuse have a current diagnosis of major depressive disorder, 40% have lifetime major depressive disorder diagnoses, and at least 30% have lifetime disruptive disorder diagnoses (ODD or CD). These prevalence rates are several times higher than those found in community samples of children and adolescents (Kaplan et al. 1999). Depression may be a consequence of abuse or may result in a child being more vulnerable to abuse. Studies also report an association

between abuse in childhood and subsequent suicidal behavior and risk taking (Kaplan et al. 1999). Furthermore, Green (1997) reported increased self-mutilation and suicidal ideation and attempts in children subjected to parental beatings or threatened abandonment by their adult caretakers. Sexually abused girls may be particularly at risk for suicide attempts, independent of other psychopathology (Bergen et al. 2003). Sexual risk taking leads to increased teenage parenthood and exposure to HIV and sexually transmitted diseases (Kaplan et al. 1999; Wozencraft et al. 1991). Depression and suicidal behavior are overrepresented among adolescent inpatients with a history of sexual abuse (Brand et al. 1996; Rew et al. 2001).

■ Dissociative Disorders

Dissociative disorders may result from abuse. Children who dissociate may experience brief psychotic symptoms (for example, hearing command auditory hallucinations). It is relatively common for severely physically abused children to hear voices commanding them to harm themselves or others. As a result, they may be misdiagnosed with a psychotic disorder such as schizophrenia. A dissociating child may also be misdiagnosed with an externalizing disorder—ADHD, ODD, or impulse control disorder. A study of a group of severely abused youngsters in residential treatment found that 23% of the boys met DSM-IV (American Psychiatric Association 1994) criteria for dissociative identity disorder (Yeager and Lewis 2000). Dissociative disorders are difficult to discern in younger children, especially before age 7 when faculties of concrete reasoning are less well developed. It is important to discern the subject of the dissociation. Dissociation may be present in victims of sexual abuse more often than in victims of physical abuse (Kisiel and Lyons 2001). Some children may have dissociative experiences as defense mechanisms or as a manner of reexperiencing or gaining understanding and mastery over the abusive experience.

■ Anxiety Disorders and Posttraumatic Stress Disorder

Anxiety disorders may take many forms, including phobias, social anxiety, generalized anxiety disorder, and PTSD. Symptoms of PTSD include fear reactions, reexperiencing phenomena, flashbacks, sleep disruption, exaggerated startle response, and hyperacuity, as well as general anxiety and deterioration of premorbid functioning. Studies in adolescents have shown that chronicity and severity of abuse increases the likelihood of a PTSD diagnosis (Brand et al. 1996). Famularo et al. (1992) reported that 39% of a cohort of maltreated children were given a diagnosis of PTSD. Talbott (2001) recently reported on the presentation of PTSD in children. Children often display disorganized or agitated behavior rather than the fear, helplessness, and horror described in adults. Repetitive play involving themes of the trauma is common, rather than the classic flashbacks or recurrent and intrusive recollections of the trauma. In her review of trauma leading to PTSD, Terr (1996) wrote that traumatic events, including physical abuse, cause psychic trauma when the child understands that something terrible is happening and that he or she is in danger, senses his or her own helplessness, and registers and stores an implicit or explicit traumatic memory. Soon after a traumatic event, play can be "grim, monotonous, and at times, dangerous." The child often does not make a connection between the play and the trauma. Terr cited protective factors, including intelli-

gence, humor, and relatedness. Only later does the clinician typically see more clearly intrusive thoughts, fears, and repeated dreams. A foreshortened sense of the future is common in abused children and can lead to reckless risk taking. Unconscious reenactment of the trauma can lead to retraumatization of the child. In some cases, this reenactment can be dangerous to the child or to others. Pelcovitz et al. (1994) studied the prevalence of PTSD in physically abused adolescents and found that these youths may be more at risk for behavioral, emotional, and social difficulties than for clear PTSD. This is in contrast to the previous work of Green (1997), who found that physically abused adolescents were at risk for developing PTSD. Pelcovitz et al. (1994) suggested that physically abused adolescents may "enact" the results of their victimization rather than express their reactions to the abuse via symptoms of PTSD. The authors point out the differences between physical and sexual assaults, with sexual abuse often accompanied by a higher level of secrecy and shame, which may reinforce the emergence of PTSD symptoms. External signs of physical abuse, such as bruises and fractures, may lead to more support, facilitating integration of the trauma. Pelcovitz et al. (1994) added that an alternative possibility is that the physically abused youths in their study did not manifest PTSD symptoms because they remained in an abusive environment. There can be a delay in the onset of PTSD symptoms until after the trauma has ended.

Treatment

■ Prevention

The cornerstone of treatment of children who are victims of abuse is first to make certain that the child is protected from further injury. The next step is generally to ensure the safety of the child both from becoming victimized by further abuse and from potential sequelae of the abuse. Reporting to child protective services needs to occur as soon as possible, preferably in the context of the initial evaluation or first disclosure. Even more important is to prevent abuse from occurring at all. Kaplan (1996) reviewed three types of child abuse primary prevention strategies: 1) competency enhancement with parent education programs; 2) media campaigns, hotlines, and parent socialization programs; and 3) targeting high-risk groups, such as single parents and teenage parents. Other high-risk groups of parents include those of low socioeconomic status and those with neurocognitively compromised children. Research has shown that maltreated children with healthier ego resiliency, ego overcontrol, and self-esteem fared better in their overall adjustment compared with abused peers lacking these strengths (Glaser 2000). A focus of treatment should therefore be helping abused youths gain better control over their urges and actions and better self-awareness, ultimately creating a coherent narrative of their life story. This is a complex undertaking, due in part to the likelihood that ego control and ego resilience are at least in part temperamentally determined and that self-esteem is influenced by nurturance (Glaser 2000). Because brain development is related to environmental forces, intense and early intervention offers the greatest hope for healthier outcomes. Leventhal (2001) described two home-based models for preventing child abuse and neglect: Research on the effectiveness of these two models has shown that families can be helped and that the effects are sustained over many years. However, home visiting does not cure all difficulties. When high levels of domestic violence are present, it

is difficult for parents to improve their parenting by the use of home visits.

The Centers for Disease Control and Prevention developed important summary recommendations to raise awareness of and improve efforts for primary prevention (McMahon and Puett 1999). This includes educating children about "bad touch" and empowering them to resist abusers (Durfee 1989). School-based primary prevention programs have been shown to be effective in raising awareness, particularly when used over a long term and with older as well as younger children (Adler and McCain 1994; Davis and Gidycz 2000; Hebert et al. 2001; MacIntyre and Carr 1999). Recent efforts have included providing outreach to adults who are abusers or victims themselves (Chasan-Taber and Tabachnick 1999).

Leventhal (2001) wrote that fathers need specific attention, because as much as two-thirds of serious physical abuse is caused by males in the family. Typically, these men have little experience caring for young children, have difficulties with their own impulse control, and tend to be violent toward their partners. One strategy is to empower women to leave their partners and to make better future decisions. Another strategy is to help men be more nurturing and effective as parents. Prevention strategies based on attachment theory focus on improving the caregiver–child relationship, which in turn buffers the child against life stressors. A number of studies have attempted to change insecure attachment relationships to secure ones (Morton and Browne 1998). Interventions focusing on enhancing parental sensitivity were more successful in changing attachment status than were more in-depth interventions that focused on the intrapsychic representational model.

Lyons-Ruth et al. (1990) examined attachment patterns among infants at social risk, measuring development, mother–infant interaction, and maternal depression and social contacts while also evaluating the efficacy of home visits in improving the security of a child's attachment to the caregiver. The home visiting service had four goals: 1) providing an accepting relationship; 2) increasing the family's competence in accessing resources; 3) modeling and reinforcing more interactive, positive, and developmentally appropriate exchanges between mother and infant, emphasizing the mother's dual role as teacher and source of emotional security for her infant; and 4) decreasing social isolation with a weekly parenting group or a monthly social hour. Psychodynamic interventions, based on the work of Fraiberg (1980), and behavioral interventions were used. The authors reported that "at 18 months of age, infants of depressed mothers who received home visiting services outperformed unserved infants of depressed mothers by a mean of 10 points on the Bayley Mental Development Index, and were twice as likely to be classified as securely attached in their relationships with their mothers" (Lyons-Ruth et al. 1990, p. 95). Because a secure attachment has been associated with lower risk of abuse, this could be a powerful intervention to decrease the risk of physical maltreatment.

■ Child and Parent Treatment

The major goals of treatment are first to protect the child and strengthen the family, and then to address the impact of past abuse in treatment of the child and the family. The ecological model calls for a focus on the multidimensional aspects of child abuse, rather than just on the abusive parent (as has been done in traditional child abuse programs). Attachment theory has emphasized the interactive aspects of maltreatment and the importance of intervening in changing the parent–child relationship, with the hope of

facilitating a more secure attachment between child and parent. Therapeutic techniques vary depending on the developmental level of the child.

Family-based therapy needs to improve the parents' devalued self-image, reverse distortions of their child that can lead to scapegoating, interpret any links between the current abuse and the parent's own abuse history, and provide the parent with a positive model of raising children. Green (1997) has suggested using therapeutic nurseries to treat infants and pathological parent–child interactions, with dyadic parent–child therapy serving as the foundation of treatment. Psychotherapy of the child should include creating a therapeutic environment, either in individual or group settings, that allows the child to master the trauma. According to Green (1997), "The retrieval and integration of traumatic memories will gradually enable the child to verbalize memories and feelings associated with the abuse rather than acting them out in a repetitive manner. Impulse control is strengthened by imposing limits on the direct expression of aggression, such as hitting or destroying play materials, and encouraging the verbalization of anger. Self-esteem gradually improves during the child's exposure to the climate of acceptance generated by the therapist, which gradually neutralizes the child's mistrust and hypervigilance" (p. 694). The child must be told that the abuse is not his or her fault and that he or she is not to be blamed. Terr (1996) reminded clinicians of the need to explore issues of betrayal, overexcitement, and personal responsibility, especially in children who have been abused within their own families. Play therapy is useful in the treatment of a traumatized child (Pynoos and Eth 1986; Terr 1996). Play and drawing allow for safe displacement of the complex thoughts and feelings stemming from the abuse and help the child to use nonverbal and symbolic expressions of events that are too painful to be expressed in words. A goal of therapy should be helping the child use healthier coping responses.

Clinicians should be sensitive to the consequences that may ensue following the results of disclosure and should not make impossible promises regarding reporting events to the appropriate authorities. A successful therapeutic alliance is important and this may mean selecting therapists of the same gender and avoiding undue physical similarity to perpetrators. Adolescent girls may be more resistant to discussing certain topics of abuse with a male counselor (Moon et al. 2000). Individual cases merit specific consideration in terms of the mode, duration, and frequency of therapy; flexibility on the part of the therapist is essential. The overall goals of treatment must be clearly focused on behavioral and functional areas that need improvement.

Group therapy may benefit older adolescents who have relatively positive self-esteem. Ideal candidates for group therapy have emotional and cognitive capacities both to benefit from the experience and not to impair the treatment of others (Sturkie 1994). Specific activities, including role-playing and games to improve communication skills, can be effective in group settings (Celano 1990). When recommending group treatment, consideration also depends on pending legal proceedings (Faller 1994). It may be inadvisable to involve a victim in group treatment before the individual is to give legal testimony because the information may be rejected or perceived as having been contaminated by suggestion from others. Family therapy or individual therapy for a parent is often necessary to assist caregivers in coming to terms with their own responses to the child's victimization (Grosz et al. 2000). Nonoffending

parents often have issues of guilt or depression regarding the fact that they were unable to prevent the child's victimization. Treatment that includes individual therapy for nonoffending parents can improve the psychosocial functioning of the abused child (Celano et al. 1996). Furthermore, a parent's own issues of childhood sexual abuse may emerge and may ultimately be disclosed coincidentally with the child's treatment. Family therapy can help to establish appropriate boundaries and roles for family members and can help avoid scapegoating the victim (Hilton and Mezey 1996).

Pharmacotherapy can also improve the outcome of abused children, especially if they are manifesting symptoms of PTSD. According to anecdotal reports (Kaplan et al. 1999; Terr 1991), propranolol decreased hyperarousal and hypervigilance in abused children. Clonidine has also helped to reduce symptoms of hyperarousal, aggression, and insomnia in abused preschool children with PTSD (Harmon and Riggs 1996).

Guanfacine was found to help alleviate sleep disturbances in boys with PTSD (Leonard 1999). Individual child and parental vulnerability, family dysfunction, and environmental stress variables all need to be addressed if the treatment is to be successful. In most states, abused and neglected children who are involved in court proceedings receive court-appointed guardians. Kaplan and colleagues (1999) noted that children and parents in maltreatment cases are often not routinely screened for psychopathology and substance abuse. These authors recommend that psychiatrists should be routinely involved as members of hospital child protection committees.

Cognitive-behavioral therapy has been shown to be superior to supportive counseling in a 12-month follow-up study (Cohen and Mannarino 1998). Cognitive-behavioral treatment may have particular utility in children who have PTSD symptoms (Deblinger et al. 1999). A recent randomized, controlled trial reported that trauma-focused cognitive-behavioral therapy not only improves PTSD symptoms, but also attributions of abuse, shame, depression, and other behavior problems (Cohen et al. 2004). In any abuse-specific therapy it is important to consider the notion of retraumatization. Therapists must be exceedingly sensitive to issues of resistance and the pace that is necessary for successful treatment. Many victims may not directly confront the realities of their abuse but instead may benefit sufficiently from a problem-oriented approach or supportive approach. Despite this fact, it is prudent for the therapist early on to make clear the reason for the initiation of the therapy and to point out behavior patterns that may be maladaptive as a result.

Positive outcomes can be enhanced with rapid, early, and effective psychotherapeutic interventions. Positive outcomes are possible despite egregious abuse scenarios. Prognosis after abuse depends on many factors, including familial, demographic, and treatment characteristics. A degree of stability within the family plays an important role. In general, parent support and involvement in treatment along with the affected child yields a significantly better outcome (Cohen and Mannarino 1996, 1998; Tremblay et al. 1999).

Heller and colleagues(1999) reviewed the literature on resilience to the effects of child maltreatment. Dispositional or temperamental attributes of the child include above-average intelligence, high self-esteem, internal locus of control, external attribution of blame, presence of spirituality, ego resilience, and high ego control. Familial cohesion including competent foster care has been related to developing resilience in children. Extrafamilial support such as a positive school experience promotes resilience, which in turn likely increases individual self-worth and sense of control over one's destiny. Rutter (1990) has suggested that resilience is probably not a fixed state but is rather a malleable and organic trait, which can be enhanced with a nurturing environment and may buffer the impact of abuse and promote a positive sense of one's worth.

Legal Considerations

Legal considerations are important in the initial stages of evaluation. Physicians and mental health clinicians are mandated by all 50 states to report suspected cases of child sexual abuse. The specific requirements in terms of timing, level of suspicion, and other details vary according to state guidelines. Most important is prompt referral to a child protective services organization to ensure appropriate collection and validation of forensic information. The forensic evaluation should be performed by a clinician who is trained in forensic assessment; this individual usually should not be the physician or therapist who is involved in ongoing treatment. Confidentiality issues must be clarified before a forensic evaluation. The fact that an evaluation is being done for purposes of court proceedings needs to be made clear to the parents and child from the outset. Treating clinicians should document direct statements of disclosure in the medical record, preferably as quotations. Depending on specific legal circumstances, such information may obviate the need for direct testimony from the child victim (Kermani 1993). Guidelines for forensic evaluation of children have been published by the American Academy of Child and Adolescent Psychiatry (1988, 1997,

1999) and by the American Professional Society on the Abuse of Children (1990).

Conclusion

Future research will need to expand the current understanding of the etiology of maltreatment. As Ertem et al. (2000) have noted, widespread assumptions about abuse—such as the adage "once abused, an abuser you will become"—need to be challenged, and when they are found to be fictitious should be discarded. Resilience, a major protective factor, needs to be better studied and better understood. Future studies could examine how resilience can be fostered and supported to minimize the impact of an adverse environment. A better understanding is needed of the complex interactions between risk and protective factors and the protective role of the caregiving relationship in mediating both extrinsic and intrinsic risk factors (Glaser 2000). Neurodevelopmental research must continue to explore the impact of abuse and neglect on the developing child's brain and the subsequent emotional and behavioral dysregulation and derailment of social development. This understanding can support the development of more effective psychotherapeutic interventions. The role of dissociation in the symptoms displayed by the abused child also needs to be better understood. Stress has been shown to have a suppressive effect on hippocampal neurogenesis, which in turn likely negatively affects the consolidation of memory and may play a role in the development of dissociation. Juvenile victimization would greatly benefit from assessment instruments that are comprehensive, methodologically sound, and relevant to settings such as health and mental health clinics, criminal justice institutions, and child protection agencies (Hamby and Finkelhor 2000).

Finally, early intervention and preventive programs must be developed to work with at-risk parents to promote a secure attachment pattern, which has been associated with later psychological well-being.

References

Adler NA, McCain JL: Prevention of child abuse: issues for the mental health practitioner. Child Adolesc Psychiatr Clin N Am 3:679–693, 1994

Ainsworth MDS, Blehar MC, Waters E, et al: Patterns of Attachment: A Psychological Study of the Strange Situation. Hillsdale, NJ, Lawrence Erlbaum, 1978

American Academy of Child and Adolescent Psychiatry: Guidelines for the clinical evaluation of child and adolescent sexual abuse. J Am Acad Child Adolesc Psychiatry 27:655–657, 1988

American Academy of Child and Adolescent Psychiatry: Practice parameters for the forensic evaluation of children and adolescents who may have been physically or sexually abused. J Am Acad Child Adolesc Psychiatry 36:423–442, 1997

American Academy of Child and Adolescent Psychiatry: Practice parameters for the assessment and treatment of children and adolescents who are sexually abusive of others. J Am Acad Child Adolesc Psychiatry 38 (12 suppl):55S–76S, 1999

American Academy of Pediatrics, Committee on Child Abuse and Neglect: Guidelines for the evaluation of sexual abuse of children: subject review. Pediatrics 103:186–191, 1999

American Academy of Pediatrics, Committee on Child Abuse and Neglect: Shaken baby syndrome: rotational cranial injuries—technical report. Pediatrics 108:206–210, 2001

American Professional Society on the Abuse of Children: Guidelines for Psychosocial Evaluation of Suspected Sexual Abuse in Young Children. Chicago, IL, American Professional Society on the Abuse of Children, 1990

American Psychiatric Association: Diagnostic and Statistical Manual of Mental Disorders, 4th Edition. Washington, DC, American Psychiatric Association, 1994

Anderson S, Lauderdale M: Characteristics of abusive parents: a look at self-esteem. Child Abuse Negl 6:285–293, 1982

Atabaki S, Paradise JE: The medical evaluation of the sexually abused child: lessons from a decade of research. Pediatrics 104 (1 suppl):178–186, 1999

Beardslee WR, Salt P, Versage EM, et al: Sustaining change in parents receiving preventive interventions for families with depression. Am J Psychiatry 154:510–515, 1997

Bell K: Female offenders of sexual assault. J Emerg Nurs 25:241–243, 1999

Belsky J: Child maltreatment: an ecological integration. Am Psychol 35:320–335, 1980

Bergen HA, Martin G, Richardson AS, et al: Sexual abuse and suicidal behavior: a model constructed from a large community sample of adolescents. J Am Acad Child Adolesc Psychiatry 42:1301–1309, 2003

Berkowitz L: Physical pain and the inclination to aggression, in Biological Perspectives on Aggression. Edited by Flannelly KJ, Blanchard RJ, Blanchard DC. New York, Alan R Liss, 1984, pp 27–47

Bowlby J: Attachment and Loss, 2nd Edition, Vol 1: Attachment. London, Hogarth Press, 1982

Brand EF, King CA, Olson E, et al: Depressed adolescents with a history of sexual abuse: diagnostic comorbidity and suicidality. J Am Acad Child Adolesc Psychiatry 35:34–41, 1996

Bremner JD, Randall P, Scott TM, et al: Deficits in short-term memory in adult survivors of childhood abuse. Psychiatry Res 59:97–107, 1995

Bremner JD, Randall P, Vermetten E, et al: MRI-based measurement of hippocampal volume in PTSD related to childhood physical and sexual abuse: a preliminary report. Biol Psychiatry 41:23–32, 1997

Bremner JD, Vythilingam M, Vermetten E, et al: MRI and PET study of deficits in hippocampal structure and function in women with childhood sexual abuse and posttraumatic stress disorder. Am J Psychiatry 160:924–932, 2003

Bulloch B, Schubert CJ, Brophy PD, et al: Cause and clinical characteristics of rib fractures in infants. Pediatrics 105:148, 2000

Cadzow SP, Armstrong KL: Rib fractures in infants: red alert! The clinical features, investigation, and child protection outcomes. J Paediatr Child Health 36:322–326, 2000

Cahill LT, Kaminer RK, Johnson PG: Developmental, cognitive, and behavioral sequelae of child abuse. Child Adolesc Psychiatr Clin N Am 8:827–843, 1999

Castro-Alamancos MA, Connors BW: Short-term plasticity of a thalamocortical pathway dynamically modulated by behavioral state. Science 272:274–276, 1996

Celano MP: Activities and games for group psychotherapy with sexually abused children. Int J Group Psychother 40:419–429, 1990

Celano M, Hazzard A, Webb C, et al: Treatment of traumagenic beliefs among sexually abused girls and their mothers: an evaluation study. J Abnorm Child Psychol 24:1–17, 1996

Chasan-Taber L, Tabachnick J: Evaluation of a child sexual abuse prevention program. Sex Abuse 11:279–292, 1999

Cheung KK: Identifying and documenting findings of physical child abuse and neglect. J Pediatr Health Care 13:142–143, 1999

Cicchetti D, Toth SL: A developmental psychopathology perspective on child abuse and neglect. J Am Acad Child Adolesc Psychiatry 34:541–565, 1995

Cohen JA, Mannarino AP: Factors that mediate treatment outcome of sexually abused preschool children. J Am Acad Child Adolesc Psychiatry 34:1402–1410, 1996

Cohen JA, Mannarino AP: Factors that mediate treatment outcome of sexually abused preschool children: six and 12 month follow-up. J Am Acad Child Adolesc Psychiatry 37:44–51, 1998

Cohen JA, Deblinger E, Mannarino AP, et al: A multisite, randomized controlled trial for children with sexual abuse–related PTSD symptoms. J Am Acad Child Adolesc Psychiatry 43:393–402, 2004

Coster WJ, Gersten MS, Beeghly M, et al: Communicative functioning in maltreated toddlers. Dev Psychol 25:777–793, 1989

Crowell JA: A review of adult attachment measures: implications for theory and research. Social Development 4:294–327, 1995

Davis MK, Gidycz CA: Child sexual abuse prevention programs: a meta-analysis. J Clin Child Psychol 29:257–265, 2000

DeAngelis C: Clinical indicators of child abuse, in Clinical Handbook of Child Psychiatry and the Law. Edited by Schetky DH, Benedek EP. Baltimore, MD, Williams & Wilkins, 1992, pp 104–118

Deblinger E, Steer RA, Lippman J: Two-year follow-up study of cognitive behavioral therapy for sexually abused children suffering posttraumatic stress symptoms. Child Abuse Negl 23:1371–1378, 1999

Dodge KA, Bates JE, Pettit GS: Mechanisms in the cycle of violence. Science 250:1678–1683, 1990

Durfee M: Prevention of child sexual abuse. Psychiatr Clin North Am 12:445–453, 1989

Egeland B, Jacobvitz D, Sroufe LA: Breaking the cycle of abuse. Child Dev 59:1080–1088, 1988

Egeland B, Carlson E, Sroufe LA: Resilience as process. Dev Psychopathol 5:517–528, 1993

Elders JM, Albert AE: Adolescent pregnancy and sexual abuse. JAMA 280:648–649, 1998

English DJ, Marshall DB, Brummer S, et al: Characteristics of repeated referrals to child protective services in Washington State. Child Maltreatment 4:297–307, 1999

Ertem IO, Leventhal JM, Dobbs S: Intergenerational continuity of child physical abuse: how good is the evidence? Lancet 356:814–819, 2000

Evans A: Personality characteristics and disciplinary attitudes of child-abusing mothers. Child Abuse Negl 4:179–187, 1980

Faller KC: Extrafamilial sexual abuse. Child Adolesc Psychiatr Clin North Am 3:713–727, 1994

Famularo R, Kinscherff R, Fenton T: Psychiatric diagnoses of maltreated children: preliminary findings. J Am Acad Child Adolesc Psychiatry 31:863–867, 1992

Fergusson DM, Horwood LJ, Lynskey MT: Childhood sexual abuse and psychiatric disorder in young adulthood, II: psychiatric outcomes of childhood sexual abuse. J Am Acad Child Adolesc Psychiatry 34:1365–1374, 1996

Finkelhor D, Berliner L: Research on the treatment of sexually abused children: a review and recommendations. J Am Acad Child Adolesc Psychiatry 34:1408–1423, 1995

Finkelhor D, Browne A: Initial and long-term effects: conceptual framework, in Sourcebook on Child Sexual Abuse. Edited by Finkelhor D. Beverly Hills, CA, Sage, 1986, pp 180–198

Finkelhor D, Hotaling G, Lewis IA, et al: Sexual abuse in a national survey of adult men and women: prevalence, characteristics, and risk factors. Child Abuse Negl 14:19–28, 1990

Fisher AJ, Kramer RA, Hoven CW, et al: Psychosocial characteristics of physically abused children and adolescents. J Am Acad Child Adolesc Psychiatry 36:123–131, 1997

Fox L, Long SH, Anglois A: Patterns of language comprehension deficit in abused and neglected children. J Speech Hear Disord 53:239–244, 1988

Fraiberg S (ed): Clinical Studies in Infant Mental Health. New York, Basic Books, 1980

Friedrich WN, Fisher J, Broughton D, et al: Normative sexual behavior in children: a contemporary sample. Pediatrics 101(4):E9, 1998

Fromuth ME, Burkhart BR: Long-term psychological correlates of childhood sexual abuse in two samples of college men. Child Abuse Negl 13:533–542, 1989

Glaser D: Child abuse and neglect and the brain: a review. J Child Psychol Psychiatry 41(1):97–116, 2000

Glasser M, Kolvin I, Campbell D, et al: Cycle of child sexual abuse: links between being a victim and becoming a perpetrator. Br J Psychiatry 179:482–494, 2001

Glod CA, Teicher MH, Hartman CR, et al: Increased nocturnal activity and impaired sleep maintenance in abused children. J Am Acad Child Adolesc Psychiatry 36:1236–1243, 1997

Green AH: Child sexual abuse: immediate and long-term effects and intervention. J Am Acad Child Adolesc Psychiatry 32:890–902, 1993

Green AH: Physical abuse of children, in Textbook of Child and Adolescent Psychiatry, 2nd Edition. Edited by Weiner JM. Washington DC, American Psychiatric Press, 1997, pp 687–697

Grosz CA, Kempe RS, Kelly M: Extrafamilial sexual abuse: treatment for child victims and their families. Child Abuse Negl 24:9–23, 2000

Gunnar M: Quality of early care and buffering of neuroendocrine stress reactions: potential effects on the developing human brain. Prev Med 27:208–211, 1998

Hamby SL, Finkelhor D: The victimization of children: recommendations for assessment and instrument development. J Am Acad Child Adolesc Psychiatry 39:829–840, 2000

Harmon RJ, Riggs PD: Clonidine for posttraumatic stress disorder in preschool children. J Am Acad Child Adolesc Psychiatry 35:1247–1249, 1996

Haugaard JJ: The challenge of defining child sexual abuse. Am Psychol 55:1036–1039, 2000

Hebert M, Lavoie F, Piche C, et al: Proximate effects of a child sexual abuse prevention program in elementary school children. Child Abuse Negl 25:505–522, 2001

Heller SS, Larrieu JA, D'Imperio R, et al: Research on resilience to child maltreatment: empirical considerations. Child Abuse Negl 23:321–338, 1999

Herman JL: Trauma and Recovery. New York, Basic Books, 1992

Herrenkohl RC, Egolf BP, Herrenkohl EC: Preschool antecedents of adolescent assaultive behavior: a longitudinal study. Am J Orthopsychiatry 67:422–432, 1997

Hilton MR, Mezey GC: Victims and perpetrators of child sexual abuse. Br J Psychiatry 169:408–421, 1996

Hobbs CJ, Wynne JM, Thomas AJ: Colposcopic genital findings in prepubertal girls assessed for sexual abuse. Arch Dis Child 73:465–469, 1995

Holmes WC, Slap GB: Sexual abuse of boys: definition, prevalence, correlates, sequelae, and management. JAMA 280:1855–1862, 1998

Ito Y, Teicher MH, Glod CA, et al: Increased prevalence of electrophysiological abnormalities in children with psychological, physical and sexual abuse. J Neuropsychiatry Clin Neurosci 5:401–408, 1993

Ito Y, Teicher MH, Glod CA, et al: Preliminary evidence for aberrant cortical development in abused children: a quantitative EEG study. J Neuropsychiatry Clin Neurosci 10:298–307, 1998

Kaplan SJ: Physical abuse and neglect, in Child and Adolescent Psychiatry: A Comprehensive Textbook, 2nd Edition. Edited by Lewis M. Baltimore, MD, Williams & Wilkins 1996, pp 1033–1041

Kaplan SJ, Pelcovitz D, Weiner M: Adolescent physical abuse. Child Adolesc Psychiatr Clin N Am 3:695–711, 1994

Kaplan SJ, Pelcovitz D, Salzinger S, et al: Adolescent physical abuse: risk for adolescent psychiatric disorders. Am J Psychiatry 155:954–959, 1998

Kaplan SJ, Pelcovitz D, Labruna V: Child and adolescent abuse and neglect research: a review of the past 10 years, I: physical and emotional abuse and neglect. J Am Acad Child Adolesc Psychiatry 38:1214–1222, 1999

Kaufman J, Zigler E: Do abused children become abusive parents? Am J Orthopsychiatry 57:186–192, 1987

Keenan HT, Runyan DK, Marshall SW, et al: A population-based study of inflicted traumatic brain injury in young children. JAMA 290:621–626, 2003

Kempe CH: Sexual abuse, another hidden pediatric problem: the 1977 C. Anderson Aldrich Lecture. Pediatrics 62:382–389, 1978

Kempe CH, Silverman FN, Steele BF, et al: The battered child syndrome. JAMA 181:17–24, 1962

Kermani EJ: Child sexual abuse revisited by the U.S. Supreme Court. J Am Acad Child Adolesc Psychiatry 32:971–974, 1993

Kisiel CL, Lyons JS: Dissociation as a mediator of psychopathology among sexually abused children and adolescents. Am J Psychiatry 158:1034–1039, 2001

Klimes-Dougan B, Kistner J: Physically abused preschoolers' responses to peers' distress. Dev Psychol 26:599–602, 1990

Kuntz J, Bahr SJ: A profile of parental homicide against children. J Fam Violence 11:347–362, 1996

LeDoux JE, Romanski L, Xagoraris A: Indelibility of subcortical emotional memories. J Cogn Neurosci 1:238–243, 1989

Leonard H: Guanfacine alleviates sleep disorders in boys with PTSD. Brown University Child and Adolescent Psychopharmacology Update, October 1999, p 1

Leventhal JM: The prevention of child abuse and neglect: successfully out of the blocks. Child Abuse Negl 25:431–439, 2001

Lewis DO: From abuse to violence: psychophysiological consequences of maltreatment. J Am Acad Child Adolesc Psychiatry 31:383–391, 1992

Lewis DO: Development of the symptom of violence, in Child and Adolescent Psychiatry: A Comprehensive Textbook, 2nd Edition. Edited by Lewis M. Baltimore, MD, Williams & Wilkins, 1996, pp 334–344

Livingston R, Lawson L, Jones JG: Predictors of self-reported psychopathology in children abused repeatedly by a parent. J Am Acad Child Adolesc Psychiatry 32:948–953, 1993

Lyons-Ruth K, Connell DB, Grunebaum H: Infants at social risk: maternal depression and family support services as mediators of infant development and security of attachment. Child Dev 61:85–98, 1990

MacIntyre D, Carr A: Evaluation of the effectiveness of the stay safe primary prevention programme for child sexual abuse. Child Abuse Negl 23:1307–1325, 1999

Main M, Hesse E: Parents' unresolved traumatic experiences are related to infant disorganized attachment status: is frightened and/or frightening parent behavior the linking mechanism? In Attachment in the Preschool Years: Theory, Research, and Intervention. Edited by Greenberg M, Cicchetti D, Cummings E. Chicago, IL, University of Chicago Press, 1990, pp 161–182

Martin JA, Elmer E: Battered children grown up: a follow-up study of individuals severely maltreated as children. Child Abuse Negl 16:75–87, 1992

Mathews R, Hunter JA, Vuz J: Juvenile female sexual offenders: clinical characteristics and treatment issues. Sex Abuse 9:187–199, 1997

McFadyen RG, Kitson WJH: Language comprehension and expression among adolescents who have experienced childhood physical abuse. J Child Psychol Psychiatry 37:551–562, 1996

McMahon PM, Puett RC: Child sexual abuse as a public health issue: recommendations of an expert panel. Sex Abuse 11:257–266, 1999

Moody CW: Male child sexual abuse. J Pediatr Health Care 13:112–119, 1999

Moon LT, Wagner WG, Kazelskis R: Counseling sexually abused girls: the impact of counselor. Child Abuse Negl 24:753–765, 2000

Morton N, Browne KD: Theory and observation of attachment and its relation to child maltreatment: a review. Child Abuse Negl 22:1093–1104, 1998

Mrazek DA, Mrazek PB: Psychosexual development within the family, in Sexually Abused Children and Their Families. Edited by Mrazek PB, Kempe CH. Oxford, UK, Pergamon, 1981, pp 17–32

Muram D: The medical evaluation in cases of child sexual abuse. J Pediatr Adolesc Gynecol 14:55–64, 2001

Oliver JE: Intergenerational transmission of child abuse: rattles, research, and clinical implications. Am J Psychiatry 150:1315–1324, 1993

Palusci VJ, Cox EO, Cyrus TA, et al: Medical assessment and legal outcome in child sexual abuse. Arch Pediatr Adolesc Med 153:388–392, 1999

Pelcovitz D, Kaplan S, Goldenberg B, et al: Posttraumatic stress disorder in physically abused adolescents. J Am Acad Child Adolesc Psychiatry 33:305–312, 1994

Peluso E, Putman N: Case study: sexual abuse of boys by females. J Am Acad Child Adolesc Psychiatry 35:51–54, 1996

Perez CM, Widom CS: Childhood victimization and long-term intellectual and academic outcomes. Child Abuse Negl 18:617, 1994

Perry BD, Pollard R: Homeostasis, stress, trauma and adaptation—a neurodevelopmental view of childhood trauma. Child Adolesc Psychiatr Clin N Am 7:33–51, 1998

Phillips RG, LeDoux JE: Differential contribution of amygdala and hippocampus to cued and contextual fear conditioning. Behav Neurosci 106:274–285, 1992

Putnam FW: Ten-year research update review: child sexual abuse. J Am Acad Child Adolesc Psychiatry 42:269–278, 2003

Pynoos R, Eth S: Witness to violence: the child interview. J Am Acad Child Adolesc Psychiatry 25:306–319, 1986

Rew L, Taylor-Seehafer M, Fitzgerald ML: Sexual abuse, alcohol and other drug use, and suicidal behaviors in homeless adolescents. Issues Compr Pediatr Nurs 24:225–240, 2001

Rosen B, Stein M: Women who abuse their children. Am J Dis Child 134:947–950, 1980

Rutter M: Psychosocial resilience and protective mechanisms, in Risk and Protective Factors in the Development of Psychopathology. Edited by Rolf J, Masten AS, Cicchetti K, et al. New York, Cambridge University Press, 1990, pp 181–214

Ryan G: Childhood sexuality: a decade of study, I: research and curriculum development. Child Abuse Negl 24:33–48, 2000

Ryan G, Miyoshi TJ, Metzner JL, et al: Trends in a national sample of sexually abusive youths. J Am Acad Child Adolesc Psychiatry 35:17–25, 1996

Sapolsky R: Why stress is bad for your brain. Science 273:749–750, 1996

Sato Y, Yuh WT, Smith WL, et al: Head injury in child abuse: evaluation with MR imaging. Radiology 173:653–657, 1989

Scherl SA, Miller L, Lively N, et al: Accidental and nonaccidental femur fractures in children. Clin Orthop Rel Res 376:96–105, 2000

Schetky D, Green A: Child Sexual Abuse: A Handbook for Health Care and Legal Professionals. New York, Brunner/Mazel, 1988

Sedlak AJ, Broadhurst DD: The Third National Incidence Study of Child Abuse and Neglect. Washington, DC, U.S. Department of Health and Human Services, 1996

Shaw JA, Applegate B, Rothe E: Psychopathology and personality disorders in adolescent sex offenders. Am J Forensic Psychiatry 17:19–37, 1996

Singer W: Development and plasticity of cortical processing architectures. Science 270:758–764, 1995

Smith SM, Hanson R, Noble S: Parents of battered babies: a controlled study. BMJ 4:388–391, 1973

Straus M, Gelles R, Steinmets S: Behind Closed Doors: Violence in the American Family. New York, Anchor Press, 1980

Sturkie K: Group treatment for sexually abused children: clinical wisdom and empirical findings. Child Adolesc Psychiatr Clin N Am 3:813–829, 1994

Talbott JA: Look beyond classic symptoms to spot PTSD in affected kids. Clinical Psychiatry News, October 2001, p 26

Terr LC: Childhood traumas: an outline and overview. Am J Psychiatry 148:10–20, 1991

Terr LC: Acute responses to external events and posttraumatic stress disorder, in Child and Adolescent Psychiatry: A Comprehensive Textbook, 2nd Edition. Edited by Lewis M. Baltimore, MD, Williams & Wilkins, 1996, pp 753–763

Thompson MP, Kingree JB, Desai S: Gender differences in long-term health consequences of physical abuse of children: data from a nationally representative survey. Am J Public Health 94:599–604, 2004

Thompson RA: Social support and the prevention of child maltreatment, in Protecting Children From Abuse and Neglect: Foundations for a New National Strategy. Edited by Melton GB, Barry FD. New York, Guilford, 1994, pp 40–130

Toomey S, Bernstein H: Child abuse and neglect: prevention and intervention. Curr Opin Pediatr 13:211–215, 2001

Tremblay C, Hebert M, Piche C: Coping strategies and social support as mediators of consequences in child sexual abuse victims. Child Abuse Negl 23:929–945, 1999

U.S. Department of Health and Human Services: Abuse and neglect (section HC 210), in Trends in the Well-Being of America's Children and Youth 2001. Washington, DC, Office of the Assistant Secretary for Planning and Evaluation, U.S. Department of Health and Human Services, 2001, pp 142–143

U.S. Department of Health and Human Services: HHS reports new child abuse and neglect statistics. HHS News, April 2, 2001. Available at: http://www.hhs.gov/news/press/2001pres/20010402.html. Accessed July 21, 2003.

Vondra JI, Barnett D, Cicchetti D: Self-concept, motivation, and competence among preschoolers from maltreating and comparison families. Child Abuse Negl 14:525–540, 1990

Weinstein D, Staffelbach D, Biaggio M: Attention-deficit hyperactivity disorder and post-traumatic stress disorder: differential diagnosis in childhood sexual abuse. Clin Psychol Rev 20:359–378, 2000

Weiss EL, Longhurst JG, Mazure CM: Childhood sexual abuse as a risk factor for depression in women: psychosocial and neurobiological correlates. Am J Psychiatry 156:816–828, 1999

Widom CS: Child abuse, neglect, and adult behavior. Criminology 27:251–271, 1989

Wissow LS: Child abuse and neglect. N Engl J Med 332:1425–1431, 1995

Wodarski JS, Kurtz PD, Gaudin JM Jr, et al: Maltreatment and the school age child: major academic, socioemotional, and adaptive outcomes. Soc Work 35:506–513, 1990

Wolfe DA, Wekerle C, Reitzel-Jaffe D, et al: Factors associated with abusive relationships among maltreated and nonmaltreated youth. Dev Psychopathol 10:61–85, 1998

Wozencraft H, Wagner W, Pellegrin A: Depression and suicidal ideation in sexually abused children. Child Abuse Negl 15:505–511, 1991

Wyatt GE, Loeb TB, Solis B, et al: The prevalence and circumstances of child sexual abuse: changes across a decade. Child Abuse Negl 23:45–60, 1999

Yates A: Sexual abuse of children, in Textbook of Child and Adolescent Psychiatry, 2nd Edition. Edited by Wiener JM. Washington, DC, American Psychiatric Press, 1997, pp 699–709

Yeager CA, Lewis DO: Mental illness, neuropsychological deficits, child abuse, and violence. Child Adolesc Psychiatr Clin N Am 9:793–813, 2000

Self-Assessment Questions

Select the single best response for each question.

27.1 Which of the following statements concerning the epidemiology of physical abuse of children is *false?*

    A. Younger children (less than 3 years of age) have the greatest risk of fatal maltreatment.

    B. Homicides occurring during the first week of life are almost exclusively perpetrated by mothers.

    C. Fathers are more likely to fatally injure their children ages 1 week to 13 years.

    D. Fathers committed the majority of parent-perpetrated homicides of children 13–19 years of age.

    E. None of the above.

27.2 Which of the following statements concerning sexual abuse of boys is *false?*

    A. Perpetrators of abuse against boys are most likely to be related to the victim.

    B. Boys are less likely than girls to disclose abuse.

    C. Surveys indicate that as many as 18% of males older than 18 years report having been victims of childhood sexual abuse.

    D. Perpetrators of abuse against boys are most likely to be male.

    E. Sexual abuse of boys may be significantly underreported and untreated.

27.3 Risk factors that may predict recurrence of physical abuse in children include which of the following?

    A. Young age of the child.

    B. Number of previous referrals to child protective services.

    C. History of childhood abuse in the caretaker.

    D. Prematurity, mental retardation, or physical handicaps in the child.

    E. All of the above.

27.4 Perpetrators of sexual abuse

    A. Are often children and adolescents.

    B. Are gender-specific regarding their choice of victims.

    C. Often associate themselves with events or activities in which they have access to children.

    D. May seek to "groom" victims with gifts or money.

    E. All of the above.

27.5 Which of the following characteristics in children should increase a clinician's suspicion of possible physical abuse?

    A. A child who is afraid to leave home.

    B. A child who craves physical contact.

    C. A child with excessive needs for being comforted.

    D. A child who is on the alert for danger.

    E. All of the above.

27.6 Physical findings in an injured child suggestive of physical abuse include which of the following?

    A. Bruises or lacerations in the shape of an object.
    B. Posterior rib fractures.
    C. Anogenital lacerations.
    D. Twisting injuries of the ear lobe.
    E. All of the above.

Suicide and Suicidality

Cynthia R. Pfeffer, M.D.

This chapter reviews risk and protective factors of childhood and adolescent suicidal behavior, assessment and identification of those at risk, and strategies for intervention and prevention.

Diagnostic Criteria, Course, and Prognosis

Suicidal behavior is a psychiatric symptom defined as a preoccupation or act that intentionally aims to inflict injury or death to oneself. Although intent to cause self-injury or to die is essential in the definition, it is not necessary that a child have a mature concept of the finality of death.

Clinicians should evaluate the objective and perceived lethality of an intended suicidal act. Objective lethality involves actual potential for death or serious injury if a self-destructive method is enacted. Children may not appreciate the outcome of self-destructive intent because they may lack an understanding of the effects of a suicidal method. A child who considers a suicide plan to be lethal may be considered at high risk even if the objective lethality is low. Lethality of im-

pulsive suicide attempts is most associated with the availability of lethal suicide methods (e.g., firearms); but lethality of nonimpulsive suicide attempts is most associated with distinct suicide intent and severity of mood and/or substance abuse disorders (Brent 1997).

The diagnosis of suicidal behavior is made by direct inquiry of the child and other informants to ascertain whether the child wishes to kill him- or herself and has a plan for enacting suicide intent. Suicide risk assessment may be complicated by children's immature understanding of cause and effect and inability to discuss suicidal thinking because of anhedonia, psychomotor retardation, psychosis, impulsivity, or poor concentration (Jacobsen et al. 1994). Parents may not report reliably about children's suicidal intent or acts because of their perceived culpability for their children's emotional distress, lack of knowledge of their children's suicidal condition, and stigma of suicidal behavior (Jacobsen et al. 1994).

The best predictor of suicidal behavior is past suicidal acts. Prospective research suggests that prepubertal children who report suicidal ideation or a suicide attempt are three and six times more likely, respectively, to attempt suicide in adolescence (Pfeffer et al. 1993). Psychological autopsy studies suggest that 26% to 33% of children and adolescents who commit suicide attempted suicide previously (Brent et al. 1993; Shaffer et al. 1996). Suicide is 17-fold more likely if there is a history of attempted suicide (Brent et al. 1993).

Differential Diagnosis and Comorbidity

Differential diagnosis for suicidal behavior involves self-mutilation involving superficially cutting oneself or pulling out hair or eyelashes, sexual asphyxiation, and high-risk behaviors, including eating disorders, substance abuse, motor vehicle accidents, and homicide. When superficial cutting is associated with suicidal intent, it is a suicidal act. However, self-mutilation involving superficial cutting of the arms, legs, and other body areas is often associated with stress, dissociative phenomena, and anger. Self-mutilation is not associated with suicidal intent and it is not considered a suicidal act. Trichotillomania, involving pulling out hair or eyelashes or eyebrows, does not involve suicidal intent and is not considered a suicidal act. Sexual asphyxiation occurs when the airway is obstructed while a person is involved in sexual self-stimulation. Adolescents, especially males, have hung themselves during acts of sexual self-stimulation. Sexually stimulating pictures or other objects often are found at the scene of death, and this enables differentiation of suicide from sexual asphyxiation behavior. High-risk behaviors, such as driving above a speed limit or promiscuous sexual behavior, should be differentiated from suicidal behavior by determining whether such behaviors involved suicidal intent.

Suicidal ideation and/or acts are criterion items only for the diagnoses of major depressive and borderline personality disorders (American Psychiatric Association 1994). Although suicidal ideation and acts are integral diagnostic criteria for these disorders, not all individuals with these disorders exhibit suicidal ideation or acts. Furthermore, suicidal behavior is often comorbid with anxiety, conduct, substance abuse, developmental, and personality disorders.

Epidemiology

High suicide rates among 15- to 24-year-olds peaked at a rate of 13.6 per 100,000 in 1977 (Pfeffer 1986). In 2002, 4,010 youth (rate: 9.9 per 100,000), ages 15–24 years, committed suicide (Kochanek et al. 2004). In 2002, 264 children and young adolescents (rate: 0.6 per 100,000), ages 5–14 years, committed suicide (Kochanek et al. 2004).

From 1986 to 1991, suicide among black youth increased more rapidly than that among white youth (Shaffer et al. 1994). The increase in rates of youth suicide is associated with greater availability and use of firearms, the most lethal method of suicide (Boyd and Moscicki 1986). Eighty-six children and young adolescents (rate: 0.2 per 100,000), ages 5–14 years, and 2,088 adolescents (rate: 5.1 per 100,000), ages 15–24 years, died by self-inflicted firearm injuries in 2004 (Kochanek et al. 2004). Compliance of relatives in removing firearms from the home is problematic and a challenge to strategies for suicide prevention (Brent et al. 2000).

The Youth Risk Behavior Surveillance System surveyed health-risk behaviors among a nationally representative sample of 1,270 high school students in ninth through twelfth grades in the United States (Kann et al. 2000). In 1999, 19.3% of students had serious suicidal ideation, with females (24.9%) having significantly higher rates than males (13.7%) (Kann et al. 2000). Approximately 8.3% of the students attempted suicide at least once in the year prior to this survey. Females (10.8%) attempted suicide more often than did males (5.7%). Approximately 2.6% of students' suicide attempts caused serious injury or a need for medical attention. Other reports suggested that approximately 1% of preadolescents in the general population reported a recent suicide attempt (Pfeffer et al. 1984). Approximately 34% of adolescent psychiatric inpatients are hospitalized because of a recent suicide attempt (Pfeffer et al. 1988).

Etiological Risk Factors

Efforts to understand the genetics of suicidal behavior, thought to be the etiological elements of suicidal behavior, focused on abnormalities in the serotonergic neurotransmitter system, believed to be partly under genetic control (Mann et al. 2001). Candidate genes for suicide risk include the 5-HT$_{1B}$ gene and receptor, the tryptophan hydroxylase gene, the serotonin transporter gene, the 5-HT$_{2A}$ receptor and gene, the 5-HT$_{1A}$ receptor and gene, and the monoamine oxidase A gene (Mann et al. 2001).

It is hypothesized also that intermediate phenotypes involving impulsivity, pathological aggression, psychomotor change, and abnormalities of gene products may be related to genetic variants that increase risk for suicidal behavior (Mann et al. 2001). A study of 75 prepubertal psychiatric inpatients and 35 prepubertal nonsuicidal children in the community offered information about intermediate phenotypes for childhood suicidal behavior (Pfeffer et al. 1998). It suggested that mean whole-blood tryptophan content was significantly lower among children with a recent suicide attempt than among nonsuicidal community children or inpatients with recent suicidal ideation. Inpatients with a mood disorder had significantly higher platelet serotonin content than inpatients without a mood disorder.

Childhood environmental stresses were identified as suicide risk factors in a study of 120 adolescent suicide victims and 147 age-, gender-, and race/ethnicity-matched adolescents (Gould et al. 1996). It suggested that risk for suicide was increased by adolescent unemployment or not being a student (odds ratio [OR] = 44.1, 95% confidence interval [CI]=4.5–432.0), adolescent suspension from school (OR=6.1, 95% CI=1.6–23.4), adolescent school dropout (OR=5.1, 95% CI=1.2–20.7), adolescent disciplinary crises (OR=5.1, 95% CI=2.7–9.5), family history of suicidal behavior (OR=4.6, 95% CI=1.8–11.7), poor communication with mother (OR=4.3, 95% CI=1.6–11.6) or father (OR=4.0, 95% CI=1.8–9.0), father's problems with police (OR=4.0, 95% CI=1.5–10.9), adolescent failure of school grade (OR=3.3, 95% CI=1.4–7.7), mother with history of mood disorder (OR=2.0, 95% CI=1.1–3.7), lack of intact family (OR=1.9, 95% CI=1.1–3.3), and loss (OR=1.9, 95% CI=1.1–3.3). In addition, history of physical or sexual abuse, significant risk factors for youth suicidality, should be evaluated, especially among youth with symptoms of depression and hopelessness (Martin et al. 2004).

The National Institute of Mental Health Methods for the Epidemiology of Child and Adolescent Mental Disorders (MECA) Study of a representative sample of 1,285 randomly selected children and adolescents, ages 9–17 years suggested environmental risk factors for nonfatal suicidal behavior. Forty-two adolescents (3.3%) attempted suicide and 67 (5.2%) reported only suicidal ideation (King et al. 2001). After adjusting for demographic features

and psychiatric disorders, those with suicidal ideation or attempts, compared with
those without suicidality, had significantly
higher rates of low parental monitoring
(OR = 5.0, 95% CI=2.4–10.4) and poor
family environment (OR=3.6, 95% CI =
2.2–5.8).

The interactive effects of environmental adversity and a polymorphism in the
promoter region of the serotonin transporter gene was reported to increase risk
for suicidal behavior and major depressive disorder (Caspi et al. 2003). This prospective study of children who were followed into young adulthood suggested
that those young adults who were homo-
zygous or heterozygous for the short (s)
allele in the promoter region of the serotonin transporter gene and who had
heightened childhood adverse events
were at increased risk for suicidal behavior and depression. Those with the long
(l) allele, regardless of the degree of
childhood adverse events, were at lowest
risk for depression and suicidal behavior.
Those who had low childhood adverse
events and the short allele were intermediate in risk for depression and suicidal
behavior.

Other Risk Factors

Multiple research methods have been
utilized to identify youth suicide risk factors. Among prospective studies was a
6- to 8-year follow-up of 69 prepubertal
psychiatric inpatients and 64 nonsuicidal
prepubertal children living in the community (Pfeffer et al. 1993). Prepubertal
mood disorder (relative risk [RR]=5.28,
95% CI=1.76–15.82), prepubertal poor
social adjustment (RR=4.32, 95% CI =
2.15–8.66), adolescent substance abuse
disorder (RR=2.84, 95% CI=1.1–86.83),
and life event stresses (RR=1.71, 95% CI =
1.11–2.64) were all risk factors for adolescent suicide ideation or attempts. A

5-year follow-up study to assess suicide
risk during the transition from adolescence to young adulthood included a
representative sample of 1,709 adolescents, ages 14–18 years (Lewinsohn et al.
2001). Adolescent suicide attempts predicted suicide attempts in young adulthood for females but not for males. Suicide attempt risk was higher for females;
but by age 19 years, it was equal for males
and females. Suicide attempts were predicted for young adult males and females
also by major depression (OR=3.04, 95%
CI=1.15–8.04), negative cognitions (OR =
2.12, 95% CI=1.18–3.81), and poor coping skills (OR=1.07, 95% CI=1.01–1.13).

The significance of major depressive
disorder as a suicide risk factor also was
highlighted in a longitudinal study of 73
adolescents with major depression and 37
adolescents without psychopathology who
were reevaluated 10–15 years later (Weissman et al. 1999). Among the adolescents
with major depression, 7.7% committed
suicide but no adolescent without psychopathology committed suicide. The adolescents with major depressive disorder, compared with those without psychopathology, were significantly more likely to
attempt suicide at least once in their lifetimes (OR=14.3, 95% CI=3.1–65.4) and
at least once during the follow-up period
(OR=5.6, 95% CI=1.2–25.2). A 3-year longitudinal study of 138 children, ages 7–17
years, suggested that adolescent suicide
attempters with major depressive disorder
and impulsivity may be a subgroup of
youngsters with major depression (Myers
et al. 1991).

The significance of psychopathology
as a suicide risk factor was identified in a
4- to 15-year follow-up of 1,331 child psychiatric inpatients that suggested a nine-
fold higher rate of suicide among the inpatients than expected in the general
population (Kuperman et al. 1988). In
general, except for gender, psychiatric

risk factors for youth suicide and serious suicide attempts are similar (Beautrais 2003).

A psychological autopsy study of 67 adolescent suicide victims and 67 demographically matched community selected adolescents suggested relative risks for suicide imparted by major depression (RR=27.0, 95% CI=3.6–199.8), drug abuse (RR=9.0, 95% CI=1.1–71.0), alcohol abuse (RR=7.5, 95% CI=1.7–32.8), and conduct disorder (RR=6.0, 95% CI=1.8–20.4) (Brent et al. 1993). Presence of any psychiatric disorder increased risk by 35-fold (95% CI=4.8–255.4). Another psychological autopsy study of 120 adolescent suicide victims and 147 demographically matched nonsuicidal adolescents suggested that mood disorders (RR= 12.10, 95% CI=5.12–28.57) were risk factors for suicide in males and females (Shaffer et al. 1996). Among males, a prior suicide attempt (RR=19.39, 95% CI=2.32–162.13) and substance abuse (RR=5.76, 95% CI=1.61–20.6) were suicide risk factors.

Personality traits and cognitive styles in individuals younger than 25 years were identified in the Canterbury Suicide Project in Christchurch, New Zealand (Beautrais et al. 1999). Among the 129 youths who attempted suicide, compared with the 153 youths who reported no suicidal behavior, significant risk factors for suicide attempts included hopelessness (OR = 18.5, 95% CI = 4.9–10.0), neuroticism (OR = 5.4, 95% CI = 3.9–7.6), and external locus of control (OR = 2.9, 95% CI = 2.1–4.0). Other studies have suggested that poor self-esteem is correlated with hopelessness in adolescent suicide attempters (Donaldson et al. 2000).

A psychological autopsy study of 58 adolescent suicide victims and 55 demographically matched nonsuicidal adolescents suggested that increased rates of suicide and suicide attempts among first-degree relatives (OR = 5.3, 95% CI = 2.0–14.3) and second-degree relatives (OR = 3.7, 95% CI = 1.6–8.7) of suicide victims, compared with those among relatives of nonsuicidal adolescents, were independent of family rates of psychiatric disorders (Brent et al. 1996a). A comparative family study of 488 first- and 1,062 second-degree relatives of 69 prepubertal psychiatric inpatients and 54 nonsuicidal prepubertal children selected from the community reported that children's suicidal ideation and suicide attempts were significantly associated with suicidal acts of the first-degree relatives (Pfeffer et al. 1994). The first-degree relatives of the suicidal children, compared with those of the nonsuicidal community selected children, also had higher rates of antisocial personality disorder, assaultive behavior, and substance abuse. These studies imply that history of family suicidal behavior and psychopathology should be evaluated in assessments of childhood and adolescent suicidal risk.

A study of 56 lesbian, gay, or bisexual youth, ages 16–21 years, and age- and gender-matched heterosexual youth suggested that sexual orientation was not associated with higher risk for suicidal behavior when severity of depression, hopelessness, substance abuse, and social support were controlled in the statistical analyses (Safren and Heimberg 1999). However, 30% of the minority sexually oriented youth, compared with 13% of the heterosexual youth reported a past suicide attempt. Other studies did not support these findings. A 21-year follow-up study of 1,265 children identified 28 (2.8%) participants who reported being gay, lesbian or bisexual (Fergusson et al. 1999). These sexual minority adolescents were at increased risk for suicidal ideation (OR=5.4, 95% CI=2.4–12.2) and suicide attempts (OR=6.2, 95% CI=2.7–14.3). Higher risk for suicidal ideation

(OR=3.61, 95% CI=1.40–9.36) and suicide attempts (OR=7.10, 95% CI=3.05–16.53) among sexual minority adolescents also was suggested by a study of 394 sexual minority adolescents, compared with 336 gender- and age-matched heterosexual adolescents (Remafedi et al. 1998). Additional research is needed to clarify these risk issues.

Treatment

Two important documents, The Surgeon General's "call to action" report (U.S. Public Health Service 1999) and the "Practice Parameters for the Assessment and Treatment of Children and Adolescents with Suicidal Behavior" (American Academy of Child and Adolescent Psychiatry 2001) summarize for clinicians important principles for treatment and prevention of youth suicidal behavior.

A barrier to suicide prevention is the lack of consistent use of treatment services. This may be affected by the degree of depression and hopelessness of suicidal youths (Barbe et al. 2004). It may be affected also by parental perceptions of their children's mental health treatment as identified in a representative community sample of 206 children and adolescents, ages 9–17 years, who had diagnoses of major depression or dysthymia (Wu et al. 2001). In this study, 36% of children never received professional care, and of those who were treated, only 31% were treated with antidepressants (Wu et al. 2001). Mothers' level of education, children's health insurance, and whether the children had suicidal or other severe psychiatric symptoms were associated with whether the children received antidepressant treatment.

An 18-month follow-up of the outcomes of 140 adolescent female suicide attempters, who received an experimental emergency service intervention that pro-

vided psychoeducation to the family and staff, was compared with follow-up outcomes of female suicide attempters who received emergency service treatment as usual (Rotheram-Borus et al. 2000). The experimental emergency service intervention improved outcomes of adolescent suicide attempters, lowered parental emotional distress, and enhanced family cohesion.

A randomized study of an experimental home-based family intervention, compared with routine treatment, suggested that reduction of suicidal ideation occurred for adolescents who received the experimental family treatment and who did not have mood disorders (Harrington et al. 2000). However, among adolescents with mood disorders, there was no difference in outcome between those who received the experimental family intervention and those who received routine treatment.

It has been recommended that treatments for suicidal youth should focus on decreasing coexisting psychopathology, remediate social and problem-solving deficits, and provide family psychoeducation and intervention (Brent 1997). Cognitive-behavior therapy (CBT) (Brent 1997), dialectical behavior therapy (Katz et al. 2004), and interpersonal psychotherapy (Mufson and Fairbanks 1996) utilize techniques that aim to improve dysfunctional cognitions and decrease impulsive behaviors. Results of a recent empirical treatment trial of depressed adolescents suggested that treatment with fluoxetine medication combined with CBT was significantly more effective than placebo in reducing symptoms of major depressive disorder (Treatment for Adolescents With Depression Study [TADS] Team 2004). This combined treatment was more effective than fluoxetine alone or CBT alone. Additional research is needed to evaluate the efficacy of such treatments for adolescent suicide attempters.

Few psychopharmacological treatment studies for suicidal youth have been conducted. Many classes of medications, including antidepressants, mood stabilizers, and atypical antipsychotic medications have been used to reduce symptoms of mood, anxiety, and psychotic disorders. Empirical research suggests that a negative relationship exists between the number of antidepressant medication prescriptions for children and adolescents and rates of youth suicide (Olfson et al. 2003). However, the risk–benefit ratio of selective serotonin reuptake inhibitor (SSRI) medications is low, because a higher risk for suicidal ideation and acts with these drugs, compared with placebo, has been demonstrated in controlled clinical trials (Whittington et al. 2004). In 2004, the U.S. Food and Drug Administration placed a black box warning on all antidepressants used to treat children and adolescents. It does not contraindicate use of these medications, but it mandates close monitoring of treated children. It is imperative that additional empirical research be conducted to identify the most effective psychopharmacological agents for treatment of suicidality in children and adolescents.

Research Issues

Short-term prospective studies have not identified significant associations between childhood or adolescent suicide attempts and exposure to suicide of relatives or friends (Brent et al. 1996b; Mercy et al. 2001; Pfeffer et al. 1997, 2000a). Although such bereaved adolescents suffer traumatic grief reactions (Melhem et al. 2004), additional research is necessary to elucidate the developmental course of youth who are bereaved after the suicide of a relative or friend.

Screening for risk of suicidal behavior by reliable and valid measures is one of the initial aspects of suicide prevention (Larzelere et al. 2004; Pfeffer et al. 2000b; Shaffer et al. 2004). As with all self-report measures of a low prevalence behavior, such as suicidal behavior, there is a high rate of false positive findings. Therefore, additional research is needed to identify whether the utilization of screening approaches that combine self-report and direct interview methods are more specific for youth suicide risk assessment.

Research is needed to develop effective education strategies for parents and school, medical and other professionals who work with children on ways of identifying children and adolescents at risk for suicidal behavior and methods of referring them to a trained health professional for definitive assessment and treatment. Additional research is necessary to develop effective prevention strategies that enhance help-seeking behaviors of suicidal adolescents (Gould et al. 2004).

Research is needed to define effective psychosocial and psychopharmacological treatments to reduce suicidal behavior in children and adolescents (American Academy of Child and Adolescent Psychiatry 2001). Treatment studies should focus on decreasing the effects of aberrant neurobiological factors that may increase risk for suicidal behavior.

References

American Academy of Child and Adolescent Psychiatry: Practice parameters for the assessment and treatment of children and adolescents with suicidal behavior. J Am Acad Child Adolesc Psychiatry 40 (7 suppl):24S–51S, 2001

American Psychiatric Association: Diagnostic and Statistical Manual of Mental Disorders, 4th Edition. Washington, DC, American Psychiatric Association, 1994

Barbe RP, Bridge J, Birhamer B, et al: Suicidality and its relationship to treatment outcome in depressed adolescents. Suicide Life Threat Behavior 34:44–55, 2004

Beautrais AL: Suicide and serious suicide attempts in youth: a multiple-group comparison study. Am J Psychiatry 160:1093–1099, 2003

Beautrais AL, Joyce PR, Mulder RT: Personality traits and cognitive styles as risk factors for serious suicide attempts among young people. Suicide Life Threat Behav 29:37–47, 1999

Boyd JH, Moscicki EK: Firearms and youth suicide. Am J Public Health 76:1240–1242, 1986

Brent DA: Practitioner review: the aftercare of adolescents with deliberate self-harm. J Child Psychol Psychiatry 38:277–286, 1997

Brent DA, Perper JA, Moritz G, et al: Psychiatric risk factors for adolescent suicide: a case-control study. J Am Acad Child Adolesc Psychiatry 32:521–529, 1993

Brent DA, Bridge J, Johnson BA, et al: Suicidal behavior runs in families: a controlled family study of adolescent suicide victims. Arch Gen Psychiatry 53:1145–1152, 1996a

Brent DA, Moritz G, Bridge J, et al: Long-term impact of exposure to suicide: a three-year controlled follow-up. J Am Acad Child Adolesc Psychiatry 35:646–653, 1996b

Brent DA, Baugher M, Birmaher B, et al: Compliance with recommendations to remove firearms in families participating in a clinical trial for adolescent depression. J Am Acad Child Adolesc Psychiatry 39:1220–1226, 2000

Caspi A, Sugden K, Moffitt TE, et al: Influence of life stress on depression: moderation by a polymorphism in the 5-HTT gene. Science 301: 386–389, 2003

Donaldson D, Spirito A, Farnett E: The role of perfectionism and depressive cognitions in understanding the hopelessness experienced by adolescent suicide attempters. Child Psychiatry Hum Dev 31:99–111, 2000

Fergusson DM, Horwood LJ, Beautrais AL: Is sexual orientation related to mental health problems and suicidality in young people? Arch Gen Psychiatry 56:876–880, 1999

Gould MS, Fisher P, Parides M, et al: Psychosocial risk factors of child and adolescent completed suicide. Arch Gen Psychiatry 53:1155–1162, 1996

Gould MS, Velting D, Kleinman M, et al: Teenagers' attitudes about coping strategies and help-seeking behavior for suicidality. J Am Acad Child Adolesc Psychiatry 43:1124–1133, 2004

Harrington R, Kerfoot M, Dyer E, et al: Deliberate self-poisoning in adolescence: why does a brief family intervention work in some cases and not others? J Adolescence 23:13–20, 2000

Jacobsen LK, Rabinowitz I, Popper MS, et al: Interviewing prepubertal children about suicidal ideation and behavior. J Am Acad Child Adolesc Psychiatry 33:439–452, 1994

Kann L, Kinchen SA, Williams BI, et al: Youth Risk Behavior Surveillance—United States, 1999. J Sch Health 70:271–285, 2000

Katz LY, Cox BJ, Gunasekara S, et al: Feasibility of dialectical behavior therapy for suicidal adolescent inpatients. J Am Acad Child Adolesc Psychiatry 43:276–282, 2004

King RA, Schwab-Stone M, Flisher AJ, et al: Psychosocial and risk behavior correlates of youth suicide attempts and suicidal ideation. J Am Acad Child Adolesc Psychiatry 40:837–846, 2001

Kochanek KD, Murphy SL, Anderson RN, et al: Deaths: final data for 2002. National Vital Statistics Reports, Vol 53, No 5. Hyattsville, MD: National Center for Health Statistics, 2004

Kuperman S, Black DW, Burns TL: Excess suicide among formerly hospitalized child psychiatry patients. J Clin Psychiatry 49:88–93, 1988

Larzelere RE, Andersen JJ, Ringle JL, et al: The child suicide risk assessment: a screening measure of suicide risk in pre-adolescents. Death Studies 28:809–827, 2004

Lewinsohn PM, Rohde P, Seeley JR, et al: Gender differences in suicide attempts from adolescence to young adulthood. J Am Acad Child Adolesc Psychiatry 40:427–434, 2001

Mann JJ, Brent DA, Arango V: The neurobiology and genetics of suicide and attempted suicide: a focus on the serotonergic system. Neuropsychopharmacology 24:467–477, 2001

Martin G, Bergen HA, Richardson AS, et al: Sexual abuse and suicidality: gender differences in a large community sample of adolescents. Child Abuse Negl 28:491–503, 2004

Melhem NM, Day N, Shear MK, et al: Traumatic grief among adolescents exposed to a peer's suicide. Am J Psychiatry 161:1411–1416, 2004

Mercy JA, Kresnow MJ, O'Carroll PW, et al: Is suicide contagious? A study of the relation between exposure to the suicidal behavior of others and nearly lethal suicide attempts. Am J Epidemiol 154:120–127, 2001

Mufson L, Fairbanks J: Interpersonal psychotherapy for depressed adolescents: a one-year naturalistic follow-up study. J Am Acad Child Adolesc Psychiatry 35:1145–1155, 1996

Myers K, McCauley E, Calderon R, et al: The 3-year longitudinal course of suicidality and predictive factors for subsequent suicidality in youths with major depressive disorder. J Am Acad Child Adolesc Psychiatry 30:804–810, 1991

Olfson M, Shaffer D, Marcus SC, et al: Relationship between antidepressant medication treatment and suicide in adolescents. Arch Gen Psychiatry 60:978–982, 2003

Pfeffer CR: The Suicidal Child. New York, Guilford, 1986

Pfeffer CR, Zuckerman S, Plutchik R, et al: Suicidal behavior in normal school children: a comparison with child psychiatric inpatients. J Am Acad Child Psychiatry 23:416–423, 1984

Pfeffer CR, Newcorn J, Kaplan G, et al: Suicidal behavior in adolescent psychiatric inpatients. J Am Acad Child Adolesc Psychiatry 27:357–361, 1988

Pfeffer CR, Klerman GL, Hurt SW, et al: Suicidal children grow up: rates and psychosocial risk factors for suicide attempts during follow-up. J Am Acad Child Adolesc Psychiatry 32:106–113, 1993

Pfeffer CR, Normandin L, Kakuma T: Suicidal children grow up: suicidal behavior and psychiatric disorders among relatives. J Am Acad Child Adolesc Psychiatry 33:1087–1097, 1994

Pfeffer CR, Martins P, Mann J, et al: Child survivors of suicide: psychosocial characteristics. J Am Acad Child Adolesc Psychiatry 36:65–74, 1997

Pfeffer CR, McBride A, Anderson GM, et al: Peripheral serotonin measures in prepubertal psychiatric inpatients and normal children: associations with suicidal behavior and its risk factors. Biol Psychiatry 44:568–577, 1998

Pfeffer CR, Jiang H, Kakuma T: Child-Adolescent Suicidal Potential Index (CASPI): a screen for risk for early onset suicidal behavior. Psychol Assess 12:304–318, 2000a

Pfeffer CR, Karus D, Siegel K, et al: Child survivors of parental death from cancer or suicide: depressive and behavioral outcomes. Psychooncology 9:1–10, 2000b

Remafedi G, French S, Story M, et al: The relationship between suicide risk and sexual orientation: results of a population-based study. Am J Public Health 88:57–60, 1998

Rotheram-Borus MJ, Piacentini J, Cantwell C, et al: The 18-month impact of an emergency room intervention for adolescent female suicide attempters. J Consult Clin Psychol 68:1081–1093, 2000

Safren SA, Heimberg RG: Depression, hopelessness, suicidality, and related factors in sexual minority and heterosexual adolescents. J Consult Clin Psychol 67:859–866, 1999

Shaffer D, Gould M, Hicks RC: Worsening suicide rate in black teenagers. Am J Psychiatry 151:1810–1812, 1994

Shaffer D, Gould MS, Fisher P, et al: Psychiatric diagnosis in child and adolescent suicide. Arch Gen Psychiatry 53:339–348, 1996

Shaffer D, Scott M, Wilcox H, et al: The Columbia Suicide Screen: validity and reliability of a screen for youth suicide and depression. J Am Acad Child Adolesc Psychiatry 43:71–79, 2004

TADS Team: Fluoxetine, cognitive-behavioral therapy, and their combination for adolescents with depression: Treatment for Adolescents with Depression Study (TADS) randomized controlled trial. JAMA 292:807–820, 2004

U.S. Public Health Service: The Surgeon General's Call to Action to Prevent Suicide. Washington, DC, U.S. Public Health Service, 1999

Weissman MM, Wolk S, Goldstein RB, et al: Depressed adolescents grown up. JAMA 281: 1707–1713, 1999

Whittington CJ, Kendall T, Fonagy P, et al: Selective serotonin reuptake inhibitors in childhood depression: systematic review of published versus unpublished data. Lancet 363:1341–1345, 2004

Wu P, Hoven CW, Cohen P, et al: Factors associated with use of mental health services for depression by children and adolescents. Psychiatr Serv 52:189–195, 2001

Self-Assessment Questions

Select the single best response for each question.

28.1 Self-mutilation

    A. Is defined as superficial cutting of the arms, legs, and other body areas.

    B. Is rarely associated with stress.

    C. Always involves a clear intention to kill oneself.

    D. Is never associated with suicidal intent.

    E. Is rarely associated with dissociative phenomena.

28.2 Which of the following statements concerning epidemiological findings in youth suicide is *false?*

    A. Suicide among black youth has increased more rapidly than that among white youth.

    B. Increased rates of youth suicide are associated with greater availability of firearms.

    C. Male youths are more likely to attempt suicide than are females.

    D. Approximately 1% of preadolescents in the general population report having made a suicide attempt.

    E. None of the above.

28.3 Which of the following childhood environmental stressors has been identified as a suicide risk factor?

    A. Adolescent unemployment.

    B. Family history of suicidal behavior.

    C. Poor communication with the mother or the father.

    D. Adolescent suspension from school.

    E. All of the above.

28.4 A "psychological autopsy" study of 67 adolescent suicide victims found greatly elevated risks for suicide associated with certain psychiatric disorders (Brent et al. 1993). Which of the following disorders imparted the greatest increase in risk?

    A. Attention-deficit/hyperactivity disorder.

    B. Alcohol abuse.

    C. Schizophrenia.

    D. Major depression.

    E. Conduct disorder.

28.5 The use of antidepressants in children and adolescents has recently received a great deal of scrutiny from the U.S. Food and Drug Administration (FDA) and from investigators. Which of the following statements is correct?

     A. A positive relationships exists between the number of antidepressant medication prescriptions for children and adolescents and rates of youth suicide.

     B. Selective serotonin reuptake inhibitors (SSRIs) are associated with a higher risk of suicidal ideation and acts compared with placebo.

     C. SSRI antidepressants are contraindicated in children and adolescents.

     D. A black-box warning has been placed on SSRI-type antidepressants, but not on other antidepressants, for their use in children and adolescents.

     E. None of the above.

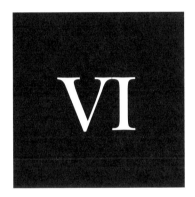

Treatment

29

Psychopharmacology

Joseph Biederman, M.D.

Thomas Spencer, M.D.

Timothy Wilens, M.D.

In modern pediatric psychopharmacology, diagnostic hypotheses guide intervention. Diagnostic information should be gathered from the child, the parents or caretakers, and, whenever possible, the teachers, and a diagnosis based on DSM-IV-TR (American Psychiatric Association 2000) criteria should be made. Careful attention should be paid to comorbidity and differential diagnosis, including both medical/neurological and psychosocial factors contributing to the clinical presentation. Because psychiatric disorders of children and adolescents can be associated with additional cognitive deficits (e.g., learning disabilities), which may not respond to psychotropics, it is important to pinpoint these deficits to help define appropriate remedial interventions. Pharmacotherapy should be part of a treatment plan in which consideration is given to all aspects of the child's or adolescent's life. It should not be used instead of other interventions or after other interventions have failed. Realistic expectations of pharmacotherapy based on knowledge of what it can and cannot

do, as well as careful definition of target symptoms, are major ingredients for a successful intervention.

Therapeutic intervention should be started early—before the occurrence of complications, chronicity, and social incapacitation, which can make treatment and restabilization of functional life habits more difficult. In addition to pharmacotherapy, treatment of behavioral and emotional disorders of youths may need to involve a variety of psychosocial methods, such as individual psychotherapy, family and group therapy, behavioral and cognitive-behavioral therapy, and parental counseling. These interventions should also be based on diagnostic hypotheses and careful selection of target symptoms. The closer the match between the treatment and the spectrum of difficulties the child and his or her family face, the more successful the intervention will be. In severe cases, hospitalization may be required.

Before treatment with a psychotropic is initiated, the family and the child need to be made familiar with the risks and benefits of the intervention, the availability of alternative treatments, and the likely adverse effects, including short-term, long-term, and withdrawal adverse effects. Certain adverse effects can be anticipated on the basis of known pharmacological properties of the drug (e.g., the anticholinergic effects of tricyclic antidepressants [TCAs]); other adverse effects, generally rare, are unexpected (idiosyncratic) and are difficult to anticipate. Short-term adverse effects can be minimized by introducing the medication at low doses and titrating slowly. Patients receiving drugs with known adverse effects should be monitored for long-term adverse effects (e.g., patients taking lithium carbonate should be monitored for changes in kidney and thyroid functions). Idiosyncratic adverse effects require drug discontinuation and selection of alternative treatment modalities.

Treatment should be started at the lowest possible dose, usually the lowest manufactured dose. Frequent (e.g., weekly) contact with the patient and family is necessary during the initial phase of treatment, to monitor response to the intervention and adverse effects. Evaluation of adverse effects should include subjective reports by the patient and family (e.g., reports of stomachaches or appetite changes) as well as objective measurements (e.g., measurement of heart rate and blood pressure). After a sufficient period of clinical stabilization (e.g., 6–12 months), it is prudent to evaluate the need for continued psychopharmacological intervention. Withdrawal symptoms should be distinguished from exacerbation of symptoms of the disorder for which the psychotropic was prescribed. To minimize withdrawal reactions, it is important to discontinue medications gradually. Because most psychiatric disorders are chronic or recurrent, timely follow-up after drug discontinuation is necessary. Despite recent progress, insufficient information exists regarding the efficacy, safety, and pharmacology of most psychotropics in children and adolescents, a situation that necessitates continued reliance on adult data to guide pediatric psychopharmacology.

Major Classes of Drugs Used in Pediatric Psychiatry

■ Stimulants (Tables 29–1 and 29–2)

Stimulant drugs were the first class of compounds reported to be effective in the treatment of behavioral disturbances in children with attention-deficit/hyperactivity disorder (ADHD). Stimulants are sympathomimetic drugs that are structurally similar to endogenous catecholamines. The most commonly used compounds in this class include methylphenidate, dextroamphetamine, and the mixed amphetamine salts product Adderall. These drugs are thought to act both in the central nervous system (CNS) and peripherally by enhancing dopaminergic and noradrenergic neurotransmission. Because the various stimulants have somewhat different mechanisms of action, some patients may respond preferentially to one or another (Greenhill et al. 1999).

Because of their short half-lives, the short-acting stimulants (methylphenidate and dextroamphetamine) are given in divided doses throughout the day, typically 4 hours apart. The total daily dose ranges from 0.3 to 2 mg/kg (0.3–1.0 mg/kg for dextroamphetamine). The starting dosage is generally 2.5–5 mg/day, given once daily in the morning. If necessary, the dose is increased every few days by 2.5–5 mg in a divided-dose schedule. Given the anorexigenic effects of the stimulants, it may be beneficial to administer the medicine after meals. The therapeutic effects of Adderall (a mixed amphetamine salts formulation) last through most or all of

Table 29–1. Stimulants

Drug	Daily dose (mg/kg)	Dosage schedule	Main indications	Adverse effects and comments
Dextroamphetamine			• ADHD • Mental retardation + ADHD	*Stimulants:* • Insomnia, decreased appetite, weight loss • Depression, psychosis (rare, with very high doses) • Mild increase in heart rate and blood pressure • Possible reduction in growth velocity with long-term use • Withdrawal effects and rebound phenomena • *Adderall:* 6 hours of action; rare potential cardiovascular risk with preexisting cardiovascular abnormalities
Dexedrine	0.3–1.0	bid–tid		
Mixed amphetamine salts formulation			• ADHD • Adjunct therapy in refractory depression	
Adderall	0.5–1.5	Once daily or bid		
Methylphenidate			• ADHD	
Focalin	0.5–1.0	bid–tid		
Methylin	1.0–2.0	bid–tid		
Ritalin	1.0–2.0	bid–tid		

Note. Doses are general guidelines. All doses must be individualized, and appropriate monitoring should be performed. Weight-corrected doses are less appropriate for obese children. ADHD = attention-deficit/hyperactivity disorder.

Table 29–2. New long-acting stimulants

Drug	Daily dose (mg/kg)	Dosage schedule	Duration of behavioral effect (hours)	Comments
Methylphenidate				
Concerta	1.0–2.0	Once daily or bid	10–12	Ascending profile, OROS technology
Metadate CD	1.0–2.0	Once daily or bid	8–9	Capsule with 3:7 ratio of IR beads to DR beads
Ritalin LA	1.0–2.0	Once daily or bid	8–9	Capsule with 1:1 ratio of IR beads to DR beads
Mixed amphetamine salts formulation				
Adderall XR	0.5–1.5	Once daily or bid	10–12	Capsule with 1:1 ratio of IR beads to DR beads

Note. Doses are general guidelines. All doses must be individualized, and appropriate monitoring should be performed. Weight-corrected doses are less appropriate for obese children. DR=delayed-release; IR=immediate-release; OROS=osmotic release oral system.

the school day. For full-day coverage, Adderall is usually administered twice a day (e.g., at 8:00 A.M. and 2:00 P.M.), with total daily doses ranging from 0.5 to 1.5 mg/kg. Typically, stimulants have a rapid onset of action; therefore, a clinical response will be evident when a therapeutic dose has been achieved.

A new generation of highly sophisticated, well-developed, safe, effective, and long-acting stimulants has reached the market and revolutionized the treatment of ADHD. These compounds use novel delivery systems to overcome acute tolerance (tachyphylaxis). The methylphenidate preparation Concerta uses an osmotic pump mechanism that creates an ascending profile of methylphenidate in the blood, providing effective treatment for 10–12 hours. Concerta is available in 18-, 36-, and 54-mg tablets, approximating the 5-, 10-, and 15-mg thrice-daily doses of immediate-release (IR) methylphenidate. The methylphenidate preparations Metadate CD and Ritalin LA both take the form of capsules containing a mixture of immediate- and delayed-release beads, providing effective treatment for 8–9 hours. In Metadate CD capsules, 30% of the beads are immediate release and 70% are delayed release. Metadate CD is available in 20-mg capsules, approximating the 10-mg twice-daily doses of IR methylphenidate. In Ritalin LA capsules, there is a 1:1 ratio of IR beads to delayed-release beads. Ritalin LA is available in 20-, 30-, and 40-mg capsules, approximating 10-, 15-, and 20-mg twice-daily doses of IR methylphenidate. Adderall XR is manufactured as capsules with a 1:1 ratio of IR beads to delayed-release beads, providing effective amphetamine (Adderall) treatment for 10–12 hours. Adderall XR is available in 10-, 20-, and 30-mg capsules, approximating 5-, 10-, and 15-mg twice-daily doses (at 0 and 4 hours) of Adderall. Formulations consisting of beads in capsules (i.e., all the aforemen-

tioned drugs but Concerta) may be used as sprinkle preparations for children unable to swallow pills.

Methylphenidate as a secondary amine gives rise to four optical isomers: D-*threo*, L-*threo*, D-*erythro*, and L-*erythro*. There is stereoselectivity in receptor site binding and its relationship to response. The standard preparation is composed of the D,L-*threo* racemate, the form apparently active in the CNS. Moreover, recent data suggest that the D-methylphenidate isomer is the active form (Ding et al. 1995). This has led to the development of a purified D-*threo*-methylphenidate compound, Focalin. Studies have shown Focalin to be at least as effective as the racemate, at half the dose (Conners et al. 2001; Novartis, data on file). Focalin is available in 2.5-, 5-, and 10-mg doses, approximating the 5-, 10-, and 20-mg doses of D,L-methylphenidate.

The early concern that optimal clinical efficacy is attained at the cost of impaired learning ability has not been confirmed (Gittelman-Klein 1987). In fact, studies indicate that both behavior and cognitive performance improve with stimulant treatment, in a dose-dependent fashion (Douglas et al. 1988; Klein 1987; Kupietz et al. 1988; Pelham et al. 1985; Rapport et al. 1987, 1989a, 1989b; Tannock et al. 1989). Findings on the association between clinical benefits in ADHD and plasma levels of stimulants have been equivocal and complicated by wide inter- and intraindividual variability in plasma levels at constant oral doses (Gittelman-Klein 1987).

The most commonly reported side effects of stimulant medications are appetite suppression and sleep disturbances. The sleep disturbance commonly reported is delay of sleep onset; this side effect is usually associated with late-afternoon or early-evening administration of stimulant medications. Although less often reported, mood disturbances ranging from increased tearfulness to a full-blown major depression–like syndrome can be associated with stimulant treatment (Wilens and Biederman 1992). Other infrequent side effects include headaches, abdominal discomfort, increased lethargy, and fatigue.

Although the adverse cardiovascular effects of stimulants—beyond effects on heart rate and blood pressure—have not been examined, mild increases (of unclear clinical significance) in pulse and blood pressure have been observed (Brown et al. 1984). Increases in blood pressure that can occur with stimulant therapy may be of greater clinical significance in adults with ADHD than in children with the disorder. A stimulant-associated toxic psychosis has also been (very rarely) observed, usually in the context of either a rapid increase in dose or very high doses. The reported psychosis in children in response to stimulant medications resembles a toxic phenomenon (e.g., visual hallucinosis) and is dissimilar to the exacerbation of psychotic symptoms in schizophrenia. Development of psychotic symptoms in a child exposed to stimulants necessitates careful evaluation to rule out a preexisting psychotic disorder.

Early reports indicated that children with a personal or family history of tic disorders were at greater risk of developing a tic disorder when exposed to stimulants (Lowe et al. 1982). However, more recent work has challenged this view (Comings and Comings 1988; Gadow et al. 1992, 1995). For example, in a controlled study involving 34 children with ADHD and tics, methylphenidate effectively suppressed ADHD symptoms and had only a weak effect on the frequency of tics (Gadow et al. 1995). In a study involving 128 boys with ADHD, there was no evidence of earlier onset, higher rates, or worsening of tics in the subgroup exposed to stimulants (Spencer et al. 1999a). Al-

though this work is reassuring, more information is needed, obtained in a larger number of subjects over a longer time period. Until more is known, it seems prudent to weigh risks and benefits on a case-by-case basis. The physician should discuss with the child and family the benefits and pitfalls of the use of stimulants in children with ADHD and tics.

Similar uncertainties remain about the abuse potential of stimulants in ADHD children. Despite the concern that ADHD may increase the risk of abuse by adolescents and young adults (or their associates), there is no clear evidence to date of abuse of prescribed stimulant medication by children with appropriately diagnosed ADHD who are carefully monitored. The most commonly abused substance among adolescents and adults with ADHD is marijuana, not stimulant medication (Biederman et al. 1995c). Furthermore, the use of stimulants and other pharmacological treatments for ADHD was recently found to significantly decrease the risk of subsequent substance use disorders among ADHD youth (Biederman et al. 1999c).

Although concerns continue regarding the effect of long-term administration of stimulants on growth, investigators have begun to question this issue. Stimulants are known to routinely produce anorexia and weight loss, but their effect on growth in height is much less certain. Although initial reports suggested that a persistent stimulant-associated decrease in growth in height occurred in children (Mattes and Gittelman 1983; Safer et al. 1972), other reports have failed to substantiate this claim (Gross 1976; Satterfield et al. 1979). Moreover, several studies showed that ultimate height appears to be unaffected if treatment is discontinued in adolescence (Klein and Mannuzza 1988). A more recent study suggested that deficits in growth in height are transient maturational delays associated with ADHD, rather than stunting of growth (Spencer et al. 1998b). If this hypothesis is confirmed, the common practice of drug holidays for ADHD children would appear unnecessary. However, it seems prudent to institute drug holidays or alternative treatment in the case of children suspected of stimulant-associated growth deficits. This recommendation should be carefully weighed against the risk of exacerbation of symptoms due to drug discontinuation. A transient behavioral deterioration occurs in some children after abrupt discontinuation of stimulant medications. The prevalence of this phenomenon and the etiology are unclear. Rebound phenomena also occur between doses in some children, creating an uneven, often disturbing clinical course. In those cases, consideration should be given to alternative treatments.

■ Antidepressants (Table 29–3)

There are several main families of antidepressant medications: tricyclic antidepressants (TCAs) (mixed neurotransmitter profile); selective serotonin reuptake inhibitors (SSRIs); monoamine oxidase inhibitors (MAOIs) (mixed neurotransmitter profile); and atypical antidepressants such as bupropion (dopaminergic/noradrenergic profile), venlafaxine (serotonergic/noradrenergic profile), mirtazapine (serotonergic/noradrenergic profile), noradrenergic-specific reuptake inhibitors, and reboxetine.

In open and controlled studies involving children and adolescents, noradrenergic antidepressant medications and TCAs were beneficial in treating ADHD (Biederman et al. 1989a, 1989b), SSRIs were beneficial in treating obsessive-compulsive disorder (OCD) (DeVeaugh-Geiss et al. 1992; D. A. Geller et al. 1995) and depression (Emslie et al. 1997; Wagner et al. 1998), and TCAs were beneficial in treating en-

uresis (Gittelman 1980). Other childhood conditions that may benefit from antidepressant treatment include anxiety (serotonergic drugs) and tic disorders (TCAs, possibly other noradrenergic compounds) (Singer et al. 1994; Spencer 1997).

Antidepressant drugs appear to act by exerting various effects on pre- and postsynaptic receptors, affecting the release and reuptake of brain neurotransmitters, including norepinephrine, serotonin, and dopamine. The effect and adverse-effect profiles of the various classes of antidepressant drugs differ greatly. Because a substantial interindividual variability in metabolism and elimination has been demonstrated in children, doses should always be individualized. Studies have begun to document striking similarities between children and adults in terms of pharmacokinetic profiles of sertraline (Alderman et al. 1998), venlafaxine (Derivan 1995), and paroxetine (Findling et al. 1999).

In October 2004, the U.S. Food and Drug Administration (FDA) issued the following statement regarding the use of antidepressants in juveniles:

> The Food and Drug Administration (FDA) directed manufacturers of all antidepressant drugs to revise the labeling for their products to include a boxed warning and expanded warning statements that alert health care providers to an increased risk of suicidality (suicidal thinking and behavior) in children and adolescents being treated with these agents...The risk of suicidality for these drugs was identified in a combined analysis of short-term (up to 4 months) placebo-controlled trials of nine antidepressant drugs...The analysis showed a greater risk of suicidality during the first few months of treatment in those receiving antidepressants. The average risk of such events on drug was 4%, twice the placebo risk of 2%. No suicides occurred in these trials. Based on these data, FDA has

Table 29–3. Antidepressants

Drug	Daily dose (mg/kg)	Dosage schedule	Main indications	Adverse effects and comments
All antidepressants				• Infrequent potential increase in suicidality, or self-harm behavior.
Tricyclic antidepressants (TCAs)			• ADHD • Enuresis • Tic disorder • ?Anxiety disorders • OCD (clomipramine)	• Mixed mechanism of action (noradrenergic and serotonergic); secondary amines more noradrenergic; clomipramine primarily serotonergic • Narrow therapeutic index • Overdoses can be fatal • Anticholinergic symptoms (dry mouth, constipation, blurred vision) • Weight loss • Serum level and electrocardiographic monitoring needed • At daily doses >3.5 mg/kg, electrocardiographic and blood pressure monitoring needed • No known long-term side effects • Possible withdrawal effects (severe gastrointestinal symptoms, malaise) • Risk of seizures
Tertiary amines				
Amitriptyline	2.0–5.0[a]	Once daily or bid		
Clomipramine	2.0–5.0[a]	Once daily or bid		
Imipramine	2.0–5.0[a]	Once daily or bid		
Secondary amines				
Desipramine	2.0–5.0[a]	Once daily or bid		
Nortriptyline	1.0–3.0[b]	Once daily or bid		

Table 29–3. Antidepressants (*continued*)

Drug	Daily dose (mg/kg)	Dosage schedule	Main indications	Adverse effects and comments
Monoamine oxidase inhibitors (MAOIs)			• Atypical depression • Refractory depression	• Difficult to use in juvenile patients • Reserved for refractory cases • Severe dietary restrictions (high-tyramine foods) • Drug–drug interactions • Hypertensive crisis with dietetic transgression or with certain drugs • Weight gain • Drowsiness • Changes in blood pressure • Insomnia • Rare hepatotoxicity
Phenelzine	0.5–1.0	bid–tid		
Selegiline	0.2–0.4	bid–tid		
Tranylcypromine	0.5–1.0	bid–tid		
Selective serotonin reuptake inhibitors (SSRIs)			• MD • Dysthymia • OCD • Anxiety disorders • Eating disorders • ?PTSD	• Serotonergic • Large margin of safety • No cardiovascular effects • Irritability • Insomnia • Gastrointestinal symptoms • Headaches • Sexual dysfunction • Withdrawal symptoms more common with short-acting SSRIs • Potential drug–drug interactions (P450 enzymes)
Citalopram	0.3–0.9	Once daily (in A.M.)		
Fluoxetine	0.3–0.9	Once daily (in A.M.)		
Fluvoxamine	1.0–4.5	Once daily (in A.M.)		
Paroxetine	0.3–0.9	Once daily (in A.M.)		
Sertraline	1.5–3.0	Once daily (in A.M.)		

Table 29–3. Antidepressants *(continued)*

Drug	Daily dose (mg/kg)	Dosage schedule	Main indications	Adverse effects and comments
Bupropion (SR)	3–6	bid	• ADHD • MD • Smoking cessation • ?Bipolar depression	• Mixed mechanism of action (dopaminergic and noradrenergic) • Irritability • Insomnia • Drug-induced seizures at doses >6 mg/kg • Contraindicated in bulimic patients
Mirtazapine	0.2–0.9	Once daily (in P.M.)	• MD • Anxiety disorders • ?Stimulant-induced insomnia • ?Bipolar depression	• Mixed mechanism of action (serotonergic and noradrenergic) • Sedation • Weight gain • Dizziness • ?Less likely to induce mania
Venlafaxine (XR)	1–3	Once daily	• MD • Anxiety disorders • ?ADHD • ?OCD	• Mixed mechanism of action (serotonergic and noradrenergic) • Adverse effects similar to SSRIs • Irritability • Insomnia • Gastrointestinal symptoms • Headaches • Potential withdrawal symptoms • Blood pressure changes

Note. Doses are general guidelines. All doses must be individualized, and appropriate monitoring should be performed. Weight-corrected doses are less appropriate for obese children. When high doses are used, serum levels may be obtained to avoid toxicity. ADHD = attention-deficit/hyperactivity disorder; MD = major depression; OCD = obsessive-compulsive disorder; PTSD = posttraumatic stress disorder; SR = sustained-release; XR = extended-release.
[a]Dose adjusted according to serum levels.
[b]Dose adjusted according to serum levels; therapeutic window.

determined that the following points are appropriate for inclusion in the boxed warning:

- Antidepressants increase the risk of suicidal thinking and behavior (suicidality) in children and adolescents with major depressive disorder and other psychiatric disorders.
- Anyone considering the use of an antidepressant in a child or adolescent for any clinical use must balance the risk of increased suicidality with the clinical need.
- Patients who are started on therapy should be observed closely for clinical worsening, suicidality, or unusual changes in behavior.
- Families and caregivers should be advised to closely observe the patient and to communicate with the prescriber.
- A statement regarding whether the particular drug is approved for any pediatric indication(s) and, if so, which one(s).

Among the antidepressants, only Prozac is approved for use in treating major depressive disorder in pediatric patients. Prozac, Zoloft, Luvox, and Anafranil are approved for OCD in pediatric patients. None of the drugs is approved for other psychiatric indications in children. (U.S. Food and Drug Administration 2004)

In reviewing these warnings, the American Psychiatric Association (APA) and the American Academy of Child and Adolescent Psychiatry agreed with the recommendation for increased education, caution and monitoring with the use of these compounds but were concerned that the warnings and medication guides did not adequately address potential benefits or the risks of not treating. The APA issued the following statement:

The American Psychiatric Association believes antidepressants save lives. As part of a comprehensive treatment plan, antidepressants can be extremely helpful for many young people struggling with depression, an illness with significant long-term consequences, including an increased risk for suicide. We believe the biggest threat to a depressed child's well-being is to receive no care at all. (American Psychiatric Association 2004)

In understanding the FDA statement, it is important to note three important qualifiers:

1. The increased suicidality noted in the FDA report included general symptoms of anger and not specifically suicidality (there were no suicides).
2. There has been a significant (33%) decline in worldwide youth suicide rates during a period of rapidly increasing use of SSRIs (American College of Neuropsychopharmacology 2004).
3. Although a number of studies did not document the superiority of SSRIs over placebo in the treatment of depression, most did not prove that the drugs were ineffective because of methodological limitations. There are daunting hurdles to conducting depression trials in children. For ethical reasons, such trials are hard to conduct without considerable psychosocial support for children and their families. The ensuing high placebo response rates make it difficult to show superiority of any effective treatment. Thus, many pediatric studies are considered failed trials rather than negative trials.

An important addition to the debate on the use of antidepressants has been provided by a non-industry-sponsored (National Institute of Mental Health) study (March et al. 2004). This large, randomized multisite investigation, known as the Treatment for Adolescents With Depression (TADS) study, examined the effectiveness of medication and cognitive-behavioral therapy (CBT) in depressed adolescents. Rates of response defined as much or very much improved were 71.0% for the combination of fluoxetine and CBT, 60.6% for fluoxetine alone, 43.2% for CBT alone, and 34.8% for placebo. Thus, fluoxetine alone was effective and more effective than CBT alone. Fluoxetine-related adverse events were mostly mild and consistent with previous studies. Almost 30% of TADS participants had suicidal ideation at the start of the study, and fluoxetine did not increase suicidal ideation. By contrast, harm-related behavioral events, although uncommon, were more common in patients receiving fluoxetine as follows: fluoxetine alone (11.9%), the combination of fluoxetine and CBT (8.4%), CBT alone (4.5%), and placebo (5.4%). Thus, consistent with its impact on suicidal ideation, CBT may protect against these events in patients taking fluoxetine. Only 1.6% of patients (7 of 439) made a suicide attempt; there were no completed suicides. The authors concluded that "despite calls to restrict access to medications, medical management of major depression with fluoxetine, including careful monitoring for adverse events, should be made widely available, not discouraged" (March et al. 2004, p. 819). Given its role in effectiveness and decrease in harm-related events, they also recommended that CBT be available as part of comprehensive treatment for depressed adolescents.

In clinical practice, antidepressants are essential options for patients with unipolar depression or anxiety. Care must be taken to assess for a previous history of mania-like symptoms and to monitor fluctuations in suicidality with treatment. With careful administration, it is clear that these medications provide relief from depression that may be lifesaving.

TCAs include tertiary (imipramine and amitriptyline) and secondary (desipramine and nortriptyline) amine compounds. Treatment with a TCA should be initiated with a 10-mg or 25-mg dose, and the dose should be increased by 20%–30% every 4–5 days. When a daily dose of 3.0 mg/kg (or a lower effective daily dose, or, in the case of nortriptyline, a daily dose of 1.5 mg/kg) is reached, steady-state serum levels and an electrocardiogram (ECG) should be obtained. Typical dose ranges for TCAs are 2.0–5.0 mg/kg (for nortriptyline, 1.0–3.0 mg/kg). Common short-term adverse effects of TCAs include anticholinergic effects, such as dry mouth, blurred vision, and constipation. However, chronic administration of these drugs has no known deleterious effects. Gastrointestinal symptoms and vomiting may occur when TCAs are discontinued abruptly; thus, slow tapering of these medications is recommended. Because the anticholinergic effects of TCAs limit salivary flow, the drugs may promote tooth decay.

Evaluations of short- and long-term effects of therapeutic doses of TCAs on the cardiovascular system in children have shown TCAs to be generally well tolerated, with only minor electrocardiographic changes associated with daily oral doses as high as 5.0 mg/kg. TCA-induced electrocardiographic abnormalities (conduction defects) have been consistently reported in children receiving doses higher than 3.5 mg/kg (Biederman et al. 1989a) (nortriptyline dose, 1.0 mg/kg). Although of unclear hemodynamic significance, the development of conduction defects in children receiving TCAs merits closer electrocardiographic and clinical monitoring, especially when relatively high doses of these medicines are used. In the context of cardiac disease, conduction defects may have more serious clinical implications. When there is doubt about the cardiovascular state of a patient, a more comprehensive cardiac evaluation is suggested—including cardiac consultation and 24-hour electrocardiographic monitoring—before initiation of treatment with a TCA, to help determine the risk–benefit ratio of such an intervention. In a recent controlled study of heart rate variability, investigators examined the cardiac risk associated with use of desipramine in children (Prince et al., unpublished data, May 2003). Although changes in individual markers of heart rate variability were noted in ADHD youths treated with desipramine, the agent did not appear to adversely affect the overall balance of sympathetic or parasympathetic input into the myocardium.

In the 1980s, several case reports of sudden death in children being treated with desipramine raised concern about the potential cardiotoxic risk associated with TCA therapy in the pediatric population (Riddle et al. 1991). Despite uncertainty and imprecise data, an epidemiological evaluation suggested that the risk of desipramine-associated sudden death is slightly increased but is not significantly greater than the baseline risk of sudden death among children not taking medication (Biederman et al. 1995b). Nevertheless, treatment with a TCA should be preceded by a baseline ECG, with serial ECGs taken at regular intervals throughout treatment. Because of the potential lethality of TCA overdose, parents should be advised to store the medication in a place that is inaccessible to children.

SSRIs include fluoxetine, paroxetine, sertraline, fluvoxamine, and citalopram. The SSRIs are structurally dissimilar to each other and vary in their pharmacokinetics and side-effect profiles. Because of their pharmacological profiles, these medications have fewer anticholinergic, sedative, cardiovascular (in terms of blood pressure and electrocardiographic

changes) (Leonard et al. 1998; Wilens et al. 1996b), and weight-related adverse side effects than do TCAs.

Fluoxetine comes in capsules of 10 and 20 mg and in a scored 10-mg tablet. Fluoxetine and its active metabolite have long half-lives (approximately 7–9 days). In contrast, paroxetine, sertraline, and citalopram have medium half-lives (approximately 24 hours), as does fluvoxamine (approximately 15 hours). Paroxetine comes in 10-, 20-, 30-, and 40-mg tablets, and citalopram comes in 20- and 40-mg tablets. Fluoxetine, paroxetine, and citalopram are all available in liquid form. Fluoxetine, paroxetine, and citalopram have similar potencies, and suggested daily doses range from 0.3 to 0.9 mg/kg. Sertraline comes in 25-, 50-, and 100-mg scored tablets, and the usual daily dose range is 1.5–3.0 mg/kg (≤ 200 mg/day). Fluvoxamine comes in 25-, 50-, and 100-mg scored tablets, and the usual daily dose range is 1.0–4.5 mg/kg (≤ 300 mg/day). Among the common adverse effects of SSRIs are agitation, gastrointestinal symptoms, irritability, insomnia, and sexual dysfunction, including decreased libido and anorgasmia.

The atypical antidepressants include venlafaxine, bupropion, and mirtazapine. Venlafaxine is chemically unrelated to other antidepressants and has both SSRI and TCA properties (i.e., is serotonergic and noradrenergic). IR venlafaxine has a short half-life (approximately 5 hours; the half-life of O-desmethylvenlafaxine is approximately 11 hours), but venlafaxine was recently reformulated into a long-acting compound that allows once-daily administration. The long-acting preparation of venlafaxine comes in 37.5, 75, 150, and 225 mg. Venlafaxine lacks significant activity at muscarinic, cholinergic, α-adrenergic, and histaminergic sites and therefore has fewer side effects (sedation, anticholinergic effects) than other antidepressants. Because ven-lafaxine therapy has been associated with changes in blood pressure in adults, it is advisable to monitor blood pressure when using this antidepressant.

Mirtazapine is an atypical mixed anti-depressant with complex and unique pre- and postsynaptic effects affecting both serotonergic and noradrenergic neurotransmission. Because of its strong effects on histaminergic neurotransmis-sion, it has potent hypnotic effects. Use of the agent has been also associated with weight gain. Mirtazapine is available in 15-, 30-, and 45-mg tablets.

Bupropion is a novel-structured anti-depressant of the aminoketone class and is related to the phenylisopropylamines but pharmacologically distinct from known antidepressants. Although its spe-cific site or mechanism of action remains unknown, bupropion seems to have an in-direct mixed agonist effect on dopamine and norepinephrine neurotransmission. Bupropion is indicated for depression and smoking cessation in adults (Hurt et al. 1997). It is rapidly absorbed, with peak plasma levels usually achieved after 2 hours, and its average elimination half-life is 14 hours (range, 8–24 hours). The usual dose range is 3.0–6.0 mg/kg/day, given in divided doses. Side effects in-clude irritability, anorexia, insomnia, and, rarely, edema, rashes, and nocturia. Exac-erbation of tic disorders has also been re-ported with bupropion therapy. Com-pared with use of other antidepressants, use of bupropion appears to be associated with a somewhat higher rate (0.4%) of drug-induced seizures, particularly at daily doses greater than 6.0 mg/kg, as well as in patients with preexisting seizure dis-order and patients with bulimia. Bupro-pion is also formulated as a long-acting (sustained-release) preparation that can be administered twice daily, and this form of the drug appears to be associated with a lower risk of seizures than the IR com-pound. A once-daily (extended-release) formulation of bupropion has been devel-oped.

MAOIs include hydrazine (phenel-zine) and nonhydrazines (tranylcypro-mine), and selegiline. In adults, MAOIs have been found to be helpful in the treat-ment of atypical depressive disorders with reverse endogenous features and depres-sive disorders with prominent anxiety fea-tures (Quitkin et al. 1991). Daily doses of phenelzine and tranylcypromine, which range from 0.5 to 1.0 mg/kg/day (and of selegiline, 0.2–0.4 mg/kg/day) should be carefully titrated according to response and adverse effects. Short-term adverse effects include orthostatic hypotension, weight gain, drowsiness, and dizziness. Major limitations for the use of MAOIs in children and adolescents are the severe dietetic restrictions (patients must not eat tyramine-containing foods, including most cheeses) and severe drug interactions (e.g., with pressor amines, most cold med-icines, and amphetamines); incorrect use of MAOIs can induce a hypertensive crisis and a serotonergic syndrome. A new fam-ily of reversible inhibitors of monoamine oxidase A, used in Europe and Canada but not currently available in the United States, may be free of these difficulties. Currently being developed is a new gener-ation of MAOIs, administered transder-mally to avoid dietetic and drug–drug in-teractions.

Antidepressants and many other psy-chotropic agents are metabolized in the liver by the cytochrome P450 system (see the section "Combined Therapy" below) (DeVane 1998; Greenblatt et al. 1998; Nemeroff et al. 1996). Because of genetic polymorphism, patients may be slow or extensive (rapid) metabolizers. In addi-tion, exogenous compounds can dramati-cally affect the efficacy of these enzymes and lead to drug–drug interactions. Coadministration of a TCA and an SSRI (parox-etine, fluoxetine, or sertraline; fluvoxa-mine) may result in increased levels of the TCA. Some compounds metabolized by the P450 enzyme 3A4 have been associated with QT prolongations when combined with drugs that inhibit 3A4, and such co-administration could lead to potentially lethal ventricular arrhythmias (torsade de pointes). Thus, great caution should be exercised when using the drugs that affect 3A4 activity (i.e., fluvoxamine and, to a lesser degree, fluoxetine and sertraline). Citalopram, venlafaxine, and mirtazapine minimally inhibit P450 enzymes. Caution should be exercised when using combina-tion treatments, because an increase to dangerous levels is possible with any drug that is metabolized by a P450 enzyme whose activity is inhibited by another drug (DeVane 1998; Greenblatt et al. 1998; Nemeroff et al. 1996).

■ Antipsychotics (Table 29–4)

On the basis of their mechanisms of action, antipsychotics can be divided into typical (blocking dopamine D_2 receptors) and atypical (having mixed dopaminer-gic and serotonergic [5-HT_2]) activity). Typical antipsychotic drugs include low-potency phenothiazines (which must be given at high daily doses), high-potency phenothiazines (given at low daily doses), butyrophenones (haloperidol and pimo-zide), thioxanthenes (thiothixene), and indole derivatives (molindone). Low-potency phenothiazines (e.g., chlorpro-mazine, thioridazine) are particularly likely to have unwanted autonomic side effects, such as hypotension and sedation, whereas high-potency compounds are as-sociated with a higher risk of extrapyra-midal adverse effects. Their in vitro recep-tor binding properties and their in vivo effects confirm that the typical antipsy-chotic drugs in current use block the

binding of dopamine at the dopamine D_2 receptor. The best evidence that the ob-served dopamine D_2 receptor antagonism is relevant to the therapeutic effects of an-tipsychotic drugs (in psychotic disorders) is the finding that their rank order of clin-ical potency (e.g., haloperidol > per-phenazine > chlorpromazine) is the same as their rank order of in vitro binding af-finity for the dopamine D_2 receptor but not for other receptors. Even if the dopamine D_2 receptor is the primary site of action of typical antipsychotic drugs, much remains to be learned. In particu-lar, the afferents and efferents of the me-solimbic dopamine projections and the role of dopaminergic transmission in healthy as well as psychotic individuals must be better understood before an un-derstanding of what dopamine D_2 recep-tor blockade actually accomplishes can be gained. Because most psychotic patients improve over a period of days to weeks, it is likely that blockade of the dopamine D_2 receptor initiates a slow-onset change in some other component of the synaptic machinery or in the postsynaptic neuron (Hyman and Nestler 1993).

The atypical antipsychotics include dibenzazepines (loxapine, clozapine), ris-peridone, olanzapine, quetiapine, and ziprasidone. These chemically varied drugs differ in clinical activity and adverse effects. Atypical antipsychotic agents have relatively strong antagonistic interactions with serotonergic (5-HT_2) receptors and perhaps more variable activity at central α_1-adrenergic, cholinergic, and hista-minic (H_1) sites, which may account for the varying adverse-effect profiles of these compounds. Although clozapine exerts only weak antagonism of dopaminergic (D_2) transmission, it has a high affinity for dopamine D_4 receptors, with a greater specificity for mesolimbic and mesocor-tical tracts. Thus, these compounds are associated with a low risk of acute extrapy-

Table 29–4.   Antipsychotics

Drug	Daily dose (mg/kg)	Dosage schedule	Main indications	Adverse effects and comments
Typical antipsychotics			• Psychosis	• Primarily dopaminergic (D_2) antagonism
Butyrophenones			• Mania	• Anticholinergic effects (dry mouth,
Haloperidol, others	0.1–0.3	Once daily or bid	• Tourette's disorder	constipation, blurred vision); more common
Indole derivatives			• Hyperaggressive behavior, severe	with low-potency agents
Molindone, others	0.1–0.5	Once daily or bid	agitation, severe insomnia, severe	• Weight gain (lower risk associated with
Phenothiazines			self-injurious behavior	molindone)
Low-potency				• Extrapyramidal reactions (dystonia, rigidity,
Chlorpromazine,	3.0–6.0	Once daily or bid		tremor, akathisia); higher risk associated with
thioridazine, others				high-potency agents
High-potency				• Drowsiness
Fluphenazine,	0.1–0.5	Once daily or bid		• Risk of TD with chronic administration
perphenazine, others				• Withdrawal dyskinesia
Thioxanthenes				
Thiothixene, others	0.1–0.5	Once daily or bid		
Atypical antipsychotics			• Psychosis	• Dopaminergic- and serotonergic-like typical
Loxapine[a]	0.5–2.0	Once daily or bid	• Positive and negative symptoms	antipsychotics
Olanzapine	0.1–0.2	Once daily or bid	• Mania	• Lower incidence of extrapyramidal adverse
Quetiapine	0.7–4.0	Once daily or bid		effects than associated with typical
Risperidone	0.01–0.1	Once daily or bid		antipsychotics
Ziprasidone	0.5–1.5	Once daily or bid		• With ziprasidone, QTc monitoring needed

Table 29–4. Antipsychotics (continued)

Drug	Daily dose (mg/kg)	Dosage schedule	Main indications	Adverse effects and comments
Atypical antipsychotics (continued)				
Clozapine	3.0–7.0	bid–tid	• Refractory psychosis • Refractory mania	• Serotonergic, adrenergic, histaminergic • Low incidence of extrapyramidal adverse effects; does not induce dystonia • Low risk of TD • Granulocytopenia or agranulocytosis (treatment involves constant monitoring of blood count) • Seizure risk is dose related

Note. Doses are general guidelines. All doses must be individualized, and appropriate monitoring should be performed. Weight-corrected doses are less appropriate for obese children. When high doses are used, serum levels may be obtained to avoid toxicity. TD = tardive dyskinesia.
[a]Loxapine has features similar to atypicals.

ramidal adverse effects and can be effective in treatment-resistant cases or in children who develop tardive dyskinesia. Risperidone, olanzapine, and quetiapine are novel atypical antipsychotic medications that combine dopaminergic (D_2) and serotonergic (5-HT_2) antagonist properties and are also associated with a lower incidence of acute extrapyramidal adverse effects and perhaps a lower risk of tardive dyskinesia.

Target symptoms that most commonly respond to typical antipsychotics are so-called positive symptoms (see "Psychotic Disorders"). In contrast, atypical antipsychotics are more effective agents for "negative symptoms." In addition to use in childhood psychotic disorders, antipsychotics have been used to control symptoms of agitation, aggression, and self-injurious behaviors that occur in children with mental retardation and pervasive developmental disorders (autistic and autistic-like disorders). Because of their serotonergic (5-HT_2) antagonist activity, atypical antipsychotics possess thymoleptic properties that are helpful in mood regulation. In recent years, atypical antipsychotics have been found to be efficacious in the treatment of adult and pediatric mania, having beneficial effects on both manic and depressive symptoms (Frazier et al. 1999). However, because of this thymoleptic activity, these agents may also precipitate or worsen mania.

The typical antipsychotic drugs haloperidol and pimozide have been widely used in the treatment of Tourette's disorder, with equivocal results (Shapiro et al. 1988). QTc prolongations of unclear clinical significance have been reported with pimozide treatment. Pimozide at doses up to 0.3 mg/kg is recommended for use in patients with Tourette's disorder who fail to respond to more conventional treatments. In addition to typical antipsychotics, clonidine and guanfacine have been found to be useful in the treatment of some children with this disorder (Leckman et al. 1991).

The usual oral dose of antipsychotic drugs ranges between 3.0 and 6.0 mg/kg/day for low-potency phenothiazines and between 0.1 and 0.3 (up to 1.0) mg/kg/day for high-potency phenothiazines, butyrophenones, thioxanthenes, and indole derivatives. The daily dose range of clozapine is 3.0–7.0 mg/kg; that of risperidone is up to 85 µg/kg. Antipsychotic medications have relatively long half-lives and therefore should be administered not more than twice daily. Most antipsychotic preparations are available in either tablet or capsule form. In addition, at least one compound from each class of antipsychotics is available in a liquid concentrate form, including risperidone (1 mg/mL). Several compounds, including chlorpromazine, haloperidol, and fluphenazine, are available in injectable form for intramuscular administration.

Common short-term adverse effects of antipsychotic drugs are drowsiness, increased appetite, and weight gain. It is not entirely clear why weight gain, a particularly thorny adverse effect, is associated with use of atypical antipsychotics. Anticholinergic effects such as dry mouth, nasal congestion, and blurred vision are more commonly seen with use of low-potency phenothiazines. Extrapyramidal effects such as acute dystonia, akathisia (motor restlessness), and parkinsonism (bradykinesia, tremor, facial inexpressiveness) are more commonly seen with administration of high-potency compounds (phenothiazines, butyrophenones, and thioxanthenes). Treatment with thioridazine and with ziprasidone has been associated with increases in QTc and may necessitate electrocardiographic monitoring.

Although children appear generally less vulnerable to tardive dyskinesia (and tardive dystonia) than adults, long-term administration of typical antipsychotic drugs in children and adolescents may be associated with tardive dyskinesia. Tardive dyskinesia should be distinguished from the more common, generally benign, withdrawal dyskinesia that is associated with abrupt cessation of antipsychotic drugs and tends to subside several months after drug discontinuation. In children with mental retardation and pervasive developmental disorders, tardive dyskinesia should be differentiated from the commonly occurring stereotypies. One approach to minimize withdrawal reactions is to taper antipsychotic drugs very slowly over several months. Early detection with regular monitoring is the only available approach for tardive dyskinesia. It appears that treatment with atypical antipsychotics is less likely to be associated with tardive dyskinesia.

Increases in prolactin levels have occurred with the use of typical antipsychotics because of dopamine D_2 receptor–blocking effects on prolactin release, but the risk of hyperprolactinemia appears to be particularly high with the use of the atypical antipsychotic risperidone. The clinical implications of hyperprolactinemia remain unknown, but given the potential for disruption of the pituitary–gonadal axis, more efforts are needed to evaluate this problem in children and adolescents. In a recent case series, antipsychotic-induced hyperprolactinemia was successfully treated with cabergoline (Cohen and Biederman 2001). The serum prolactin levels normalized in all four subjects at a mean cabergoline dose of 2 mg/week. The cabergoline dose was reduced to 1 mg/week in three of four subjects. Cabergoline was well tolerated and had no adverse effects.

The atypical antipsychotic clozapine is associated with an increased risk of leukopenia and agranulocytosis, necessitating weekly monitoring of blood counts for the first 6 months and biweekly thereafter.

Another serious idiosyncratic reaction to antipsychotics is neuroleptic malignant syndrome, which is potentially lethal and consists of muscle rigidity, delirium, and autonomic instability (instability of blood pressure and pulse, diaphoresis, and hyperpyrexia), often accompanied by high creatine phosphokinase levels and less commonly accompanied by rhabdomyolysis. Preliminary evidence indicates that its presentation in juvenile patients is similar to that in adult patients. This syndrome may be difficult to distinguish from primary CNS pathology, concurrent infection, or other, more benign side effects of antipsychotic treatment, including extrapyramidal involvement or anticholinergic toxicity. Treatment of neuroleptic malignant syndrome involves intensive medical surveillance, immediate discontinuation of the antipsychotic, symptomatic treatment, and aggressive treatment of concomitant medical conditions, such as rhabdomyolysis. Although there is no general agreement about specific pharmacological treatment for neuroleptic malignant syndrome, dantrolene and bromocriptine have been used.

Short-term adverse effects of antipsychotics are more easily managed. Excessive sedation can be avoided by using less sedating antipsychotics and managed by prescribing most of the daily dose at night. Drowsiness should not be confused with impaired cognition and can usually be eliminated by adjusting the dose and the timing of administration. In fact, there is no evidence that antipsychotics adversely affect cognition when given at low doses. Anticholinergic adverse effects can be minimized by choosing a medium- or high-potency compound or atypical antipsychotics. Extrapyramidal reactions can be avoided in most cases by slowly titrating the antipsychotic dose. Antiparkinsonian agents (i.e., anticholinergic drugs, antihistamines, amantadine) should be avoided unless strictly necessary, because of the added adverse effects that these drugs may produce. Extrapyramidal reactions can be prevented in many cases by avoiding rapid increase in neuroleptic dose or the use of high-potency typical antipsychotics such as haloperidol. When a child or adolescent taking antipsychotics develops an acutely agitated clinical picture with associated inability to sit still and aggressive outbursts, akathisia should be rapidly considered in the differential diagnosis. If akathisia is suspected, the dose of the antipsychotic may need to be decreased. β-Blockers (e.g., propranolol) and high-potency benzodiazepines have been found helpful in relieving symptoms of antipsychotic-induced akathisia in adults and may help relieve similar symptoms in juvenile patients (Ananth and Lin 1986).

■ Mood Stabilizers (Table 29–5)

Lithium Carbonate

Lithium is a simple solid element, and it bears chemical similarities to sodium, potassium, calcium, and magnesium. As with other psychotropic agents, the precise cellular mechanism of action by which lithium produces its beneficial effects is not known. Lithium has diverse cellular actions that alter hormonal, metabolic, and neuronal systems. Proposed theories for lithium's mechanism of action relate to neurotransmission (i.e., interaction with catecholamine, indolamine, cholinergic, and endorphin systems; inhibition of β-adrenoreceptors), endocrine effects (i.e., blocking of testosterone synthesis and the release of thyroid hormone), circadian rhythm (i.e., normalization of altered sleep–wake cycles), and cellular processes (i.e., ionic substitution, inhibition of adenylate cyclase).

In children, the elimination half-life of lithium is approximately 18 hours, and it takes 5–7 days to reach steady state (Alessi et al. 1994). Aside from a shorter elimination half-life and a higher total clearance, the pharmacokinetics of lithium in children seem to be the same as in adults. Because work done to determine therapeutic ranges of lithium has been based on a 12-hour sampling interval, blood samples for determination of serum lithium levels should be obtained 12 hours after the last dose. Micromethods permit use of the finger-stick technique to obtain samples. A recent finding that lithium levels in saliva correlate with serum lithium levels (Weller et al. 1987) could facilitate monitoring of lithium therapy in young children, in whom venipuncture may be problematic.

The usual lithium starting dose ranges from 10 to 30 mg/kg, given once a day or in divided doses twice a day. There is no established therapeutic serum lithium level in pediatric psychiatry. Suggested guidelines, based on the adult literature, include serum levels of 0.8–1.5 mEq/L for acute episodes and 0.6–0.8 mEq/L for maintenance or prophylactic therapy. Nonetheless, as with any other intervention, the lowest effective dose or serum level should always be chosen. Slow- and controlled-release lithium carbonate preparations are available. Lithium is also available in a liquid form, lithium citrate, which contains 8 mEq of lithium per 5 mL, equivalent to the amount in 300 mg of lithium carbonate.

Common short-term adverse effects include gastrointestinal symptoms such as nausea and vomiting, renal symptoms such as polyuria and polydipsia, and CNS symptoms such as tremor, sleepiness, and memory impairment. Chronic administration of lithium may be associated with metabolic (weight gain, decreased calcium metabolism), endocrine (decreased thyroid functioning), and possible renal damage. Data collected over the last 10 years, however,

Table 29–5. Mood stabilizers

Drug	Daily dose (mg/kg)	Dosage schedule	Main indications	Adverse effects and comments
Lithium carbonate	10–30[a]	Once daily or bid	• Bipolar disorder • Bipolar disorder prophylaxis • Hyperaggressive behavior	• *Lithium:* Polyuria, polydipsia; tremor, nausea, diarrhea; weight gain, drowsiness, skin abnormalities; possible effects on thyroid and renal functioning with chronic administration; monitoring of lithium levels and thyroid and renal function needed; lithium toxicity (level>2 mEq/L) can be life-threatening
Typical antiepileptic drugs			• Adjunct therapy in refractory MD • ?Dysphoric conduct disorder	• *Antiepileptic drugs:* Sedation, nausea, dizziness, rashes • *Carbamazepine:* Bone marrow suppression (monitoring of blood counts and levels needed, initially and during treatment); may increase metabolism of low-dose oral contraceptives; rare liver toxicity
Carbamazepine	10–20[a]	bid		• *Oxcarbazepine:* Little effect on P450 system, few drug–drug interactions
Oxcarbazepine	15–35	bid		• *Valproic acid:* Rare liver toxicity; monitoring of blood counts and liver and renal function needed, initially and during treatment
Valproic acid	15–60[a]	bid–tid		

Table 29–5. Mood stabilizers *(continued)*

Drug	Daily dose (mg/kg)	Dosage schedule	Main indications	Adverse effects and comments
Atypical antiepileptic drugs				
Gabapentin	10–30	bid–tid	• Bipolar disorder	• *Gabapentin, tiagabine, and topiramate:* Renally excreted; little effect on P450 system, few drug–drug interactions, large margin of safety; laboratory monitoring usually not necessary
Lamotrigine	3–7	bid	• Bipolar disorder prophylaxis	
Tiagabine	0.3–0.8	bid–qid	• Hyperaggressive behavior	
Topiramate	3–6	bid	• Adjunct therapy in refractory MD	• *Lamotrigine:* Hepatically metabolized; interactions with typical antiepileptic drugs; associated with potentially life-threatening toxic epidermal necrolysis (Stevens-Johnson syndrome) in 2% of children
			• ?Dysphoric conduct disorder	• *Tiagabine:* Risk of kidney stones (weak carbonic anhydrase inhibitor)

Note. Doses are general guidelines. All doses must be individualized, and appropriate monitoring should be performed. Weight-corrected doses are less appropriate for obese children. When high doses are used, serum levels may be obtained to avoid toxicity. MD = major depression.
[a]Dose adjusted according to serum levels.

suggest that maintenance lithium therapy does not lead to serious nephrotoxicity, at least in adults. Nevertheless, renal function (blood urea nitrogen and creatinine levels) and thyroid function should be measured in children before lithium treatment is started, and these tests should be repeated at least every 6 months. Particular caution should be exercised when lithium is used in patients with neurological, renal, or cardiovascular disorders. In addition, nonsteroidal anti-inflammatory agents, certain diuretics, and angiotensin-converting enzyme inhibitors may increase plasma lithium levels. Concomitant use of these drugs necessitates closer monitoring of plasma lithium levels.

Anticonvulsants

Alternative mood-stabilizing antimanic agents include the typical antiepileptic drugs carbamazepine, oxcarbazepine, and valproic acid, as well as atypical antiepileptic drugs.

Carbamazepine.   Carbamazepine is structurally related to TCAs. The plasma half-life after chronic administration is between 13 and 17 hours. The therapeutic plasma concentration is variably reported at 4–12 μg/mL, and recommended daily doses in children range from 10 to 20 mg/kg, administered twice a day. Because the relationship between dose and plasma level is variable and uncertain, with marked interindividual variability, close plasma level monitoring is recommended. Common short-term side effects include dizziness, drowsiness, nausea, vomiting, and blurred vision. Idiosyncratic reactions such as bone marrow suppression, liver toxicity, and skin disorders (including Stevens-Johnson syndrome) have been reported but appear to be rare. However, given the seriousness of these reactions, careful monitoring of blood counts and liver and renal function is warranted, initially and during treat-

ment. Carbamazepine should be used with care in females because it is teratogenic and may increase the metabolism of low-dose oral contraceptives, resulting in an increased risk of unwanted pregnancy. Carbatrol is a carbamazepine formulation that consists of immediate-release, extended-release, and enteric-release beads, allowing twice-daily dosing. It is available in 200- and 300-mg capsules that can be opened and used as a sprinkle preparation.

Oxcarbazepine.   Oxcarbazepine is chemically similar to carbamazepine, with some important differences. Because there is little interaction between oxcarbazepine and the P450 system, few drug–drug interactions are associated with administration, and the drug does not induce its own metabolism. It also does not share the hepatic and hematological liability of carbamazepine, and thus laboratory monitoring is not required. The drug is given twice daily. In adults, the maximum suggested dose is 2,400 mg/day. Controlled trials of oxcarbazepine in pediatric epilepsy led to development of weight-based dosing guidelines. Oxcarbazepine is available in 150-, 300-, and 600-mg scored tablets.

Valproic acid.   Valproic acid is another anticonvulsant with well-documented efficacy in adult mania, particularly the mixed or dysphoric subtype of mania (Pope et al. 1991). Valproic acid is primarily metabolized by the liver and has a plasma half-life of 8–16 hours. The therapeutic plasma concentration range is 50–100 μg/mL. The recommended initial daily dose is 15 mg/kg, gradually increased to a maximum of 60 mg/kg, administered three times a day. Common short-term side effects include sedation, thinning of hair, anorexia, nausea, and vomiting. Idiosyncratic reactions such as bone marrow suppression and liver toxicity have been reported but appear to be rare. Asymptomatic increases in aspartate aminotransferase (AST) levels usually resolve spontaneously. Although hepatic fatalities have been reported in children less than 10 years old who were receiving monotherapy, most of these children were less than 2 years old. The risk of serious hepatic involvement is increased by concomitant use of other antiseizure medications and may be dose related. Careful monitoring of blood counts and liver and renal function is warranted, initially and during treatment. Valproate should be used with care in females because it is teratogenic.

Atypical antiepileptic drugs.   A generation of atypical antiepileptic drugs with potential mood-stabilizing effects has emerged. These drugs include gabapentin (available in 100, 300, and 400 mg), tiagabine (4, 12, 16, and 20 mg), topiramate (25, 100, and 200 mg), and lamotrigine (25, 100, 150, and 200 mg). Their roles in the treatment of mania are being actively investigated, and initial case reports and published case series are encouraging. Gabapentin, tiagabine, and topiramate are postulated to act on γ-aminobutyric acid (GABA) levels, with little effect on the P450 system. Considering their wide margin of safety, the lack of a need for laboratory monitoring, and their renal excretion, they may represent major additions to the therapeutic armamentarium if they are found to be effective in the treatment of pediatric mania. Topiramate may be anorectic and therefore may be helpful as an adjunct to atypical antipsychotics, with their associated weight gain side effects. Unlike other atypical antiepileptic drugs, lamotrigine acts by inhibiting use-dependent sodium channels and is hepatically metabolized; therefore, serum levels are affected by coadministration of lamotrigine and typical antiepileptic drugs. Lamotrigine has been associated with a high risk of potentially life-

threatening toxic epidermal necrolysis (Stevens-Johnson syndrome) and should be used with extreme caution in children and be titrated extremely slowly over several weeks.

■ Antianxiety Drugs (Table 29–6)

The major agents in the antianxiety drug class are the benzodiazepines. Related compounds include barbiturates, several compounds structurally related to alcohol (i.e., chloral hydrate, paraldehyde, meprobamate), and sedative antihistamines (i.e., diphenhydramine, hydroxyzine, promethazine). The first nonbenzodiazepine antianxiety medicine to come on the market was buspirone. Buspirone is a novel nonbenzodiazepine anxiolytic without anticonvulsant, sedative, or muscle relaxant properties. The anxiolytic effects of buspirone may relate to reduction in serotonergic neurotransmission (Eison 1989). Clinical experience suggests that this drug has limited antianxiety efficacy. The daily dose is estimated to range from 0.2 to 0.65 mg/kg. Buspirone may be effective in the treatment of aggressive behaviors in children with pervasive developmental disorders (Realmuto et al. 1989).

Benzodiazepines (along with other sedatives, hypnotics, and antihistamines) are widely used in children, mostly to treat poorly diagnosed symptoms of agitation and insomnia, because of their pharmacological properties (clinical effects), toxicological properties (comfortable margin of safety), and minimal pharmacokinetic interactions with other drugs (D. M. Quinn 1986). Most benzodiazepines are lipophilic and are highly bound to plasma membranes; most have active metabolites that dominate their course of activity. Most benzodiazepines are absorbed at an intermediate rate, with peak plasma levels appearing 1–3 hours after ingestion. Benzodiazepines

Table 29–6. Antianxiety drugs

Drug	Daily dose (mg/kg)	Dosage schedule	Main indications	Adverse effects and comments
High-potency benzodiazepines			• Anxiety disorders	• Drowsiness, disinhibition, agitation
Long-acting			• Adjunct in refractory psychosis	• Confusion
Clonazepam	0.01–0.04	Once daily or bid	• Adjunct in mania	• Depression
Short- to intermediate-acting			• Severe agitation	• Potential risk of abuse and dependence
Alprazolam	0.02–0.06	tid	• Tourette's disorder	• Risk of rebound and withdrawal reactions greater with short-acting benzodiazepines
Lorazepam	0.04–0.09	tid	• Severe insomnia	
			• MD+anxiety	
Nonbenzodiazepines			• Anxiety disorders	• Large margin of safety, laboratory monitoring usually not necessary
Buspirone	0.20–0.65	bid	• ?Agitated states	

Note. Doses are general guidelines. All doses must be individualized, and appropriate monitoring should be performed. Weight-corrected doses are less appropriate for obese children. MD = major depression.

and related sedative drugs can produce tolerance (and cross-tolerance with other benzodiazepines), physiological dependence (addiction), and psychological dependence (habituation).

GABA A receptors are the primary sites of action of benzodiazepines and barbiturates in the CNS. Some of the intoxicating effects of ethanol also occur at GABA A receptors. Benzodiazepines and barbiturates act at separate binding sites on the receptor, to potentiate the inhibitory action of GABA. Barbiturates and ethanol, but not benzodiazepines, can also independently open the chloride ion channel within the receptor. The fact that benzodiazepines, barbiturates, and ethanol all have related actions on a common receptor type explains their pharmacological synergy and cross-tolerance. It is not yet clear how benzodiazepines function as anxiolytics. The general belief, based on animal models, is that the anxiolytic properties of benzodiazepines reflect their actions on the limbic system, including the hippocampus and amygdala. The drugs' anticonvulsant actions may be primarily cortical, and their sedative actions may be primarily mediated in the brain stem. Neurons inhibited by benzodiazepines to produce anxiolysis may include serotonin (5-HT) and noradrenergic neurons. The pharmacological effects of buspirone include inhibition of serotonin neurons and the decrease of striatal levels of serotonin binding sites.

Because the pharmacological profiles of antianxiety drugs include behavioral disinhibition, and because many childhood psychiatric disorders are characterized by behavioral disinhibition, use of these agents in the absence of a specific indication may worsen the clinical picture (Wilens et al. 1998). Possible indications for use of antianxiety agents in pediatric psychiatry include childhood anxiety symptoms and disorders (Leonard and Rapoport 1989). The high-potency benzodiazepines alprazolam and clonazepam have received increasing attention as effective and safe agents for the treatment of adult panic disorder with or without agoraphobia (Biederman 1990; Herman et al. 1987). Reports suggest that children also may manifest adult-type anxiety disorders such as panic disorder and agoraphobia, which may respond to treatment with high-potency benzodiazepines (Biederman 1987). Possible additional uses of benzodiazepines include adjunct treatment of acute psychotic episodes, treatment of refractory schizophrenia, and treatment of antipsychotic-induced akathisia (Kutcher et al. 1989). The chlorinated benzodiazepines clonazepam and clorazepate may be particularly helpful in the treatment of complex partial seizures. Lorazepam and oxazepam do not have active metabolites and do not tend to accumulate in tissue; this makes them preferable for short-term symptomatic use. When long-term use is anticipated, longer-acting benzodiazepines (such as clonazepam) are preferable. It has been suggested that buspirone is beneficial in agitated states such as those occurring in patients with developmental disorders (Realmuto et al. 1989).

In general, the clinical toxicity of benzodiazepines is low. The most commonly encountered short-term adverse effects are sedation, drowsiness, and decreased mental acuity. When these drugs are given at high doses, patients can become confused. In adults, benzodiazepines have been reported to be associated with depressogenic adverse effects. With the exception of the potential risk of tolerance and dependence (this risk is suspected but not well studied in adults and is unknown in children), benzodiazepines have no known long-term adverse effects. Adverse withdrawal effects can occur, and benzodiazepines should always be tapered slowly.

In recent years, however, serotonergic antidepressants (including paroxetine, sertraline, and venlafaxine) have been increasingly found to have strong antianxiety effects in juvenile patients with OCD or other anxiety disorders. Clomipramine, sertraline, and fluvoxamine underwent large-scale, multisite clinical trials, and positive results were achieved in children and adolescents. Considering the safety profiles of serotonergic drugs, their long half-lives, the absence of addictive potential, and their antidepressant properties, serotonergic antidepressants should be considered first-line agents in the treatment of juvenile anxiety disorders.

The P450 enzyme 2C19 is involved in the biotransformation of diazepam and is inhibited by fluoxetine, sertraline, and fluvoxamine. In addition, 3A4 is involved in the biotransformation of triazolobenzodiazepines (triazolam, alprazolam, and midazolam) and is affected by fluoxetine, sertraline, and fluvoxamine. Thus, administration of benzodiazepines with these other drugs could affect serum levels of the benzodiazepines.

■ Other Drugs (Table 29–7)

Alpha-Adrenergic Agonists

Clonidine. Clonidine, a presynaptic α_2-adrenergic agonist, has been widely used in pediatric psychiatry, despite extremely limited safety and efficacy data supporting its use. Clonidine is an imidazoline derivative with α-adrenergic agonist properties that has been primarily used in the treatment of hypertension. At low doses, the drug appears to stimulate inhibitory, presynaptic autoreceptors in the CNS. In pediatric psychiatry, clonidine is most commonly used in the treatment of Tourette's disorder and other tic disorders (Leckman et al. 1991), ADHD, and ADHD-associated sleep disturbances (Hunt et al. 1990; Prince et al. 1996). In addition, the agent has been reported to be useful in controlling aggression toward self and others in patients with developmental disorders.

Clonidine is a relatively short-acting compound with a plasma half-life ranging from approximately 5.5 hours (in children) to 8.5 hours (in adults). Daily doses should be titrated and individualized. Usual daily doses range from 3 to 10 μg/kg, given generally in two, three, or sometimes four divided doses. Therapy is usually initiated with a full or half 0.1-mg tablet (the lowest manufactured dose), depending on the size of the child (for a dose of approximately 1–2 μg/kg), and the dose is increased depending on clinical response and adverse effects. Because of clonidine's sedative effect, initial doses are best given in the evening hours or before bed.

Sedation is the most common short-term adverse effect. Hypotension, dry mouth, depression, and confusion may also occur. Clonidine is not known to have long-term adverse effects. In hypertensive adults, abrupt withdrawal of clonidine has been associated with rebound hypertension. Thus, slow tapering must precede discontinuation of the drug. Clonidine should not be administered concomitantly with β-blockers because adverse interactions have been reported with this combination. Recent reports of death in several children taking the combination of methylphenidate and clonidine have generated new concerns about clonidine's safety. Although more work is needed to determine whether an increased risk exists with this combination, a cautious approach is advised, including increased surveillance and cardiovascular monitoring.

Guanfacine. There has been anecdotal evidence that the more selective α-adrenergic agonist guanfacine (an α_{2a}-adrenergic agonist) has benefits similar to those of clonidine, with less sedation and longer duration of action (Chappell et al. 1995;

Table 29–7.   Other drugs

Drug	Daily dose	Dosage schedule	Main indications	Adverse effects and comments
α_2-**Adrenergic agonists**				
Clonidine	3–10 µg/kg	bid–qid	• Tourette's disorder	• Sedation (very frequent)
Guanfacine	15–90 µg/kg	Once daily or bid	• ADHD	• Hypotension (rare)
			• Aggression, self-abuse	• Dry mouth
			• Severe agitation	• Confusion (with high dose)
			• Withdrawal syndromes	• Depression
				• Rebound hypertension
				• Localized irritation with transdermal preparation
				• *Guanfacine:* Same effects as above, but less sedation and less hypotension
β-**Blockers**				
Propranolol	1–7 mg/kg	bid	• Aggression, self-abuse	• Sedation
			• Severe agitation	• Depression
			• Akathisia	• Risk of bradycardia and hypotension (dose dependent) and rebound hypertension
				• Bronchospasm (propranolol contraindicated in asthmatic patients)
				• Rebound hypertension with abrupt withdrawal
Naltrexone	1–2 mg/kg	Once daily or bid	• Self-injurious behavior	• Long-acting opioid antagonist
			• Addiction	• Minimal adverse effects
				• Hepatotoxicity (rare)
DDAVP (Desmopressin)	20–40 µg intranasally	Once daily hs	• Enuresis	• Headache
	0.2–0.4 mg orally	Once daily hs		• Nausea

Table 29–7. Other drugs (continued)

Drug	Daily dose	Dosage schedule	Main indications	Adverse effects and comments
Noradrenergic-specific reuptake inhibitors				
Atomoxetine	0.5–1.8 mg/kg	Once daily or bid	• ADHD with or without comorbidity	• Mild increase in pulse and diastolic blood pressure • Mild decrease in appetite • No insomnia • No cardiac conduction or repolarization delays • Not abusable • Rare serious hepatotoxicity

Note. Doses are general guidelines. All doses must be individualized, and appropriate monitoring should be performed. Weight-corrected doses are less appropriate for obese children. ADHD=attention-deficit/hyperactivity disorder; DDAVP=1-desamino-8-D-arginine-vasopressin.

Horrigan and Barnhill 1995; Hunt et al. 1995). Usual daily doses range from 15 to 90 μg/kg, given generally in two or three divided doses.

Propranolol

Propranolol is a nonselective (i.e., affecting both β_1 and β_2 receptors) β-adrenergic antagonist. It has received considerable attention for its potential efficacy in psychiatric disorders, including drug-induced akathisia, anxiety disorders, and schizophrenia, as well as in aggressive and self-abusive behavior disorders (Ananth and Lin 1986; Sorgi et al. 1986). Propranolol's effects are mediated through the drug's blocking of β-adrenergic receptors at multiple sites in the body. Propranolol also crosses the blood–brain barrier, a circumstance that probably accounts for some of its efficacy in psychiatric disorders but that also contributes to concerns regarding its potential CNS toxicity. It is unclear whether the benefits of propranolol therapy are primarily due to peripheral or to central effects of the drug. In pediatric psychiatry, propranolol has been used in the management of severe aggressive and self-injurious behaviors (the drug is administered in daily doses of 2–5 mg/kg).

Short-term adverse effects of propranolol include nausea, vomiting, constipation, and mild diarrhea. Propranolol can cause bradycardia and hypotension as well as increased airway resistance, and it is contraindicated in asthmatic and certain cardiac patients. Chronic administration of propranolol has no known long-term effects. Because abrupt cessation of propranolol has been associated with rebound hypertension, gradual tapering of the drug is recommended. Coadministration of β-blockers such as propranolol with SSRIs could affect serum levels of β-blockers.

Naltrexone

Naltrexone is a potent, long-acting opioid antagonist with a rapid onset of action. It has been administered in daily doses of 1–2 mg/kg to children with pervasive developmental disorders and to children with self-abuse (Lienemann and Walker 1989). Although naltrexone is relatively free of serious adverse effects, there have been some rare reports of hepatotoxicity. Naltrexone has been used in the treatment of alcohol craving (O'Malley et al. 1996).

Desmopressin

Desmopressin (1-desamino-8-D-arginine-vasopressin; DDAVP), a synthetic antidiuretic hormone peptide analogue, is approved by the FDA for the treatment of enuresis. Daily doses are 0.1–0.2 mL by intranasal spray, given at bedtime. A tablet formulation is now also available. Although desmopressin suppresses urine production for 7–10 hours, it lacks the pressor effects of antidiuretic hormone. Adverse effects are minimal. The drug's safety has been established in patients requiring long-term therapy (Rew and Rundle 1989).

Atomoxetine

Atomoxetine is a potent noradrenergic-specific reuptake inhibitor that has been studied in more than 1,800 children and more than 250 adults and has been submitted for FDA approval (Michelson et al. 2001; Spencer et al. 2002). Atomoxetine has been shown to be effective for ADHD at all ages and has a favorable adverse-effect profile, consisting of mild appetite suppression and no insomnia. As with TCAs, there are mild increases in diastolic blood pressure and heart rate. Unlike tricyclics, atomoxetine does not affect electrocardiographic intervals. In a study involving children and adolescents, response to atomoxetine was best at 1.2 or 1.8 mg/kg/day and superior to 0.5 mg/kg/day; all three doses were superior to placebo (Kratochvil et al. 2001). Safety and efficacy data at 1 year revealed that atomoxetine continued to be effective and well tolerated. The acute mild increases in diastolic blood pressure and heart rate persisted but did not worsen. Growth in height and weight was normal, and there were no significant differences between atomoxetine and placebo in terms of laboratory parameters and electrocardiographic intervals.

Although no evidence of adverse hepatic effects were evident in an extensive clinical trial program involving thousands of patients, postmarketing surveillance identified two cases of liver injury out of more than 2 million patients who have received atomoxetine since its approval in 2003. Despite the rarity of these events and the fact that both patients fully recovered after discontinuing atomoxetine, Eli Lilly decided to add a bolded warning to the product label for atomoxetine because of concerns that potential atomoxetine-related liver injuries might progress to acute liver failure if the drug were not discontinued. The black-box warning recommends that atomoxetine be discontinued promptly in patients who develop clinical evidence of liver injury, including pruritus, jaundice, dark urine, light-colored stools, or upper-right-sided abdominal tenderness.

Main Diagnostic Categories and Clinical Considerations

■ Attention-Deficit/Hyperactivity Disorder (Table 29–8)

ADHD is one of the major clinical and public health problems in the United States in terms of morbidity and disability in children and adolescents. ADHD is estimated to affect at least 5% of school-age children. Its effect on society is enormous in terms of financial cost, stress on families, effect on schools, and damaging effects on self-esteem. Although the etiology of ADHD remains unknown, data from family, genetic, twin, adoption, and segregation analyses strongly suggest a genetic etiology. Indeed, the genetic contribution appears to be substantial, as suggested by the very high heritability coefficients (mean, 0.8) associated with this disorder. Preliminary molecular genetic studies have implicated several candidate genes, including the dopamine D_2 receptor gene (*DRD2*) and the dopamine D_4 receptor gene (*DRD4*), as well as the dopamine transporter gene (*DAT1*) (Faraone and Biederman 1999). Both dopamine and norepinephrine, neurotransmitters thought to mediate the response to anti-ADHD medications, are potent agonists of the dopamine D_4 receptor.

Data from follow-up studies indicate that children with ADHD are at risk of maintaining and developing new psychiatric disorders in adolescence and adulthood, including antisocial and substance use (tobacco, alcohol, drugs) disorders. Follow-up data also indicate that the disorder persists into adulthood in a substantial number of individuals and may be a common adult diagnosis (Spencer et al. 1998a). In recent years, ADHD has been increasingly recognized as highly heterogeneous, occurring at high levels in conjunction with psychiatric disorders (conduct and oppositional defiant disorders, unipolar and bipolar mood disorders, and anxiety disorders), cognitive problems (learning disability), and social problems (social disability, nonverbal learning disability). Neuroimaging studies have identified subtle anomalies in the frontal cortex and in projecting subcortical structures (Faraone and Biederman 1999), and it has been posited that dysregulation of catecholamine neurotransmission under-

Table 29–8.   Pharmacotherapy for disruptive behavior disorders

Disorder	Main characteristics	Pharmacotherapy
Attention-deficit/ hyperactivity disorder (ADHD)	• Inattentiveness, impulsivity, hyperactivity • Persists into adulthood in 50% of individuals	*First-line* • Stimulants (70% response; for uncomplicated ADHD; caution advised in patients with tic disorders) • Atomoxetine *Second-line* • TCAs (70% response; consider for patients with comorbid MD or anxiety disorders and for patients with ADHD+tics; serum level and cardiovascular monitoring needed) • Bupropion *Third-line* • Clonidine, guanfacine (consider for patients with ADHD+tics) *Fourth-line* • MAOIs • Combined pharmacotherapy for treatment-resistant cases
Conduct disorder (CD)	• Persistent and pervasive patterns of aggressive and antisocial behaviors • Often associated with ADHD, MD, and bipolar disorder	• No specific pharmacotherapy available for core disorder • Behavior therapy • Conduct disorder in conjunction with other Axis I disorders (e.g., ADHD, MD, mania, psychosis, anxiety): treat underlying disorder (α-adrenergic agents and β-blockers for agitation, aggression, and self-abuse)

Note.   MAOI = monoamine oxidase inhibitor; MD = major depression; SSRI = selective serotonin reuptake inhibitor; TCA = tricyclic antidepressant.

lies ADHD's pathophysiology (Zametkin and Rapoport 1987).

Stimulants

There is extensive, clear documentation of the short-term efficacy of methylphenidate treatment, mostly in latency-age Caucasian boys (Spencer et al. 1997). The literature on stimulants administered at other ages or to females or ethnic minorities is more limited. The few studies of stimulants in adolescents found rates of response highly consistent with response rates among latency-age children. In contrast, the few studies involving preschoolers appear to indicate that young children respond less well to stimulant therapy, which suggests that ADHD in preschoolers may be more refractory. It has been clearly documented that treatment with stimulants improves not only abnormal behaviors of ADHD but also self-esteem and cognitive, social, and family function, findings that support the importance of treating ADHD patients beyond school or work hours. Two controlled clinical trials indicated the efficacy of methylphenidate and Adderall in adults with ADHD (Spencer et al. 1995, 1999b). In these trials, there was a highly clinically and statistically significant difference between study drug and placebo, and the magnitude of effects was consistent with that in pediatric trials.

New long-acting stimulant preparations have revolutionized ADHD treatment. An analogue classroom paradigm was used to test the fine-grained pharmacodynamic and pharmacokinetic profiles of some of these medications. Developed by Swanson et al. (2000), these settings simulate real-life demands and distractions of a typical classroom. Trained observers hourly record frequencies of behaviors as well as academic production and accuracy. Sequential serum sampling from catheters allows correlation of blood levels to behavioral activity.

The first medication developed was the methylphenidate preparation Concerta. Concerta uses an osmotic pump mechanism that creates an ascending profile of methylphenidate in the blood, providing effective treatment for 10–12 hours. Concerta is available in 18-, 36-, and 54-mg tablets, approximating the 5-, 10-, and 15-mg thrice-daily doses of IR methylphenidate. A laboratory classroom study involving 68 children found that a single morning dose of Concerta was effective for 12 hours with regard to social and task behaviors and academic performance (Pelham et al. 2001). A large multicenter, randomized clinical trial was used to determine the safety and efficacy of Concerta in an outpatient setting (Wolraich et al. 2001). Two hundred eighty-two children with ADHD (ages 6–12 years) were randomized to placebo administration (n=90), IR methylphenidate three times a day (n=97), or Concerta once a day (n=95) in a double-blind, 28-day trial. Throughout the study, children in the Concerta and IR methylphenidate treatment groups showed significantly greater reductions in core ADHD symptoms than did children receiving placebo. Concerta was well tolerated; there was mild appetite suppression, but study subjects experienced no sleep abnormalities. A 1-year follow-up study involving 407 children treated with Concerta found no marked effects on weight, height, blood pressure, or pulse and no tic exacerbation (Wilens and Group 2000).

A new extended-release form of the methylphenidate preparation Ritalin (Ritalin LA) provides effective methylphenidate treatment for 8–9 hours. Ritalin LA's bimodal release system produces, in single-dose administration, pharmacokinetic characteristics that resemble those of two doses of Ritalin administered 4–5 hours apart. Ritalin LA consists of a mixture of immediate- and delayed-release beads in a 1:1 ratio. The delayed-release beads are coated with an absorption-delaying polymer. Ritalin LA is available in 20-, 30-, and 40-mg capsules, approximating 10-, 15-, and 20-mg twice-daily doses of IR methylphenidate. Ritalin LA may be used as a sprinkle preparation for children unable to swallow pills. The initial analogue classroom study evaluated the pharmacodynamic (efficacy) profile, safety, and tolerability of Ritalin LA (Spencer et al. 2000). Compared with placebo, single doses of all variants of Ritalin LA improved classroom behavior and academic productivity over the 9-hour period after dosing. Ritalin LA had a rapid onset of effect, and the improvement relative to placebo was statistically significant during both the morning (0–4 hours after dosing) and the afternoon (4–9 hours after dosing).

Ritalin LA was further tested in a multicenter, double-blind trial involving 160 children (Biederman et al. 2001). There was a 2- to 4-week titration to optimal dose, followed by a 1-week placebo washout period. A total of 137 subjects with persistent ADHD symptoms during the washout were randomized to treatment with Ritalin LA or placebo. Compared with children taking placebo, children taking Ritalin LA were rated (by teachers and parents) on the Conners ADHD/DSM-IV Scale as greatly improved. Scores on the subscales of inattention and hyperactivity indicated equally robust improvements. Significant drug-specific improvement was also noted by clinicians in scores on the Clinical Global Impression Scale. Ritalin LA was well tolerated, having minimal side effects. Rates of mild appetite suppression and mild insomnia were both low (3.1%).

Metadate CD comes in capsules with a mixture of immediate- and delayed-release beads containing methylphenidate. In Metadate CD capsules, 30% of the beads are immediate release and 70%

are delayed release, to provide effective methylphenidate treatment for 8–9 hours. The efficacy and safety of Metadate CD were tested in a multicenter, randomized, double-blind, placebo-controlled trial conducted at 32 sites and involving 316 children with ADHD (Greenhill et al. 2002). The trial consisted of a 1-week single-blind, placebo run-in, followed by a 3-week double-blind titration and treatment period. Improvement compared with placebo was equally good morning and afternoon as measured by teachers on the Conners Global Index. The medication was well tolerated, with relatively low rates of decreased appetite (9.7% in the treated group vs. 2.5% in the placebo group) and insomnia (7.1% vs. 2.5%). Metadate CD is available in 20-mg capsules, approximating the 10-mg twice-daily doses of IR methylphenidate. Recently, a study found that the bioavailability and tolerability of Metadate CD are not altered when the capsule is opened and the beads are sprinkled on food (Pentikis et al. 2002).

Adderall XR (a mixed amphetamine salts formulation) comes in capsules with a 1:1 ratio of IR beads to delayed-release beads, to release drug content in a time course similar to that of Adderall given twice daily (at 0 and 4 hours). Adderall XR is available in 10-, 20-, and 30-mg capsules. An analogue classroom study compared various doses of Adderall XR with Adderall given twice daily and placebo (McCracken et al. 2000). Behavioral and academic improvement were documented to 12 hours after dosing. The efficacy and safety of Adderall XR were further tested in a multicenter, randomized, double-blind, placebo-controlled trial conducted at 47 sites (Biederman et al. 2002). A total of 584 children with ADHD were randomized to administration of once-daily morning doses of placebo or Adderall XR 10 mg, 20 mg, or 30 mg for

3 weeks. Continuous, significant improvement was determined in morning and afternoon assessments by teachers (using the Conners Global Index Scale for Teachers) and in morning, afternoon, and late-afternoon assessments by parents (using the Conners Global Index Scale for Parents). All active-treatment groups showed significant dose-related improvement in behavior from baseline. The medication was well tolerated, with rates of adverse events similar for active treatments and placebo. A 1-year follow-up study involving 411 children taking Adderall XR examined long-term safety and efficacy (Chandler et al. 2001). Efficacy was maintained for 12 months, as measured by the Conners Global Index. The medication was safe and well tolerated, with a low frequency of mild adverse events and no evidence of untoward cardiovascular effects.

In February 2005, the FDA issued the following public health advisory:

> Health Canada, the Canadian drug regulatory agency, has suspended the sale of Adderall XR in the Canadian market.... The Canadian action was based on U.S. postmarketing reports of sudden deaths in pediatric patients... When one considers the rate of sudden death in pediatric patients treated with Adderall products based on the approximately 30 million prescriptions written between 1999 and 2003 (the period of time in which these deaths occurred), it does not appear that the number of deaths reported is greater than the number of sudden deaths that would be expected to occur in this population without treatment. For this reason, the FDA has decided not to take any further regulatory action at this time. However, because it appeared that patients with underlying heart defects might be at increased risk for sudden death, the labeling for Adderall XR was changed in August 2004 to include a warning that these patients might be at particular risk, and that these patients should ordinarily not be treated with Adderall products. (U.S. Food and Drug Administration 2005)

Although at present there is limited concern about the general cardiovascular safety of Adderall or other psychostimulants, caution should be used in the treatment of patients presenting with a family history of early cardiac death or arrhythmias, a personal history of structural abnormalities, chest pain, palpitations, or fainting episodes of unclear etiology either before or during treatment with this compound. In such cases, consultation with a cardiologist is recommended.

Methylphenidate as a secondary amine gives rise to four optical isomers: D-*threo*, L-*threo*, D-*erythro*, and L-*erythro*. There is stereoselectivity in receptor site binding and its relationship to response. The standard preparation is composed of the D,L-*threo* racemate, the form apparently active in the CNS. Moreover, recent data suggest that the D-methylphenidate isomer is the active form. In a positron emission tomography study, D-*threo*-methylphenidate was found to bind specifically to the basal ganglia, rich in dopamine transporter receptors, whereas L-*threo*-methylphenidate widely distributed with only nonspecific binding (Ding et al. 1995). These findings led to the development of a purified D-*threo*-methylphenidate compound, Focalin. When given in equimolar doses, D-*threo*-methylphenidate and D,L-*threo*-methylphenidate were found to have similar pharmacokinetic profiles. That is, the maximum concentration, the time to maximum concentration, and the half-life of D-methylphenidate were the same for the two racemates.

The efficacy of Focalin was established in two controlled studies. In the first trial, 132 children and adolescents were randomized to administration of D-*threo*-methylphenidate, D,L-*threo*-methylphenidate, or placebo at 8 A.M. and noon for 4 weeks (Conners et al. 2001). At week 4, teacher ratings on the Swanson, Nolan, and Pelham, version IV (SNAP-IV), scale revealed robust improvement with active treatment. The average improvement from baseline was equivalent to one standard deviation on the SNAP-IV scale—a clinically important change. Parent ratings on the SNAP-IV scale revealed superiority of both treatments over placebo 3 hours after dosing, but only superiority of D-methylphenidate (not D,L-methylphenidate) 6 hours after dosing. In a second controlled study, investigators tested the specificity of response to D-*threo*-methylphenidate (data on file, Novartis). A total of 116 patients were treated openly with D-*threo*-methylphenidate to determine the optimal dose. At the end of 6 weeks, 75 responders were randomized to blinded treatment with D-*threo*-methylphenidate or placebo over 2 weeks. Subjects randomized to placebo administration had a high rate of relapse (62%) compared with those who continued taking D-*threo*-methylphenidate (17%). In addition, the parent SNAP-IV scale ratings indicated persistent effect 6 hours after D-*threo*-methylphenidate dosing. In both studies, adverse effects of D-*threo*-methylphenidate were consistent with those of D,L-*threo*-methylphenidate. These studies showed Focalin to be as effective as the racemate at half the dose. Focalin is available in 2.5-, 5-, and 10-mg doses, approximating the 5-, 10-, and 20-mg doses of D,L-methylphenidate.

Treatment with stimulants improves a wide variety of cognitive abilities (Barkley 1977; Klein 1987; Rapport et al. 1988), increases school-based productivity (Famularo and Fenton 1987), and improves performance on academic tests (H. Abikoff, personal communication, June

1965). Patients with ADHD may also manifest learning disabilities that are not responsive to pharmacotherapy (Bergman et al. 1991; Faraone et al. 1993) but respond to educational remediation.

It is estimated that at least 30% of individuals with ADHD do not respond adequately to or cannot tolerate stimulant treatment (Barkley 1977; Gittelman 1980; Spencer et al. 1996). In addition, stimulants are short-acting drugs that must be administered multiple times during the day, necessitating treatment during school or work hours and affecting compliance. Although this problem may be offset by the development of an effective long-acting stimulant, that class of drugs often affects sleep, making use in evening hours difficult when children and adults need to be able to concentrate in order to deal with daily demands and interact with family members and friends. In addition to these problems, the fact that stimulants are controlled substances continues to create worries in children, families, and the treating community, further inhibiting their use. These feelings are based on lingering concerns about the potential for abuse of stimulant drugs by the child or his or her family members or associates; concerns about the possibility of diversion; and safety concerns regarding the use of a controlled substance by patients who are impulsive and frequently have antisocial tendencies (Goldman et al. 1998). Similarly, the controlled nature of stimulant drugs creates important medicolegal concerns for the treating community that further increase the barriers to treatment.

In addition to these unresolved problems, it is increasingly evident that ADHD frequently occurs with mood or anxiety disorders, conditions that may affect response to stimulant drugs. Stimulants are poorly effective in the treatment of ADHD in the context of coexisting manic symptomatology, and their use in such patients may result in increased mood instability (Biederman et al. 1999b).

Antidepressants

Noradrenergic and dopaminergic active antidepressants such as MAOIs (Zametkin et al. 1985), secondary amine TCAs (Biederman et al. 1989a; Donnelly et al. 1986; Wilens et al. 1993), and bupropion (Barrickman et al. 1995; Casat et al. 1989; Conners et al. 1996) have been found to be superior to placebo in controlled clinical trials. (See "Antidepressants" for details on specific drugs and Table 29–3 for doses and side effects.) Possible advantages of these compounds over stimulants include a longer duration of action without symptom rebound or insomnia, greater flexibility in dosage, the option (with TCAs) of monitoring plasma drug levels, minimal risk of abuse or dependence, and potential treatment of comorbid internalizing symptoms. Little clinical or scientific evidence implicates serotonergic systems in the pathophysiology of ADHD.

Perhaps the best established of the second-line agents for ADHD are the TCAs. Of 33 studies (21 controlled, 12 open) evaluating TCA therapy in children, adolescents (N=1,139), and adults (N=78), 91% found that TCAs had positive effects on ADHD symptoms (Spencer et al. 1997). Of the studies of TCA therapy in ADHD, the studies of imipramine treatment and of desipramine treatment are the most numerous; a handful of studies focusing on other TCAs have been conducted. Although most TCA studies (73%) were relatively brief, lasting a few weeks to several months, 9 studies (27%) found enduring effects of up to 2 years. Outcomes in both short- and long-term studies were equally positive. Although one study found that the drop-out rate after 1 year was 50%, it is noteworthy that subjects who continued taking imipramine experienced sustained improvement (P.O. Quinn and Rapoport 1975). More recent studies using aggressive doses of TCAs found sustained improvement for up to 1 year with desipramine therapy (>4 mg/kg) (Biederman et al. 1986; Gastfriend et al. 1985) and nortriptyline therapy (2.0 mg/kg) (Wilens et al. 1993). Although response was equally positive at all the dose ranges, it was more sustained in studies in which higher doses were administered. A high interindividual variability in serum TCA levels has been consistently reported for imipramine and desipramine, with little relationship between serum level and daily dose, response, or side effects. In contrast, dose and serum level appear to be positively associated in nortriptyline therapy (Wilens et al. 1993).

In the largest controlled study of TCA therapy in children, our group reported favorable results with desipramine in 62 clinically referred children with ADHD, most of whom had previously failed to respond to psychostimulant treatment (Biederman et al. 1989a). The study was a randomized, placebo-controlled, parallel-design, 6-week clinical trial. Clinically and statistically significant differences in behavioral improvement were found for desipramine over placebo, at an average daily desipramine dose of 5 mg/kg. Although the presence of comorbidity increased the likelihood of a placebo response, neither comorbidity with conduct disorder (CD), depression, or anxiety nor a family history of ADHD yielded differential responses to desipramine treatment. In addition, desipramine-treated patients with ADHD showed a substantial reduction in depressive symptoms compared with placebo-treated patients.

In a recent prospective, placebo-controlled discontinuation trial, we demonstrated the efficacy of nortriptyline at doses of up to 2 mg/kg/day in 35 school-age youths with ADHD (Prince et al. 1999). In that study, 80% responded by week 6 in the open phase. During the discontinuation phase, subjects randomized to placebo administration lost the anti-ADHD effect, whereas those receiving nortriptyline maintained a robust anti-ADHD effect. Youths receiving nortriptyline also were found to have more modest but statistically significant reductions in oppositionality and anxiety. Nortriptyline was well tolerated, with some weight gain. (Weight gain is frequently considered a desirable side effect in this population.) Less favorable results were obtained in a systematic study involving 14 youths with refractory ADHD who received protriptyline (mean dose, 30 mg). Because of adverse effects, only 45% of subjects responded to or could tolerate protriptyline (Wilens et al. 1996a).

Thirteen (40%) of the 33 TCA studies compared TCAs and stimulants. Five studies found stimulants to be superior to TCAs (Garfinkel et al. 1983 [studied two TCAs]; Gittelman-Klein 1974; Greenberg et al. 1975; Rapoport et al. 1974), five studies found stimulants to be equal to TCAs (Gross 1973; Huessy and Wright 1970; Kupietz and Balka 1976; Rapport et al. 1993; Yepes et al. 1977), and three studies found TCAs to be superior to stimulants (Watter and Dreyfuss 1973; Werry 1980; Winsberg et al. 1972). Analyses of response profiles indicate that TCAs more consistently improve behavioral symptoms—as rated by clinicians, teachers, and parents—than they affect cognitive function as measured through neuropsychological testing (Gualtieri and Evans 1988; P. O. Quinn and Rapoport 1975; Rapport et al. 1993; Werry 1980). Studies of TCAs have uniformly found a robust rate of response of ADHD symptoms in ADHD subjects with comorbid depression or anxiety (Biederman et al. 1993; Cox 1982; Wilens et al. 1993,

1995a). In addition, studies of TCAs have consistently found a robust rate of response in ADHD subjects with comorbid tic disorders (Dillon et al. 1985; Hoge and Biederman 1986; Riddle et al. 1988; Singer et al. 1994; Spencer et al. 1993a, 1993b). For example, in a controlled study, Spencer (1997) replicated data from a retrospective chart review indicating that desipramine has a robust beneficial effect on ADHD and tic symptoms. The potential benefits of TCAs in the treatment of ADHD have been clouded by safety concerns stemming from reports of sudden unexplained death in four ADHD children treated with desipramine ("Sudden Death in Children Treated With a Tricyclic Antidepressant" 1990), although the causal link between desipramine and these deaths remains uncertain.

The mixed dopaminergic/noradrenergic antidepressant bupropion was shown to be effective in treating ADHD in children in a controlled multisite study ($N=72$) (Casat et al. 1987, 1989; Conners et al. 1996) and in a comparison with methylphenidate ($N=15$) (Barrickman et al. 1995). Although bupropion has been associated with a slightly increased risk (0.4%) of drug-induced seizures relative to other antidepressants, this risk has been linked to high doses, a history of seizures, and eating disorders.

Although a small number of studies suggested that MAOIs may be effective in juvenile and adult ADHD, the potential for hypertensive crisis associated with use of irreversible MAOIs (e.g., phenelzine, tranylcypromine), with dietetic transgressions (consumption of tyramine-containing foods [e.g., most cheeses]), and with drug interactions (interactions with pressor amines, most cold medicines, and amphetamines) seriously limits their use. The "cheese effect" might be obviated with reversible MAOIs such as moclobemide (not available in the United States), which has shown promise in one open trial (Trott et al. 1991, 1992). The usefulness of SSRIs in the treatment of core ADHD symptoms is not supported by clinical experience or research. Similarly uncertain is the usefulness of the mixed serotonergic/noradrenergic atypical antidepressant venlafaxine in the treatment of ADHD. Although a response rate of 77% was reported for subjects who completed treatment in four open studies involving 61 adults with ADHD, 21% of subjects dropped out because of side effects (Adler et al. 1995; Findling et al. 1996; Hornig-Rohan and Amsterdam 1995; Reimherr et al. 1995). Additionally, in a single open study of venlafaxine therapy in 16 children with ADHD, the response rate for subjects who completed therapy was 50%, and the rate of dropping out because of side effects (most prominently, increased hyperactivity) was 25% (Olvera et al. 1996).

Atomoxetine

Atomoxetine, a potent noradrenergic-specific reuptake inhibitor, has been studied in more than 1,800 children and more than 250 adults and has been submitted for FDA approval. Three acute, randomized, double-blind, placebo-controlled studies have been conducted: two involving children, and two involving children and adolescents (Michelson et al. 2001; Spencer et al. 2002). A total of 291 ADHD children, ages 7 through 13, were randomized in two trials (combined: atomoxetine therapy, $n=129$; placebo treatment, $n=124$; and methylphenidate therapy, $n=38$) (Spencer et al. 2002). The acute treatment period was 9 weeks. The stimulant-naive patients were randomized to double-blind treatment with atomoxetine ($n=56$), placebo ($n=53$), or methylphenidate ($n=38$). Patients with previous exposure to stimulants were randomized to double-blind treatment with

atomoxetine ($n=73$) or placebo ($n=71$). Atomoxetine significantly reduced total scores on an investigator-rated DSM-IV (American Psychiatric Association 1994) ADHD rating scale. Response was defined as a $\geq 25\%$ decrease in scores on the ADHD rating scale. Response rates were greater in the atomoxetine treatment group than in the placebo treatment group (61.4% vs. 32.3%, $P<0.05$). In the stimulant-naive stratum, 69.1% of atomoxetine-treated patients, 73% of methylphenidate-treated patients, and 31.4% of placebo-treated patients were considered responders. Atomoxetine was well tolerated. Mild appetite suppression was reported in 22% of patients receiving atomoxetine, compared with 32% of methylphenidate-treated patients and 7% of placebo-treated patients. Less insomnia was associated with atomoxetine treatment than with methylphenidate treatment (7.0% vs. 27.0%, $P<0.05$). Mild increases in diastolic blood pressure and heart rate were noted in the atomoxetine treatment group, with no significant differences in electrocardiographic intervals or laboratory parameters between the atomoxetine and placebo treatment groups.

In an additional controlled study, 297 children and adolescents were randomized to different doses of atomoxetine or placebo for 8 weeks (Michelson et al. 2001). Atomoxetine was associated with a graded dose response: response was best at 1.2 or 1.8 mg/kg/day, poorer at 0.5 mg/kg/day, and poorer still with placebo. There was also a dose-dependent enhancement of social and family function. The Child Health Questionnaire was used to assess the well-being of the child and the family. Parents of children taking atomoxetine reported fewer emotional difficulties and behavioral problems, as well as greater self-esteem, in their children and less emotional worry and fewer limitations on their personal time in themselves.

Safety and efficacy data were evaluated in a year-long, open follow-up study involving atomoxetine-treated children and adolescents (N=325) (Kratochvil et al. 2001). Atomoxetine treatment continued to be effective and well tolerated. The acute mild increases in diastolic blood pressure and heart rate persisted without a change in severity. Growth in height and weight were normal, and there were no significant differences between atomoxetine and placebo treatment groups in laboratory parameters and electrocardiographic intervals.

Alpha-Adrenergic Agents

Despite clonidine's wide use in children with ADHD, only four studies (N=122 children; two studies were controlled) have supported this agent's efficacy (Gunning 1992; Hunt 1987; Hunt et al. 1985; Steingard et al. 1993). Clonidine appears to have mostly behavioral effects on disinhibited and agitated youth; the drug has limited effect on cognition. Several cases of sudden death have been reported in children treated with clonidine plus methylphenidate, raising concerns about the safety of this combination (see "Clonidine") (Wilens et al. 1999b).

Only three small open studies of guanfacine in children and adolescents with ADHD have been conducted (Chappell et al. 1995; Horrigan and Barnhill 1995; Hunt et al. 1995). In these studies, beneficial effects on hyperactive behaviors and attentional abilities were noted.

Other Drugs

Use of β-adrenergic blockers in ADHD has also been studied. An open study of propranolol in ADHD adults with temper outbursts found improvement at daily doses of up to 640 mg (Mattes 1986). Another report indicated that β-blockers may be helpful in combination with stimulants (Ratey et al. 1991). In a controlled study of pindolol in 52 children with ADHD, symptoms of behavioral dyscontrol and hyperactivity were improved, with less apparent cognitive benefit (Buitelaar et al. 1996). However, prominent adverse effects such as nightmares and paresthesias led to discontinuation of the drug in all test subjects. An open study of nadolol in aggressive, developmentally delayed children with ADHD symptoms found effective diminution of aggression, with little apparent effect on ADHD symptoms (Connor et al. 1997).

The nonbenzodiazepine anxiolytic buspirone has a high affinity for 5-HT$_{1A}$ receptors, both pre- and postsynaptic, as well as a modest effect on the dopaminergic system and α-adrenergic activity. However, in a recent multisite, controlled clinical trial involving a large number of children with ADHD, the response to transdermal buspirone was not different from the response to placebo (Bristol-Myers Squibb, unpublished data, June 1996).

Although old literature suggested that typical antipsychotics are effective in the treatment of children with ADHD, the drugs' short-term (extrapyramidal reactions) and long-term (tardive dyskinesia) adverse effects greatly limit their usefulness.

Evidence has emerged that nicotinic dysregulation may contribute to the pathophysiology of ADHD. This is not surprising, given that nicotinic activation enhances dopaminergic neurotransmission (Mereu et al. 1987; Westfall et al. 1983). Independent lines of investigation have demonstrated that ADHD is associated with an increased risk and earlier age at onset for cigarette smoking (Milberger et al. 1997; Pomerleau et al. 1996); that maternal smoking during pregnancy increases the risk of ADHD in the offspring (Milberger et al. 1996); and that in animals, in utero exposure to nicotine confers a heightened risk of an ADHD-like syndrome in the newborn (Fung 1988; Fung and Lau 1989; Johns et al. 1982). In subjects without ADHD, central nicotinic activation has been shown to improve temporal memory (Meck and Church 1987), attention (Jones et al. 1992; Peeke and Peeke 1984; Wesnes and Warburton 1984), cognitive vigilance (Jones et al. 1992; Parrott and Winder 1989; Wesnes and Warburton 1984), and executive function (Wesnes and Warburton 1984).

Support for a "nicotinic hypothesis" for ADHD is derived from a study of the therapeutic effects of nicotine in adults with ADHD (Levin et al. 1996). Although this controlled clinical trial found that use of a commercially available transdermal nicotine patch significantly improved ADHD symptoms, working memory, and neuropsychological functioning (Levin et al. 1996), the trial was short (2 days long) and included only a handful of patients. The usefulness of nicotinic drugs in ADHD was more substantially demonstrated in a recent controlled clinical trial of ABT-418 in adults with ADHD (Wilens et al. 1999a). ABT-418 is a CNS cholinergic nicotinic activating agent that is structurally similar to nicotine. Phase 1 studies of this compound in humans indicated its low abuse liability, as well as adequate safety and tolerability in elderly adults (Abbott Laboratories, unpublished data, June 1998). In a double-blind, placebo-controlled, randomized, crossover trial comparing a transdermal patch of ABT-418 (75 mg daily) and placebo in adults with a DSM-IV diagnosis of ADHD, a significantly higher proportion of the ADHD adults were much improved while receiving ABT-418 than while receiving placebo (40% vs. 13%; χ^2=5.3, P=0.021) (Wilens et al. 1999a). Although preliminary, these results suggest that nicotinic analogues may have utility in the treatment of ADHD.

Several other compounds have been evaluated and found to be ineffective in the treatment of ADHD; they include dopamine agonists (amantadine and L-dopa) (Gittelman-Klein 1987) and amino acid precursors (DL-phenylalanine and L-tyrosine) (Reimherr et al. 1987). In addition, a controlled study of the antiserotonergic, anorectic drug fenfluramine failed to find therapeutic benefits in patients with ADHD (Donnelly et al. 1989).

■ Other Disruptive Behavior Disorders: Conduct Disorder (see Table 29–8) and Oppositional Defiant Disorder

In DSM-IV-TR, conduct disorder is conceptualized as a childhood-onset disorder characterized by antisocial and aggressive behaviors. Children with CD are at high risk of developing adult antisocial personality disorder and substance use disorders. Oppositional defiant disorder (ODD) is characterized by oppositional and obstinate behaviors. Although very taxing to families, ODD does not share CD's serious adult outcome. There is no specific pharmacotherapy for CD or ODD, but several controlled investigations have found mood stabilizers and antipsychotics to be effective in reducing aggression and explosiveness (but not sociopathy) in children with CD (Campbell et al. 1992; Platt et al. 1984). These findings are consistent with mounting evidence linking some forms of CD and ODD with bipolar and nonbipolar mood disorders (hence "dysphoric") (Biederman et al. 1999a; Frazier et al. 1999). Studies have also shown a significant decrease in aggressive behaviors with the use of behavioral management techniques, whether focused on the child's coping skills or the parents' management skills (Greene 1998; Quay 1986). When CD or ODD occurs with ADHD, mood disorders, or anxiety disorders, treatment of the comorbid disorder can result in substantial clinical stabilization and facilitate psychosocial treatment of CD or ODD.

■ Tic Disorders (Table 29–9)

Tic disorders are common and may occur in 5%–10% of children. The best known of these disorders is Tourette's disorder, a rare but more severe neuropsychiatric syndrome of childhood onset and lifelong duration that consists of multiform motor and phonic tics and associated behavioral and psychological symptoms. Affected patients commonly have spontaneous waxing, waning, and symptomatic fluctuation. Tourette's disorder is commonly associated with ADHD (in about 50% of cases) and OCD (in about 30% of cases) (Pauls et al. 1986). In many cases, the comorbid disorder, rather than the tic disorder, is the major source of distress and disability. The association with ADHD is particularly problematic, because ADHD appears earlier in life than the tics and because the use of stimulants may be detrimental in some cases.

The noradrenergic modulators clonidine (Leckman et al. 1991) and guanfacine (Chappell et al. 1995) have proven effective in some children with Tourette's disorder. For severe or treatment-resistant conditions, antipsychotic drugs—particularly haloperidol, pimozide, and, more recently, risperidone (Lombroso et al. 1995)—appear to be the most effective medications. However, antipsychotics have limited effects on the frequently associated comorbid disorders, and antipsychotic drugs carry a risk of development of tardive dyskinesia when they are administered chronically (Riddle et al. 1987). In addition, clonazepam, β-blockers, nortriptyline, and desipramine (Singer et al. 1994; Spencer 1997) have been reported to be helpful in some children with Tourette's disorder. Clonidine, guanfacine, and TCAs may be particularly helpful in patients with Tourette's disorder and ADHD. Patients with comorbid OCD may need additional pharmacotherapy, in the form of serotonergically active drugs such as clomipramine or SSRIs.

Table 29–9. Pharmacotherapy for tic disorders

Disorder	Main characteristics	Pharmacotherapy
Tourette's disorder	• Multiple motor tics and one or more vocal tics • Frequently associated with ADHD or obsessive-compulsive disorder	*First-line* • Treatment unclear • Atypical (blocking dopamine D_2 receptors) and typical antipsychotics • α-Adrenergic agents • TCAs *Second-line* • High-potency benzodiazepines • β-Blockers • Cholinergic agents • Combined pharmacotherapy for treatment-resistant cases

Note. ADHD = attention-deficit/hyperactivity disorder; TCA = tricyclic antidepressant.

■ Childhood Anxiety Disorders (Table 29–10)

The category of childhood anxiety disorders includes a subclass of disorders in which anxiety that is not due to psychosocial stressors is the predominant feature. In addition to separation anxiety disorder and selective mutism, the family of anxiety disorders affecting the young also includes panic disorder, agoraphobia (Biederman 1990; Leonard and Rapoport 1989), social and specific phobias, generalized anxiety disorder, OCD, posttraumatic stress disorder, and the atypical anxiety disorders termed *anxiety disorders not otherwise specified.* This continuity of adult- and childhood-onset anxiety disorders is recognized in DSM-IV-TR; disorders formerly coded as childhood disorders (overanxious disorder and avoidant disorder) are now subsumed under the corresponding adult diagnoses (generalized anxiety and social phobia, respectively).

Although childhood anxiety disorders are common disorders that bear striking similarities to the adult anxiety disorders and in many cases persist into adult life, not much is known about their treatment, with the notable exception of treatment of OCD. TCAs and MAOIs can be effective in the treatment of anxiety disorders, but their adverse-effect profiles, multiple drug–drug interaction problems, and narrow margins of safety, as well as the dietetic restrictions of MAOIs, make these compounds less desirable for use in management of anxiety disorders in youths. Similarly, although the high-potency benzodiazepines clonazepam, lorazepam, and alprazolam are important therapeutic agents in the management of anxiety disorders (Bernstein et al. 1987; Biederman 1987), their sedative properties, their potential for addiction and misuse, and their potential for negative cognitive adverse effects make them less desirable agents in the management of pediatric anxiety disorders. Of the high-potency benzodiazepines, clonazepam may be particularly useful in the treatment of children and adolescent patients, because of the drug's high potency and long duration of action. Although it has not been tested in youth, the non-benzodiazepine anxiolytic buspirone may also have a role to play in the management of some forms of juvenile anxiety disorders.

Several controlled clinical trials have clearly demonstrated that the serotonergic-specific antidepressants clomipramine, sertraline, and fluvoxamine are superior to placebo in the treatment of juvenile OCD, and the responses achieved in those studies were strikingly similar to documented responses in adults with this disorder. Because of the findings of these investigations, use of clomipramine, sertraline, fluoxetine, and fluvoxamine in pediatric OCD has FDA approval. Although not yet tested in children and adolescents, the serotonergic antidepressants have been found to be superior to placebo in the treatment of panic disorder and agoraphobia in adults, and paroxetine and venlafaxine have been found to be superior to placebo in the treatment of social phobia and generalized anxiety disorder in adults. Thus, serotonergic antidepressants may play a similarly beneficial therapeutic role in the treatment of pediatric forms of generalized anxiety disorder, social phobia, panic disorder, agoraphobia, and perhaps posttraumatic stress disorder. Because of their favorable adverse-effect profiles and large margins of safety, serotonergic antidepressants should be considered first-line agents in the treatment of anxiety disorders.

Table 29–10.　Pharmacotherapy for anxiety disorders

Disorder	Main characteristics	Pharmacotherapy
Separation anxiety disorder	• Excessive anxiety on separation from caretakers or familial surroundings • Inability to separate from the parent or from major attachment figures • Similar to agoraphobia	*First-line* • SSRIs (particularly when MD is present) • Atypical antidepressants (serotonergic) *Second-line* • Benzodiazepines *Third-line* • Buspirone for mild anxiety • Combined pharmacotherapy for refractory illness or patients with comorbid diagnoses (e.g., ADHD)
Selective mutism	• Persistent failure to speak in specific social situations • Similar to social phobia	
Panic disorder (with or without agoraphobia)	• Recurrent discrete periods of intense fear (panic attacks) • Frequent comorbidity with MD (50%) and ADHD (30%)	
Agoraphobia	• Fear of being in places or situations with limited escape possibilities (e.g., school); because of this fear, adolescent restricts travel or needs a companion or caretaker when away from home	
Social phobia	• Fear of social situations in which individual may be exposed to scrutiny or endure humiliation	
Generalized anxiety disorder	• Excessive or unrealistic worry about future events	
Adjustment disorder with anxiety (severe)	• Maladaptive short-term reaction to a severe stressor	
Obsessive-compulsive disorder	• Recurrent, severe, and distressing obsession and/or compulsion	• SSRIs, clomipramine • Combined pharmacotherapy for refractory illness or patients with comorbid diagnoses (e.g., MD, ADHD, psychosis)

Note.　ADHD = attention-deficit/hyperactivity disorder; MD = major depression; SSRI = selective serotonin reuptake inhibitor.

■ Mood Disorders (Table 29–11)

Depressive Disorders

Pediatric depression is recognized in DSM-IV-TR as a family of conditions with core symptoms similar to those found in adult depression. Core features of depression in youths include a sad or irritable mood, a persistent loss of interest or pleasure in favorite activities, physiological disturbances such as changes in appetite and weight, abnormal sleep patterns, psychomotor abnormalities, fatigue, diminished ability to think and concentrate, feelings of worthlessness or guilt, and suicidal preoccupation. Also recognized in DSM-IV-TR are developmentally specific associated features in depression affecting youth, including academic difficulties, school refusal, negativism, aggression, and antisocial behavior. In addition, emerging evidence indicates that depression in youths may have unique features, compared with adult depression, that can complicate its identification. These include dysphoria and irritability as predominant mood disturbances, rather than sadness and melancholia (Biederman et al. 1995a); "mood reactivity" as seen in atypical forms of adult depression (Nierenberg et al. 1998); insidious onset and a chronic course rather than acuteness and an episodic course (Biederman et al. 1995a; Kovacs et al. 1984); male preponderance or equal gender representation (Angold and Costello 1993), rather than female preponderance; and an increased personal and familial risk of bipolar disorder (B. Geller et al. 1994). In addition, pediatric depression is characterized by a much larger spectrum of comorbidity than is seen in adult depression (Angold and Costello 1993; Biederman et al. 1995a); comorbid conditions in juvenile patients with depression include not only anxiety disorders but also ADHD, CD, and ODD (Angold and Costello 1993; Biederman et al. 1995a, 1996).

Controlled clinical trials failed to document efficacy for TCAs in pediatric depression (Bostic et al. 1999). In contrast, a number of studies have obtained more promising results with SSRIs. In a controlled study, Emslie et al. (1997) found that improvement with fluoxetine (in 57% of subjects) was significantly superior to placebo (33%) in a sample of nearly 100 depressed youths. Important features of this study were that 1) children with comorbid ADHD were not excluded as in previous investigations and 2) both children and adolescents were included. A very large multisite trial of paroxetine in 275 adolescents with depression also found that although paroxetine (improvement in 66%) was superior to placebo (43%), imipramine (57%) was not (Wagner et al. 1998). Furthermore, 32% of subjects receiving imipramine dropped out of the study because of adverse events, compared with 10% of the paroxetine treatment group and 7% of the placebo treatment group ($P<0.05$). Finally, in a recent open but prospective trial of sertraline in a sample of depressed adolescents, there was a positive response to sertraline therapy (Ambrosini et al. 1999). These studies, plus the more advantageous adverse-effect profiles and large margins of safety of these compounds, suggest that SSRIs should be considered first-line agents in the treatment of depression in the young.

Pediatric Mania

There is emerging evidence that children not only have unipolar depressions but also develop mania. Recent studies have begun to challenge the long-held notion that mania is nonexistent or rare in children. In fact, a recent report documented that mania was diagnosed in 15% of preadolescents referred to a pediatric psychopharmacology clinic (Wozniak et al.

Table 29–11.   Pharmacotherapy for mood disorders

Disorder	Main characteristics	Pharmacotherapy
Major depression	• Sad or irritable mood and associated cognitive, psychological, and vegetative symptoms occurring together for a time	*First-line* • SSRIs *Second-line* • Atypical antidepressants (serotonergic) *Third-line* • TCAs • Combined pharmacotherapy for refractory illness or patients with comorbid diagnoses (e.g., ADHD) • ECT for refractory illness
Bipolar disorder Manic	• Elevated or severely irritable or angry mood with or without associated psychotic symptoms • Often violent • Frequent comorbidity with conduct disorder • Very dysfunctional	• Atypical antipsychotics (risk of weight gain and hyperprolactinemia necessitate monitoring) • Mood stabilizers (lithium, oxcarbazepine, carbamazepine, valproic acid, atypical AEDs) • Combined therapy for refractory illness (i.e., atypical antipsychotics+mood stabilizers) • ECT for refractory illness
Depressed	• Potential for worsening of mania or induction of rapid cycling	• Antidepressants that may be less likely to induce mania: bupropion, paroxetine, mirtazapine
Mixed	• Mixed depressive and manic symptoms • Most common presentation of bipolar disorder in juvenile patients • Very severe clinical picture	• Atypical antipsychotics and/or mood stabilizers+antidepressants

Note.   ADHD=attention-deficit/hyperactivity disorder; AED=antiepileptic drug; ECT=electroconvulsive therapy; SSRI=selective serotonin reuptake inhibitor; TCA=tricyclic antidepressant.

1995), indicating that mania may be far more common than previously thought. When diagnosed, mania was characterized by extreme and persistent irritability and explosiveness, a mixed presentation (symptoms of mania and depression, dysphoric mania), and a chronic course (Wozniak et al. 1995). In addition, a high degree of comorbidity (ADHD, CD, anxiety disorders, and psychosis) characterized these manic children.

There is a paucity of information on pharmacological treatment of juvenile mania. Although mood stabilizers (lithium, carbamazepine, valproic acid) are generally considered the mainstays of treatment for adult bipolar disorders, their therapeutic role is less certain in pediatric mania. A recent systematic review of records of youths with mania confirmed that mood stabilizers are selectively associated with improvement of manic symptoms, but their beneficial effects were exceedingly slow to unfold, and children who improved rapidly deteriorated (Biederman et al. 1998a). In contrast, a systematic exploration of the effectiveness of the atypical antipsychotic risperidone revealed that this compound had a more effective, rapid, and sustained response in pediatric mania than previously observed with mood stabilizers (Frazier et al. 1999). A particularly thorny issue in the treatment of youths with bipolar disorders is the management of comorbid ADHD, which is very prevalent in children with juvenile mania (Biederman et al. 1998b). In a recent report, we documented that in the treatment of patients who have bipolar disorder and ADHD, mood stabilization must precede attempts to treat ADHD (Biederman et al. 1999b). Children with active manic symptoms failed to respond to anti-ADHD treatments until mood was stable. Because bipolar disorder with or without comorbid disorders (depression, ADHD) must commonly be treated aggressively, with several therapeutic agents targeting the various comorbid disorders, special attention should be given to potential drug–drug interactions.

■ Psychotic Disorders (Table 29–12)

The term *psychosis* is used in DSM-IV to describe abnormal behaviors of individuals with grossly impaired reality testing. The term is also used when the individual's behavior is grossly disorganized and it can be inferred that reality testing is impaired. A diagnosis of psychosis involves the presence of either delusions, false implausible beliefs, or hallucinations (i.e. false perceptions that may be visual, auditory, or tactile). Psychotic disorders in children, as in adults, can be functional or organic. Functional psychotic syndromes include schizophrenia and related disorders and the psychotic forms of mood disorders. Organic psychosis can develop as a result of lesions in the CNS as a consequence of

Table 29–12. Pharmacotherapy for psychotic disorders

Disorder	Main characteristics	Pharmacotherapy
Psychotic disorders	• Delusions and hallucinations • Negative symptoms	• Atypical antipsychotics (risk of weight gain and hyperprolactinemia necessitate monitoring) • Typical antipsychotics (risk of tardive dyskinesia) • Combined therapy for treatment-resistant cases • Clozapine for treatment-resistant cases

medical illnesses, trauma, or drug use, both licit and illicit.

The early literature on childhood schizophrenia overlapped with that on autism, and hallucinations or delusions were not requirements (McClellan and Werry 1994). Beginning with DSM-III (American Psychiatric Association 1980), the criteria for childhood- and adult-onset schizophrenia were identical, and psychotic symptoms became the hallmark of the disorder. In DSM-IV-TR, a diagnosis of schizophrenia now involves a 1-month period of two symptoms (or a single symptom, if very bizarre) such as delusions, hallucinations, disorganized speech or behavior, or negative symptoms. It continues to be a problem to distinguish, in children, true psychotic phenomena from nonpsychotic idiosyncratic thinking and perceptions caused by developmental delays or language disorders. However, psychotic features such as hallucinations and delusions are required for a diagnosis of schizophrenia to be made, and these features are usually associated with a marked change in mental status and lowered level of function (McClellan and Werry 1994).

Antipsychotics are indicated in the treatment of childhood psychotic disorders. Positive symptoms are the target symptoms most likely to respond to antipsychotics. These symptoms include hallucinations, delusions, formal thought disorder (incoherence), catatonic symptoms (stupor, negativism, rigidity, excitement, and posturing), and bizarre affect. In contrast, negative symptoms include affective blunting, poverty of speech and thought, apathy, anhedonia, and poor social functioning. Negative symptoms are associated with 1) insidious onset, positive premorbid history, and chronic deterioration and 2) atrophy as shown by computed tomography, abnormalities indicated by neuropsychological testing, and poor response to or worsening during treatment with typical antipsychotics. The atypical antipsychotics clozapine and risperidone appear to be more effective agents for negative symptoms.

When the psychotic process occurs in the context of a mood disorder, concomitant use of specific treatments for mood disorders is crucial for clinical stabilization. When psychosis is associated with severe agitation, adjunctive use of high-potency benzodiazepines, such as lorazepam or clonazepam, can facilitate management of the patient and may lead to use of lower doses of antipsychotics. The extent to which antiparkinsonian agents should be used prophylactically when antipsychotics are introduced is controversial. Whenever possible, use of antiparkinsonian agents should be reserved until extrapyramidal symptoms emerge. Extrapyramidal reactions can be prevented in many cases by avoiding rapid increase in neuroleptic dose or the use of high-potency typical antipsychotics such as haloperidol. When a child or adolescent taking antipsychotics develops an acutely agitated clinical picture with associated inability to sit still and aggressive outbursts, akathisia should be rapidly considered in the differential diagnosis. If akathisia is suspected, the dose of the antipsychotic may need to be decreased. β-Blockers (e.g., propranolol) and high-potency benzodiazepines have been found helpful in relieving symptoms of antipsychotic-induced akathisia in adults and may help relieve similar symptoms in juvenile patients (Ananth and Lin 1986).

In recent years, postpsychotic depression has received increasing attention. Initial trials of antidepressant drugs added to the antipsychotic treatment appear to be promising in terms of elimination of associated depression, thus fostering rehabilitation efforts. Postpsychotic depression should be distinguished from akinesia, an adverse extrapyramidal effect that may respond to treatment with antiparkinsonian agents.

■ Developmental Disorders
(Table 29–13)

In DSM-IV-TR, the developmental disorders are mental retardation (Axis II), pervasive developmental disorders (autistic and autistic-like disorders), and learning disorders. Autism is discussed in Chapter 11 ("Autistic Disorder") of this volume. The learning disorders represent a mixed group of cognitive dysfunctions in the context of no overall intelligence deficit and adequate educational opportunities.

Children with mental retardation or pervasive developmental disorders often have other psychiatric disorders and behavioral problems, including hyperactive, aggressive, distractible, and self-abusive behaviors. They also often manifest multiple neurological abnormalities. Psychotropics are primarily used in this population for the treatment of agitation, aggression, and self-injurious behaviors. Antipsychotics have been commonly used to control these symptoms. In recent years, the atypical antipsychotics have been used in the management of affective dysregulation, manic-like symptoms, and aggressive symptoms in this population. β-Blockers and clonidine have also been used in the management of aggression and dyscontrol in patients with developmental disorders.

Antidepressant drugs and antimanic agents can also be effective in controlling mood dysregulation of the bipolar and nonbipolar types, and stimulants may improve symptoms of ADHD in children and adolescents with mental retardation or pervasive developmental disorders. With the increasing popularity of serotonergic-specific drugs in recent years, there has been rising interest in their use in patients with pervasive developmental disorders. This interest stems in part from the hypothesis linking repetitive stereotypical behaviors in these patients to OCD shown to be responsive to serotonergic-specific drugs. Gordon et al. (1993) reported results of a controlled clinical trial evaluating the efficacy and tolerability of the serotonergic TCA clomipramine, the noradrenergic tricyclic desipramine, and placebo in patients with pervasive developmental disorders. They found that clomipramine was superior to placebo and desipramine in terms of ratings of autistic symptoms including stereotypies, anger, and compulsive ritualized behaviors. However, clomipramine and desipramine were equally effective in controlling symptoms of hyperactivity in this group.

Antianxiety agents should be used with caution in children with developmental disorders because these drugs tend to produce disinhibition, which may result in increased restlessness and more disturbed behavior. In an open study, Campbell et al. (1988) evaluated the efficacy and safety of naltrexone, a potent and long-acting opioid antagonist, in the treatment of autistic children; daily doses of 1–2 mg/kg were administered. In this open trial, naltrexone was associated with improvement in social and language behaviors and was well tolerated.

The treatment of learning disorders is largely remedial and supportive. Psychotropics have not been effective in altering the basic course of the disorder. Children with learning disabilities and ADHD or major depression can benefit from treatments directed at the associated psychiatric disorder.

Children with functional enuresis usually respond to nonpharmacological therapies (e.g., behavior modification), and these treatments should be considered first. When an immediate therapeutic effect is necessary, an antidepressant drug, commonly imipramine, may be used. In most cases, symptoms reappear

Table 29–13.   Pharmacotherapy for developmental disorders

Disorder	Main characteristics	Pharmacotherapy
Mental retardation (MR)	• Significant subaverage global intellectual functioning and deficits in adaptive functioning	• No specific pharmacotherapy for core disorder • Nonspecific treatment for aggression and self-abuse: β-blockers (e.g., propranolol), α-adrenergic agents, antimanic agents, opioid antagonist (naltrexone), typical and atypical antipsychotics • SSRIs for OCD-like repetitive behaviors • MR in conjunction with Axis I disorders (e.g., ADHD, mania, psychosis, anxiety): treat underlying disorder
Pervasive developmental disorders (PDDs)	• Qualitative impairment of social interactions and acquisition of cognitive, language, and motor skills • Can be global or exist in specific or multiple areas	• Same as for MR
Specific developmental disorders (learning disabilities)	• Inadequate development of specific academic, language, and motor skills that is not due to physical or neurological disorders, PDDs, or deficient educational opportunities	• No specific pharmacotherapy for core disorder • Remedial help and special education remain main treatments • Specific developmental disorders in conjunction with other Axis I disorders (e.g., ADHD, major depression, anxiety): treat underlying disorders
Enuresis	• Bed-wetting	• Behavior therapy • DDAVP (Desmopressin) • TCAs (low doses)

Note.   ADHD=attention-deficit/hyperactivity disorder; DDAVP=1-desamino-8-D-arginine-vasopressin; OCD=obsessive-compulsive disorder; SSRI=selective serotonin reuptake inhibitor; TCA=tricyclic antidepressant.

after the drug is withdrawn. Antidepressant therapy should not be continued for more than 6 months, because enuresis may remit spontaneously. In addition, the FDA has approved the use of the synthetic antidiuretic hormone desmopressin for the treatment of enuresis.

Combined Therapy

Although in clinical practice, many juvenile patients receive multiple treatments, the literature on combined pharmacotherapy is sparse and thus does not permit development of clear therapeutic guidelines. In contrast to polypharmacy, rational combined pharmacological approaches can be used for the treatment of psychiatric comorbidity, as augmentation strategies for patients with insufficient response to a single agent, and for the management of treatment-emergent adverse effects. Examples of the rational use of combined treatment include the use of an antidepressant plus a stimulant for ADHD and comorbid depression, the use of clonidine to ameliorate stimulant-induced insomnia, and the use of lithium plus an anti-ADHD agent to treat ADHD occurring with bipolar disorder (Wilens et al. 1995b). All psychotropics except lithium are metabolized by the P450 system. When multiple medications are used, there must be monitoring for drug–drug interactions, with careful evaluation of adverse effects and serum levels.

The hepatic P450 system consists of more than 40 enzymes that metabolize psychotropics and similar compounds. Because of genetic polymorphism, 5%–10% of Caucasians have innate deficiencies in this metabolic capacity and thus are slow metabolizers. Likewise, 5%–10% of Caucasians have duplicate copies and are extensive (rapid) metabolizers (DeVane 1998; Greenblatt et al. 1998; Nemeroff et al. 1996). Efficiency of these enzymes can be affected by competing substrates or by inhibition or enhancement (induction) by exogenous compounds, which often leads to drug–drug interactions in which serum levels of psychotropics are dramatically increased (or decreased).

The P450 enzyme 1A2 is involved in the demethylation of tertiary TCAs to secondary TCAs and is inhibited by fluvoxamine. 2C19 is involved in the demethylation of tertiary TCAs and biotransformation of diazepam and is inhibited by fluoxetine, sertraline, and fluvoxamine. 2D6 is involved in the hydroxylation of secondary TCAs (desipramine and nortriptyline) (Preskorn et al. 1994) and is affected by paroxetine, fluoxetine, and sertraline; thus, coadministration of these SSRIs and TCAs results in increased levels of the TCAs. In addition, 2D6 is involved in the metabolism of antipsychotics (haloperidol, thioridazine, perphenazine, clozapine, risperidone) and hydroxylation of β-blockers; thus, serum levels could be affected if any of the following are coadministered: an antipsychotic, β-blocker, TCA, or SSRI (paroxetine, fluoxetine, sertraline). 3A4 is involved in the demethylation of tertiary TCAs and biotransformation of benzodiazepines (triazolam, alprazolam, midazolam, carbamazepine), and the nonsedating antihistamine loratadine (Claritin) is affected by fluvoxamine and, to a lesser degree, fluoxetine and sertraline (DeVane 1998; Greenblatt et al. 1998; Nemeroff et al. 1996). Citalopram, venlafaxine, and mirtazapine minimally inhibit P450 enzymes. Similarly, there is little drug–drug interaction between lithium and TCAs or SSRIs, or between stimulants and antidepressants (Cohen et al. 1999).

Conclusion

Although the origins of pediatric psychopharmacology date from more than 50 years ago, the long-term outlook for pediatric psychopharmacology is dependent on careful clinical applications and future research. It is essential to apply a careful differential diagnostic assessment that considers psychiatric, social, cognitive, educational, and medical or neurological factors, all of which may contribute to the child's clinical presentation. It is therefore also essential to consider the use of pharmacotherapy as part of a broader treatment plan that encompasses all aspects of a child's life. Major ingredients of a successful pharmacological intervention include realistic expectations regarding the intervention, careful definition of target symptoms, and careful assessment of the potential risks and benefits of this type of intervention for psychiatrically disturbed children. The lack of FDA approval for pediatric use of many of the medications, although it imposes a restriction on general use, does permit the careful introduction of innovative therapy. It is to be hoped that an increasing number of referral centers will explore the appropriate use of psychopharmacological agents in pediatric psychiatry through high-quality research protocols.

References

Adler LA, Resnick S, Kunz M, et al: Open-label trial of venlafaxine in adults with attention deficit disorder. Psychopharmacol Bull 31:785–788, 1995

Alderman J, Wolkow R, Chung M, et al: Sertraline treatment of children and adolescents with obsessive-compulsive disorder or depression: pharmacokinetics, tolerability, and efficacy. J Am Acad Child Adolesc Psychiatry 37:386–394, 1998

Alessi N, Naylor M, Ghaziuddin M, et al: Update on lithium carbonate therapy in children and adolescents. J Am Acad Child Adolesc Psychiatry 33:291–304, 1994

Ambrosini PJ, Wagner KD, Biederman J, et al: Multicenter open-label sertraline study in adolescent outpatients with major depression. J Am Acad Child Adolesc Psychiatry 38:566–572, 1999

American College of Neuropsychopharmacology: Executive Summary, Preliminary Report of the Task Force on SSRIs and Suicidal Behavior in Youth, January 21, 2004. Available at: http://www.acnp.org/exec_summary.pdf. Accessed July 2005.

American Psychiatric Association: Diagnostic and Statistical Manual of Mental Disorders, 3rd Edition. Washington, DC, American Psychiatric Association, 1980

American Psychiatric Association: Diagnostic and Statistical Manual of Mental Disorders, 4th Edition. Washington, DC, American Psychiatric Association, 1994

American Psychiatric Association: Diagnostic and Statistical Manual of Mental Disorders, 4th Edition, Text Revision. Washington, DC, American Psychiatric Association, 2000

American Psychiatric Association: Press Release: APA Responds to FDA's New Warning on Antidepressants (Release No 04-55). Arlington, VA, American Psychiatric Association, October 15, 2004. Available at: www.psych.org/news_room/press_releases/04-55apaonfdablackboxwarning.pdf. Accessed July 2005.

Ananth H, Lin K: Propranolol in psychiatry. Neuropsychobiology 15:20–27, 1986

Angold A, Costello EJ: Depressive comorbidity in children and adolescents: empirical, theoretical and methodological issues. Am J Psychiatry 150:1779–1791, 1993

Barkley RA: A review of stimulant drug research with hyperactive children. J Child Psychol Psychiatry 18:137–165, 1977

Barrickman L, Perry P, Allen A, et al: Bupropion versus methylphenidate in the treatment of attention-deficit hyperactivity disorder. J Am Acad Child Adolesc Psychiatry 34:649–657, 1995

Bergman A, Winters L, Cornblatt B: Methylphenidate: effects on sustained attention, in Ritalin: Theory and Patient Management. Edited by Greenhill L, Osman B. New York, Mary Ann Liebert, 1991, pp 223–231

Bernstein GA, Garfinkel B, Borchart C: Imipramine versus alprazolam for school phobia. Paper presented at the annual meeting of the American Academy of Child and Adolescent Psychiatry, Washington, DC, October 1987

Biederman J: Clonazepam in the treatment of prepubertal children with panic-like symptoms. J Clin Psychiatry 48:38–41, 1987

Biederman J: The diagnosis and treatment of adolescent anxiety disorders. J Clin Psychiatry 51:20–26, 1990

Biederman J, Gastfriend DR, Jellinek MS: Desipramine in the treatment of children with attention deficit disorder. J Clin Psychopharmacol 6:359–363, 1986

Biederman J, Baldessarini RJ, Wright V, et al: A double-blind placebo-controlled study of desipramine in the treatment of attention deficit disorder, I: efficacy. J Am Acad Child Adolesc Psychiatry 28:777–784, 1989a

Biederman J, Baldessarini RJ, Wright V, et al: A double-blind placebo-controlled study of desipramine in the treatment of attention deficit disorder, II: serum drug levels and cardiovascular findings. J Am Acad Child Adolesc Psychiatry 28:903–911, 1989b

Biederman J, Baldessarini RJ, Wright V, et al: A double-blind placebo controlled study of desipramine in the treatment of ADD, III: lack of impact of comorbidity and family history factors on clinical response. J Am Acad Child Adolesc Psychiatry 32:199–204, 1993

Biederman J, Faraone S, Mick E, et al: Psychiatric comorbidity among referred juveniles with major depression: fact or artifact? J Am Acad Child Adolesc Psychiatry 34:579–590, 1995a

Biederman J, Thisted R, Greenhill L, et al: Estimation of the association between desipramine and the risk for sudden death in 5- to 14-year-old children. J Clin Psychiatry 56:87–93, 1995b

Biederman J, Wilens T, Mick E, et al: Psychoactive substance use disorder in adults with attention deficit hyperactivity disorder: effects of ADHD and psychiatric comorbidity. Am J Psychiatry 152:1652–1658, 1995c

Biederman J, Faraone SV, Mick E, et al: Child behavior checklist (CBCL) findings further support comorbidity between ADHD and major depression in a referred sample. J Am Acad Child Adolesc Psychiatry 35:734–742, 1996

Biederman J, Mick E, Bostic J, et al: The naturalistic course of pharmacological treatment of children with manic-like symptoms: a systematic chart review. J Clin Psychiatry 59:628–637, 1998a

Biederman J, Russell R, Soriano J, et al: Clinical features of children with both ADHD and mania: does ascertainment source make a difference? J Affect Disord 51:101–112, 1998b

Biederman J, Faraone S, Chu M, et al: Further evidence of a bidirectional overlap between juvenile mania and conduct disorder in children. J Am Acad Child Adolesc Psychiatry 38:468–476, 1999a

Biederman J, Mick E, Prince J, et al: Systematic chart review of the pharmacological treatment of comorbid attention deficit hyperactivity disorder in youth with bipolar disorder. J Child Adolesc Psychopharmacol 9:247–256, 1999b

Biederman J, Wilens T, Mick E, et al: Pharmacotherapy of attention-deficit/hyperactivity disorder reduces risk for substance use disorder. Pediatrics (serial online) 104:20, 1999c. Available at: http://www.pediatrics.org/cgi/content/full/104/2/e20. Accessed May 12, 2003.

Biederman J, Quinn D, Weiss M, et al: Methylphenidate HCl extended-release capsules (Ritalin LA): a new once-daily therapy for ADHD, in Scientific Proceedings of the 48th Annual Meeting of the American Academy of Child and Adolescent Psychiatry. Edited by Villani S. Honolulu, HI, American Academy of Child and Adolescent Psychiatry, October 2001, p A41

Biederman J, Lopez FA, Boellner SW, et al: A randomized, double-blind, placebo-controlled, parallel-group study of SLI381 (Adderall XR) in children with attention-deficit/hyperactivity disorder. Pediatrics 110:258–266, 2002

Bostic J, Wilens T, Spencer T, et al: Pharmacological treatment of juvenile depression. Psychiatr Clin North Am 6:175–191, 1999

Brown RT, Wynne ME, Slimmer LW: Attention deficit disorder and the effect of methylphenidate on attention, behavioral, and cardiovascular functioning. J Clin Psychiatry 45:473–476, 1984

Buitelaar JK, van der Gaag RJ, Swaab-Barneveld H, et al: Pindolol and methylphenidate in children with attention-deficit hyperactivity disorder: clinical efficacy and side-effects. J Child Psychol Psychiatry 37:587–595, 1996

Campbell M, Adams P, Small AM, et al: Naltrexone in infantile autism. Psychopharmacol Bull 24:135–139, 1988

Campbell M, Gonzalez NM, Silva RR: The pharmacological treatment of conduct disorders and rage outbursts. Psychiatr Clin North Am 15:69–85, 1992

Casat CD, Pleasants DZ, Van Wyck Fleet J: A double-blind trial of bupropion in children with attention deficit disorder. Psychopharmacol Bull 23:120–122, 1987

Casat CD, Pleasants DZ, Schroeder DH, et al: Bupropion in children with attention deficit disorder. Psychopharmacol Bull 25:198–201, 1989

Chandler M, Lopez F, Boeliner S: Long-term safety of SLI381 in children with ADHD, in Scientific Proceedings of the 48th Annual Meeting of the American Academy of Child and Adolescent Psychiatry. Edited by Villani S. Honolulu, HI, American Academy of Child and Adolescent Psychiatry, October 2001, p B12

Chappell P, Riddle M, Scahill L, et al: Guanfacine treatment of comorbid attention-deficit hyperactivity disorder and Tourette's syndrome. J Am Acad Child Adolesc Psychiatry 34:1140–1146, 1995

Cohen LG, Biederman J: Treatment of risperidone-induced hyperprolactinemia with a dopamine agonist in children. J Child Adolesc Psychopharmacol 11:435–440, 2001

Cohen LG, Prince J, Biederman J, et al: Absence of effect of stimulants on the pharmacokinetics of desipramine in children. Pharmacotherapy 19:746–752, 1999

Comings DE, Comings BG: Tourette's syndrome and attention deficit disorder, in Tourette's Syndrome and Tic Disorders: Clinical Understanding and Treatment. Edited by Cohen DJ, Bruun RD, Leckman JF. New York, Wiley, 1988, pp 119–136

Conners CK, Casat CD, Gualtieri CT, et al: Bupropion hydrochloride in attention deficit disorder with hyperactivity. J Am Acad Child Adolesc Psychiatry 35:1314–1321, 1996

Conners CK, Casat C[D], Coury D, et al: Randomized trial of dex-methylphenidate (D-MPH) and D,L-MPH in children with ADHD, in Scientific Proceedings of the 48th Annual Meeting of the American Academy of Child and Adolescent Psychiatry. Edited by Villani S. Honolulu, HI, American Academy of Child and Adolescent Psychiatry, October 2001, p C49

Connor D, Ozbayrak K, Benjamin S, et al: A pilot study of nadolol for overt aggression in developmentally delayed individuals. J Am Acad Child Adolesc Psychiatry 36:826–834, 1997

Cox W: An indication for the use of imipramine in attention deficit disorder. Am J Psychiatry 139:1059–1060, 1982

Derivan A: Venlafaxine metabolism in children and adolescents, in Scientific Proceedings, American Academy of Child and Adolescent Psychiatry, XI, New Orleans, LA, 1995, NR162 p 128

DeVane CL: Differential pharmacology of newer antidepressants. J Clin Psychiatry 59 (suppl 20):85–93, 1998

DeVeaugh-Geiss J, Moroz G, Biederman J, et al: Clomipramine hydrochloride in childhood and adolescent obsessive-compulsive disorder: a multicenter trial. J Am Acad Child Adolesc Psychiatry 31:45–49, 1992

Dillon DC, Salzman IJ, Schulsinger DA: The use of imipramine in Tourette's syndrome and attention deficit disorder: case report. J Clin Psychiatry 46:348–349, 1985

Ding YS, Fowler JS, Volkow ND, et al: Carbon-11-D-*threo*-methylphenidate binding to dopamine transporter in baboon brain. J Nucl Med 36:2298–2305, 1995

Donnelly M, Zametkin AJ, Rapoport JL, et al: Treatment of childhood hyperactivity with desipramine: plasma drug concentration, cardiovascular effects, plasma and urinary catecholamine levels, and clinical response. Clin Pharmacol Ther 39:72–81, 1986

Donnelly M, Rapoport JL, Potter WZ, et al: Fenfluramine and dextroamphetamine treatment of childhood hyperactivity. Clinical and biochemical findings. Arch Gen Psychiatry 46:205–212, 1989

Douglas V, Barr R, Amin K, et al: Dosage effects and individual responsivity to methylphenidate in attention deficit disorder. J Child Psychol Psychiatry 29:453–475, 1988

Eison MS: The new generation of serotonergic anxiolytics: possible clinical roles. Psychopathology 22:13–20, 1989

Emslie GJ, Rush AJ, Weinberg WA, et al: A double-blind, randomized, placebo-controlled trial of fluoxetine in children and adolescents with depression. Arch Gen Psychiatry 54:1031–1037, 1997

Famularo R, Fenton T: The effect of methylphenidate on school grades in children with attention deficit disorder without hyperactivity: a preliminary report. J Clin Psychiatry 48:112–114, 1987

Faraone SV, Biederman J: The neurobiology of attention deficit hyperactivity disorder, in Neurobiology of Mental Illness. Edited by Charney DS, Nestler EJ, Bunney BS. New York, Oxford University Press, 1999, pp 788–801

Faraone SV, Biederman J, Lehman BK, et al: Intellectual performance and school failure in children with attention deficit hyperactivity disorder and in their siblings. J Abnorm Psychol 102:616–623, 1993

Findling RL, Schwartz MA, Flannery DJ, et al: Venlafaxine in adults with attention-deficit/hyperactivity disorder: an open trial. J Clin Psychiatry 57:184–189, 1996

Findling RL, Reed MD, Myers C, et al: Paroxetine pharmacokinetics in depressed children and adolescents. J Am Acad Child Adolesc Psychiatry 38:952–959, 1999

Frazier JA, Meyer MC, Biederman J, et al: Risperidone treatment for juvenile bipolar disorder: a retrospective chart review. J Am Acad Child Adolesc Psychiatry 38:960–965, 1999

Fung YK: Postnatal behavioural effects of maternal nicotine exposure in rats. J Pharm Pharmacol 40:870–872, 1988

Fung YK, Lau YS: Effects of prenatal nicotine exposure on rat striatal dopaminergic and nicotinic systems. Pharmacol Biochem Behav 33:1–6, 1989

Gadow KD, Nolan EE, Sverd J: Methylphenidate in hyperactive boys with comorbid tic disorder, II: short-term behavioral effects in school settings. J Am Acad Child Adolesc Psychiatry 31:462–471, 1992

Gadow KD, Sverd J, Sprafkin J, et al: Efficacy of methylphenidate for attention-deficit hyperactivity disorder in children with tic disorder. Arch Gen Psychiatry 52:444–455, 1995

Garfinkel BD, Wender PH, Sloman L, et al: Tricyclic antidepressant and methylphenidate treatment of attention deficit disorder in children. J Am Acad Child Adolesc Psychiatry 22:343–348, 1983

Gastfriend DR, Biederman J, Jellinek MS: Desipramine in the treatment of attention deficit disorder in adolescents. Psychopharmacol Bull 21:144–145, 1985

Geller B, Fox L, Clark K: Rate and predictors of prepubertal bipolarity during follow-up of 6- to 12-year-old depressed children. J Am Acad Child Adolesc Psychiatry 33:461–468, 1994

Geller DA, Biederman J, Reed ED, et al: Similarities in response to fluoxetine in the treatment of children and adolescents with obsessive-compulsive disorder. J Am Acad Child Adolesc Psychiatry 34:36–44, 1995

Gittelman R: Childhood disorders, in Drug Treatment of Adult and Child Psychiatric Disorders. Edited by Klein D, Quitkin F, Rifkin A, et al. Baltimore, MD, Williams & Wilkins, 1980, pp 576–756

Gittelman-Klein R: Pilot clinical trial of imipramine in hyperkinetic children, in Clinical Use of Stimulant Drugs in Children. Edited by Conners C. The Hague, The Netherlands, Excerpta Medica, 1974, pp 192–201

Gittelman-Klein R: Pharmacotherapy of childhood hyperactivity: an update, in Psychopharmacology: The Third Generation of Progress. Edited by Meltzer HY. New York, Raven, 1987, pp 1215–1224

Goldman L, Genel M, Bezman R, et al: Diagnosis and treatment of attention-deficit/hyperactivity disorder in children and adolescents. JAMA 279:1100–1107, 1998

Gordon C, State R, Nelson J, et al: A double-blind comparison of clomipramine, desipramine, and placebo in the treatment of autistic disorder. Arch Gen Psychiatry 50:441–447, 1993

Greenberg L, Yellin A, Spring C, et al: Clinical effects of imipramine and methylphenidate in hyperactive children. International Journal of Mental Health 4:144–156, 1975

Greenblatt D, Moltke L, Harmatz J, et al: Drug interactions with newer antidepressants: role of human cytochromes P450. J Clin Psychiatry 59:19–27, 1998

Greene R: The Explosive Child: A New Approach for Understanding and Parenting Easily Frustrated, "Chronically Inflexible" Children, 1st Edition. New York, HarperCollins, 1998

Greenhill LL, Halperin JM, Abikoff H: Stimulant medications. J Am Acad Child Adolesc Psychiatry 38:503–512, 1999

Greenhill LL, Findling RL, Swanson JM: A double-blind, placebo-controlled study of modified-release methylphenidate in children with attention-deficit/hyperactivity disorder. Pediatrics (serial online) 109:39, 2002. Available at: http://www.pediatrics.org/cgi/content/full/109/3/e39. Accessed May 12, 2003.

Gross M: Imipramine in the treatment of minimal brain dysfunction in children. Psychosomatics 14:283–285, 1973

Gross M: Growth of hyperkinetic children taking methylphenidate, dextroamphetamine, or imipramine/desipramine. J Pediatr 58:423–431, 1976

Gualtieri CT, Evans RW: Motor performance in hyperactive children treated with imipramine. Percept Mot Skills 66:763–769, 1988

Gunning B: A controlled trial of clonidine in hyperkinetic children. Unpublished thesis, Department of Child and Adolescent Psychiatry, Academic Hospital Rotterdam–Sophia Children's Hospital Rotterdam, Rotterdam, The Netherlands, 1992

Herman JB, Rosenbaum JF, Brotman AW: The alprazolam to clonazepam switch for the treatment of panic disorder. J Clin Psychopharmacol 7:175–178, 1987

Hoge SK, Biederman J: A case of Tourette's syndrome with symptoms of attention deficit disorder treated with desipramine. J Clin Psychiatry 47:478–479, 1986

Hornig-Rohan M, Amsterdam J: Venlafaxine vs stimulant therapy in patients with dual diagnoses of ADHD and depression. Poster 92, presented at the New Clinical Drug Evaluation Unit Program, Orlando, FL, June 1995

Horrigan JP, Barnhill LJ: Guanfacine for treatment of attention-deficit hyperactivity disorder in boys. J Child Adolesc Psychopharmacol 5:215–223, 1995

Huessy HR, Wright AL: The use of imipramine in children's behavior disorders. Acta Paedopsychiatr 37:194–199, 1970

Hunt RD: Treatment effects of oral and transdermal clonidine in relation to methylphenidate: an open pilot study in ADD-H. Psychopharmacol Bull 23:111–114, 1987

Hunt RD, Minderaa RB, Cohen DJ: Clonidine benefits children with attention deficit disorder and hyperactivity: report of a double-blind placebo-crossover therapeutic trial. J Am Acad Child Psychiatry 24:617–629, 1985

Hunt RD, Capper L, O'Connell P: Clonidine in child and adolescent psychiatry. J Child Adolesc Psychopharmacol 1:87–102, 1990

Hunt RD, Arnsten AF, Asbell MD: An open trial of guanfacine in the treatment of attention-deficit hyperactivity disorder. J Am Acad Child Adolesc Psychiatry 34:50–54, 1995

Hurt RD, Sachs DP, Glover ED, et al: A comparison of sustained-release bupropion and placebo for smoking cessation. N Engl J Med 337:1195–1202, 1997

Hyman SE, Nestler EJ: The Molecular Foundations of Psychiatry, 1st Edition. Washington, DC, American Psychiatric Press, 1993

Johns JM, Louis TM, Becker RF, et al: Behavioral effects of prenatal exposure to nicotine in guinea pigs. Neurobehav Toxicol Teratol 4:365–369, 1982

Jones GM, Sahakian BJ, Levy R, et al: Effects of acute subcutaneous nicotine on attention, information processing and short-term memory in Alzheimer's disease. Psychopharmacology (Berl) 108:485–494, 1992

Klein RG: Pharmacotherapy of childhood hyperactivity: an update, in Psychopharmacology: The Third Generation of Progress. Edited by Meltzer HY. New York, Raven, 1987, pp 1215–1225

Klein RG, Mannuzza S: Hyperactive boys almost grown up, III: methylphenidate effects on ultimate height. Arch Gen Psychiatry 45:1131–1134, 1988

Kovacs M, Feinberg TL, Crouse-Novak M, et al: Depressive disorders in childhood, I: a longitudinal prospective study of characteristics and recovery. Arch Gen Psychiatry 41:229–237, 1984

Kratochvil C, Wernicke J, Michelson D, et al: Long-term study of atomoxetine in the treatment of ADHD, in Scientific Proceedings of the 48th Annual Meeting of the American Academy of Child and Adolescent Psychiatry. Edited by Villani S. Honolulu, HI, American Academy of Child and Adolescent Psychiatry, October 2001, p 119

Kupietz SS, Balka EB: Alterations in the vigilance performance of children receiving amitriptyline and methylphenidate pharmacotherapy. Psychopharmacology (Berl) 50:29–33, 1976

Kupietz SS, Winsberg BG, Richardson E, et al: Effects of methylphenidate dosage in hyperactive reading-disabled children, I: behavior and cognitive performance effects. J Am Acad Child Adolesc Psychiatry 27:70–77, 1988

Kutcher S, Williamson P, MacKenzie S, et al: Successful clonazepam treatment of neuroleptic-induced akathisia in older adolescents and young adults: a double-blind, placebo-controlled study. J Clin Psychopharmacol 9:403–406, 1989

Leckman JF, Hardin MT, Riddle MA, et al: Clonidine treatment of Gilles de la Tourette's syndrome. Arch Gen Psychiatry 48:324–328, 1991

Leonard H, Rapoport J: Anxiety disorders in childhood and adolescence, in American Psychiatric Press Review of Psychiatry, Vol 9. Edited by Tasman A, Hales R, Frances A. Washington, DC, American Psychiatric Press, 1989, pp 162–179

Leonard H, March J, Rickler K, et al: Pharmacology of the selective serotonin reuptake inhibitors in children and adolescents. J Am Acad Child Adolesc Psychiatry 36:725–736, 1998

Levin E, Conners C, Sparrow E, et al: Nicotine effects on adults with attention-deficit/hyperactivity disorder. Psychopharmacology (Berl) 123:55–63, 1996

Lienemann J, Walker F: Naltrexone for treatment of self-injury (letter). Am J Psychiatry 146:1639–1640, 1989

Lombroso P, Scahill L, King R, et al: Risperidone treatment of children and adolescents with chronic tic disorders: a preliminary report. J Am Acad Child Adolesc Psychiatry 34:1147–1152, 1995

Lowe TL, Cohen DJ, Detlor J: Stimulant medications precipitate Tourette's syndrome. JAMA 247:1168–1169, 1982

March J, Silva S, Petrycki S, et al: Fluoxetine, cognitive-behavioral therapy, and their combination for adolescents with depression: Treatment for Adolescents With Depression Study (TADS) randomized controlled trial. JAMA 292:807–820, 2004

Mattes JA: Propranolol for adults with temper outbursts and residual attention deficit disorder. J Clin Psychopharmacol 6:299–302, 1986

Mattes JA, Gittelman R: Growth of hyperactive children on maintenance regimen of methylphenidate. Arch Gen Psychiatry 40:317–321, 1983

McClellan J, Werry J: Practice parameters for the assessment and treatment of children and adolescents with schizophrenia. J Am Acad Child Adolesc Psychiatry 33:616–635, 1994

McCracken JT, Biederman J, Greenhill LL, et al: Analog classroom assessment of SLI381 for treatment of ADHD, in Scientific Proceedings of the 47th Annual Meeting of the American Academy of Child and Adolescent Psychiatry. Edited by Villani S. New York, American Academy of Child and Adolescent Psychiatry, October 2000, Poster 114

Meck W, Church R: Cholinergic modulation of the content of temporal memory. Behav Neurosci 101:457–464, 1987

Mereu G, Yoon K, Gessa G, et al: Preferential stimulation of ventral tegmental area dopaminergic neurons by nicotine. Eur J Pharmacol 141:395–399, 1987

Michelson D, Faries D, Wernicke J, et al: Atomoxetine in the treatment of children and adolescents with attention-deficit/hyperactivity disorder: a randomized, placebo-controlled, dose-response study. Pediatrics (serial online) 108:83, 2001. Available at: http://www.pediatrics.org/cgi/content/full/108/5/e83. Accessed May 12, 2003.

Milberger S, Biederman J, Faraone SV, et al: Is maternal smoking during pregnancy a risk factor for attention deficit hyperactivity disorder in children? Am J Psychiatry 153:1138–1142, 1996

Milberger S, Biederman J, Faraone SV, et al: ADHD is associated with early initiation of cigarette smoking in children and adolescents. J Am Acad Child Adolesc Psychiatry 36:37–43, 1997

Nemeroff CB, DeVane CL, Pollock BG: Newer antidepressants and the cytochrome P450 system. Am J Psychiatry 153:311–320, 1996

Nierenberg A, Alpert J, Pava J, et al: Course and treatment of atypical depression. J Clin Psychiatry 59:5–9, 1998

Olvera RL, Pliszka SR, Luh J, et al: An open trial of venlafaxine in the treatment of attention-deficit/hyperactivity disorder in children and adolescents. J Child Adolesc Psychopharmacol 6:241–250, 1996

O'Malley SS, Jaffe AJ, Chang G, et al: Six-month follow-up of naltrexone and psychotherapy for alcohol dependence. Arch Gen Psychiatry 53:217–224, 1996

Parrott AC, Winder G: Nicotine chewing gum (2 mg, 4 mg) and cigarette smoking: comparative effects upon vigilance and heart rate. Psychopharmacology (Berl) 97:257–261, 1989

Pauls DL, Towbin KE, Leckman JF, et al: Gilles de la Tourette's syndrome and obsessive-compulsive disorder: evidence supporting a genetic relationship. Arch Gen Psychiatry 43:1180–1182, 1986

Peeke S, Peeke H: Attention, memory, and cigarette smoking. Psychopharmacology (Berl) 84:205–216, 1984

Pelham WE, Bender ME, Caddell J, et al: Methylphenidate and children with attention deficit disorder. Arch Gen Psychiatry 42:948–952, 1985

Pelham WE, Gnagy EM, Burrows-Maclean L, et al: Once-a-day Concerta methylphenidate versus three-times-daily methylphenidate in laboratory and natural settings. Pediatrics (serial online) 107:105, 2001. Available at: http://www.pediatrics.org/cgi/content/full/107/6/e105. Accessed May 12, 2003.

Pentikis HS, Simmons RD, Benedict MF, et al: Methylphenidate bioavailability in adults when an extended-release multiparticulate formulation is administered sprinkled on food or as an intact capsule. J Am Acad Child Adolesc Psychiatry 41:443–449, 2002

Platt JE, Campbell M, Green WH, et al: Cognitive effects of lithium carbonate and haloperidol in treatment-resistant aggressive children. Arch Gen Psychiatry 41:657–662, 1984

Pomerleau O, Downey K, Stelson F, et al: Cigarette smoking in adult patients diagnosed with ADHD. J Subst Abuse 7:373–378, 1996

Pope HG, McElroy SL, Keck PE Jr, et al: Valproate in the treatment of acute mania. Arch Gen Psychiatry 48:62–68, 1991

Preskorn S, Alderman J, Chung M, et al: Pharmacokinetics of desipramine coadministered with sertraline or fluoxetine. J Clin Psychopharmacol 14:90–98, 1994

Prince J, Wilens T, Biederman J, et al: Clonidine for ADHD related sleep disturbances: a systematic chart review of 62 cases. J Am Acad Child Adolesc Psychiatry 35:599–605, 1996

Prince J, Wilens T, Biederman J, et al: A controlled study of nortriptyline in children and adolescents with attention deficit hyperactivity disorder, in Scientific Proceedings, American Academy of Child and Adolescent Psychiatry, XV. Chicago, IL, May 1999

Quay HC: Conduct disorder, in Psychopathologic Disorders of Childhood. Edited by Quay HC, Werry JS. New York, Wiley, 1986, pp 35–73

Quinn DM: Prevalence of psychoactive medication in children and adolescents. Can J Psychiatry 31:575–580, 1986

Quinn PO, Rapoport JL: One-year follow-up of hyperactive boys treated with imipramine or methylphenidate. Am J Psychiatry 132:241–245, 1975

Quitkin FM, Harrison W, Stewart JW, et al: Response to phenelzine and imipramine in placebo nonresponders with atypical depression. Arch Gen Psychiatry 48:319–323, 1991

Rapoport JL, Quinn P, Bradbard G, et al: Imipramine and methylphenidate treatment of hyperactive boys: a double-blind comparison. Arch Gen Psychiatry 30:789–793, 1974

Rapport MD, Jones JT, DuPaul GJ, et al: Attention deficit disorder and methylphenidate: group and single-subject analyses of dose effects on attention in clinic and classroom settings. J Clin Child Psychol 16:329–338, 1987

Rapport MD, Stoner G, DuPaul GJ, et al: Attention deficit disorder and methylphenidate: a multilevel analysis of dose-response effects on children's impulsivity across settings. J Am Acad Child Adolesc Psychiatry 27:60–69, 1988

Rapport MD, DuPaul GJ, Kelly KL: Attention deficit hyperactivity disorder and methylphenidate: the relationship between gross body weight and drug response in children. Psychopharmacol Bull 25:285–290, 1989a

Rapport MD, Quinn SO, DuPaul GJ, et al: Attention deficit disorder with hyperactivity and methylphenidate: the effects of dose and mastery level on children's learning performance. J Abnorm Child Psychol 17:669–689, 1989b

Rapport MD, Carlson GA, Kelly KL, et al: Methylphenidate and desipramine in hospitalized children, I: separate and combined effects on cognitive function. J Am Acad Child Adolesc Psychiatry 32:333–342, 1993

Ratey JJ, Greenberg MS, Lindem KJ: Combination of treatments for attention deficit hyperactivity disorder in adults. J Nerv Ment Dis 179:699–701, 1991

Realmuto GM, August GJ, Garfinkel BD: Clinical effect of buspirone in autistic children. J Clin Psychopharmacol 9:122–125, 1989

Reimherr FW, Wender PH, Wood DR, et al: An open trial of L-tyrosine in the treatment of attention deficit disorder, residual type. Am J Psychiatry 144:1071–1073, 1987

Reimherr F[W], Hedges D, Strong R, et al: An open-trial of venlafaxine in adult patients with attention deficit hyperactivity disorder. Paper presented at the New Clinical Drug Evaluation Unit Program, Orlando, FL, May 1995

Rew DA, Rundle JS: Assessment of the safety of regular DDAVP therapy in primary nocturnal enuresis. Br J Urol 63:352–353, 1989

Riddle MA, Hardin MT, Towbin KE, et al: Tardive dyskinesia following haloperidol treatment in Tourette's syndrome (letter). Arch Gen Psychiatry 44:98–99, 1987

Riddle MA, Hardin MT, Cho SC, et al: Desipramine treatment of boys with attention-deficit hyperactivity disorder and tics: preliminary clinical experience. J Am Acad Child Adolesc Psychiatry 27:811–814, 1988

Riddle MA, Nelson JC, Kleinman CS, et al: Sudden death in children receiving Norpramin: a review of three reported cases and commentary. J Am Acad Child Adolesc Psychiatry 30:104–108, 1991

Safer DJ, Allen RP, Barr E: Depression of growth in hyperactive children on stimulant drugs. N Engl J Med 287:217–220, 1972

Satterfield JH, Cantwell DP, Schell A, et al: Growth of hyperactive children treated with methylphenidate. Arch Gen Psychiatry 36: 212–217, 1979

Shapiro AK, Shapiro ES, Young JG, et al: Gilles de la Tourette Syndrome. New York, Raven, 1988

Singer S, Brown J, Quaskey S, et al: The treatment of attention-deficit hyperactivity disorder in Tourette's syndrome: a double-blind placebo-controlled study with clonidine and desipramine. Pediatrics 95:74–81, 1994

Sorgi PJ, Ratey JJ, Polakoff S: Beta-adrenergic blockers for the control of aggressive behavior in patients with schizophrenia. Am J Psychiatry 143:775–776, 1986

Spencer T: A double-blind, controlled study of desipramine in children with ADHD and tic disorders, in Scientific Proceedings, 44th annual meeting of the American Academy of Child and Adolescent Psychiatry, Toronto, Ontario, Canada, October 1997

Spencer T, Biederman J, Kerman K, et al: Desipramine treatment of children with attention-deficit hyperactivity disorder and tic disorder or Tourette's syndrome. J Am Acad Child Adolesc Psychiatry 32:354–360, 1993a

Spencer T, Biederman J, Wilens T, et al: Nortriptyline treatment of children with attention-deficit hyperactivity disorder and tic disorder or Tourette's syndrome. J Am Acad Child Adolesc Psychiatry 32:205–210, 1993b

Spencer T, Wilens T, Biederman J, et al: A double-blind, crossover comparison of methylphenidate and placebo in adults with childhood-onset attention-deficit hyperactivity disorder. Arch Gen Psychiatry 52:434–443, 1995

Spencer T, Biederman J, Wilens T, et al: Pharmacotherapy of attention-deficit hyperactivity disorder across the life cycle. J Am Acad Child Adolesc Psychiatry 35:409–432, 1996

Spencer T, Biederman J, Wilens T: Pharmacotherapy of ADHD: a life span perspective, in American Psychiatric Press Review of Psychiatry, Vol 16. Edited by Oldham J, Riba M. Washington, DC, American Psychiatric Press, 1997, pp 87–128

Spencer T, Biederman J, Wilens TE, et al: Adults with attention-deficit/hyperactivity disorder: a controversial diagnosis. J Clin Psychiatry 59 (suppl 7):59–68, 1998a

Spencer T, Biederman J, Wilens T[E]: Growth deficits in children with attention deficit hyperactivity disorder. Pediatrics 102:501–506, 1998b

Spencer T, Biederman J, Coffey B, et al: The 4-year course of tic disorders in boys with attention-deficit/hyperactivity disorder. Arch Gen Psychiatry 56:842–847, 1999a

Spencer T, Wilens T, Biederman J, et al: Efficacy and tolerability of a mixed amphetamine salts compound in adults with attention deficit hyperactivity disorder, in Scientific Proceedings of the American Academy of Child and Adolescent Psychiatry, XV. Chicago, IL, May 1999b

Spencer T, Swanson J, Weidenman M, et al: Pharmacodynamic profile of Ritalin LA, a new extended-release dosage form of Ritalin, in children with ADHD, in Scientific Proceedings of the 47th Annual Meeting of the American Academy of Child and Adolescent Psychiatry. Edited by Villani S. New York, American Academy of Child and Adolescent Psychiatry, October 2000

Spencer T, Heiligenstein J, Biederman J, et al: Results from two proof-of-concept, placebo-controlled studies of atomoxetine in children with ADHD. J Clin Psychiatry 63:1140–1147, 2002

Steingard R, Biederman J, Spencer T, et al: Comparison of clonidine response in the treatment of attention deficit hyperactivity disorder with and without comorbid tic disorders. J Am Acad Child Adolesc Psychiatry 32:350–353, 1993

Sudden death in children treated with a tricyclic antidepressant. Med Lett Drugs Ther 32:53, 1990

Swanson J, Agler D, Fineberg E, et al: University of California, Irvine, laboratory school protocol for pharmacokinetic and pharmacodynamic studies, in Ritalin: Theory and Practice, 2nd Edition. Edited by Greenhill L, Osman B. Larchmont, NY, Mary Ann Liebert, 2000, pp 405–430

Tannock R, Schachar RJ, Carr RP, et al: Dose-response effects of methylphenidate on academic performance and overt behavior in hyperactive children. Pediatrics 84:648–657, 1989

Trott GE, Menzel M, Friese HJ, et al: Effectiveness and tolerance of the selective MAO-A inhibitor in children with hyperkinetic syndrome (in German). Z Kinder Jugendpsychiatr 19:248–253, 1991

Trott GE, Friese HJ, Menzel M, et al: Use of moclobemide in children with attention deficit hyperactivity disorder. Psychopharmacology (Berl) 106 (suppl):S134–S136, 1992

U.S. Food and Drug Administration: Press Release: FDA Launches a Multi-Pronged Strategy to Strengthen Safeguards for Children Treated With Antidepressant Medications, October 15. 2004. Available at: http://www.fda.gov/bbs/topics/news/2004/NEW01124.html. Accessed July 2005.

U.S. Food and Drug Administration: Public Health Advisory for Adderall and Adderall XR, February 9, 2005. Available at: www.fda.gov/cder/drug/advisory/adderall.htm. Accessed July 2005.

Wagner K, Birmaher B, Carlson G, et al: Safety of paroxetine and imipramine in the treatment of adolescent depression. Paper presented at the New Clinical Drug Evaluation Unit Program, Boca Raton, FL, June 1998

Watter N, Dreyfuss FE: Modifications of hyperkinetic behavior by nortriptyline. Virginia Medical Monthly 100:123–126, 1973

Weller EB, Weller RA, Fristad MA, et al: Saliva lithium monitoring in prepubertal children. J Am Acad Child Adolesc Psychiatry 26:173–175, 1987

Werry J: Imipramine and methylphenidate in hyperactive children. J Child Psychol Psychiatry 21:27–35, 1980

Wesnes K, Warburton DM: The effects of cigarettes of varying yield on rapid information processing performance. Psychopharmacology (Berl) 82:338–342, 1984

Westfall TC, Grant H, Perry H: Release of dopamine and 5-hydroxytryptamine from rat striatal slices following activation of nicotinic cholinergic receptors. Gen Pharmacol 14:321–325, 1983

Wilens TE, on behalf of the Concerta study group: Prospective one-year study of OROS MPH, dosed qd in children with ADHD. Paper presented at the annual meeting of the American Academy of Neurology, San Diego, CA, June 2000

Wilens T[E], Biederman J: The stimulants. Psychiatr Clin North Am 15:191–222, 1992

Wilens TE, Biederman J, Geist DE, et al: Nortriptyline in the treatment of ADHD: a chart review of 58 cases. J Am Acad Child Adolesc Psychiatry 32:343–349, 1993

Wilens TE, Biederman J, Mick E, et al: A systematic assessment of tricyclic antidepressants in the treatment of adult attention-deficit hyperactivity disorder. J Nerv Ment Dis 183:48–50, 1995a

Wilens TE, Spencer T, Biederman J, et al: Combined pharmacotherapy: an emerging trend in pediatric psychopharmacology. J Am Acad Child Adolesc Psychiatry 34:110–112, 1995b

Wilens TE, Biederman J, Abrantes AM, et al: A naturalistic assessment of protriptyline for attention-deficit hyperactivity disorder. J Am Acad Child Adolesc Psychiatry 35:1485–1490, 1996a

Wilens TE, Biederman J, Baldessarini RJ, et al: Cardiovascular effects of therapeutic doses of tricyclic antidepressants in children and adolescents. J Am Acad Child Adolesc Psychiatry 35:1491–1501, 1996b

Wilens TE, Wyatt D, Spencer TJ: Disentangling disinhibition. J Am Acad Child Adolesc Psychiatry 37:1225–1227, 1998

Wilens TE, Biederman J, Spencer TJ, et al: A pilot controlled clinical trial of ABT-418, a cholinergic agonist, in the treatment of adults with attention deficit hyperactivity disorder. Am J Psychiatry 156:1931–1937, 1999a

Wilens TE, Spencer TJ, Swanson JM, et al: Combining methylphenidate and clonidine: a clinically sound medication option. J Am Acad Child Adolesc Psychiatry 38:614–619, 1999b

Winsberg BG, Bialer I, Kupietz S, et al: Effects of imipramine and dextroamphetamine on behavior of neuropsychiatrically impaired children. Am J Psychiatry 128:1425–1431, 1972

Wolraich ML, Greenhill LL, Pelham W, et al: Randomized, controlled trial of OROS methylphenidate once a day in children with attention-deficit/hyperactivity disorder. Pediatrics 108:883–892, 2001

Wozniak J, Biederman J, Kiely K, et al: Mania-like symptoms suggestive of childhood onset bipolar disorder in clinically referred children. J Am Acad Child Adolesc Psychiatry 34:867–876, 1995

Yepes LE, Balka EB, Winsberg BG, et al: Amitriptyline and methylphenidate treatment of behaviorally disordered children. J Child Psychol Psychiatry 18:39–52, 1977

Zametkin AJ, Rapoport JL: Noradrenergic hypothesis of attention deficit disorder with hyperactivity: a critical review, in Psychopharmacology: The Third Generation of Progress. Edited by Meltzer HY. New York, Raven, 1987, pp 837–842

Zametkin A[J], Rapoport JL, Murphy DL, et al: Treatment of hyperactive children with monoamine oxidase inhibitors, I: clinical efficacy. Arch Gen Psychiatry 42:962–966, 1985

Self-Assessment Questions

Select the single best response for each question.

29.1 Commonly reported and well-substantiated side effects of stimulant medications include all of the following *except*

A. Appetite suppression.
B. Sleep disturbance.
C. Mild increases in pulse and blood pressure.
D. Stunting of growth in height.
E. Weight loss.

29.2 A number of studies have evaluated the short- and long-term effects of therapeutic doses of tricyclic antidepressants (TCAs) on the cardiovascular system in children. Which of the following statements is *incorrect?*

A. TCAs are generally well tolerated.
B. TCAs may produce electrocardiographic abnormalities at doses between 1 and 2 mg/kg.
C. Patients should be carefully monitored at higher TCA doses (> 3.5 mg/kg).
D. Before initiating TCAs, a baseline electrocardiogram is recommended.
E. None of the above.

29.3 Some compounds metabolized by the cytochrome P450 enzyme 3A4 have been associated with QT prolongations when combined with drugs that inhibit 3A4. Antidepressants that affect 3A4 activity include all of the following *except*

A. Fluvoxamine.
B. Venlafaxine.
C. Nefazodone.
D. Fluoxetine.
E. Sertraline.

29.4 Novel atypical antipsychotic medications exert their therapeutic effects through antagonism of which of the following receptors?

A. Dopaminergic (D_1).
B. Histaminic (H_1).
C. Serotonergic ($5\text{-}HT_2$).
D. Alpha$_1$-adrenergic.
E. None of the above.

29.5 Oxcarbazepine is chemically similar to carbamazepine with some important differences, which include all of the following *except*

A. Laboratory monitoring is still required with oxcarbazepine.
B. Oxcarbazepine has little interaction with the cytochrome P450 system.
C. Oxcarbazepine lacks the hepatic liability of carbamazepine.
D. Oxcarbazepine does not induce its own metabolism.
E. Oxcarbazepine lacks the hematological liability of carbamazepine.

29.6   In child psychiatry, clonidine is commonly used in the treatment of all of the following *except*

     A.   Attention-deficit/hyperactivity disorder (ADHD).

     B.   Tourette's disorder.

     C.   Aggression.

     D.   Sleep disturbance in ADHD children.

     E.   Major depressive disorder.

29.7   Side effects associated with the use of atomoxetine in children include which of the following?

     A.   Increased appetite.

     B.   Cardiac conduction delays.

     C.   Insomnia.

     D.   Increase in pulse and diastolic blood pressure.

     E.   Abuse.

Appendix

Answer Guide to Self-Assessment Questions

The self-assessment questions in this Appendix, as well as additional questions covering all topics in *The American Psychiatric Publishing Textbook of Child and Adolescent Psychiatry*, are available for purchase online at cme.psychiatryonline.org. Purchase the online version and receive instant scoring and CME credits.

Chapter 1—Overview of Development From Infancy Through Adolescence

Select the single best response for each question.

1.1   Theories of development formulated by Freud, Erikson, and Piaget share which of the following characteristics?

  A. They postulate a genetically determined capacity for the development of patterns or systems of behavior by the child.
  B. They propose that the overall behavior patterns that emerge are qualitatively similar to one another.
  C. They are all structural theories of development that imply that reorganization within the child is unnecessary.
  D. They postulate that the child reacts in particular ways to environmental stimuli.
  E. None of the above.

The correct response is option A.

Psychoanalysis (Freud), psychosocial development (Erikson), and cognitive development (Piaget), the theories of development known as structural theories, postulate a genetically determined capacity for the development of patterns or systems of behavior in which the child acts on the environment from the beginning. The overall behavior patterns that emerge are qualitatively different from one another but exhibit continuity. Structural theories imply that reorganization within the child is required. Option D characterizes reactive theories, not structural theories. **(pp. 3–4)**

1.2   By age 5 years, a child will have attained all of the following motor developmental milestones *except*

  A. Can stand on one foot.
  B. Can dance and jump.
  C. Manifests firmly established leg, eye, and ear dominance.
  D. Can copy a square.
  E. Can build a tower of 10 cubes.

The correct response is option C.

Leg, eye, and ear dominance may not become firmly established until the seventh, eight, or ninth year of life, respectively. By age 3 years, children can stand on one foot, dance and jump, and build a tower of 10 cubes. At age 5 years, they can copy a square. **(pp. 4–5)**

1.3   Piaget conceptualized four major stages of cognitive development. Which of the
       following states the correct sequence in which these stages normally occur, from
       birth to adolescence?

    A. Preoperational, sensorimotor, concrete operational, formal operational.
    B. Concrete operational, sensorimotor, preoperational, formal operational.
    C. Sensorimotor, concrete operational, formal operational, preoperational.
    D. Formal operational, concrete operational, sensorimotor, preoperational.
    E. Sensorimotor, preoperational, concrete operational, formal operational.

The correct response is option E.

Piaget's four major stages of development are sensorimotor (from birth to
2 years), preoperational (from 2 years to 7 years), concrete operational (from
7 years to adolescence), and formal operational (adolescence). **(p. 7)**

1.4   *Chunking* is

    A. A process by which representations, procedures, and memories that occur
        together are automatically accessed simultaneously.
    B. A type of long-term memory.
    C. A form of procedural knowledge.
    D. All of the above.
    E. None of the above.

The correct response is option A.

Chunking, which occurs in *short-term memory,* is the process by which representations, procedures, and memories that occur together are automatically accessed
simultaneously. *Long-term memory* involves two types of knowledge: declarative
knowledge and procedural knowledge. *Declarative knowledge* is knowledge of facts,
concepts, and ideas. Amnesia due to brain damage usually results in loss of declarative knowledge. *Procedural knowledge* is knowledge of how to perform certain
acts. This kind of knowledge is usually unconscious and is not lost in amnesia due
to brain damage. **(p. 11)**

1.5   According to Spitz (1965), organizers that govern the process of transition from
       one level to the next in the development of attachment include all of the follow-
       ing *except*

    A. Sustained eye contact in response to an interaction.
    B. The smiling response.
    C. Eight-month anxiety.
    D. Achievement of the sign of negation.
    E. None of the above.

The correct response is option A.

Spitz (1965) described three "organizers" in the development of attachment: the
smiling response, the 8-month anxiety, and the use of negation and of the word
no. Spitz did not include sustained eye contact as an organizer. **(p. 15)**

1.6   In psychoanalytic theory, the *anal phase* of psychosexual development is characterized by

    A. The child's focus on autoerotic activities.

    B. The child's experience of intense sexual and aggressive urges toward both parents.

    C. The child's development of concepts of inevitability regarding birth, death, and sex differences.

    D. The child's experience of feelings of separateness and worth.

    E. The child's sequential development of play.

The correct response is option D.

According to psychoanalytic theory, the four phases of psychosexual development are oral, anal, phallic–oedipal, and latency. During the *anal phase,* the child begins to experience feelings about separateness and worth. The focus on autoerotic activities (self-stimulating) occurs during the *oral phase;* the sequential development of play and intense sexual and aggressive urges occurs during the *phallic–oedipal phase;* and clarification of the inevitability of birth, death, and sex differences occurs during the *latency phase.* **(pp. 16–17)**

■ Reference

Spitz R: The First Year of Life. New York, International Universities Press, 1965

Chapter 2—Classification of Child and Adolescent Psychiatric Disorders

Select the single best response for each question.

2.1   A number of changes were made in DSM-IV (American Psychiatric Association 1994) that apply to childhood. Which of the following is one of these changes?

    A. A new category of pervasive developmental disorders was to be coded on Axis II.

    B. Motor skills disorders were moved from Axis II to Axis I.

    C. Learning disorders were moved from Axis I to Axis II.

    D. Communications disorders were moved from Axis I to Axis II.

    E. None of the above.

The correct response is option B.

In DSM-IV, pervasive developmental disorders and learning disorders, motor skills disorder, and communication disorders were moved from Axis II to Axis I. **(p. 33)**

2.2   Pervasive developmental disorders include all of the following *except*

    A. Childhood schizophrenia.

    B. Autistic disorder.

    C. Rett's disorder.

    D. Asperger's disorder.

    E. Childhood disintegrative disorder.

The correct response is option A.

Childhood schizophrenia is not a pervasive developmental disorder. **(p. 33)**

2.3   In DSM-IV, the new category *feeding and eating disorders of infancy or early childhood* included all of the following *except*

    A. Feeding disorder of infancy or early childhood (persistent failure to eat adequately, with weight loss or failure to gain weight).

    B. Pica.

    C. Anorexia nervosa.

    D. Rumination disorder.

    E. None of the above.

The correct response is option C.

The new DSM-IV category *feeding and eating disorders of infancy or early childhood* included pica, rumination disorder, and feeding disorder of infancy or early childhood—the persistent failure to eat adequately and to gain weight. Anorexia nervosa and bulimia nervosa were moved to a separate eating disorders section. **(p. 34)**

2.4 The tic disorders category of DSM-IV was left essentially unchanged from that in DSM-III-R (American Psychiatric Association 1987) except for which of the following?

A. The addition of Tourette's disorder.
B. The elimination of chronic motor or vocal tic disorder.
C. The lowering of the upper limit of age at onset to 18 years.
D. The addition of transient tic disorder.
E. None of the above.

The correct response is option C.

The tic disorders category remained essentially unchanged in DSM-IV, with only a drop in the upper limit of age at onset from 21 to 18 years. The category includes Tourette's disorder, chronic motor or vocal tic disorder, transient tic disorder, and tic disorder not otherwise specified. **(p. 34)**

2.5 In DSM-IV, the category *other disorders of infancy, childhood, or adolescence* was reorganized to include which of the following disorders?

A. Separation anxiety disorder.
B. Selective mutism.
C. Reactive attachment disorder of infancy or early childhood.
D. Stereotypic movement disorder.
E. All of the above.

The correct response is option E.

In addition to all of the disorders listed above, the category *other disorders of infancy, childhood, or adolescence* contains a *not otherwise specified* diagnosis. **(p. 34)**

■ References

American Psychiatric Association: Diagnostic and Statistical Manual of Mental Disorders, 3rd Edition, Revised. Washington, DC, American Psychiatric Association, 1987

American Psychiatric Association: Diagnostic and Statistical Manual of Mental Disorders, 4th Edition. Washington, DC, American Psychiatric Association, 1994

Chapter 3—The Clinical Interview of the Child

Select the single best response for each question.

3.1   The Mental Health Assessment Form (MHAF)

   A. May be used with children between the ages of 3 and 6 years.
   B. Usually requires about 3 hours to complete.
   C. Employs questionnaires.
   D. Consists of 54 items.
   E. Obtains information on all areas of a child's life and functioning.

The correct response is option E.

The MHAF (Kestenbaum and Bird 1978) was developed to provide a bridge between the structured questionnaire and the open-ended clinical interview. It consists of 189 items, can be used with children between the ages of 6 and 12 years,
does not employ questionnaires or cards, and is designed to gather information on
all areas of the child's life and functioning. **(pp. 40–41)**

3.2   The MHAF consists of two parts. Part II ("Content of the Interview") deals with
        all of the following areas *except*

   A. Motoric behavior and speech.
   B. Interpersonal relations.
   C. Self-concept.
   D. Feeling states.
   E. Symbolic representation.

The correct response is option A.

Motoric behavior and speech are addressed in Part I ("Mental Status"), not Part II,
of the MHAF. In addition to the areas listed above, Part II also deals with con-
science/moral judgment and the child's general level of adaptation. **(pp. 41–42, Table 3–1)**

3.3   When interviewing the younger child (ages 5–9 years), the examiner should do
        all of the following *except*

   A. Interview one or both parents before meeting the child.
   B. Allow the child to examine the environment.
   C. Explain the nature of the interview to the parents.
   D. Refrain from explaining the reason for the interview to the child, because
      such information may be upsetting.
   E. Provide reassurance if necessary.

The correct response is option D.

The clinician should interview one or both parents before meeting the child, in
order to ascertain the nature of the presenting problem and to obtain pertinent
information; should allow the child to examine the surroundings; and should explain to the child the reason for the interview, providing reassurance if necessary.
(pp. 41–42)

3.4   When interviewing the older child (ages 10–12 years), the examiner should

    A. Begin with general questions to avoid having a child get defensive about the chief complaint.
    B. Start by using the MHAF designed for older children.
    C. Obtain some idea about the child's development of empathy.
    D. End with the chief complaint.
    E. Refrain from having a parents-only meeting after the initial interview so that the child will not feel excluded.

The correct response is option C.

The interviewer should begin with the chief complaint and should attempt to assess the extent of the child's development of empathy by asking questions about family pets and other animals. There is no specific age cutoff at which the "older children" version of MHAF should be used; the decision depends on the child's cognitive level as assessed by the interviewer. The treatment plan may or may not include separate parents-only or child-only meetings. However, older children should be told of the expected plan either way. **(pp. 44–45)**

3.5   The MHAF semistructured interview can be used to accomplish all of the following *except*

    A. Assess for the signs and symptoms of a psychiatric disorder.
    B. Identify positive attributes of the patient.
    C. Conduct a formal assessment of the patient's cognitive functioning.
    D. Establish a relationship with the patient.
    E. Evaluate the strengths of the patient.

The correct response is option C.

The MHAF is not designed to obtain a formal assessment of cognitive functioning. (p. 45)

■ Reference

Kestenbaum CJ, Bird HR: A reliability study of the Mental Health Assessment Form for school-age children. J Am Acad Child Psychiatry 17:338–347, 1978

Chapter 4—The Clinical Interview of the Adolescent

Select the single best response for each question.

4.1 Which of the following statements concerning the initial interview of an adolescent is *false?*

   A. Seeing the adolescent first highlights the patient's active participation in the process.
   B. Seeing the adolescent first may allay fears that the parents and therapist will gang up on the patient.
   C. The therapeutic alliance between the clinician and adolescent may be harmed if the clinician meets alone with the parents; such an approach is therefore discouraged.
   D. The clinician should make clear to the adolescent that he or she is not out to assign blame.
   E. None of the above.

The correct response is option C.

Several factors must be considered when deciding whether the initial meeting should be with the adolescent, the parents, or all together. In most cases, the adolescent should be present at the first meeting, preferably alone, in order to encourage his or her active participation. However, it is also important to meet with the parents alone at some point so that the clinician can obtain information that would be difficult to obtain with the adolescent present. **(pp. 49–50)**

4.2 Characteristic adolescent patterns of responding to interviews with a therapist include which of the following?

   A. Anxiety about revealing problems that they may regard as weaknesses.
   B. Externalization of one side or another of conflicted feelings.
   C. Counterphobic measures to deal with painful affects.
   D. An unrealistic faith in the "omnipotence of thought."
   E. All of the above.

The correct response is option E.

In addition to all of the above considerations, it is good to remember that the adolescent's relationship with most adults is colored by a strong push toward autonomy and a great wariness of feeling vulnerable, dependent, or controlled. **(pp. 50–51)**

4.3 To interview an adolescent effectively, which of the following are important qualities for a clinician?

   A. Having experienced similar problems in adolescence.
   B. Possessing a sense of humor.
   C. Being informal and familiar.
   D. Being close in age to the adolescent so that he or she can identify with the clinician.
   E. All of the above.

The correct response is option B.

Of the qualities listed, only a sense of humor is important. Having experienced similar struggles is not helpful unless the clinician has actually come to terms with the problems of his or her own adolescence. A skilled clinician can be effective regardless of his or her age. **(p. 51)**

4.4   When should a formal mental status examination be conducted with an adolescent?

    A. When there is a concern about psychosis.
    B. When the disorder may be severe.
    C. When precise documentation is required.
    D. When there is a possibility of dementia.
    E. All of the above.

The correct response is option E.

A formal mental status exam should be conducted when the disorder is severe, when precise documentation is required, or when there are concerns about psychosis, dementia, or an organic brain syndrome. **(p. 52)**

4.5   In interviewing adolescents, the therapist should

    A. Limit the interview to areas of difficulty.
    B. Demonstrate his or her familiarity with any topic that the adolescent may bring up, such as rock groups.
    C. Make early interpretations to assist the adolescent with the session.
    D. Avoid asking about dating or sexual relationships.
    E. Ask about friends and peers.

The correct response is option E.

An important area of exploration with adolescents is that of friends and peers, which will lead naturally to the topic of dating and sexual relationships. The interview should not be limited to areas of difficulty. It is better to simply let the adolescent express his or her particular interests, rather than attempting to demonstrate one's own familiarity with the topics. In addition, the clinician should resist the temptation to make early interpretations—such communications are more likely to scare the patient away than to be helpful. **(pp. 52–53)**

Chapter 5—The Parent Interview

Select the single best response for each question.

5.1 Mednick and Shaffer (1963) found that when maternal interviews were compared with pediatric records, the mothers' reports were discrepant what percentage of the time?

A. 0–6%.
B. 7%–15%.
C. 16%–20%.
D. 21%–62%.
E. 63%–75%.

The correct response is option D.

When maternal interviews were compared with pediatric records, the mothers' reports were found to be discrepant 21%–62% of the time for facts about discrete experiences, such as breast-feeding, childhood illnesses, and the age at completion of toilet training (Mednick and Shaffer 1963). **(p. 58)**

5.2 A number of investigators have studied the parent interview. Which of the following descriptions of their findings is *incorrect*?

A. Weissman et al. (1987) found that parents reported far more information about their children's disorders than did the children themselves.
B. Orvaschel et al. (1981) found that parents were more accurate in providing factual time-related information.
C. Edelbrock et al. (1985) found that the reliability of a child's report increased with the child's age.
D. Edelbrock et al. (1985) found that in children 10 years of age and older, parent and child reports showed little or no difference in reliability.
E. None of the above.

The correct response is option A.

Weissman at al. (1987) found that children reported far *more* information about their disorders than did their parents. **(p. 58)**

5.3 Which of the following is a function of the parent interview?

A. Gathering information about the child's history.
B. Assessing the child's present functioning.
C. Identifying the child's strengths and weaknesses.
D. Giving parents information about normal child development.
E. All of the above.

The correct response is option E.

All of the above are important functions of the parent interview. **(p. 59)**

5.4   The parent interview may be divided into five phases: preliminaries, prologue, interview proper, closing, and epilogue. What is the primary purpose of the *closing* phase?

     A. Assess the parents' and the clinician's expectations for the interview.

     B. Establish an alliance or empathetic relationship with the parents while collecting data and making the appropriate interventions.

     C. Reassure the parents and reinforce their control and competence.

     D. Review the interview, the validity of the plans, and the next step.

     E. None of the above.

The correct response is option C.

The purpose of the *closing* phase is to reassure the parents and reinforce their control and competence. The purpose of the *preliminaries* phase is to identify the patient and the purpose of the interview. During the *prologue*, it is useful to assess both the parents' and the clinician's expectations for the interview. The *interview proper* provides the opportunity to establish an alliance with the parents while collecting data and making the appropriate interventions. During the *epilogue*, the clinician can review the validity of the plans and the next step. **(pp. 59–61)**

5.5   In emergency settings, the focus of the parent interview is

     A. Directly related to the parents' sense of control, frustration, and incompetence in the clinical situation.

     B. To assess the risk of danger and to establish a safe and protective environment for the child.

     C. To assess the child's medical care.

     D. To obtain factual and impressionistic information.

     E. All of the above.

The correct response is option B.

In emergency settings, the focus of the interview must be on assessing the risk of danger and establishing a safe and protective environment for the child. **(pp. 61–62)**

■ References

Edelbrock C, Costello AJ, Dulcan NM, et al: Age differences in the reliability of the psychiatric interview of the child. Child Dev 56:265–275, 1985

Mednick SA, Shaffer JBP: Mothers' retrospective reports in child-rearing research. Am J Orthopsychiatry 33:457–461, 1963

Orvaschel H, Weissman MM, Padian N, et al: Assessing psychopathology in children of psychiatrically disturbed parents: a pilot study. J Am Acad Child Psychiatry 20:112–122, 1981

Weissman MM, Wickramaratne P, Warner V, et al: Assessing psychiatric disorders in children: discrepancies between mothers' and children's reports. Arch Gen Psychiatry 44:747–753, 1987

Chapter 6—Diagnostic Interviews

Select the single best response for each question.

6.1   According to Angold and Fisher (1999), clinician diagnoses are potentially fraught with numerous biases. All of the following are examples of such biases *except*

    A. Making diagnoses before all relevant information is collected.

    B. Collecting information selectively when confirming and/or ruling out a diagnosis.

    C. Not systematically collecting and organizing information.

    D. Not permitting one's special expertise to influence diagnostic assessment.

    E. Assuming correlations in symptoms and illnesses that in reality are spurious or nonexistent.

The correct response is option D.

By allowing his or her own special expertise to influence diagnostic assessment, a clinician would potentially bias the diagnosis. **(p. 68)**

6.2   *Construct validity* is defined as

    A. How well a category as defined appears to describe a recognized illness.

    B. Whether a category has meaning in terms of what it is designed to describe.

    C. How well a category predicts a pertinent aspect of care.

    D. How internally consistent a measure is.

    E. How often different interviewers assign the same diagnosis.

The correct response is option B.

Construct validity refers to whether a category has meaning in terms of what it is designed to describe. *Face validity* is how well a category appears to describe an illness. Predictive validity is how well the category predicts a pertinent aspect of care. *Reliability* is how internally consistent the measure is, and *interrater reliability* is how often different interviewers assign the same diagnosis. **(p. 69)**

6.3   Which of the statements concerning reliability is *false?*

    A. Reliability includes how often different interviewers assign the same diagnosis.

    B. Diagnostic tools need to be reliable in order to be useful.

    C. Reliability ensures validity.

    D. Reliability includes how internally consistent the measure is.

    E. Reliability encompasses how consistently respondents report the same symptoms or diagnoses over time.

The correct response is option C.

Reliability does not ensure validity. A diagnostic category may be reliably defined but not valid. Conversely, a disorder may be valid, but the diagnostic criteria or the instruments used to assess for its presence may not be reliable. **(p. 70)**

6.4   Which of the following statements concerning assessment of a diagnostic instrument's ability to detect cases is *true*?

A. *Sensitivity* is the percentage of individuals in a sample who have the disorder who are accurately identified by the interview.

B. *Predictive value positive* is the percentage of individuals in the defined sample positively identified by the interview who actually have the disorder.

C. *Specificity* is the percentage of individuals in a sample who do not have the disorder who are accurately identified by the interview as not having the disorder.

D. *Predictive value negative* is the percentage of individuals in the defined sample identified as not having the disorder by the interview who in fact do not have the disorder.

E. All of the above.

The correct response is option E.

All of the above definitions are correct. **(pp. 70–71)**

6.5   Although a number of structured diagnostic interviews are available for assessment of psychiatric illnesses in youth, these instruments have limitations. Examples of such limitations include all of the following *except*

A. Children may underreport new or unusual phenomena.

B. Children may lack the requisite attention span.

C. Children may lack the abstract awareness to understand the concepts.

D. Children may not be aware of the concept being described.

E. Children may lack the necessary verbal skills.

The correct response is option A.

Children tend to overreport, not underreport, rare or unusual phenomena, such as obsessive-compulsive, psychotic, or manic symptoms. **(p. 76)**

■ Reference

Angold A, Fisher PW: Interviewer-based interviews, in Diagnostic Assessment in Child and Adolescent Psychopathology. Edited by Shaffer D, Lucas CP, Richters JE. New York, Guilford, 1999, pp 34–64

Chapter 7—Rating Scales

Select the single best response for each question.

7.1 The *reliability* of a rating instrument

    A. Is equivalent to random error.

    B. Refers to the consistency with which an instrument measures a construct in the same way every time.

    C. Pertains to whether the instrument accurately assesses what it was designed to measure.

    D. Is inversely proportional to the validity of the instrument.

    E. Is reduced when the measured construct changes over time.

The correct response is option B.

Reliability refers to the consistency with which a scale's items measure the same construct every time. **(p. 82)**

7.2 Which of the following is the best example of a broad-band rating scale?

    A. Conners Rating Scale—Revised.

    B. Children's Depression Inventory.

    C. Hopelessness Scale for Children.

    D. Child Behavior Checklist.

    E. ADHD Rating Scale—IV.

The correct response is option D.

The Child Behavior Checklist (Achenbach and Rescorla 2000, 2001) is the most popular broad-band rating scale and has been considered the "gold standard" since the 1960s. **(p. 82)**

7.3 All of the following statements pertaining to broad-band rating scales are correct *except*

    A. They include measurements of both internalizing and externalizing behaviors.

    B. They assess a variety of clinical problems.

    C. They may be lengthy and cumbersome to complete.

    D. They assess for both breadth and depth of pathology in all clinical domains.

    E. They are best used to identify problems that will require further evaluation.

The correct response is option D.

Broad-band scales tend to sacrifice depth of assessment for breadth. **(p. 82)**

7.4 The Conners Rating Scale—Revised

    A. Includes parent, teacher, and youth self-report versions.

    B. Mostly assesses internalizing behaviors.

    C. Includes some abbreviated versions, but only for youth self-report.

    D. Has no mechanism for assessing common comorbid conditions.

    E. Is most useful for initial assessment in its abbreviated version.

The correct response is option A.

The Conners Rating Scale—Revised (Conners 1997), the primary attention-deficit/hyperactivity disorder (ADHD) rating scale, includes parent, teacher, and youth self-report versions. **(pp. 84–85, Table 7–2)**

7.5   Which of the following scales measuring internalizing symptoms is clinician-administered rather than self-reported?

A. Beck Depression Inventory.
B. Children's Depression Inventory.
C. Children's Depression Rating Scale.
D. Beck Hopelessness Scale.
E. Hopelessness Scale for Children.

The correct response is option C.

The Children's Depression Rating Scale—Revised (Poznanski and Mokros 1999) is administered by a clinician, a feature thought to provide greater accuracy than is possible with self-report or adult-report instruments. **(pp. 89, 92; Table 7–2)**

■ References

Achenbach TM, Rescorla LA: Manual for the ASEBA school-age forms & profiles. Burlington, VT, University of Vermont, Research Center for Children, Youth, and Families, 2000. Available from the Achenbach System of Empirically Based Assessment (ASEBA), 1 South Prospect Street, room 6436, Burlington, VT 05401-3456; phone: (802) 656-8313 or (802) 656-2608; http://www.aseba.org. Accessed May 1, 2003.

Achenbach TM, Rescorla LA: Manual for the ASEBA preschool forms & profiles. Burlington, VT, University of Vermont, Research Center for Children, Youth, and Families, 2001. Available from the Achenbach System of Empirically Based Assessment (ASEBA), 1 South Prospect Street, room 6436, Burlington, VT 05401-3456; phone: (802) 656-8313 or (802) 656-2608; http://www.aseba.org. Accessed May 1, 2003.

Conners CK: Conners Rating Scales—Revised, Technical Manual. North Tonawanda, NY, Multi-Health Systems, 1997. Available from Multi-Health Systems, Inc., 908 Niagara Falls Boulevard, North Tonawanda, NY 14120-2060; (800) 456-3003; http://www.mhs.com. Accessed April 30, 2003.

Poznanski EO, Mokros HB: Children's Depression Rating Scale—Revised (CDRS-R). Los Angeles, CA, Western Psychological Services, 1999. Available from Western Psychological Services, 12031 Wilshire Boulevard 90025-1251; phone: (800) 648-8857; http://www.wpspublish.com. Accessed May 2, 2003.

Chapter 8—Laboratory and Diagnostic Testing

Select the single best response for each question.

8.1   In a study conducted by Sheline and Kehr (1990), the use of screening tests in psychiatric inpatients led to changes in clinical management in what percentage of cases?

   A. 1%.
   B. 6%.
   C. 10%.
   D. 14%.
   E. None of the above.

The correct response is option B.

Although 49% of the patients had coexisting medical illnesses, laboratory tests led to changes in clinical management for only 6% of these patients (Sheline and Kehr 1990). **(p. 100)**

8.2   Laboratory tests recommended as part of a comprehensive examination or pre-medication workup include all of the following *except*

   A. Complete blood count (CBC).
   B. Urinalysis.
   C. Thyroid panel.
   D. Liver function tests.
   E. Blood urea nitrogen (BUN).

The correct response is option C.

A thyroid panel is not part of the recommended workup. The following tests are recommended: CBC, differential and hematocrit; urinalysis; BUN level; serum electrolytes; liver function tests; and lead level in children younger than 7 years of age when risk factors are present or in older children when indicated. **(p. 100)**

8.3   Which of the following thyroid disorders has been reported to be associated with attention-deficit/hyperactivity disorder (ADHD)–like symptoms?

   A. Hyperthyroidism.
   B. Syndrome of resistance to thyroid hormone.
   C. Hypothyroidism.
   D. All of the above.
   E. None of the above.

The correct response is option D.

All three thyroid disorders listed above have been reported to be associated with ADHD-like symptoms. **(pp. 101–102)**

8.4   For patients who attempt suicide by drug overdose, recommended medical/laboratory tests depend on the specific substance taken. Which of the following recommendations is *incorrect*?

    A. Blood toxicology workup for overdose on illegal substances.

    B. Liver function test for acetaminophen overdose.

    C. Serum electrolytes for aspirin overdose.

    D. Electrocardiogram (ECG) for selective serotonin reuptake inhibitor (SSRI) overdose.

    E. None of the above.

The correct response is option D.

An ECG should be obtained for patients who have overdosed with tricyclic antidepressants (TCAs), not necessarily SSRIs, unless the patient has a history of underlying cardiac problems. Blood toxicology workups should be ordered for patients who have overdosed on prescribed drugs or illegal substances. Liver function tests are important for assessing acetaminophen overdose, and serum electrolyte values are needed to assess anion gap in cases of aspirin overdose. **(pp. 102–103)**

8.5   Peer-reviewed articles support the use of single-photon emission computed tomography (SPECT) to rule out which of the following disorders in children?

    A. ADHD.

    B. Wilson's disease.

    C. Seizure disorder.

    D. Prader-Willi syndrome.

    E. None of the above.

The correct response is option E.

The peer-reviewed scientific literature contains no analyses of the validity of SPECT in the diagnosis and treatment of neurodevelopmental disorders. **(p. 105)**

■ Reference

Sheline Y, Kehr C: Cost and utility of routine admission laboratory testing for psychiatric inpatients. Gen Hosp Psychiatry 12:329–334, 1990

Chapter 9—Presentation of Findings and Recommendations

Select the single best response for each question.

9.1 The main purposes of the postassessment or "informing" interview in regard to a child or adolescent patient include which of the following?

A. Sharing the clinician's observation with the child's parents.
B. Elaborating further on parental feelings and perceptions.
C. Discussing the clinician's recommendations.
D. Arriving at a plan that will be helpful to the child and the family.
E. All of the above.

The correct response is option E.

The postassessment interview is a crucial aspect of the diagnostic process in child and adolescent psychiatry. Its main purposes are to share the clinician's observation with the child's parents, to elaborate further on parental feelings and perceptions, and to discuss the clinician's recommendations so as to arrive collaboratively at a treatment plan. **(p. 113)**

9.2 Which of the following statements concerning confidentiality in children and adolescents is *false?*

A. Confidentiality is qualitatively different for younger children than for adolescents.
B. The clinician can promise confidentiality to a child with the proviso that information that is potentially self-destructive or destructive to others will be shared with those who may protect the child.
C. It is usually necessary to include younger children in the postdiagnostic interview.
D. The issues of confidentiality are of greater importance to adolescent patients than they are for adult patients.
E. None of the above.

The correct response is option C.

It usually is not necessary to include younger children in the postdiagnostic interview. **(pp. 115–116)**

9.3 Factors that are relevant to a family's remaining in therapy include all of the following *except*

A. The therapist's activity and directiveness.
B. The family's ability to influence the consultation.
C. The congruence between the family's expectations and the therapist's response.
D. The severity of the child's psychiatric disorder.
E. The family's perception that they are active participants in the therapeutic process.

The correct response is option D.

The family's relationship with the therapist and the therapist's directedness, not the severity of the child's disorder, usually determine whether the family remains in therapy. **(p. 117)**

Chapter 10—Mental Retardation

Select the single best response for each question.

10.1 DSM-IV-TR (American Psychiatric Association 2000) criteria require an IQ score in which of the following ranges for a diagnosis of "severe mental retardation"?

    A. Below 20–25.
    B. Between 20–25 and 35–40.
    C. Between 35–40 and 50–55.
    D. Between 50–55 and 70.
    E. None of the above.

The correct response is option B.

The diagnosis of severe mental retardation requires an IQ score between 20–25 and 35–40. **(pp. 122–123, Table 10–1)**

10.2 Data from the National Health Interview Survey for 1994–1995 (University of Minnesota 2000) indicate that the combined prevalence of mental retardation and developmental disabilities in the United States during that period was approximately what percentage of the population?

    A. 1.5%.
    B. 3%.
    C. 5%.
    D. 7%.
    E. 9%.

The correct response is option A.

The prevalence of mental retardation and developmental disabilities in the United States in 1994–1995 was 1.58% (University of Minnesota 2000). **(p. 124)**

10.3 Prader-Willi syndrome in children is characterized by all of the following *except*

    A. Obesity.
    B. Hypogonadism in males.
    C. Spasticity.
    D. Dysmorphic features.
    E. Hyperphagia.

The correct response is option C.

Prader-Willi syndrome is not characterized by spasticity, but rather by hypotonia, obesity, developmental and behavioral problems (including mental retardation), hyperphagia, hypogonadism in males, and dysmorphic features. **(pp. 129–130)**

10.4 DNA probes and molecular biology analyses have identified the q11–q12 region of chromosome 15 as the abnormal region of the human genome responsible for which of the following syndromes?

  A. Prader-Willi syndrome and Angelman's syndrome.
  B. Angelman's syndrome and fragile X syndrome.
  C. Prader-Willi syndrome and fragile X syndrome.
  D. Prader-Willi syndrome and Williams syndrome.
  E. Fragile X syndrome and Rett's disorder.

  The correct response is option C.

  Abnormalities of the q11–q12 region of chromosome 15 have been implicated in Prader-Willi and Angelman's syndromes. **(p. 130)**

10.5 The most common inherited form of mental retardation is

  A. Angelman's syndrome.
  B. Rett's disorder.
  C. Williams syndrome.
  D. Prader-Willi syndrome.
  E. Fragile X syndrome.

  The correct response is option E.

  Fragile X syndrome is the most common inherited form of mental retardation. **(p. 130)**

10.6 Current estimates of the prevalence of schizophrenia in individuals with mental retardation are in the range of

  A. 1%–3%.
  B. 3%–5%.
  C. 5%–8%.
  D. 8%–10%.
  E. 10%–12%.

  The correct response is option A.

  Current estimates of the prevalence of schizophrenia in persons with mental retardation range from 1% to 2%–3%. **(p. 138)**

■ References

American Psychiatric Association: Diagnostic and Statistical Manual of Mental Disorders, 4th Edition, Text Revision. Washington, DC, American Psychiatric Association, 2000

University of Minnesota, the College of Education and Human Development: MR/DD Data Brief, Vol 2, No. 1, p 5, 2000. Available at: http://rtc.umn.edu/nhis/databrief2/index.html. Accessed July 2003.

Chapter 11—Autistic Disorders

Select the single best response for each question.

11.1 Which of the following is an essential characteristic of infantile autism, as proposed by Rutter (1968)?

A. Onset before age 30 months.
B. Bizarre motor behavior.
C. Impaired language.
D. Lack of social interest and responsiveness.
E. All of the above.

The correct response is option E.

Rutter (1968), in his critical analysis of the existing empirical evidence, identified four features present in nearly all children with autism: 1) lack of social interest and responsiveness; 2) impaired language, ranging from absence of speech to peculiar speech patterns; 3) bizarre motor behavior, ranging from rigid and limited play patterns to more complex ritualistic and compulsive behavior; and 4) early onset (before age 30 months). **(pp. 153–154)**

11.2 All of the following are pervasive developmental disorders *except*

A. Autistic disorder.
B. Mental retardation.
C. Rett's disorder.
D. Childhood disintegrative disorder.
E. Asperger's disorder.

The correct response is option B.

Mental retardation is not a pervasive developmental disorder. **(p. 154)**

11.3 A common comorbid medical condition noted in patients with autism is epilepsy. Which of the following statements is *true?*

A. The risk of epilepsy in patients with autism is highest during late adolescence.
B. A prospective study of epilepsy in children with autistic spectrum disorders found a rate of 5%.
C. The most common type of epilepsy is generalized or grand mal seizures.
D. Males with autism have seizures more frequently than do females with autism.
E. None of the above.

The correct response is option B.

A prospective study of epilepsy in children with autistic spectrum disorder found that about 5% of those with an autistic condition had epilepsy (Wong 1993). The risk of epilepsy in patients with autism seems to be highest in early childhood, not late adolescence. The most common type of seizures are partial seizures, and females have a greater risk of seizures than do males. **(p. 162)**

11.4 All of the following psychopharmacological agents have been reported to de-crease autistic symptoms *except*

A. Fluoxetine.
B. Fluvoxamine.
C. Quetiapine.
D. Venlafaxine.
E. Sertraline.

The correct response is option C.

In an open-label quetiapine treatment trial in six autistic children, Martin et al. (1999) reported that there was no significant improvement as rated on the Clinical Global Impressions Scale. Quetiapine was also poorly tolerated by many patients and was associated with serious side effects. **(pp. 182–183)**

11.5 Which of the following factors has consistently been shown to be related to out-come in autistic patients?

A. Age at onset.
B. Family history of mental illness.
C. IQ.
D. Perinatal complications.
E. Birth weight.

The correct response is option C.

Three factors have consistently been shown to be related to outcome in autistic patients: IQ, presence or absence of speech, and severity of the disorder. Outcome does not appear to be related to age at onset, family history of mental illness, peri-natal complications, or birth weight. **(p. 187)**

■ References

Martin A, Koenig K, Scahill L, et al: Open-label quetiapine in the treatment of children and ado-lescents with autistic disorder. J Child Adolesc Psychopharmacol 9:99–107, 1999
Rutter M: Concepts of autism: a review of research. J Child Psychol Psychiatry 9:1–25, 1968
Wong V: Epilepsy in children with autistic spectrum disorder. J Child Neurol 8:316–322, 1993

Chapter 12—Developmental Disorders of Communication, Motor Skills, and Learning

Select the single best response for each question.

12.1 In language, *morphology* is defined as

  A. A language's sound system and accompanying rules governing the combination of sounds.
  B. The system that governs the structure and formation of words in a language.
  C. The system that governs the order and combination of words to form sentences.
  D. The system that governs the meaning of words and sentences.
  E. The system that combines the language components into functional and socially appropriate communication.

The correct response is option B.

Morphology is the system that governs the structure and formation of words in a language. *Phonology* is a language's sound system and accompanying rules governing the combination of sounds. *Syntax* is the system that governs the order and combination of words to form sentences. *Semantics* is the system that governs the meaning of words and sentences. *Pragmatics* is the system that combines all of the above language components into functional and socially appropriate communication. **(pp. 205–206, Table 12–1)**

12.2 Which of the following communication disorders disproportionately affects males?

  A. Developmental (versus acquired) expressive language disorder.
  B. Mixed receptive–expressive language disorder.
  C. Phonological disorder.
  D. Stuttering.
  E. All of the above.

The correct response is option E.

Although there is some evidence that referral bias may contribute to the higher prevalence rates of developmental expressive language disorder and mixed receptive–expressive language disorder in boys, all of the disorders listed above are believed to affect males more often than females. **(pp. 206–207)**

12.3 Which of the following statements concerning the etiology of communication disorders is *false?*

  A. The etiology is primarily due to family environment and sociological factors.
  B. Exposure to intrauterine teratogens may adversely affect language development.
  C. Anoxia and asphyxia have been implicated in the development of communication disorders.
  D. Important environmental risk factors for the development of communication disorders include poverty and abuse or neglect.
  E. Early childhood risk factors that have been implicated in communication disorders include persistent otitis media and other childhood illnesses.

The correct response is option A.

The etiology of communication disorders is primarily biological, although family environment and sociological factors also play a role. **(pp. 211–212)**

12.4 All of the following statements concerning developmental coordination disorder are correct *except*

A. The disorder occurs in up to 6% of 5- to 11-year-olds.
B. The clumsiness associated with this disorder can lead to peer teasing.
C. Children with developmental coordination disorder seldom have associated delays of other developmental milestones.
D. Comorbid conditions such as attention-deficit/hyperactivity disorder (ADHD) are frequently seen in children with developmental coordination disorder.
E. The coordination deficits may continue throughout life.

The correct response is option C.

Developmental coordination disorder occurs in up to 6% of 5- to 11-year-olds. It is usually first diagnosed when parents notice a delay in development of specific motor skills, or difficulty with skills once attempted. The disorder often is associated with delays in other developmental milestones, and it may be comorbid with ADHD and other conditions. The clumsiness associated with this disorder often leads to peer teasing, which can have a harmful emotional impact. Although motor deficits can be remediated, in some cases problems continue throughout life. **(pp. 214–215)**

12.5 Which of the following statements concerning the clinical presentation of learning disorders is *false?*

A. Reading disorder occurs in 2%–20% of children.
B. Reading disorder accounts for up to 80% of all children diagnosed with a learning disorder.
C. An equal proportion of boys and girls are diagnosed with a reading disorder.
D. Disorder of written expression is more common in boys than in girls.
E. Mathematics disorder is reported to occur in 1%–6% of school-age children.

The correct response is option C.

Approximately 80% of children diagnosed with a reading disorder are boys (American Psychiatric Association 2000). **(p. 218)**

◼ Reference

American Psychiatric Association: Diagnostic and Statistical Manual of Mental Disorders, 4th Edition, Text Revision. Washington, DC, American Psychiatric Association, 2000

Chapter 13—Schizophrenia and Other Psychotic Disorders

Select the single best response for each question.

13.1　The diagnosis of schizophrenia with childhood onset

　　A.　Is a common presentation for this disorder.
　　B.　Is five times more likely in females than in males.
　　C.　Requires no mood disorder exclusion.
　　D.　Can be made when signs of disturbance have been present for at least 3 months.
　　E.　May have a prevalence of less than 1 in 1,000.

The correct response is option E.

Population studies have suggested that the prevalence of childhood-onset schizophrenia may be less than 1 in 1,000. Spencer and Campbell (1994) reported a male-to-female ratio of 3.8 to 1 in a sample of 24 children. In diagnosing schizophrenia, mood disorders and schizoaffective disorders must be ruled out. The diagnosis can be made when signs of the disturbance have been present for at least 6 months, with at least 1 month of active-phase symptoms. **(pp. 236–237)**

13.2　In regard to National Institute of Mental Health studies comparing patients with childhood-onset schizophrenia and patients with adult-onset schizophrenia, all of the following findings are correct *except*

　　A.　Childhood-onset patients showed greater delay in language development than did adult-onset patients.
　　B.　Childhood-onset patients evidenced more disruptive behavior disorders than did adult-onset patients.
　　C.　Childhood-onset patients evidenced more learning disorders than did adult-onset patients.
　　D.　Childhood-onset patients evidenced few motor stereotypes.
　　E.　Childhood-onset schizophrenia appears to represent a more malignant form of the disorder.

The correct response is option D.

Patients with childhood-onset schizophrenia commonly present with motor stereotypes (Alaghband-Rad et al. 1995). **(p. 237)**

13.3　Which phase of illness in schizophrenic patients is best described by the following definition: "A 1- to 6-month (or longer) period when symptoms of hallucinations, delusions, thought disorder, or disorganized behavior are predominant?"

　　A.　Prodrome.
　　B.　Acute phase.
　　C.　Recovery phase.
　　D.　Residual phase.
　　E.　Chronicity.

The correct response is option B.

During the *acute phase*, which usually lasts 1–6 months or longer, positive symptoms (i.e., hallucinations, delusions, thought disorder, and disorganized behavior) are predominant. **(p. 240)**

13.4 Which of the following statements concerning the differential diagnosis of childhood psychotic disorders is *true*?

  A. The diagnostic criteria for schizophreniform disorder require an illness duration of less than 6 months.
  B. Once a diagnosis of schizophreniform disorder is made, a diagnosis of schizophrenia can never be given.
  C. A diagnosis of schizophreniform disorder requires the presence of a decline in function.
  D. Brief psychotic disorder requires a symptom duration of at least 1 month but no more than 6 months.
  E. The diagnosis of psychotic disorder not otherwise specified is very rare in the hospitalized adolescent population.

The correct response is option A.

To qualify for a schizophreniform disorder diagnosis, a child must have an illness duration of less than 6 months. With time, a child with schizophreniform disorder may warrant a diagnosis of schizophrenia. **(pp. 243–244)**

13.5 Magnetic resonance imaging (MRI) studies in children with schizophrenia have reported all of the following findings *except*

  A. Decreases in total cerebral volume.
  B. Cerebral asymmetry.
  C. Decreases in ventricular volume.
  D. Increases in temporal lobe volume.
  E. Decreases in midsagittal thalamic area.

The correct response is option C.

MRI studies in children with schizophrenia have reported increases in ventricular volume and decreases in total cerebral volume (Rapoport et al. 1997, 1999). Other findings reported in children with childhood-onset schizophrenia were larger volumes of the superior temporal lobe gyrus (Jacobsen et al. 1996) and a smaller midsagittal thalamic area (Frazier et al. 1996). **(pp. 248–250)**

■ References

Alaghband-Rad J, McKenna K, Gordon CT: Childhood-onset schizophrenia: the severity of premorbid course. J Am Acad Child Adolesc Psychiatry 34:1273–1283, 1995

Frazier JA, Giedd JA, Hamburger SD, et al: Brain anatomic magnetic resonance imaging in childhood-onset schizophrenia. Arch Gen Psychiatry 53:617–624, 1996

Jacobsen LK, Giedd JN, Vaituzis AC, et al: Temporal lobe morphology in childhood-onset schizophrenia. Am J Psychiatry 153:355–361, 1996

Rapoport JL, Giedd J, Kumra S, et al: Childhood-onset schizophrenia. Progressive ventricular change during adolescence. Arch Gen Psychiatry 54:897–903, 1997

Rapoport JL, Giedd JN, Blumenthal J: Progressive cortical change during adolescence in childhood-onset schizophrenia: a longitudinal magnetic resonance imaging study. Arch Gen Psychiatry 56:649–654, 1999

Spencer EK, Campbell M: Children with schizophrenia: diagnosis, phenomenology, and pharmacotherapy. Schizophr Bull 20:713–725, 1994

Chapter 14—Mood Disorders

Select the single best response for each question.

14.1 Childhood mood disorders are often underdiagnosed or misdiagnosed for which of the following reasons?

A. The belief, on the part of some clinicians, that a child's immature superego and personality structure do not permit the development of a mood disorder.
B. Many children lack the capacity to express their emotions verbally.
C. Many children present with somatic complaints that are diagnosed as physical illness.
D. Parents who are bipolar are often underdiagnosed.
E. All of the above.

The correct response is option E.

All of the reasons above are contributing factors to the underdiagnosis or misdiagnosis of childhood mood disorders. **(pp. 267–268)**

14.2 Commonly presenting symptoms of depression in adolescents include

A. Poor school performance.
B. Social withdrawal.
C. Substance abuse.
D. Conduct disorder.
E. All of the above.

The correct response is option E.

Substance abuse is the presenting symptom in approximately 20% of adolescents with mood disorders (Weller and Weller 1990). Poor school performance, social withdrawal, conduct disorder, and promiscuous sexual behavior are also common among depressed adolescents. **(p. 270)**

14.3 Diagnosing bipolar disorder in adolescence may be challenging for all of the following reasons *except*

A. Presenting symptoms are often minor or major depression.
B. Severity of symptoms frequently results in hospitalization.
C. Because symptoms may build up gradually, they frequently are overlooked.
D. Inappropriate sexual behavior and other "atypical" presentations are common.
E. Serious conduct behaviors, such as vandalism, may mask underlying manic symptoms.

The correct response is option B.

In adolescents, symptoms frequently do not receive clinical attention because they may build up gradually. McGlashan (1988) noted that a delay of up to 5 years often occurs between the onset of symptoms during adolescence and an episode of sufficient severity to require hospitalization or treatment. **(pp. 272–273)**

14.4 In a study by Carlson et al. (2000) comparing patients with early-onset (between the ages of 15 and 20 years) and adult-onset bipolar disorder, which of the following findings was reported?

A. Women predominated in the early-onset group.
B. More remissions occurred during follow-up in the early-onset group than in the adult-onset group.
C. Individuals in the early-onset group were more likely than those in the adult-onset group to have a substance use disorder.
D. Patients with early-onset bipolar disorder had an increased risk of mood-incongruent psychotic symptoms.
E. Depressive episodes occurred more frequently in the early-onset group.

The correct response is option C.

Early-onset bipolar patients were more likely than adult-onset patients to have a substance use disorder at the onset of their bipolar disorder (Carlson et al. 2000). Males predominated in the early-onset group. Mood-incongruent psychotic symptoms were equally likely in early-onset and adult-onset bipolar patients. Fewer remissions were seen in early-onset patients, and manic, not depressive, episodes occurred more frequently in this group. **(pp. 273–274)**

14.5 Approximately 40%–70% of children and adolescents with major depressive disorder have a comorbid psychiatric disorder. All of the following are common comorbid conditions *except*

A. Eating disorders.
B. Anxiety disorders.
C. Dysthymic disorder.
D. Disruptive behavior disorders.
E. Substance use.

The correct response is option A.

Eating disorder are not common comorbid conditions in children and adolescents with major depressive disorder. The most frequent comorbid diagnoses are dysthymic disorder (30%–80%), anxiety disorders (30%–80%), disruptive disorders (10%–80%), and substance abuse (20%–30%). Twenty to fifty percent of children with major depressive disorder have two or more comorbid diagnoses. **(pp. 274–275)**

14.6 Common side effects of lithium treatment in children and adolescents include all of the following *except*

A. Diarrhea.
B. Tremor.
C. Leukopenia.
D. Fatigue.
E. Ataxia.

The correct response is option C.

Common lithium side effects in youth include nausea, diarrhea, tremor, enuresis, fatigue, ataxia, and leukocytosis (*not* leukopenia). **(p. 299)**

■ References

Carlson GA, Bromet EJ, Sievers S: Phenomenology and outcome of subjects with early and adult-onset psychotic mania. Am J Psychiatry 157:213–219, 2000

McGlashan TH: Adolescent versus adult onset of mania. Am J Psychiatry 145:221–223, 1988

Weller EB, Weller RA: Depressive disorders in children and adolescents, in Psychiatric Disorders in Children and Adolescents. Edited by Garfinkel BD. Philadelphia, PA, WB Saunders, 1990, pp 3–20

Chapter 15—Attention-Deficit/Hyperactivity Disorder

Select the single best response for each question.

15.1   Which of the following is *not* one of the core symptom clusters of attention-deficit/hyperactivity disorder (ADHD) as identified in DSM-IV-TR (American Psychiatric Association 2000)?

     A. Hyperactivity.
     B. Inattention.
     C. Impulsivity.
     D. Disruptive behavior.
     E. Distractibility.

The correct response is option D.

Inattention, hyperactivity, and impulsivity are the core symptom clusters in ADHD. Disruptive behavior is not a core symptom of the disorder, although it may be present. **(pp. 324–325, Table 15–1)**

15.2   Which of the following is *not* one of the DSM-IV-TR diagnostic criteria for ADHD?

     A. Symptoms must have persisted for at least 6 months.
     B. Symptoms must be evident in at least two different environments.
     C. Symptoms must have been present before age 5 years.
     D. Symptoms must be maladaptive in terms of functioning.
     E. Symptoms cannot be accounted for by another DSM-IV-TR diagnosis (e.g., a pervasive developmental disorder).

The correct response is option C.

Some symptoms that caused impairment must have been present before age 7 years. **(pp. 324–325, Table 15–1)**

15.3   Which of the following comorbid psychiatric disorders has been reported to occur most frequently in children diagnosed with ADHD?

     A. Schizophrenia.
     B. Oppositional defiant disorder.
     C. Autism.
     D. Bipolar disorder.
     E. Panic disorder.

The correct response is option B.

Oppositional defiant disorder and conduct disorder occur with a high frequency in children with ADHD (as many as 30%–50%) (Biederman et al. 1991). **(p. 330)**

15.4 Which of the following statements concerning the epidemiology of ADHD is *false?*

    A. The disorder seems to be more common in boys than in girls.

    B. The prevalence reported in DSM-IV-TR is 3%–7% of school-age children.

    C. ADHD is more common in school-age populations than in older populations.

    D. Prevalence rates show little variation across cultures, countries, and settings (urban, suburban, and rural).

    E. None of the above.

The correct response is option D.

Rates of ADHD may vary across different cultures and countries, as well as according to whether the sample studied is urban, suburban, or rural. **(p. 332)**

15.5 Which of the following statements concerning research findings on the course and duration of ADHD is *correct?*

    A. At least some impairment from the disorder is present in most adolescents who were referred for clinical treatment as school-age children.

    B. The disorder is generally episodic rather than chronic.

    C. Inattention tends to remit over time, in contrast to hyperactivity, which is remarkably persistent.

    D. Inattention symptoms may place a child at greater risk for the development of antisocial behavior.

    E. None of the above.

The correct response is option A.

Prospective studies of clinical samples report that at least some impairment from the disorder is present in most adolescents who were referred for clinical treatment as school-age children (Barkley et al. 1991; Gittelman et al. 1985). The disorder is generally chronic and enduring (Keller et al. 1992). Inattention problems are remarkably persistent and intractable, whereas hyperactivity tends to remit over time (Biederman et al. 2000). Hyperactivity and impulsivity symptoms may place a child at greater risk for the development of antisocial outcomes (Babinski et al. 1999). **(p. 336)**

15.6 The research literature supports the use of all of the following medications for ADHD *except*

    A. Tricyclic antidepressants.

    B. Psychostimulants.

    C. Clonidine.

    D. Bupropion.

    E. Benzodiazepines.

The correct response is option E.

Benzodiazepines are not recommended in the treatment of ADHD. Psychostimulants are the agents of choice for symptom suppression. Tricyclic antidepressants are considered second-line agents. Both clonidine and bupropion have shown some promise in the treatment of ADHD symptoms. **(pp. 336–340)**

■ References

American Psychiatric Association: Diagnostic and Statistical Manual of Mental Disorders, 4th Edition, Text Revision. Washington, DC, American Psychiatric Association, 2000

Babinski LM, Hartsough CS, Lambert NM: Childhood conduct problems, hyperactivity-impulsivity, and inattention as predictors of adult criminal activity. J Child Psychol Psychiatry 40:347–355, 1999

Barkley RA, Fischer M, Edelbrock C, et al: The adolescent outcome of hyperactive children diagnosed by research criteria, III: mother-child interactions, family conflicts and maternal psychopathology. J Child Psychol Psychiatry 32:233–255, 1991

Biederman J, Newcorn J, Sprich S: Comorbidity of attention deficit hyperactivity disorder with conduct, depressive, anxiety, and other disorders. Am J Psychiatry 148:564–577, 1991

Biederman J, Mick E, Faraone SV: Age-dependent decline of symptoms of attention-deficit/hyperactivity disorder: impact of remission definition and symptom type. Am J Psychiatry 157:816–818, 2000

Gittelman R, Mannuzza S, Shenker R, et al: Hyperactive boys almost grown up, I: psychiatric status. Arch Gen Psychiatry 42:937–947, 1985

Keller MB, Lavori PW, Beardslee WR, et al: The disruptive behavioral disorder in children and adolescents: comorbidity and clinical course. J Am Acad Child Adolesc Psychiatry 31:204–209, 1992

Chapter 16—Conduct Disorder and Oppositional Defiant Disorder

Select the single best response for each question.

16.1 Which of the following statements regarding the diagnoses of conduct disorder and oppositional defiant disorder (ODD) is *true*?

A. Children with these disorders are a distinct group that presents in a uniform and narrow fashion.
B. The relationship between conduct disorder and ODD is clearly defined.
C. The diagnosis of conduct disorder is controversial in child psychiatry.
D. ODD behaviors typically are preceded by more serious violations of age-appropriate behavioral norms.
E. Conduct disorder has been determined to be a biological condition.

The correct response is option C.

The classification of conduct disorder is a controversial and unsettled issue in mental health. Children with conduct disorder represent a varied group because of the myriad of manifestations of antisocial behavior and the complex factors that contribute to it. The relationship between conduct disorder and ODD remains unclear. ODD behaviors tend to precede more serious violations of age-appropriate behavioral norms. The etiology of conduct disorder is manifold, with biological, psychological, and social factors all playing a role. **(pp. 357–358)**

16.2 All of the following statements regarding the prevalence of conduct disorder are correct *except*

A. The prevalence of conduct disorder is difficult to estimate because of variations in definition.
B. The prevalence is estimated as approximately 9% for males and 2% for females younger than 18 years.
C. The childhood-onset type of the disorder (onset before 10 years of age) is clearly much more common in males.
D. Individuals with adolescent-onset conduct disorder are much more likely to develop adult antisocial personality disorder than are those with childhood-onset conduct disorder.
E. Adolescent-onset conduct disorder is less likely than childhood-onset conduct disorder to involve a preponderance of males.

The correct response is option D.

Individuals with childhood-onset conduct disorder are more likely than those with adolescent-onset conduct disorder to develop antisocial personality disorder. **(p. 358)**

16.3　Which of the following statements regarding subtypes of conduct disorder is *true?*

　　A. Subtyping aggressive behavior into predatory and affective categories is not a useful distinction.

　　B. Predatory aggression is characterized by the presence of high levels of autonomic and emotional arousal with little apparent instrumental gain.

　　C. Children who demonstrate reactive aggression tend to be more delinquent than those demonstrating proactive aggression.

　　D. The process of subclassifying conduct disorder according to age at onset, degree of aggressivity, and extent of socialization has been completely validated.

　　E. The value of subtyping conduct disorder into childhood-onset and adolescent-onset variants is related to the prognostic significance of age at onset.

The correct response is option E.

The value of subtyping conduct disorder into childhood-onset and adolescent-onset is clearly related to the prognostic significance of age at onset, with early onset being more ominous. Subtyping aggressive behavior into predatory and affective categories is a useful distinction. Predatory aggression is goal directed and involves minimal associated autonomic arousal. Affective aggression is characterized by the presence of high levels of autonomic and emotional arousal with little apparent instrumental gain. Children who manifest proactive aggression are more delinquent that those demonstrating reactive aggression. No system of subtyping conduct disorder has been completely validated. **(p. 359)**

16.4　A biological factor associated with conduct disorder is

　　A. Reduced novelty-seeking trait.

　　B. A history of maternal smoking during pregnancy.

　　C. Anxious temperament.

　　D. Reduced rates of expression of the *L/L* variant of the serotonin transporter gene.

　　E. Elevated harm-avoidance trait.

The correct response is option B.

Wakschlag et al. (1997) demonstrated that maternal smoking during pregnancy was associated with a significant increase in the rate of conduct disorder, even after adjustment for previously identified risk factors. Adolescents who showed elevations in novelty seeking and reductions in harm avoidance demonstrated increased rates of aggressive and delinquent behavior (Schmeck and Poustka 2001). Enhanced rates of expression of the *L/L* variant of the serotonin transporter gene were found in a sample of hyperactive children and adolescents both with and without conduct disorder (Seeger et al. 2001). **(pp. 362–366)**

16.5 All of the following statements concerning treatment of youngsters with conduct disorder are correct *except*

A. Treatment may take place in a variety of different long-term and short-term programs in outpatient, inpatient, and residential settings.

B. Cognitive-behavioral approaches include improvement in problem-solving skills, impulse control, and anger management.

C. Family therapy is not an effective treatment modality in conduct disorder patients.

D. Parent management training focuses on modifying coercive parent–child interactions that encourage child antisocial behaviors.

E. When used, pharmacotherapy commonly targets aggression in the conduct disorder population.

The correct response is option C.

Tolan et al. (1986), in an extensive literature review, found that family therapy was in many cases more effective than other therapeutic modalities. **(pp. 370–373)**

■ References

Schmeck K, Poustka F: Temperament and disruptive behavior disorders. Psychopathology 34:159–163, 2001

Seeger G, Schloss P, Schmidt MH: Functional polymorphism within the promoter of the serotonin transporter gene is associated with severe hyperkinetic disorders. Mol Psychiatry 6:235–238, 2001

Tolan PH, Cromwell RE, Brasswell M: Family therapy with delinquents: a critical review of the literature. Fam Process 25:619–650, 1986

Wakschlag LS, Lahey B, Loeber R, et al: Maternal smoking during pregnancy and the risk of conduct disorder in boys. Arch Gen Psychiatry 54:670–676, 1997

Chapter 17—Substance Abuse Disorders

Select the single best response for each question.

17.1 Which of the following has been reported to be a problem in applying DSM-IV-TR (American Psychiatric Association 2000) criteria to adolescents?

A. Withdrawal and drug-related medical problems are common.
B. One abuse symptom yields a diagnosis.
C. Abuse symptoms frequently precede dependence symptoms.
D. Two dependence symptoms with no abuse symptoms yields a diagnosis.
E. None of the above.

The correct response is option B.

In the DSM-IV-TR criteria, one abuse symptom yields a diagnosis. In adolescents, however, abuse symptoms often do not precede dependence symptoms. Under the DSM-IV-TR criteria, an adolescent with two dependence symptoms but no abuse symptoms would not qualify for a diagnosis, although such an individual would need therapeutic intervention. Withdrawal and drug-related medical problems are rare, not common, in youth. **(p. 390)**

17.2 In the 2001 Monitoring the Future Survey (Johnston et al. 2001), epidemiological findings concerning substance abuse in high school seniors included all of the following *except*

A. Marijuana use by about 37%.
B. Cigarette smoking during the past month by 29.5%.
C. MDMA (3,4-methylenedioxymethamphetamine; "ecstasy") use by 9.2%.
D. Anabolic steroid use by 12.4%.
E. Alcohol use by about 73%.

The correct response is option D.

In 2001, only 2.4% of high school seniors reported the use of anabolic steroids (Johnston et al. 2001). **(pp. 390–392)**

17.3 The well-known CAGE screening questions developed for adults are not useful for adolescents. The CRAFFT, a screening instrument developed for adolescents, includes all of the following questions *except*

A. "Have you ever ridden in a **C**ar driven by someone (including yourself) who was high or had been using alcohol or drugs?"
B. "Do you ever use alcohol/drugs to **R**elax, feel better about yourself, or fit in?"
C. "Do you get **A**ngry when you are told that you have a problem?"
D. "Do you ever **F**orget things you did while using alcohol/drugs?"
E. "Have you ever gotten into **T**rouble while you were using alcohol/drugs?"

The correct response is option C.

The CRAFFT screen includes all of the questions above except for that in option C. The correct question corresponding to the letter *A* in CRAFFT is "Do you ever use alcohol/drugs while you are by yourself or **A**lone?" The CRAFFT also includes a second *F* question—"Do your **F**amily or **F**riends ever tell you that you should cut down on your drinking or drug use?" Two or more "yes" answers suggest serious problems with substances and indicate the need for further evaluation (Knight et al. 1999). **(p. 394)**

17.4 Risk factors for the development of substance abuse disorders include all of the following *except*

A. Economic and social advantage.
B. School failure.
C. Friends who use drugs.
D. Psychiatric comorbidity.
E. History of parental divorce.

The correct response is option A.

Economic and social *deprivation*, rather than advantage, is a risk factor for substance abuse. **(p. 396, Table 17–3)**

17.5 A common comorbid diagnosis in male adolescents with substance abuse is

A. Conduct disorder.
B. Attention-deficit/hyperactivity disorder.
C. Avoidant personality disorder.
D. Oppositional defiant disorder.
E. None of the above.

The correct response is option A.

Conduct disorder and antisocial personality disorder are the most common comorbid diagnoses with substance abuse, particularly in males. **(p. 407)**

■ References

American Psychiatric Association: Diagnostic and Statistical Manual of Mental Disorders, 4th Edition, Text Revision. Washington, DC, American Psychiatric Association, 2000

Johnston LD, O'Malley PM, Bachman JG: National Survey Results on Drug Use From the Monitoring the Future Study, 1975–2000, Vol 1: Secondary School Students (NIH Publ No 01-4924). Rockville, MD, National Institute on Drug Abuse, 2001

Knight JR, Shrier LA, Bravender TD, et al: A new brief screen for adolescent substance abuse. Arch Pediatr Adolesc Med 153:591–596, 1999

Chapter 18—Separation Anxiety Disorder and Generalized Anxiety Disorder

Select the single best response for each question.

18.1 Separation anxiety

    A. Begins at age 18 months and peaks at age 30 months.

    B. Is a normative part of development.

    C. Usually indicates the presence of a disorder.

    D. Symptoms are seldom subclinically present in the pediatric population.

    E. Is rarely persistent and excessive.

The correct response is option B.

Separation anxiety is a normative part of development, typically beginning at around 6–7 months, peaking around 18 months, and decreasing after 30 months. Isolated subclinical separation anxiety disorder (SAD) symptoms can be reasonably common. When separation anxiety is persistent and excessive, a diagnosis of SAD should be considered. **(pp. 415–416)**

18.2 Which of the following DSM-IV-TR (American Psychiatric Association 2000) criteria is not required in order to make a diagnosis of generalized anxiety disorder (GAD) in children?

    A. Excessive anxiety and worry for at least a 6-month period.

    B. Difficulty controlling the worry.

    C. Three or more associated physiological symptoms (restlessness, fatigue, difficulty concentrating, irritability, muscle tension, or sleep disturbance).

    D. The focus of the worry is not related to another Axis I condition.

    E. Presence of clinically significant distress or impairment.

The correct response is option C.

Only one physiological symptom is required for the GAD diagnosis in children, in contrast to the three or more that are required in adults. **(p. 418, Table 18–2)**

18.3 Which of the following statements regarding the epidemiology of GAD and SAD is *true*?

    A. SAD is more prevalent among older children.

    B. GAD is more prevalent among younger children.

    C. Rates of SAD increase with age.

    D. Rates of SAD and GAD do not vary with age.

    E. Rates of GAD increase with age.

The correct response is option E.

Rates of GAD increase with age. SAD is more prevalent among younger children, GAD is more prevalent among older children. Rates of SAD decrease with age, whereas rates of SAD and GAD vary by age. **(pp. 420–421)**

18.4 Which of the following statements about temperament and its contributing role to childhood anxiety is *false?*

A. Approximately 20% of healthy infants are born with traits that predispose them to become highly reactive in novel environments (Kagan and Snidman 1999).

B. Kagan (1994) described the temperamental characteristic of behavioral inhibition as a child's tendency to approach unfamiliar or novel situations with distress, restraint, or avoidance.

C. Behavioral inhibition appears to be a highly unstable temperamental trait.

D. Children with behavioral inhibition may be differentiated from non–behaviorally inhibited children through neurophysiological markers (Kagan et al. 1988).

E. Children who are identified as shy may be more prone to anxiety symptoms than those who are not (Biederman et al. 1995).

The correct response is option C.

The tendency to approach or avoid new situations is often an enduring temperamental trait. **(pp. 421–422)**

18.5 The use of selective serotonin reuptake inhibitors (SSRIs) in the treatment of childhood anxiety disorders

A. Is considered a second-line choice (after benzodiazepines).

B. Has been supported by the results of several recent randomized, placebo-controlled trials.

C. Should usually continue indefinitely once initiated.

D. Has resulted in no documented side effects.

E. Has resulted in minimal clinical benefit over placebo.

The correct response is option B.

SSRIs are the first-line choice in the pharmacological treatment of childhood anxiety disorders, a conclusion supported by the results of three recent, randomized trials. After remission of target symptoms with SSRIs, a drug-free trial should be considered (Pine 2002). If a youth relapses during the period without medication, the SSRI should be restarted. Stomachaches and increased motor activity have been reported with the use of fluvoxamine (Research Unit on Pediatric Psychopharmacology Anxiety Study Group 2001). Children receiving fluvoxamine (or SSRIs in general) showed a significant decrease in clinician-rated anxiety, compared with the placebo group. **(pp. 425–426)**

■ References

American Psychiatric Association: Diagnostic and Statistical Manual of Mental Disorders, 4th Edition, Text Revision. Washington, DC, American Psychiatric Association, 2000

Biederman J, Rosenbaum JF, Chaloff J, et al: Behavioral inhibition as a risk factor for anxiety disorders, in Anxiety Disorders in Children and Adolescents. Edited by March JS. New York, Guilford, 1995, pp 61–81

Kagan J: Galen's Prophecy. New York, Basic Books, 1994

Kagan J, Snidman N: Early childhood predictors of adult anxiety disorders. Biol Psychiatry 46:1536–1541, 1999

Kagan J, Reznick JS, Snidman N: Biological bases of childhood shyness. Science 240:167–171, 1988

Pine DS: Treating children and adolescents with selective serotonin reuptake inhibitors: how long is appropriate? J Child Adolesc Psychopharmacol 12:189–203, 2002

Research Unit on Pediatric Psychopharmacology Anxiety Study Group: Fluvoxamine for the treatment of anxiety disorders in children and adolescents. N Engl J Med 344:1279–1285, 2001

Chapter 19—Obsessive-Compulsive Disorder

Select the single best response for each question.

19.1 According to studies conducted by Geller et al. (1998) and Swedo et al. (1989), which of the following epidemiological findings related to obsessive-compulsive disorder (OCD) is *false?*

A. Girls tended to have an earlier age at onset.

B. In young children, there was a male predominance (male-to-female ratio: 3 to 2).

C. The mean age at onset was 10 years.

D. Children with early-onset OCD were more likely to have a family member with OCD.

E. In adolescence, the gender distribution between girls and boys with OCD was about equal.

The correct response is option A.

Boys tended to have an earlier age at onset, around age 9 years, whereas girls were more likely to have an onset around puberty, at about age 11 years (Swedo et al. 1989). **(p. 442)**

19.2 Which of the following is *not* a proposed subtype of OCD in children?

A. Early-onset OCD.

B. Late-onset OCD.

C. Tic-related OCD.

D. Streptococcal-precipitated OCD.

E. None of the above.

The correct response is option B.

Late-onset OCD is not a proposed subtype of the disorder in children. **(pp. 442–443)**

19.3 Several lines of neuroscience research have implicated, as a cause for OCD, a dysfunction in which brain structure?

A. Hippocampus.

B. Amygdala.

C. Basal ganglia.

D. Dorsal lateral prefrontal cortex.

E. Substantia nigra.

The correct response is option C.

Several lines of research suggest that OCD may be the result of frontal lobe–limbic-basal ganglia dysfunction. Brain insults that result in basal ganglia damage (e.g., head injury, brain tumors) have been reported to be related to the onset of OCD. **(pp. 444–445)**

19.4 Recent research supports the addition of which of the following pharmacological agents as an appropriate augmentation to a selective serotonin reuptake inhibitor (SSRI)?

    A. Lithium.
    B. Imipramine.
    C. Lamotrigine.
    D. Bupropion.
    E. Risperidone.

The correct response is option E.

A controlled trial of SSRI augmentation (McDougle et al. 2000) demonstrated that the addition of risperidone was superior to placebo in reducing OCD symptoms. **(p. 447)**

19.5 In the largest and most recent systematic follow-up study of children with OCD being treated with SSRIs and behavior therapy (Leonard et al. 1993), what percentage still met diagnostic criteria for OCD 2–7 years after initial presentation?

    A. 17%.
    B. 28%.
    C. 43%.
    D. 68%.
    E. 82%.

The correct response is option C.

Leonard et al. (1993) found that among patients seen 2–7 years after initial presentation, 43% still met diagnostic criteria for OCD. **(p. 449)**

■ References

Geller DA, Biederman J, Jones J, et al: Is juvenile obsessive-compulsive disorder a developmental subtype of the disorder? A review of the pediatric literature. J Am Acad Child Adolesc Psychiatry 37:420–427, 1998

Leonard HL, Swedo SE, Lenane MC, et al: A 2- to 7-year follow-up study of 54 obsessive compulsive children and adolescents. Arch Gen Psychiatry 50:429–439, 1993

McDougle CJ, Naylor ST, Cohen CJ, et al; A double-blind, placebo-controlled study of risperidone addition to serotonin reuptake inhibitor–refractory obsessive-compulsive disorder. Arch Gen Psychiatry 57:794–801, 2000

Swedo S, Rapoport JL, Leonard HL, et al: Obsessive-compulsive disorder in children and adolescents: clinical phenomenology of 70 consecutive cases. Arch Gen Psychiatry 46:335–341, 1989

Chapter 20—Specific Phobia, Panic Disorder, Social Phobia, and Selective Mutism

Select the single best response for each question.

20.1 To which of the following disorders does the DSM-IV-TR (American Psychiatric Association 2000) definition "a marked and persistent fear that is excessive or unreasonable, cued by the presence or anticipation of a specific object or situation" apply?

    A. Social phobia.
    B. Selective mutism.
    C. Specific phobia.
    D. Panic disorder.
    E. Anxiety disorder not otherwise specified.

The correct response is option C.

Specific phobia is a marked and persistent fear of circumscribed objects or situations that is excessive or unreasonable. *Social phobia* is a persistent fear of one or more social situations in which a person is exposed to unfamiliar persons or to scrutiny by others. *Selective mutism* is characterized by persistent failure to speak in one or more social situations in which speaking is expected. *Panic disorder* is characterized by recurrent, unexpected panic attacks, which are discrete periods of intense fear or discomfort. **(p. 456)**

20.2 All of the following statements regarding panic disorder are correct *except*

    A. Panic attacks are the hallmark of panic disorder.
    B. Panic disorder may occur with or without agoraphobia.
    C. Children with early development of separation anxiety disorder are at increased risk of later developing panic disorder.
    D. Symptoms, course of illness, and associated complicating conditions in children with panic disorder are very different from those in adults with panic disorder.
    E. Panic disorder may develop at any age during childhood or later.

The correct response is option D.

The symptoms, course, and associated complications and comorbid conditions (agoraphobia, depression) in children and adolescents with panic disorder appear to be very similar to those observed in adults with panic disorder. **(pp. 456–457)**

20.3 Individuals with social phobia commonly fear which of the following social situations?

    A. Public speaking or performing.
    B. Attending social gatherings.
    C. Dealing with authorities.
    D. Asking for directions.
    E. All of the above.

The correct response is option E.

Individuals with social phobia fear all of the situations listed above. **(pp. 459–460)**

20.4 In regard to the prevalence of selective mutism in children, which of the following statements is *true*?

A. Prevalence estimates in children range from 3% to 5%.

B. Selective mutism symptoms that occur upon starting school are likely to be unremitting.

C. Variability in prevalence estimates may be due to vagueness in the DSM regarding the level of impairment required to meet diagnostic criteria.

D. Scandinavian prevalence studies have reported lower rates of selective mutism than have U.S. studies among school-age children.

E. Variability in prevalence estimates is unlikely to be related to differences in the consistent application of diagnostic criteria in study populations.

The correct response is option C.

Variability in prevalence estimates may be a function of the age of the children sampled, differences in the application of the diagnostic criteria, and vagueness of the DSM criteria in terms of the degree of impairment required for the diagnosis. **(pp. 462–463)**

20.5 Which of the following descriptions refers to a *top-down* family genetic study of anxiety disorders?

A. The evaluation of the prevalence of anxiety disorders in the offspring of adult probands.

B. The evaluation of the prevalence of anxiety disorders in adult relatives of child probands.

C. The longitudinal evaluation of young offspring of adult probands with anxiety disorders.

D. The comparison of rates of co-occurrence of anxiety disorders in monozygotic twins.

E. The comparison of rates of co-occurrence of anxiety disorders in dizygotic twins.

The correct response is option A.

A *top-down* family genetic study evaluates the prevalence of anxiety disorders in the offspring of adult probands. A *bottom-up* study evaluates the prevalence of anxiety disorders in adult relatives of child and adolescent probands. A *high-risk* study examines young offspring of adult probands with anxiety disorders. A *twin* study compares the rates of co-occurrence of anxiety disorders in monozygotic and dizygotic twin pairs. **(p. 464)**

■ Reference

American Psychiatric Association: Diagnostic and Statistical Manual of Mental Disorders, 4th Edition, Text Revision. Washington, DC, American Psychiatric Association, 2000

Chapter 21—Posttraumatic Stress Disorder

Select the single best response for each question.

21.1 In assessing a child for posttraumatic stress disorder (PTSD), clinicians should do all of the following *except*

A. Establish that the incident actually occurred.
B. Take children's self-reports of trauma at face value.
C. Supplement children's self-reports with histories from parents and others.
D. Remember that children's recollections may be influenced by others.
E. Use a neutral questioning stance.

The correct response is option B.

Children's self-reports of trauma cannot be taken at face value, because it is known that children may retain false details of their recollection of real trauma. **(pp. 480–482)**

21.2 Stimuli directly or indirectly related to a traumatic event that provoke conditioned responses are known as

A. Traumatic dreams.
B. Reenactment behavior.
C. Traumatic play.
D. Traumatic reminders.
E. None of the above.

The correct response is option D.

Traumatic reminders, also called trauma triggers, are stimuli that provoke conditioned responses directly or indirectly linked to the traumatic event. *Traumatic dreams* depict personal threats and they renew emotions associated with the experience. *Reenactment behavior* refers to the replication of some aspects of the traumatic experience. *Traumatic play* refers to the repetitive dramatization in play of elements or themes of the event. **(pp. 482–484)**

21.3 Traumatized children frequently have symptoms of disorders other than PTSD. In addition to true comorbidity, spurious comorbidity with PTSD can result from 1) overlap between criteria sets and 2) confounding similar symptoms of other diagnoses with those of PTSD. Which of the following disorders overlaps with or has symptoms similar to those of PTSD?

A. Attention-deficit/hyperactivity disorder (ADHD).
B. Oppositional defiant disorder.
C. Major depressive disorder.
D. Generalized anxiety disorder.
E. All of the above.

The correct response is option E.

All of the disorders above have symptoms that overlap with those of PTSD. **(pp. 487–488)**

21.4 Important principles in the psychotherapeutic treatment of children with PTSD include all of the following *except*

A. Reexposing the individual to traumatic cues under safe conditions.

B. Allowing the sessions to be unfocused so that unconscious material may be uncovered.

C. Keeping focused on the child's current dysfunction.

D. Being diligent about continually rethinking the symptom picture.

E. Directing the therapy to facilitate higher levels of adaptation and coping.

The correct response is option B.

Psychotherapeutic treatment of children with PTSD should incorporate reparative and mastery elements in a structured, supportive manner. **(p. 492)**

21.5 Which of the following antidepressants has been approved by the U.S. Food and Drug Administration (FDA) for the treatment of PTSD in adults and is often used to treat PTSD in children and adolescents?

A. Bupropion.

B. Nefazodone.

C. Imipramine.

D. Duloxetine.

E. Paroxetine.

The correct response is option E.

Paroxetine has received FDA approval for the treatment of PTSD in adults, and it is also often used in children and adolescents. **(p. 495)**

Chapter 22—Adjustment and Reactive Disorders

Select the single best response for each question.

22.1 The diagnosis of adjustment disorder in children and adolescents

    A. Has a focus similar to that in other psychiatric disorders, emphasizing observable symptoms and internalized experiences as primary components of the condition.

    B. Elevates the importance of families and outside systems because of its emphasis on psychosocial stressors.

    C. Requires that symptoms develop within 6 months of the onset of the stressors.

    D. Requires that the presenting symptoms be similar to what would be expected for any child exposed to the stressor in question.

    E. Is warranted when symptoms continue for years after the termination of the stressor.

The correct response is option B.

The diagnosis of adjustment disorder elevates the importance of involving families and outside systems in treatment, because its focus is on the connection between stressors and psychological distress. DSM-IV-TR (American Psychiatric Association 2000) criteria require that symptoms occur within 3 months of the onset of the stressor and that symptoms be beyond what would be expected in other children meeting a similar stressor. In addition, symptoms should resolve within 6 months of the termination of the stressor or its consequences. **(pp. 505–506)**

22.2 All of the following factors can likely amplify the impact of an identifiable stressor on a child *except*

    A. Cognitive immaturity.

    B. Preexisting low self-esteem.

    C. More primitive defense mechanisms.

    D. More accurate understanding of cause-and-effect relationships.

    E. Treatment side effects.

The correct response is option D.

Children are more likely than adults to link unrelated events as cause-and-effect phenomena. **(p. 506)**

22.3 In Kovacs et al.'s (1994) controlled prospective study of children with adjustment disorder, which of the following findings was reported?

    A. More than half of the study group children reported a history of suicidal ideation after the onset of the stressor.

    B. More than half of the study population had suffered the death of a parent.

    C. The median time to recovery after symptom onset was 3 months.

    D. Close to 100% recovery was reported in the study population within 12 months.

    E. The study group evidenced significantly more long-term sequelae compared with the control group.

The correct response is option A.

In the study of Kovacs et al. (1994), more than half (58%) of the children indicated a history of suicidal ideation at some point after onset of the stressor. Only 7% of the children studied had suffered the death of a parent or grandparent. The median time to recovery was 7 months, and close to 100% of the study population had resolution of symptoms within 2 years. Compared with the control group, there was no evidence of long-term sequelae over an 8-year follow-up assessment. **(p. 508)**

22.4 In Kovacs et al.'s (1995) study of children hospitalized for acute-onset diabetes, all of the following findings were reported *except*

  A. Seventy-three percent of adjustment disorder diagnoses were made during the first month after the diabetes diagnosis.
  B. The first month posthospitalization was the period of greatest psychological vulnerability.
  C. Greater vulnerability during the first month postdiagnosis may be related to physiological factors.
  D. Short-term psychiatric outcomes for the study population were poor.
  E. The presence of adjustment disorder was a risk factor for developing other psychiatric illnesses within the next 5 years.

The correct response is option D.

The short-term psychiatric outcomes for the children in this study were good (Kovacs et al. 1995). All of the children eventually recovered from the adjustment disorder, with the average time to recovery being 3 months. **(p. 509)**

■ References

American Psychiatric Association: Diagnostic and Statistical Manual of Mental Disorders, 4th Edition, Text Revision. Washington, DC, American Psychiatric Association, 2000

Kovacs M, Gatsonis C, Pollock M, et al: A controlled prospective study of DSM-III adjustment disorder in childhood: short-term prognosis and long-term predictive validity. Arch Gen Psychiatry 51:535–541, 1994

Kovacs M, Ho V, Pollock MH: Criterion and predictive validity of the diagnosis of adjustment disorder: a prospective study of youths with new-onset insulin-dependent diabetes mellitus. Am J Psychiatry 152:523–528, 1995

Chapter 23—Infant and Childhood Obesity

Select the single best response for each question.

23.1 The prevalence of obesity in early childhood is not nearly as well studied as the prevalence of obesity in adulthood. However, the few studies that have been conducted indicate the prevalence of obesity in preschool children to be in the range of

   A. 0–5%.
   B. 5%–10%.
   C. 10%–15%.
   D. 15%–20%.
   E. 20%–25%.

The correct response is option B.

The prevalence of obesity in preschool-age children has been found to be in the 5%–10% range (Maloney and Klykylo 1983). **(p. 517)**

23.2 According to a report by the Centers for Disease Control and Prevention (2002), the prevalence of obesity in children between the ages of 6 and 19 years is in the range of

   A. 2%–5%.
   B. 6%–8%.
   C. 13%–14%.
   D. 21%–23%.
   E. 30%–33%.

The correct response is option C.

The report by the Centers for Disease Control and Prevention (2002) estimated the proportion of overweight children (ages 6–11 years) at 13%, and of overweight adolescents (ages 12–19 years) at 14%. **(p. 518)**

23.3 According to the American Academy of Child and Adolescent Psychiatry (1997), if one parent is obese, children have what percentage chance of being obese?

   A. 10%.
   B. 30%.
   C. 40%.
   D. 50%.
   E. 70%.

The correct response is option D.

If one parent is obese, there is a 50% chance that the children will also be obese, and when both parents are obese, the children have an 80% chance of also being obese (American Academy of Child and Adolescent Psychiatry 1997). **(p. 519)**

23.4 Which of the following statements concerning the genetic/familial form of obesity is *true*?

A. There is evidence of psychopathology in the child or parent.
B. Evidence of nutritional misinformation is seen.
C. The family history for obesity is negative.
D. The obesity has a sudden onset, usually around ages 12–13 years.
E. The child may have characteristics associated with "difficult temperament."

The correct response is option E.

In genetic/familial obesity, the child may have characteristics associated with the so-called difficult temperament (low rhythm/predictability and low persistence/attention). In this form of obesity, there is no evidence of psychopathology or nutritional misinformation, but the family history of obesity is positive. Usually the obesity is gradual and progressive, starting by age 5 or 6 years. **(pp. 519–520)**

23.5 Which of the following statements regarding psychogenic obesity is *true*?

A. There is evidence of psychopathology in the child or parent.
B. There is no evidence of nutritional misinformation.
C. The family history for obesity is negative.
D. In one type, associated with traumatic separation from the primary caregiver, there is a sudden onset, usually before age 3 years.
E. All of the above.

The correct response is option E.

All of the statements above characterize psychogenic obesity. **(pp. 520–521)**

■ References

American Academy of Child and Adolescent Psychiatry: Obesity in children and teens. Facts for Families Series (79). Washington, DC, American Academy of Child and Adolescent Psychiatry, 1997. Available at: http://www.aacap.org/publications/factsfam/79.htm. Accessed May 4, 2003.

Centers for Disease Control and Prevention: Prevalence of overweight among children and adolescents: United States, 1999. Hyattsville, MD, National Center for Health Statistics, 2002

Maloney MJ, Klykylo WM: An overview of anorexia nervosa, bulimia, and obesity in children and adolescents. J Am Acad Child Psychiatry 22:99–107, 1983

Chapter 24—Anorexia Nervosa and Bulimia Nervosa

Select the single best response for each question.

24.1 The DSM-IV-TR (American Psychiatric Association 2000) diagnostic criteria for anorexia nervosa include which of the following?

A. Body weight less than 50% of that expected.
B. Body height less than 85% of that expected.
C. Apathy to weight change.
D. Amenorrhea in postmenarcheal females.
E. Loss of interest in body habitus.

The correct response is option D.

Amenorrhea is present in postmenarcheal females afflicted by anorexia nervosa. Patients refuse to maintain body weight at or above a minimally normal weight for age and height; they have an intense fear of gaining weight, deny the seriousness of their current low body weight, and place undue value on body weight and shape on self-evaluation. **(p. 528)**

24.2 Common signs and symptoms associated with anorexia nervosa include which of the following?

A. Heat intolerance.
B. Tachycardia.
C. Diarrhea.
D. Breast engorgement.
E. Growth of lanugo hair.

The correct response is option E.

Common signs and symptoms of anorexia nervosa include growth of lanugo hair; cold intolerance; bradycardia; constipation; breast atrophy; dental enamel erosion; lesions on the dorsal surfaces of the hands, known as Russell's sign; and dry and yellow-tinged skin. **(p. 528)**

24.3 Which of the following medical complications is not routinely associated with anorexia nervosa?

A. Arrhythmias.
B. Leukopenia.
C. Neurological abnormalities.
D. Decreased gastric motility.
E. Decreased bone mineral density.

The correct response is option C.

Neurological abnormalities are rarely found in physical examination of patients with anorexia nervosa. Electrocardiographic abnormalities, mild anemia and leukopenia, decreased gastric motility, and delayed gastric emptying are commonly found in anorexic patients. Bone mineral density is reduced at several skeletal sites in most women with anorexia nervosa. **(pp. 529–530)**

24.4 Which of the following statements regarding the use of pharmacotherapy in the treatment of anorexia nervosa is *true?*

    A. Medication has no adjunctive role.

    B. Many psychotropic medications have been shown to effectively reverse the disorder.

    C. Clomipramine and lithium have shown positive effects in clinical studies.

    D. Fluoxetine may have a role in maintaining weight in weight-recovered anorexia patients.

    E. Pharmacotherapy has been shown to be superior to combined medication–psychotherapy treatment in several studies.

The correct response is option D.

Fluoxetine has shown promise in the treatment of weight-recovered anorexic patients. Pharmacotherapy can be a useful adjunct to other treatments. To date, no psychotropic medication has been demonstrated to effectively reverse anorexia nervosa. Clomipramine and lithium have yielded negative or equivocal results in clinical studies. Psychotropic medication should be used only in the context of psychotherapy. **(pp. 540–541)**

24.5 DSM-IV-TR (American Psychiatric Association 2000) diagnostic criteria for bulimia nervosa include all of the following *except*

    A. The individual engages in recurrent episodes of binge eating.

    B. The individual engages in recurrent inappropriate compensatory behavior to prevent weight gain.

    C. Binge eating and inappropriate compensatory behaviors both occur, on average, at least weekly for 6 months.

    D. Self-evaluation is unduly influenced by body shape and weight.

    E. The disturbance does not occur exclusively during episodes of anorexia nervosa.

The correct response is option C.

Binge eating and inappropriate compensatory behaviors both occur, on average, at least twice a week for 3 months. **(p. 543)**

24.6 Compared with normal-weight individuals, persons with bulimia nervosa demonstrate elevations of which of the following neuropeptides and hormones?

    A. Neuropeptide Y.

    B. Cholecystokinin.

    C. Leptin.

    D. Cortisol.

    E. None of the above.

The correct response is option A.

Neuropeptide Y and peptide YY have been shown to be elevated in patients with bulimia nervosa. Lower levels of cholecystokinin have been found in women with bulimia. Plasma leptin concentration is significantly higher in bulimic patients than in those with anorexia nervosa, but it tends to be lower than the level found in healthy control subjects. **(p. 547)**

24.7 Which of the following antidepressants has been studied most extensively in bulimia nervosa and has been shown to be effective in its treatment?

A. Venlafaxine.
B. Mirtazapine.
C. Fluvoxamine.
D. Bupropion.
E. Fluoxetine.

The correct response is option E.

Fluoxetine is the most studied and effective antidepressant used in the treatment of bulimia nervosa. **(p. 550)**

■ Reference

American Psychiatric Association: Diagnostic and Statistical Manual of Mental Disorders, 4th Edition, Text Revision. Washington, DC, American Psychiatric Association, 2000

Chapter 25—Tic Disorders

Select the single best response for each question.

25.1 Which of the following statements regarding transient tic disorder is *true?*

  A. Transient tics are very rare among prepubertal children.
  B. Girls are more often affected than boys.
  C. Transient tics run a waxing and waning course.
  D. Transient tics most commonly involve the trunk and lower extremities.
  E. Transient vocal tics are common.

The correct response is option C.

Transient tics run a waxing and waning course, which is often exacerbated by stress, excitement, or fatigue. Transient tics are very common in prepubertal children, with boys being more often affected than girls. Transient tics most commonly involve the face, head, neck, or arms. Transient vocal tics are much more rare. **(p. 562)**

25.2 All of the following statements regarding Tourette's syndrome are correct *except*

  A. Chronic motor and phonic tic disorder was first described in 1885 by Georges Gilles de la Tourette.
  B. Initial symptoms of Tourette's syndrome most frequently appear between the ages of 5 and 8 years.
  C. Tic symptoms may wax and wane over time.
  D. Vocal tics usually precede motor tics.
  E. Children may be able to suppress tics for periods of time.

The correct response is option D.

The onset of motor tics usually precedes that of vocal tics by a year or two. **(pp. 562–563)**

25.3 The most likely neuroanatomical substrate of Tourette's syndrome is

  A. The thalamus.
  B. The pituitary.
  C. The prefrontal cortex.
  D. The basal ganglia.
  E. The amygdala.

The correct response is option D.

The basal ganglia and their connections represent the most likely neuroanatomical substrate of Tourette's syndrome. **(p. 566)**

25.4 Which of the following psychotropic agents is least likely to exacerbate tics?

    A. Haloperidol.
    B. L-dopa.
    C. Dextroamphetamine.
    D. Methylphenidate.
    E. Cocaine.

The correct response is option A.

Neuroleptics (e.g., haloperidol) are clinically useful in suppressing tics. Dopaminergic agonists (e.g., dextroamphetamine, methylphenidate, cocaine) frequently exacerbate tics. **(p. 567)**

25.5 Side effects of clonidine in the treatment of tic disorders include all of the following *except*

    A. Sedation.
    B. Irritability.
    C. Dry mouth.
    D. Cardiac arrhythmias.
    E. Hypertension.

The correct response is option E.

Hypertension is not a side effect of clonidine. Sedation is the primary side effect of clonidine, seen in about 10%–20% of patients. Other side effects include irritability, dry mouth, orthostatic hypotension, and, rarely, cardiac arrhythmias. **(p. 571)**

Chapter 26—Disorders of Elimination

Select the single best response for each question.

26.1 Which of the following statements regarding the clinical presentation of enuresis is *true*?

     A. About 80% of patients with enuresis have primary enuresis.

     B. Without treatment, the remission rate is 30%–50% per year, which decreases with age.

     C. Enuresis continues into adulthood in approximately 8% of cases.

     D. There is no identified increase prevalence of emotional–behavioral disorders in the enuretic population, when compared to the general population.

     E. Clear association between enuresis and tic disorders has been demonstrated.

The correct response is option A.

About 80% of patients with enuresis have primary enuresis. Left untreated, the remission rate is 10%–20% per year, which gradually increases with age. Enuresis continues into adulthood in 1% of patients. The prevalence of emotional–behavioral disorders in children with enuresis is greater than in the general population. No association has been demonstrated between enuresis and tics, nail biting, temper tantrums, fire setting, or cruelty to animals. **(pp. 581–582)**

26.2 Which of the following circumstances would be consistent with a child meeting DSM-IV-TR (American Psychiatric Association 2000) diagnostic criteria for enuresis?

     A. The child must be at least 3 years of age and demonstrate repeated voiding of urine in his or her bed or clothes at least twice weekly for 3 consecutive months.

     B. The child must be at least 3 years of age and demonstrate repeated voiding of urine in his or her bed or clothes at least five times weekly for 6 consecutive months.

     C. The child must be at least 3 years of age and demonstrate repeated voiding of urine in his or her bed or clothes that is not due to a physiological condition.

     D. The child must be at least 5 years of age and demonstrate repeated voiding of urine in his or her bed or clothes at least twice weekly for 3 consecutive months.

     E. The child must be at least 5 years of age and demonstrate repeated voiding of urine in his or her bed or clothes at least five times weekly for 6 consecutive months.

The correct response is option D.

The child must be at least 5 years of age and must void urine in bed or clothes at least twice a week for at least 3 consecutive months. This behavior must not be due to the direct physiological effect of a substance (e.g., a diuretic) or a general medical condition (e.g., spina bifida). **(p. 582)**

26.3 All of the statements regarding treatment of enuresis are correct *except*

   A. Enuresis is largely a self-limited, benign disorder.
   B. It is important to provide reassurance support to prevent secondary emotional effects.
   C. Treatment should be preceded by a period of observation and tracking of symptoms.
   D. The most effective treatment for primary enuresis is the enuresis alarm.
   E. Pharmacological interventions include desmopressin (DDAVP), imipramine, and methylphenidate.

The correct response is option E.

Whereas tricyclic antidepressants, especially imipramine, and DDAVP have proved beneficial in the treatment of enuresis, methylphenidate, sedatives, and anticholinergic agents have not. **(pp. 583–584)**

26.4 Which of the following statements regarding encopresis is *true?*

   A. Primary encopresis is not preceded by a period of fecal continence.
   B. Secondary encopresis may account for 10%–20% of all cases.
   C. Encopresis resulting from constipation and overflow incontinence is a rare form of the disorder.
   D. Children with encopresis characterized by intentional depositing or smearing of feces are less likely to demonstrate defiant behaviors than are children with encopresis with overflow incontinence.
   E. Most children with functional encopresis demonstrate severe behavioral problems.

The correct response is option A.

Primary encopresis is not preceded by a period of fecal continence. Secondary encopresis may account for as many as 50%–60% of all cases. Encopresis with constipation and overflow incontinence is the most common type. Children with encopresis characterized by intentional depositing or smearing of feces demonstrate more defiant behaviors than do children with encopresis with overflow incontinence. Most children with functional encopresis do not appear to have significant behavioral problems. **(pp. 585–586)**

26.5 Which of the following statements regarding the treatment of encopresis is *true?*

   A. Treatment typically includes medical interventions alone.
   B. Treatment requires little evaluation because of the ease with which encopresis is diagnosed.
   C. Treatment in children who retain feces should include education, disimpaction, and bowel training.
   D. Treatment should not include aversive consequences for soiling accidents.
   E. Biofeedback appears to be the most effective available treatment.

The correct response is option C.

The treatment principles for children who retain feces include educating the child and the parents about the problem, disimpacting the bowel, and training the child in bowel control. Medical, behavioral, and psychotherapeutic interventions should be used in the treatment of encopresis. Careful evaluation should precede any intervention. Aversive consequences for soiling accidents, such as showering and washing the soiled clothes, reinforce the child's self-monitoring. The initial promise of biofeedback therapy was not supported by subsequent studies. **(pp. 587–588)**

■ Reference

American Psychiatric Association: Diagnostic and Statistical Manual of Mental Disorders, 4th Edition, Text Revision. Washington, DC, American Psychiatric Association, 2000

Chapter 27—Physical and Sexual Abuse of Children

Select the single best response for each question.

27.1 Which of the following statements concerning the epidemiology of physical abuse of children is *false?*

A. Younger children (less than 3 years of age) have the greatest risk of fatal maltreatment.

B. Homicides occurring during the first week of life are almost exclusively perpetrated by mothers.

C. Fathers are more likely to fatally injure their children ages 1 week to 13 years.

D. Fathers committed the majority of parent-perpetrated homicides of children 13–19 years of age.

E. None of the above.

The correct response is option C.

Mothers and fathers are equally likely to fatally injure their children ages 1 week to 13 years. **(p. 596)**

27.2 Which of the following statements concerning sexual abuse of boys is *false?*

A. Perpetrators of abuse against boys are most likely to be related to the victim.

B. Boys are less likely than girls to disclose abuse.

C. Surveys indicate that as many as 18% of males older than 18 years report having been victims of childhood sexual abuse.

D. Perpetrators of abuse against boys are most likely to be male.

E. Sexual abuse of boys may be significantly underreported and untreated.

The correct response is option A.

Perpetrators of abuse against boys are most likely to be male and unrelated to the victim. **(p. 597)**

27.3 Risk factors that may predict recurrence of physical abuse in children include which of the following?

A. Young age of the child.

B. Number of previous referrals to child protective services.

C. History of childhood abuse in the caretaker.

D. Prematurity, mental retardation, or physical handicaps in the child.

E. All of the above.

The correct response is option E.

In addition to all of the above factors, a history of low birth weight or cognitive or neuropsychiatric deficits make children more vulnerable to maltreatment. **(pp. 597–598)**

27.4 Perpetrators of sexual abuse

  A. Are often children and adolescents.
  B. Are gender-specific regarding their choice of victims.
  C. Often associate themselves with events or activities in which they have access to children.
  D. May seek to "groom" victims with gifts or money.
  E. All of the above.

The correct response is option E.

Perpetrators may associate with youth group activities, schools, recreational facilities, or locations near playgrounds. They may seek to "groom" potential victims by offering gifts or money in order to gain their trust. Perpetrators are most often male and most often select female victims. They are usually gender specific in their choice of victims; those who select both male and female victims may have more severe psychopathology. Approximately 30%–50% of assaults are perpetrated by children and adolescents younger than 18 years of age. **(pp. 599–600)**

27.5 Which of the following characteristics in children should increase a clinician's suspicion of possible physical abuse?

  A. A child who is afraid to leave home.
  B. A child who craves physical contact.
  C. A child with excessive needs for being comforted.
  D. A child who is on the alert for danger.
  E. All of the above.

The correct response is option D.

Indicative characteristics include a child who is unusually fearful, docile, distrustful, or guarded; a child with no expectation of being comforted; a child who is wary of physical contact; a child who is on the alert for danger; a child who attempts to meet parents' needs by role reversal; and a child who is afraid to go home. **(p. 600)**

27.6 Physical findings in an injured child suggestive of physical abuse include which of the following?

  A. Bruises or lacerations in the shape of an object.
  B. Posterior rib fractures.
  C. Anogenital lacerations.
  D. Twisting injuries of the ear lobe.
  E. All of the above.

The correct response is option E.

Other suggestive findings include burns, head injuries, ruptured tympanic membranes, multiple fractures in different stages of healing, abdominal injuries, and chest injuries. **(pp. 600–601)**

Chapter 28—Suicide and Suicidality

Select the single best response for each question.

28.1 Self-mutilation

A. Is defined as superficial cutting of the arms, legs, and other body areas.
B. Is rarely associated with stress.
C. Always involves a clear intention to kill oneself.
D. Is never associated with suicidal intent.
E. Is rarely associated with dissociative phenomena.

The correct response is option E.

Self-mutilation involves superficial cutting of the arms, legs, and other body areas and is often associated with stress, dissociative phenomena, and anger. Although often associated with suicidal intent, self-mutilation is not in itself considered to be a suicidal act. **(p. 622)**

28.2 Which of the following statements concerning epidemiological findings in youth suicide is *false*?

A. Suicide among black youth has increased more rapidly than that among white youth.
B. Increased rates of youth suicide are associated with greater availability of firearms.
C. Male youths are more likely to attempt suicide than are females.
D. Approximately 1% of preadolescents in the general population report having made a suicide attempt.
E. None of the above.

The correct response is option C.

According to the Youth Risk Behavior Surveillance System 1999 survey (Kann et al. 2000), female adolescents were more likely to have attempted suicide than were males (10.8% vs. 5.7%). **(pp. 622–623)**

28.3 Which of the following childhood environmental stressors has been identified as a suicide risk factor?

A. Adolescent unemployment.
B. Family history of suicidal behavior.
C. Poor communication with the mother or the father.
D. Adolescent suspension from school.
E. All of the above.

The correct response is option E.

All of the above stressors have been identified as suicide risk factors (Gould et al. 1996). Other stressors include father's problem with police, mother's history of mood disorder, lack of an intact family, and loss. **(p. 623)**

28.4 A "psychological autopsy" study of 67 adolescent suicide victims found greatly elevated risks for suicide associated with certain psychiatric disorders (Brent et al. 1993). Which of the following disorders imparted the greatest increase in risk?

A. Attention-deficit/hyperactivity disorder.
B. Alcohol abuse.
C. Schizophrenia.
D. Major depression.
E. Conduct disorder.

The correct response is option D.

Major depression imparted the highest increase for suicide, followed by drug abuse, alcohol abuse, and conduct disorder (Brent et al. 1993). **(p. 625)**

28.5 The use of antidepressants in children and adolescents has recently received a great deal of scrutiny from the U.S. Food and Drug Administration (FDA) and from investigators. Which of the following statements is correct?

A. A positive relationships exists between the number of antidepressant medication prescriptions for children and adolescents and rates of youth suicide.
B. Selective serotonin reuptake inhibitors (SSRIs) are associated with a higher risk of suicidal ideation and acts compared with placebo.
C. SSRI antidepressants are contraindicated in children and adolescents.
D. A black-box warning has been placed on SSRI-type antidepressants, but not on other antidepressants, for their use in children and adolescents.
E. None of the above.

The correct response is option B.

Controlled clinical trials have demonstrated a higher risk of suicidal ideation and acts with SSRIs than with placebo. **(p. 627)**

■ References

Brent DA, Perper JA, Moritz G, et al: Psychiatric risk factors for adolescent suicide: a case–control study. J Am Acad Child Adolesc Psychiatry 32:521–529, 1993

Gould MS, Fisher P, Parides M, et al: Psychosocial risk factors of child and adolescent completed suicide. Arch Gen Psychiatry 53:1155–1162, 1996

Kann L, Kinchen SA, Williams BI, et al: Youth Risk Behavior Surveillance—United States, 1999. J Sch Health 70:271–285, 2000

Chapter 29—Psychopharmacology

Select the single best response for each question.

29.1 Commonly reported and well-substantiated side effects of stimulant medications include all of the following *except*

  A. Appetite suppression.
  B. Sleep disturbance.
  C. Mild increases in pulse and blood pressure.
  D. Stunting of growth in height.
  E. Weight loss.

The correct response is option D.

Stimulants are known to routinely produce anorexia and weight loss, but their effect on growth in height is much less certain. **(pp. 639–640)**

29.2 A number of studies have evaluated the short- and long-term effects of therapeutic doses of tricyclic antidepressants (TCAs) on the cardiovascular system in children. Which of the following statements is *incorrect?*

  A. TCAs are generally well tolerated.
  B. TCAs may produce electrocardiographic abnormalities at doses between 1 and 2 mg/kg.
  C. Patients should be carefully monitored at higher TCA doses (> 3.5 mg/kg).
  D. Before initiating TCAs, a baseline electrocardiogram is recommended.
  E. None of the above.

The correct response is option B.

TCAs are generally well tolerated, with only minor electrocardiographic changes associated with daily oral doses as high as 5.0 mg/kg. TCA-induced electrocardiographic abnormalities (conduction defects) have been consistently reported in children receiving doses higher than 3.5 mg/kg. **(pp. 646–647)**

29.3 Some compounds metabolized by the cytochrome P450 enzyme 3A4 have been associated with QT prolongations when combined with drugs that inhibit 3A4. Antidepressants that affect 3A4 activity include all of the following *except*

  A. Fluvoxamine.
  B. Venlafaxine.
  C. Nefazodone.
  D. Fluoxetine.
  E. Sertraline.

The correct response is option B.

Venlafaxine, citalopram, and mirtazapine minimally inhibit P450 enzymes. **(pp. 648–649)**

29.4 Novel atypical antipsychotic medications exert their therapeutic effects through antagonism of which of the following receptors?

    A. Dopaminergic (D_1).
    B. Histaminic (H_1).
    C. Serotonergic (5-HT_2).
    D. Alpha$_1$-adrenergic.
    E. None of the above.

The correct response is option C.

Novel atypical antipsychotic medications, such as risperidone, olanzapine, and quetiapine, combine dopaminergic (D_2) and serotonergic (5-HT_2) antagonist properties and are associated with a lower incidence of acute extrapyramidal adverse effects and possibly a lower risk of tardive dyskinesia. **(pp. 649, 652)**

29.5 Oxcarbazepine is chemically similar to carbamazepine with some important differences, which include all of the following *except*

    A. Laboratory monitoring is still required with oxcarbazepine.
    B. Oxcarbazepine has little interaction with the cytochrome P450 system.
    C. Oxcarbazepine lacks the hepatic liability of carbamazepine.
    D. Oxcarbazepine does not induce its own metabolism.
    E. Oxcarbazepine lacks the hematological liability of carbamazepine.

The correct response is option A.

Laboratory monitoring is not required, because oxcarbazepine does not share the hepatic and hematological liability of carbamazepine. **(p. 657)**

29.6 In child psychiatry, clonidine is commonly used in the treatment of all of the following *except*

    A. Attention-deficit/hyperactivity disorder (ADHD).
    B. Tourette's disorder.
    C. Aggression.
    D. Sleep disturbance in ADHD children.
    E. Major depressive disorder.

The correct response is option E.

Clonidine is not used in the treatment of major depressive disorder. **(p. 661)**

29.7 Side effects associated with the use of atomoxetine in children include which of the following?

    A. Increased appetite.
    B. Cardiac conduction delays.
    C. Insomnia.
    D. Increase in pulse and diastolic blood pressure.
    E. Abuse.

The correct response is option D.

In children, possible side effects of atomoxetine include mild increases in pulse and blood pressure and mild decreases in appetite. Atomoxetine does not cause insomnia or cardiac conduction or repolarization delays. In addition, atomoxetine is not abusable. **(pp. 663–665, Table 29–7)**

Index

*Page numbers printed in **boldface** type refer to tables or figures.*